TRAUMA MANAGEMENT
Volume III, Second Edition

Series Editors

F. William Blaisdell, M.D.
Professor and Chairman
Department of Surgery
University of California, Davis
Sacramento, California

Donald D. Trunkey, M.D.
Professor and Chairman
Department of Surgery
The Oregon Health Sciences University
Portland, Oregon

CERVICOTHORACIC TRAUMA

SECOND EDITION

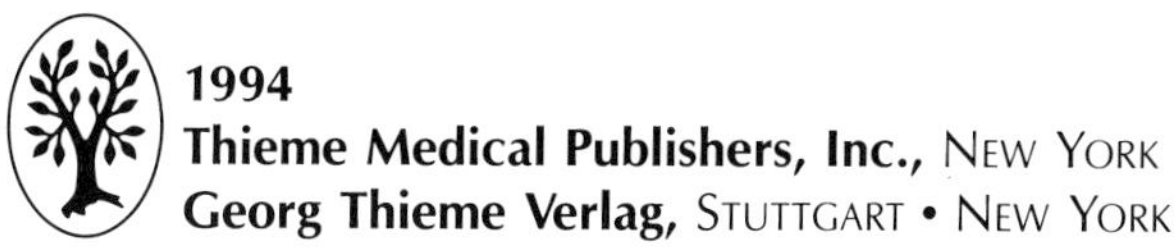

F. William Blaisdell, M.D.
Professor and Chairman
Department of Surgery
University of California, Davis
Sacramento, California

Donald D. Trunkey, M.D.
Professor and Chairman
Department of Surgery
The Oregon Health Sciences University
Portland, Oregon

1994
Thieme Medical Publishers, Inc., NEW YORK
Georg Thieme Verlag, STUTTGART • NEW YORK

Thieme Medical Publishers, Inc.
381 Park Avenue South
New York, New York 10016

CERVICOTHORACIC TRAUMA, SECOND EDITION
F. William Blaisdell
Donald D. Trunkey

Library of Congress Cataloging-in-Publication Data
Cervicothoracic trauma / edited by F. William Blaisdell, Donald D.
  Trunkey — 2nd ed.
      p.   cm. — (Trauma management ; v. 3)
    Includes bibliographic references and index.
    ISBN 0-86577-492-7. — ISBN 3-13-664602-7
    1. Chest—Wounds and injuries. 2. Neck—Wounds and injuries.
  3. Cervical vertebrae—Wounds and injuries. 4. Thoracic Surgery.
  I. Blaisdell, F. William (Frank William), 1927– . II. Trunkey,
  Donald D. III. Series.
      [DNLM: 1. Cervical Vertebrae—injuries. 2. Neck—injuries.
  3. Thoracic Injuries. WO 700 T776 1992 v.3a]
  RD536.C47 1993
  617.5'54044—dc20
  DNLM/DLC
  for Library of Congress   93-4002
                                                                                  CIP

Important note: Medicine is an ever-changing science. Research and clinical experience are continually broadening our knowledge, in particular our knowledge of proper treatment and drug therapy. Insofar as this book mentions any dosage or applications, readers may rest assured that the authors, editors, and publishers have made every effort to ensure that such references are strictly in accordance with the state of knowledge at the time of production of the book. Nevertheless, every user is requested to carefully examine the manufacturers' leaflets accompanying each drug to check on his own responsibility whether the dosage schedules recommended therein or the contraindications stated by the manufacturers differ from the statements made in the present book. Such examination is particularly important with drugs that are either rarely used or have been newly released on the market.

Some of the product names, patents, and registered designs referred to in this book are in fact registered trademarks or proprietary names even though specific reference to this fact is not always made in the text. Therefore, the appearance of a name without designation as proprietary is not to be construed as a representation by the publisher that it is in the public domain.

Printed in the United States of America.

5   4   3   2   1

TMP ISBN 0-86577-492-7
GTV ISBN 3-13-664602-7

Contents

Contributors

Felix D. Battistella, M.D.
Assistant Professor of Surgery
University of California, Davis
Sacramento, California

John R. Benfield, M.D.
Professor and Chief
Department of Cardiothoracic Surgery
University of California, Davis
Sacramento, California

Herbert A. Berkoff, M.D.
Professor of Surgery (Cardiothoracic)
University of California, Davis
Sacramento, California

F. William Blaisdell, M.D.
Professor and Chairman
Department of Surgery
University of California, Davis
Sacramento, California

Balazs Imre Bodai, M.D.
Associate Clinical Professor of Surgery
University of California, Davis

Chief of Surgery
Kaiser Hospital
Sacramento, California

Paul Capek, M.D.
Instructor in Radiology
University of California, Davis
Sacramento, California

David M. Follette, M.D.
Associate Professor of Surgery (Thoracic)
University of California, Davis
Sacramento, California

William R. Fry, M.D.
Assistant Professor of Surgery
University of California, Davis, East Bay
Oakland, California

James E. Goodnight, M.D.
Department of Surgery
University of California, Davis
Sacramento, California

James M. Guernsey, M.D.
Professor of Surgery
University of California, Davis
Sacramento, California

James W. Holcroft, M.D.
Professor and Chief
Department of Vascular Surgery and
    Critical Care
University of California, Davis
Sacramento, California

Edward J. Hurley, M.D.
Professor of Surgery (Cardiothoracic)
University of California, Davis
Sacramento, California

John P. Livoni, M.D.
Assistant Professor of Radiology
University of California, Davis
Sacramento, California

Mervin B. O'Neil, Jr., M.D.
Clinical Professor of Surgery (Thoracic)
University of California, Davis
Sacramento, California

Department of Surgery
Kaiser Hospital
Sacramento, California

John T. Owings, M.D.
Assistant Professor of Surgery
University of California, Davis
Sacramento, California

Raymond E. Parks, M.D.
Professor of Radiology
University of California, Davis
Sacramento, California

Virginia C. Poirier, M.D.
Assistant Professor of Radiology
University of California, Davis
Sacramento, California

Marc Pollock, M.D.
Assistant Professor of Surgery
(Cardiothoracic)
University of California, Davis
Sacramento, California

Amira M. Safwat, M.D.
Professor of Anesthesia
University of California, Davis
Sacramento, California

Russell W. Sawyer, M.D.
Chief Resident
Department of Surgery
University of California, Davis
Sacramento, California

Craig W. Senders, M.D.
Professor of Otorhinolaryngology
University of California, Davis
Sacramento, California

R. Stephen Smith, M.D.
Assistant Professor of Surgery
University of California, Davis, East Bay
Oakland, California

Donald D. Trunkey, M.D.
Professor and Chairman
Department of Surgery
The Oregon Health Sciences University
Portland, Oregon

David H. Wisner, M.D.
Associate Professor of Surgery
Chief, Trauma Department
University of California, Davis
Sacramento, California

Foreword

As we have pointed out in previous volumes in this series, the discipline of surgery, through the act of operating itself, inflicts trauma. Thus, the study of trauma provides special insight into surgical illness and recovery from operation. In addition, the management of trauma is an enduring surgical specialty since the treatment of injury cannot be resolved by medical measures, as is potentially true of cardiovascular disease, cancer, and gastrointestinal disorders.

The trauma surgeon must remain a generalist since, under emergency circumstances, he must be prepared to deal with unexpected problems in any area involving any body cavity. Most particularly, we do not believe in any arbitrary division of trauma at the level of the diaphragm. We sincerely believe that the general surgeon is the most appropriate person to assume leadership when injuries cross multiple specialty lines and, in particular, when any major truncal injury is involved. This volume is designed to assist the general surgeon in managing thoracic and cervical trauma. The overlap between the chest and abdominal cavity is too great to compartmentalize thoracic as opposed to abdominal injury. They are usually one and the same, and a practicing general surgeon, whether or not board certified in general or thoracic surgery, should assume primary responsibility for any patient who has any evidence of multiple injury. In life-threatening circumstances, when specialty support is not available, the surgeon should be prepared to provide definitive treatment for cardiac, pulmonary, or aortic injury. This is what general surgery training is all about and why the American Board of Surgery requires exposure to all the major surgical disciplines.

F. William Blaisdell, M.D.
Donald D. Trunkey, M.D.

Preface

This monograph, *Cervicothoracic Trauma*, the second of the *Trauma Management Series*, has been brought up-to-date to match our recent revision of *Abdominal Trauma*, the first in our series. This volume, along with *Abdominal Trauma, Extremity Trauma, Craniospinal Trauma*, and *Burn Trauma*, should provide the general surgeon and all medical and surgical specialists interested in trauma with a guide of general principles in the management of major injury.

Cervicothoracic Trauma is specifically oriented toward the general surgeon and the surgical resident. It emphasizes basic pathophysiology of cervical and chest injury, keys to assessment and diagnosis, and principles of management. It discusses complications and outcome.

In particular, it emphasizes an aggressive approach to trauma, because it is our contention that active intervention results in minimal morbidity, and undue conservatism results in significant increase in disability and mortality.

The contributors to this volume consist of our colleagues in our respective institutions, hospitals that collectively receive more than 6,000 trauma admissions each year on their active trauma services. This rich experience has resulted in certain biases with regard to the management of trauma, which we freely acknowledge. However, by limiting the contributions to colleagues with whom we work or have worked, we believe we have provided a uniform approach to trauma that we hope our readers will appreciate. Although we acknowledge that there may be many different ways in which any given problem might be successfully managed, we can say that on the basis of our experience, we know the approaches we advocate will ensure a high degree of success.

We are grateful to our secretaries who have assisted us with manuscript preparation, and especially Shirley Cable, who has assisted us with editing. We wish to thank our artists, Eric Stolting and Kathy Hirsh, whose superb illustrations have greatly contributed to the educational value of this volume. We wish to thank our editor, James Costello, at Thieme for his encouragement. Finally, and most importantly, we once again express our appreciation to our long-suffering wives, Marilyn and Jane, for their tolerance of our mistress—Surgery—who has commanded so much of our time and attention.

F. William Blaisdell, M.D.
Donald D. Trunkey, M.D.

1

Initial Assessment

DAVID H. WISNER, M.D.

HISTORY: The earliest known reference to cervicothoracic trauma is found in the Smith papyrus, which was written probably sometime before 3000 BC.[1] Of the 58 cases described in the papyrus, one was related to cervical injury and two to chest trauma. The first concerned a wound to the throat, penetrating to the esophagus. The recommended treatment was to draw the wound edges together with stitches and apply fresh meat to it the first day. Afterward it was recommended that the wound be treated with grease, honey, and lint. Another case concerned a wound of the chest that penetrated to the bone and perforated the sternum. It was recommended that this be treated with fresh meat the first day and subsequently with grease, honey, and lint. The final case was a wound associated with a break in the ribs. No treatment was recommended for this ailment.

Galen, in his treatise compiled in the second century, described a case of sternal injury.[2] Four months after treatment of the wound, infection was manifested by the development of an abscess. This was incised and the infection was found to extend down to the pericardium. A piece of the pericardium was removed and the heart could be seen beating in the depths of the wound. The patient subsequently recovered.

After the introduction of firearms, management of wounds of the chest became an important part of the surgery of trauma. The major issue with wounds of this type was dealing with open pneumothorax. The question of whether or not to close the wound was difficult to resolve. Paré quoted John Devigo of Rome who, in 1514, discussed the controversy.[3] Devigo said that there was disagreement between surgeons because "some have a mind to close a penetrating wound as soon as possible without attempting to keep it open by means of tents, for fear that the cold air would penetrate into the heart and the vital spirits would depart and vanish. Others, on the contrary, recommend keeping the wound open and if it is small, enlarge it in order to evacuate blood left in the thorax." Paré felt that those who advocated closing the wound were correct if there was no blood or only a small amount inside the chest. He also thought that it was appropriate to leave the wound open when the amount of blood in the thorax was considerable. The practice that Paré actually followed, judging from his case records, was to keep the wound open for 2 or 3 days, allowing blood to escape, and when this ceased, the wound was then closed.

It was not until the 18th century that physiologic studies and animal experiments were used to analyze function of the thoracic organs. William

Hewson[2] observed in 1767 that an open wound of the chest impaired breathing, but this was rapidly corrected when the wound was closed.

The innovation that permitted surgical treatment within the open chest was devised in 1904 by Sauerbruch, who created a negative pressure chamber.[4] This consisted of a room in which the patient and the operating team were housed with the pressure reduced so much that when the chest was opened the lung did not collapse. When this principle was first demonstrated, it was thought that it would revolutionize chest surgery. In 1905, Brauer invented an apparatus that enclosed the head of the patient to be anesthetized.[4] Air and anesthetic were introduced under positive pressure. Tiegel, Robinson, Davies, and others used tight-fitting masks instead.[4] At about this time, endotracheal intubation and anesthesia were introduced and by 1911 Ellsburg had developed a portable apparatus that provided the first intratracheal anesthesia for a chest operation, a patient with lung abscess operated on by Lilienthal.[4]

INCIDENCE

According to Besson and Saegesser's report on the epidemiology of thoracic trauma in an industrialized society, there are 12 thoracic injuries seen per day per one million population, of which four require hospital admission.[5] Associated injuries are common and account for a high mortality rate (Table 1–1).

Fifty percent of fatal accidents are associated with chest trauma and in roughly half of these the chest injury is the primary cause of death. This amounts to approximately 16,000 deaths per year in the United States.[6] According to Kemmerer and associates,[7] the distribution of injuries in 585 deaths was as noted in Table 1–2, with rib fractures, hemothorax, lung lacerations, and ruptures of great vessels being the most common. Late deaths can also occur, the most common cause being respiratory failure.[8]

The most immediately treatable causes of death relate to cardiorespiratory embarrassment. These consist of open pneumothorax, airway obstruction, flail chest, tension pneumothorax, massive hemothorax, cardiac tamponade, and air embolus. The trauma surgeon must be prepared to recognize and deal with these possibilities at the initial encounter with the patient.

Table 1–1.   Extrathoracic Injuries Associated with Chest Trauma[5]

	INCIDENCE (%) (n = 1485)	MORTALITY (%)
Encephalon	42	26
Abdominal	32	31
Orthopedic	46	24
Chest only	29	11

Table 1–2.   Thoracic Trauma[7]

	PERCENT DEATHS (n = 585)
Rib fractures	39
Hemothorax	28
Lung laceration	10
Ruptured great vessel	10
Lung contusion	6
Lacerated diaphragm	5
Myocardial injury	6
Sternal factures	5
Laceration trachea	1

INITIAL ASSESSMENT

The definitive evaluation of both blunt and penetrating trauma consists of history and physical and laboratory assessment. Although the physical examination is the key to the diagnosis of the nature and type of problem, the history should not be neglected. If not obtainable from the patient, it is often available from ambulance attendants, police, friends, relatives, or bystanders. It is important to obtain information about the mechanism of injury. Was penetrating trauma part of a fight in which there was a possibility of blunt trauma as well? Was the injury caused by an automobile accident, an automobile versus pedestrian, or a fall? In particular, the time the injury occurred relative to the patient's time of arrival in the emergency department is important to document because, if the time interval is short and the patient's condition desperate, immediate surgical intervention may be required to salvage the patient. If the time interval is long, the chances are excellent the patient will respond to resuscitation. The history can be obtained while the physical examination is being done, so that it does not necessarily result in a delay in the evaluation of the patient. Knowing whether a patient was awake and alert at the scene of an accident and knowing that he is now comatose may well change the priorities of management. What were the patient's complaints at the scene of the accident? What are they now? What was his previous state of health?

The physical examination can be carried out in a relatively short period of time (Table 1–3). One of the areas that is often neglected in the initial physical examination is the backside of the patient. All too often in a matter of moments the patient is restricted by

Table 1–3.   Examination

Breathing:	Slow, rapid, obstructed
Bleeding:	External, internal
Circulation:	Perfusion, urine output
Backside:	Inspect
Consciousness:	Level

intravenous lines, catheters, and splints. When first seen, the patient can be logrolled, with someone supporting his head and neck to prevent cervical spine injury, while the back, flanks, buttocks, and posterior aspects of the thigh and neck are inspected. Particular attention should be paid to penetrating wounds or any step-offs or other deformities of the spine. All of this should not take more than a few minutes to accomplish.

The first priority overall in assessment is the respiratory system. The presence or absence of airway obstruction should be noted. The breathing pattern should be observed, including the presence of paradoxical motion of the chest wall (flail chest). The paradoxical segment can be located either laterally as a section of ribs or anteriorly as the sternum. If the patient is comatose and has lost gag, cough, and swallowing reflex, aspiration is a possibility and endotracheal intubation should be carried out promptly. This usually should be done via the orotracheal route. If respiration is slow and shallow, there is presumption of central nervous system injury or sedation. Tachypnea is a manifestation of primary respiratory dysfunction. If the patient is tachypneic with a respiratory rate of more than 24 breaths per minute, is obtunded, or has any evidence of thoracic trauma, pulmonary injury should be assumed. In all instances in which there is evidence of chest injury, a chest radiograph should be obtained as rapidly as possible (Figs. 1–1, 1–2) and arterial blood should be drawn from the femoral artery for blood gas analysis.

The cardiovascular system is the second immediate priority. Most patients with any type of injury will have a rapid pulse as a result of apprehension or pain. The blood pressure is more reliable and should be noted initially. Young patients, by vasoconstricting, can

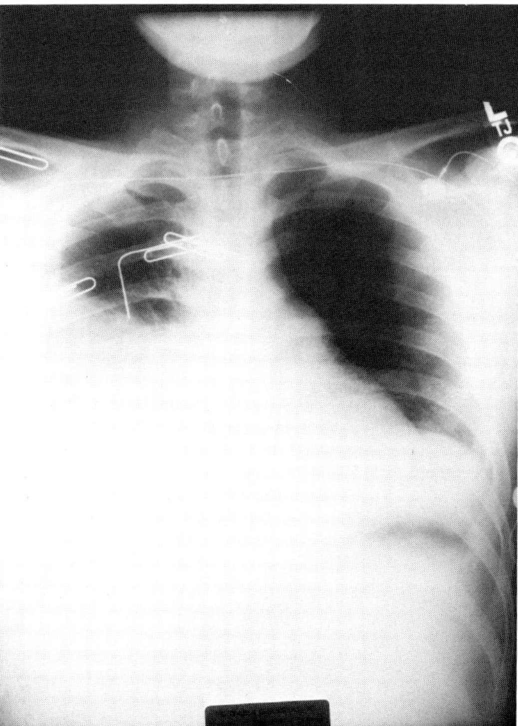

Figure 1–1. An initial chest radiograph is important for discovering intrathoracic pathology. The radiograph of this patient with multiple stab wounds to the right chest reveals a right hemothorax. Note the use of paper clips as external wound markers.

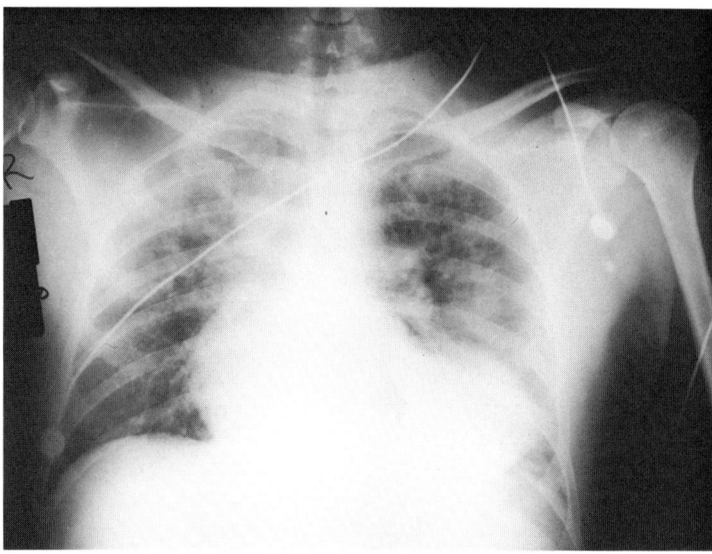

Figure 1–2. Admission chest radiographs also can reveal pathology after blunt trauma. In this patient, the radiograph demonstrated haziness of the left diaphragm, a finding of rupture of the left hemidiaphragm.

maintain a relatively normal blood pressure even though considerable blood volume has been lost. Assessment of peripheral perfusion and cardiac and cerebral function are appropriated to define the level of shock. Warm extremities, good peripheral perfusion, and a normal level of consciousness provide assurance that the cardiovascular system is intact.

Laboratory assessment can be carried out while the patient is being examined. In the initial survey of a patient with chest injury, blood should be drawn promptly for blood typing and cross-matching if there is any evidence of volume loss. A specimen should be sent for hematocrit and arterial blood gas determinations if there is any possibility of hypoxemia. Foreign objects such as bullets must be located, even if this requires extensive radiography, to try to establish the path of the bullet and to rule out bullet embolism (Fig. 1–3). The presence of pneumothorax or hemothorax should be noted and treated with tube decompression.

DEFINITIVE EXAMINATION

Once the preliminary evaluation has been done and laboratory and radiographic studies initiated, a more deliberate and complete physical examination can be performed.

Auscultation of lung and heart sounds should be done, but this is difficult in the emergency department environment. Absent breath sounds may indicate the presence of pneumothorax or hemothorax. Distant heart sounds are associated with blood in the pericardial space.

The location of penetrating injuries should be documented carefully and wounds noted with regard to their relationship to underlying structures. Examination of radiographs is improved if all wounds are marked with radiopaque markers, such as paper clips (Fig. 1–1).

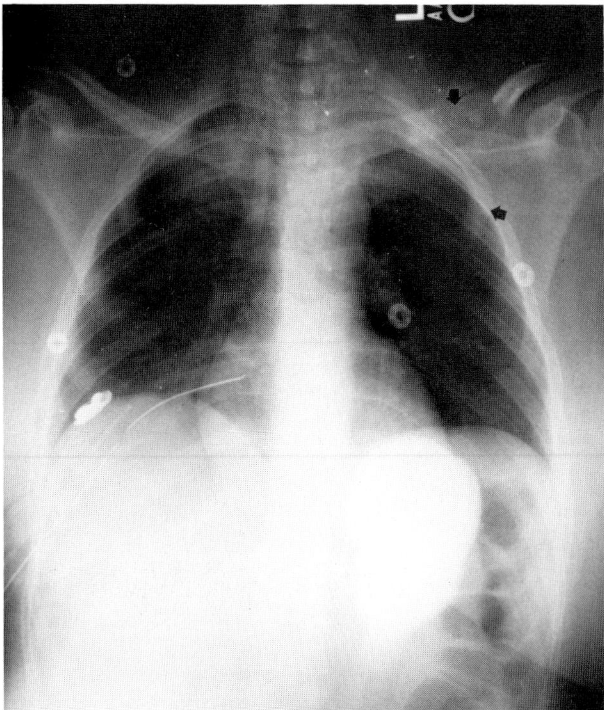

Figure 1–3. Bullets must be located. This one entered the left axilla at the lower arrow, hit the clavicle (*upper arrow*), and passed downward into the lower lobe of the right lung.

Determination of which wounds are entrance wounds and which are exit wounds is difficult; no presumptions should be made.

With blunt injury, if the patient is conscious, he should be asked to take a deep breath. The ability to do so without discomfort rules out chest wall injury and markedly decreases the likelihood of intrathoracic injury. If discomfort is manifested, the chest wall should be palpated carefully and specific rib or sternum tenderness noted. Rib fractures are a clinical, not a radiological, diagnosis and the extent of chest wall injury is best determined by examination. Radiographic studies always underestimate the number of fractures. Costochondral and sternochondral separation are not demonstrated by x-ray and sternal fracture is not seen on the usual anteroposterior view.

Blunt or penetrating injuries to the upper six ribs can involve injuries to vessels of the thoracic outlet, the lung parenchyma, or the heart. Injuries below the sixth interspace are associated with the possibility of abdominal injury[9] (Fig. 1–4). Because the diaphragm rises with normal ventilation to the sixth interspace, penetrating trauma below the sixth interspace may well penetrate the abdominal cavity. Similarly, very little volume of lung tissue lies underneath the lower six ribs, and blunt injuries associated with rib fracture are more apt to injure an underlying viscus such as liver, spleen, stomach, or kidney rather than lung. As a matter of fact, thoracic bleeding from penetrating injuries or major blunt trauma to the lower six ribs may have its source in the abdomen. Laparotomy, rather than

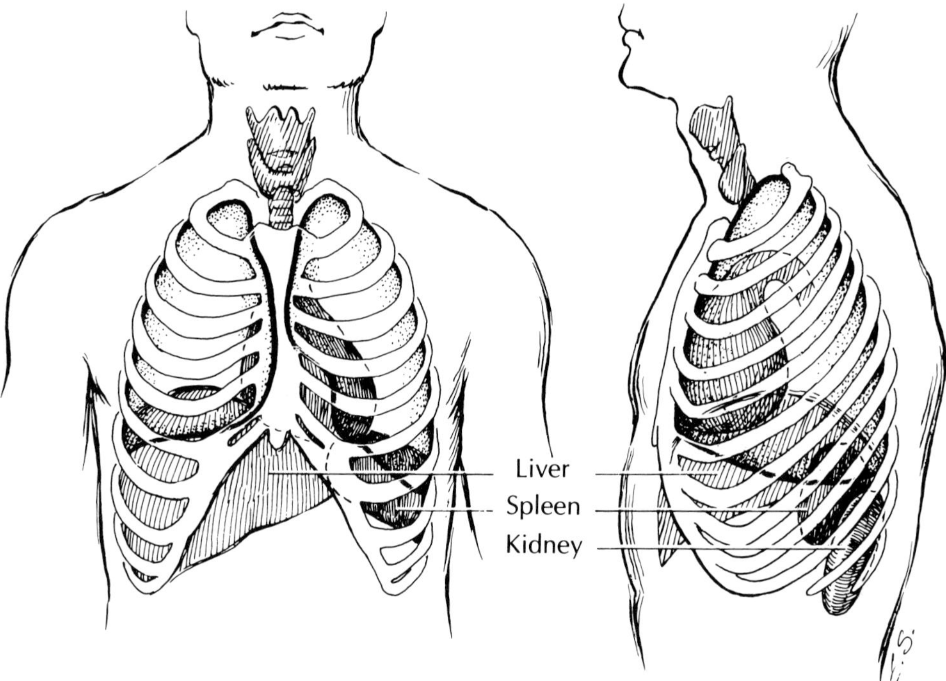

Figure 1–4.   The lower six ribs overlie abdominal structures primarily. Injuries to the lower chest are associated more frequently with abdominal rather than thoracic complications.

thoracotomy, may be necessary to control bleeding. Moreover, it has been our experience that even when the injury appears to be limited to the chest, laparotomy is indicated more commonly than thoracotomy, because injuries that require surgical treatment are much more common in the abdomen than in the chest.

Generally, diaphragmatic injuries are best treated initially by abdominal exploration, because there is greater likelihood that there will be serious abdominal injury requiring repair than there is serious thoracic injury requiring repair (Fig. 1–5). Rib fractures on the right are associated with a high incidence of liver injury and a relatively low incidence of pulmonary parenchymal injury. Injuries in the vicinity of the ninth and tenth ribs on the left suggest the possibility of splenic injury. One patient in 10 with injuries to the ninth and tenth ribs will prove subsequently to have a splenic rupture. Injuries to the 11th and 12th ribs are associated with renal injury, and urine should be assessed for blood. Shoulder pain (Kehr's sign) suggests central diaphragm tendon irritation from blood below the diaphragm.

Assessment of upper and lower extremity pulses may provide clues to localized vascular injuries. Lacerations from penetrating trauma or avulsion-type injuries that follow blunt trauma may result in a weak or absent pulse in the craniocervical vessel so affected. Discrepancy between pulse volume in the upper and lower extremities may suggest the possibility of a traumatic aortic injury. A paradoxical pulse, that is, one in which the blood pressure varies markedly with ventilation, is a finding associated with pericardial tamponade.

When evidence of impaired perfusion or cardiovascular function exists, the status of

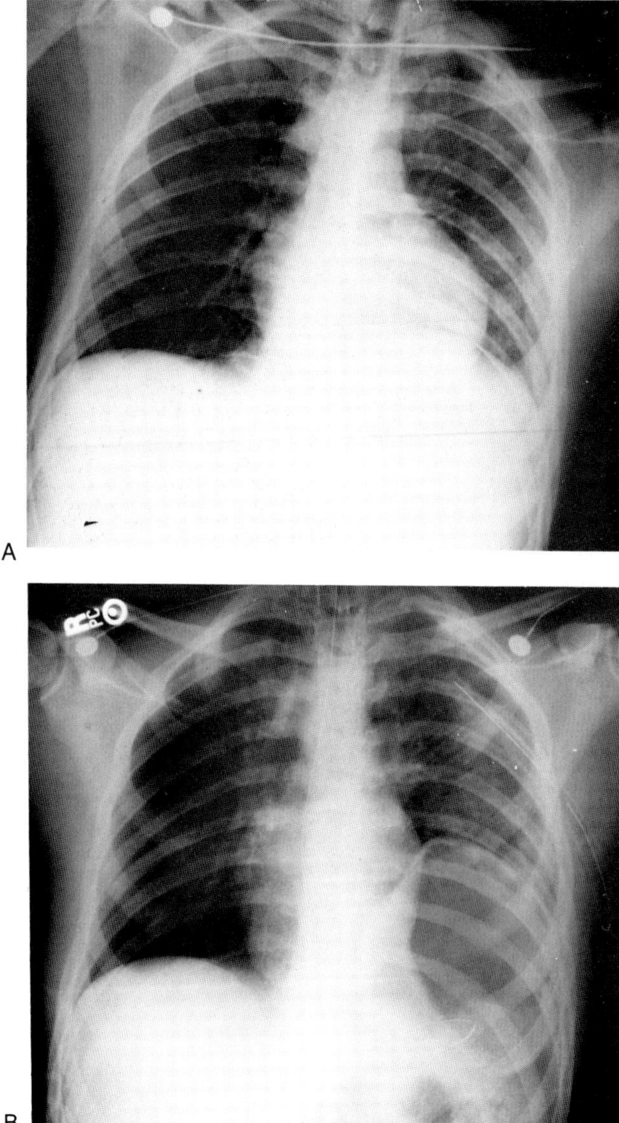

Figure 1–5.   Initial chest radiograph after a stab wound of the eighth interspace midaxillary line (**A**). Peritoneal lavage was negative. Diaphragm injury was not suspected until the patient became dyspneic 6 hr later when the stomach was found to have herniated into the chest through a diaphragm laceration (**B**).

the superficial veins should be assessed (Fig. 1–6). In most instances, shock after trauma is due to hemorrhage and is hypovolemic. In this circumstance, superficial veins are collapsed. However, when tension pneumothorax or pericardial tamponade are the causes of shock, the neck veins are distended. The former causes a relative obstruction to venous return; the latter causes an increased pericardial pressure collapsing the atria and impairing

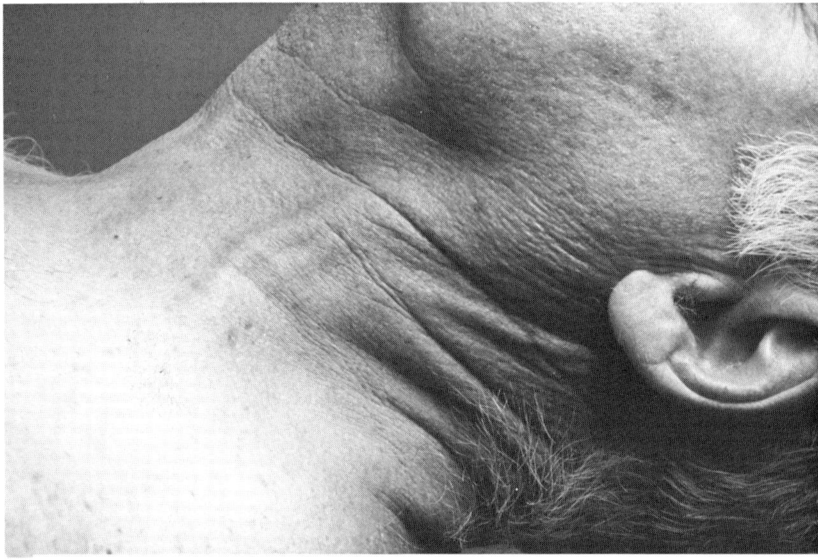

Figure 1–6.   Differentiation between hypovolemic and cardiogenic or venous obstructive shock lies in observation of neck veins. The distended jugular vein seen in this case suggests cardiogenic shock or tension pneumothorax.

filling of the heart. In these two instances, superficial veins will be distended and central venous pressure, if measured, will be high.

Although pericardial tamponade is a relatively rare complication of blunt trauma, occasional cases will be seen in any busy emergency room. The bullet in gunshot wounds in particular can go in any direction, so even an apparently remote injury may result in penetration of the heart. For this reason, the path of the bullet must be determined by examination and radiography. The following are two examples of the problems bullets can generate.

Case 1

A 45-year-old white man was admitted to the emergency room in profound shock with a story of having been shot in the right arm as he attempted to roll out of his car when held up by a hitchhiker.

On initial examination, there was one wound on the left arm. No exit wound was found. The chest, abdominal, and arm radiographs were negative for foreign body. The patient failed to respond to rapid fluid administration, with shock becoming progressively more severe, when it was observed that his neck veins were bulging. Emergency thoracotomy disclosed pericardial tamponade. The bullet was subsequently located in the vicinity of the left leg. The patient was apparently shot while in a position as shown in Figure 1–7A. The bullet passed obliquely through the body, injuring the heart en route. Failure to monitor the status of the neck veins initially very nearly cost the patient his life.

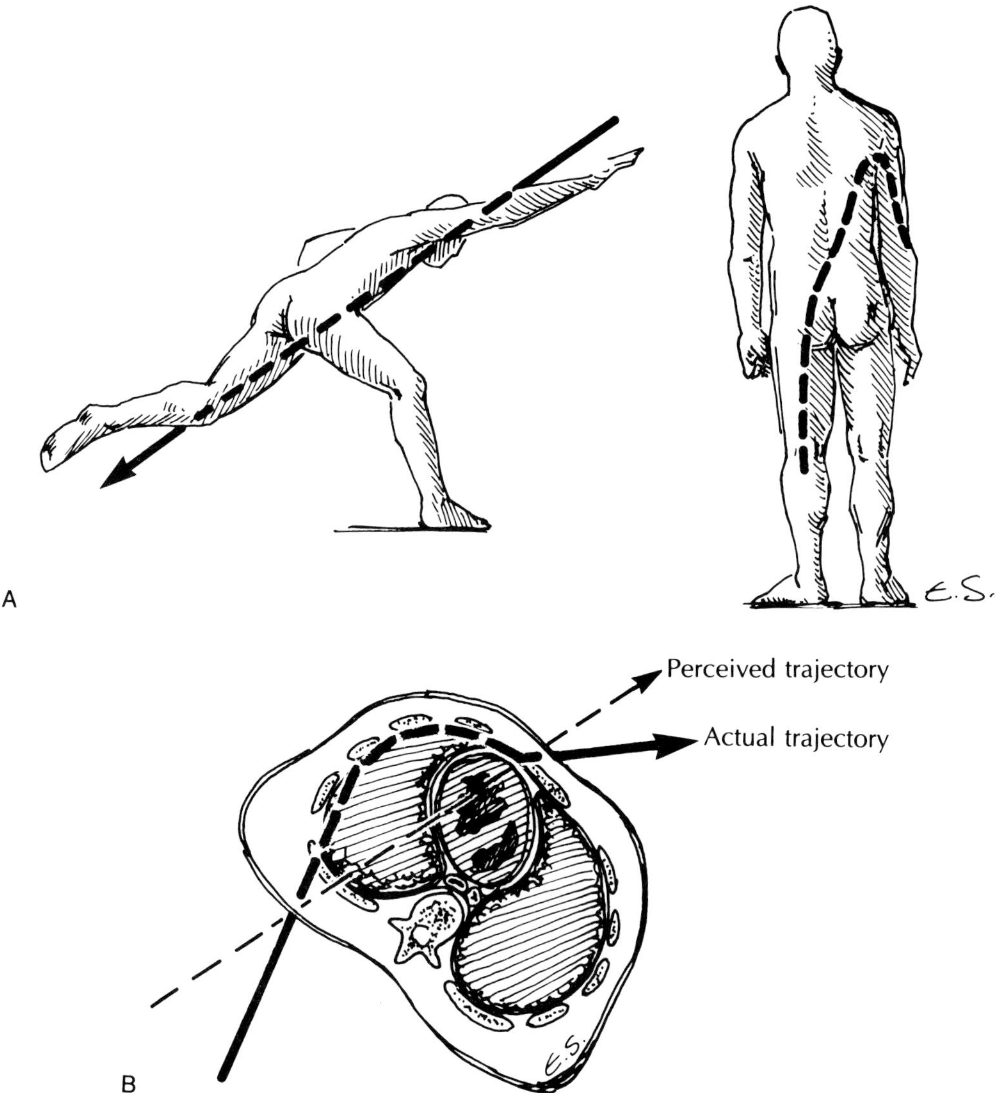

Figure 1–7.   A, B: Demonstrate, as in Fig. 1–1, the devious paths missiles can take. The path of the bullet may not be obvious even though the entrance and exit wounds of site or lodgment of the bullet are identified.

Case 2

The patient, a 23-year-old man, was admitted with evidence of a gunshot wound in the back just below the tip of the left scapula. There was a second wound two fingerbreadths below the xiphoid. Chest and abdominal films were not remarkable. An immediate thoracotomy was carried out, but no evidence of intracardiac or thoracic injury was found. The bullet apparently passed circumferentially around the chest wall (Fig. 1–7B).

FINDINGS INDICATIVE OF SERIOUS INJURY

Although any injury to the chest is potentially serious, certain findings are associated with an appreciable incidence of major injury (Table 1–4). These findings are important, as missed injuries can have dire consequences.[10] Rib fractures, particularly the first or second ribs, or flail chest document a major impact. Evidence of mediastinal blood as manifested by mediastinal widening or apical capping are additional manifestations of violence. A massive air leak, hemoptysis, major hemothorax, diaphragm laceration, or distended neck veins are likewise associated with a high probability of significant associated injuries.

The first and second ribs are short, strong ribs that overlie the subclavian arteries and veins. We have found that with fractures of the first or second rib, the incidence of underlying vascular injury is approximately 15%.[11] In two-thirds to three-fourths of cases, there will be clinical evidence of underlying vascular injury such as a bruit, impaired distal pulses, overt hemorrhage, evidence of bleeding on chest radiographs manifested by apical capping or hemothorax, or a large hematoma at the base of the neck (Fig. 1–8). In approximately 25% of cases, however, evidence of injury to vessels is minimal. Because of the force required to injure these ribs, arteriographic assessment is appropriate in most blunt traumatic injuries of the first and second ribs.

In approximately a quarter of the deaths after sudden deceleration injuries, such as automobile accidents, the cause of death is aortic rupture. Only a relatively small percentage of these patients survive to reach the emergency room. In these instances, the aortic laceration is incomplete or temporarily contained by the intact mediastinum. If the chest radiograph shows mediastinal widening or if it is at all equivocal, conventional posteroanterior chest films should be obtained if at all possible. The standard emergency chest film taken in the anteroposterior direction magnifies the contents of the anterior chest and mediastinum. Evidence of tracheal shift, apical capping, or hemothorax are all manifestations of mediastinal hemorrhage and dictate immediate arteriography. As only a third of cases of mediastinal widening are due to major vascular injury, thoracotomy is not recommended unless severe, ongoing hemorrhage is evident or the patient appears critically injured and requires urgent operation for some other reason.

Multiple rib fractures in multiple places, the "stove-in chest," is one form of flail chest. Besides compromising ventilation, there is a high incidence of major pulmonary parenchymal injury and an appreciable incidence of cardiac or major vascular injury.[8,12] The sternum also can act as a flail segment when there has been bilateral costochondral separation. This is a more benign form of flail chest with less instability and pain.

Table 1–4.   Manifestations of Major Injury

1st, 2nd rib fractures
Sternal fracture
Mediastinal widening
Flail chest
Massive air leak
Hemoptysis
Massive hemothorax
Neck vein distention
Blunt diaphragmatic injury

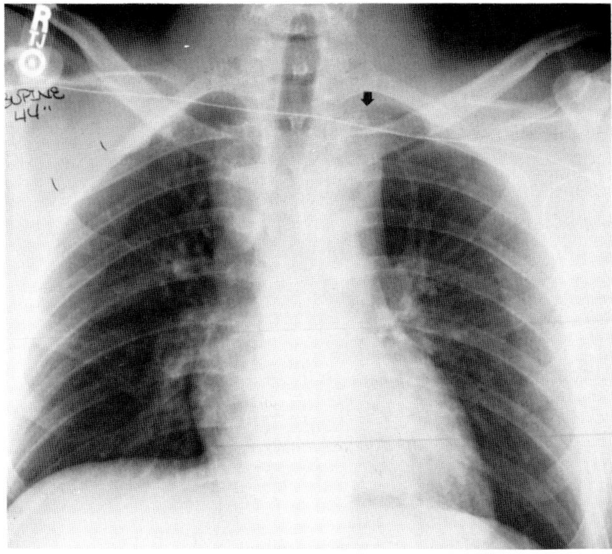

Figure 1–8.   The chest radiograph demonstrates enlargement of the upper mediastinum and apical capping (*arrow*). This suggests large vessel bleeding.

Minor air leaks are relatively common manifestations of lung lacerations. Major air leaks, such as those associated with tracheal or main stem bronchus injuries, are less common. They may present as problems of massive pulmonary collapse or subcutaneous emphysema. These manifestations often become dramatic only with the introduction of positive pressure ventilation and elevation of airway pressures well above atmospheric. With resuscitation, respiratory distress may suddenly worsen, mediastinal air and cervical or subcutaneous emphysema may develop, and a massive air leak becomes evident. In these circumstances, major airway laceration should be assumed and immediate diagnostic maneuvers or thoracotomy performed.

Hemoptysis is another manifestation of major airway laceration or extensive pulmonary parenchymal damage. If major bleeding is present, immediate operation is indicated. Airway patency may be ensured by passing a double lumen endotracheal tube that permits ventilatory isolation of the two lungs.

A large hemothorax associated with shock with no other apparent injury suggests the possibility of major intrathoracic vascular injury, especially if the time interval between injury and presentation with major hemothorax is short. Hemothorax that exceeds 1000 ml in volume, occurring within an hour of injury, suggests the possibility that major pulmonary parenchymal injury, mediastinal vascular injury, or severe chest wall injury is present. Thoracotomy usually is indicated to control bleeding and to evacuate intrapleural clot. The volume of hemothorax should be estimated by combining chest tube outputs with the radiographic appearance of the pleural cavities.

When chest trauma is associated with shock, the status of the neck veins should be assessed during resuscitation. A rapid rise in venous pressure with persistence of shock means tension pneumothorax, severe myocardial contusion, or pericardial tamponade. If doubt exists as to the cause of neck vein distention, a chest tube should be placed in the appropriate pleural space or pericardiocentesis carried out. Sometimes both procedures will be necessary.

Diaphragmatic injury secondary to blunt trauma is another sign of a potentially severe injury. There is a high incidence of associated thoracic and abdominal injuries. Also, the negative pressure in the chest will result in sucking the abdominal contents into the thoracic cavity, progressively compromising pulmonary function.

REFERENCES

1. Breasted JH. *The Edwin Smith Surgical Papyrus.* vol. I. Chicago: University of Chicago Press; 1930.
2. Hewson W. *The Works of William Hewson, F.R.S.* (Edited by George Gulliver.) London: Sydenham Society; 1846.
3. Paré A. *The Works of Ambrose Paré.* (Thomas Johnson, trans.) London; 1678.
4. Meade RH. *A History of Thoracic Surgery.* Springfield, IL: Charles C Thomas; 1961.
5. Besson A, Saegesser F. *Color Atlas of Chest Trauma and Associated Injuries.* vol. 1. Oradell, NJ: Medical Economics; 1983.
6. LoCicero J III, Mattox KL. Epidemiology of chest trauma. *Surg Clin North Am.* 1989;69(1):15.
7. Kemmerer WT, et al. Patterns of thoracic injuries in fatal traffic accidents. *J Trauma.* 1961;1:595.
8. Shorr RM, Crittenden M, Indeck M, Hartunian SL, Rodriguez A. Blunt thoracic trauma: analysis of 515 patients. *Ann Surg.* 1987.
9. Kerr TM, Sood R, Buckman RF Jr, Gelman J, Grosh J. Prospective trial of the six hour rule in stab wounds of the chest. *Surg Gynecol Obstet.* 1989;169:223.
10. Enderson BL, Maull KI. Missed injuries: the trauma surgeon's nemesis. *Surg Clin North Am.* 1991; 71(2), 399.
11. Wilson JM, Thomas AN, et al. Severe chest trauma; morbidity implications of first and second rib fracture in 120 patients. *Arch Surg.* 1978;113:846.
12. Symbas PN. Cardiothoracic trauma. *Curr Prob Surg.* 1991;XXVII(11).

2

Assessment and Treatment of Cardiopulmonary Dysfunction

JAMES W. HOLCROFT, M.D.

<hr>

HISTORY: Insofar as can be determined, the concept of shock was first recognized in the early 1700s. The term "shock" was used in 1743 by an unknown translator of the treatise of LeDran on the management of gunshot wounds. Guthrie, in 1815, as credited by Morris, used the term shock in his book on gunshot wounds of the extremities. In 1872, Samuel D. Gross referred to shock as a "rude unhinging of the machinery of life." John Collins Warren applied the term to "a momentary pause in the act of death" and postulated that shock was a reaction to major injury.

Most of the clinical observations that led to the development of the concept of shock were made on the battlefield. When external hemorrhage was massive, the cause of death was easily recognized as hemorrhage. If the patient survived the initial bleeding episode, however, the concept that the patient could still die as a consequence of the initial blood volume loss was difficult to grasp. Indeed, many illnesses were treated by bleeding to remove "toxins in the blood." In the late 1700s, John Hunter, the founder of many modern surgical concepts, assumed that toxic factors caused death after injuries and advocated bleeding to treat gunshot wounds, provided there was no overt hemorrhage. By the time of the American Civil War, phlebotomy was no longer used to treat shock, but the concept that toxic factors were the primary cause of shock still dominated. Soldiers with major wounds of the extremities died when managed nonoperatively, and extremities were amputated (amputation being the most common operation during the war) to prevent toxic and septic causes of death.

The laboratory investigations of shock by George W. Crile at the end of the 19th century demonstrated in experimental animals that the likelihood of shock increased with the magnitude of injury and that a small hemorrhage preceding injury impaired the animal's ability to survive. Crile found that the central venous pressure fell in shock and that intravenous infusions of saline improved survival rates. He hypothesized that the fluid acted to increase the venous pressure, thereby restoring cardiac filling, cardiac

14

output, blood pressure, and organ perfusion. In 1910, Yandel Henderson reiterated the importance of venous return to the heart. He, too, noted the important relationship between venous return, cardiac output, and arterial blood pressure, but he failed to recognize that internal loss of plasma or blood could deplete the blood volume and impair filling of the heart.

Recognition of interstitial fluid depletion was well established by the time of the Vietnam conflict, leading to usually successful shock resuscitation. Aggressive resuscitation and rapid transport to base hospitals enabled victims of massive injuries to survive for at least a few days. This led to the recognition of a new shock lesion, the respiratory distress syndrome. Because many of the patients had received large volumes of fluid during resuscitation and because the lungs at autopsy were noted to be edematous, it was initially believed that this lesion was caused by the excessive administration of fluid. Subsequently, through the development and use of the Swan-Ganz catheter, it was demonstrated that certain advanced forms of shock, particularly those associated with massive soft tissue injury, were followed by diffuse increase in vascular permeability and an obligatory loss of fluid from the vascular space into the interstitium. The interstitial edema found in the lung was therefore caused by shock-generated increases in vascular permeability and not by overly vigorous resuscitation.

Major trauma involving the thorax can result in serious direct injury to the heart and lungs. Blunt trauma frequently produces myocardial or pulmonary contusions that may significantly impair function of these organs; penetrating trauma, depending on the location of the injury, can have obvious serious consequences. Pneumothorax, tension pneumothorax, pericardial tamponade, and lacerations of the heart or major vessels are the resulting life-threatening injuries that require immediate treatment.

In addition to direct injuries, compromise of heart and lung function also can develop as a result of injuries located elsewhere and can be equally serious. For example, lacerations of the neck may cause venous air emboli, producing acute pulmonary artery obstruction and right heart failure, or pulmonary laceration may result in coronary air embolism with compromise of cardiac function in the absence of direct injury to this organ. Crush injuries of the extremities may result in tissue embolism and intravascular coagulation with the development of the respiratory distress syndrome.[2,3] Pulmonary embolism also may occur as a result of clot forming in the pelvic or leg veins, which is common after major injury. The development of septic complications may similarly alter pulmonary microvascular integrity with the development of, or aggravation of, preexisting pulmonary dysfunction.[4] "Vicious cycles" of cardiac and pulmonary dysfunction are frequently set up that make immediate treatment of the primary problem imperative. For example, an injury that results in pulmonary dysfunction may decrease arterial oxygen tension (Po_2) enough to impair cardiac function. Low cardiac output in turn produces venous desaturation and worsening hypoxemia, thus again compromising heart muscle function.[5] Alternatively, the cycle may be entered with a primary cardiac injury that results in pulmonary edema, pulmonary dysfunction, hypoxemia, and worsening cardiac failure.

Treatment of either the direct or indirect alterations in pulmonary and cardiac function requires an understanding of the basic pathophysiology and careful monitoring. Fluids, drugs, and mechanical ventilatory support may be indicated, and their use is dictated by certain standard criteria that also should be understood. As the patient improves and the need for intense monitoring and support resolves, criteria for discontinuing these adjuncts are equally important.

PULMONARY PATHOPHYSIOLOGY

The primary function of the lung is to exchange oxygen and carbon dioxide. This requires an unobstructed airway, adequate alveolar ventilation, a gas-permeable alveolar-capillary membrane, and well distributed pulmonary capillary perfusion. Compromise of any of these will adversely affect gas exchange (Table 2–1).

The *airway* may be compromised by maxillofacial injury with upper airway obstruction from edematous soft tissues or bleeding or, in the case of an obtunded patient, by the tongue falling back into the pharynx. The larynx can be obstructed by direct injury with edema and hemorrhage or by an aspirated foreign body. The trachea and bronchi can be obstructed by direct injury with edema and hemorrhage, by aspiration of secretions consisting of blood or gastric contents, or by major lacerations.

Alveolar ventilation results from the bellows action of the chest wall and diaphragm expanding the volume of the lung during inspiration with passive recoil during expiration. During inspiration, a negative intrathoracic pressure is generated in relation to the atmospheric pressure, resulting in filling of the lungs with air. Nonflail chest wall injuries impair ventilatory function because of pain associated with inspiration, resulting in a rapid, shallow (low tidal volume) ventilatory exchange. Because the normal anatomic dead space of the upper airway is about 150 ml and does not change, changes in tidal volume have a proportionately larger effect on alveolar ventilation. For example, a decrease from a normal breath of 600 to 300 ml represents a 50% reduction in tidal volume, whereas alveolar ventilation is reduced to one-third of normal (450–150 ml). The respiratory rate would thus have to triple to maintain the same alveolar ventilation, from, say, 12 to 36 breaths per minute.

With a flail chest wall injury, there is the same problem of pain and low tidal volumes as that associated with nonflail injuries mentioned previously and, in addition, the paradoxical motion of the chest wall results in further decreases in the efficiency of ventilation. Because the flail side is relatively underventilated, either volume expansion of the noninjured side would have to increase proportionately to compensate for failure to ventilate the injured side or respiratory rate would have to increase proportionately further. Both of these frequently occur and require further increases in the work of breathing. Furthermore, mediastinal shift that occurs with ventilation tends to have the same effect on

Table 2–1. Causes of Impaired Gas Exchange

Airway obstruction
Inadequate alveolar ventilation
Alveolar-capillary membrane dysfunction
Alveolar-capillary perfusion mismatch
Compromised pulmonary vascular patency

the noninjured side as the paradoxical chest wall movement does on the injured side. This results in difficulty in expanding the noninjured lung. Finally, the hypoventilation of the injured side results in increases in intrapulmonary shunting and hypoxia that may not be compensated for by increases in alveolar ventilation or supplemental oxygen.

In the last analysis, effective ventilation takes place in patent alveoli, and ventilation of these can be blocked by fluid accumulation in the small airways or closure of small airways (i.e., atelectasis). Fluid accumulation in alveoli can occur with aspiration of blood or gastric contents, direct injury resulting in intraalveolar bleeding (contusion), or as a result of interstitial fluid accumulation (i.e., pulmonary edema; see later). Atelectasis or progressive closure of alveoli can result from inadequate ventilation of alveoli, such as in chest wall injuries, or from lung collapse, such as occurs in pneumothorax. These problems also place increased demands on the work of breathing and, as already discussed, underventilated alveoli result in increased intrapulmonary shunting of mixed venous blood and hypoxemia that can be difficult to correct. In addition, once closed, alveoli are difficult to open even with high airway pressures. Fortunately, in most circumstances hypoxic pulmonary vaso-constriction causes the circulation to be shifted away from poorly ventilated (or collapsed) alveoli, so the defect in oxygenation is not as great as would otherwise be expected. Additionally, the phenomenon known as "absorption atelectasis" can occur when 100% oxygen is provided as the inspired gas. Nitrogen, which is normally about 80% of the volume of inspired and alveolar gas, is inert with no arteriovenous gradient and therefore can act as a stent to maintain alveolar volume even in poorly ventilated alveoli. If 100% oxygen is used as the inspired gas, complete absorption can occur in poorly perfused alveoli, resulting in alveolar collapse. Maintenance of continuous positive airway pressure (CPAP) or positive end-expiratory pressure (PEEP) helps maintain small airway patency during the entire ventilatory cycle and can prevent alveolar collapse even in poorly ventilated alveoli.[6]

The *alveolar capillary membrane* is the final barrier across which gas is exchanged. Its function can be acutely compromised by interstitial bleeding, such as might occur with pulmonary contusion, or accumulation of interstitial fluid (i.e., pulmonary edema), which develops in association with a variety of direct and indirect injuries to the lung, as well as iatrogenic fluid overload. As a result of excellent pulmonary lymphatic drainage, the normal lung is extremely resistant to the accumulation of interstitial edema caused by high pulmonary capillary pressures or severe hemodilution that can occur with the administration of large quantities of salt solution. The relatively high interstitial protein content in the lung also helps prevent pulmonary edema, because any increase in interstitial lung water tends to wash out interstitial proteins. Thus, in the case of a high hydrostatic pressure gradient (increased pulmonary capillary wedge pressure), the colloid osmotic pressure gradient increases and favors intravascular as opposed to interstitial distribution of fluid. Similarly, with hemodilution and a decreased colloid osmotic pressure gradient, the dilution of the interstitial proteins tends to return this gradient to normal, and the relative colloidal osmotic pressure between the vasculature and the interstitium of the lung is reestablished.[7]

In certain circumstances, such as those associated with the respiratory distress syndrome after shock, massive trauma, or sepsis, there may be diffuse systemic injury to *vascular endothelium* with a loss of the integrity of the vascular system.[2,3,4,8] Although this leaky microvasculature is systemic, it is manifested most profoundly in the lung, with corresponding alterations in pulmonary alveolar function as interstitial edema, alveolar flooding, and small airway collapse, resulting in alveolar-capillary perfusion mismatch

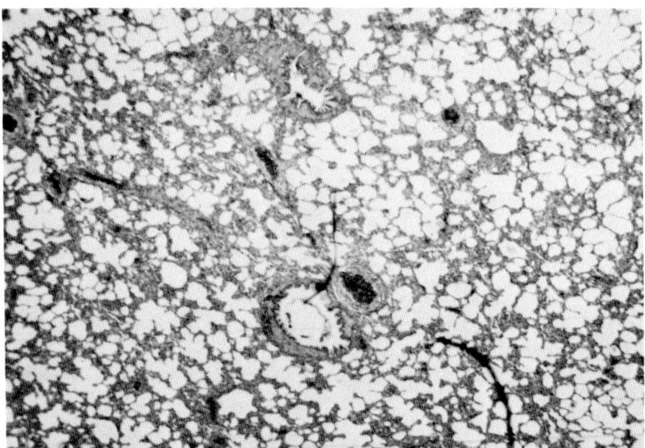

Figure 2–1.   Microscopic section of the lung 48 hr after injury reveals interstitial and alveolar edema and hemorrhage.

(Fig. 2–1). This is reflected in loss of elasticity (compliance) of the lung and increased arteriovenous shunting, as manifested by systemic arterial hypoxemia. Pulmonary contusion, which results in diffuse interstitial and alveolar hemorrhage, also results in compromise of pulmonary function by this mechanism. Again, maintaining positive airway pressure offers a means of preventing alveolar collapse and also may modify interstitial edema through alveolar counterpressure or by encouraging lymphatic drainage.[9]

Another aspect of pulmonary dysfunction relating to alveolar-capillary mismatch occurs when there is compromise of *vascular patency* and perfusion. Vascular patency is rarely severely compromised and, when major vascular obstruction results, such as with pulmonary embolism, the primary impact is on the heart; however, high flows at high pressures through a limited patent vascular bed can result in pulmonary edema (see next section). Moreover, the shock state associated with tissue trauma or sepsis is frequently accompanied by intravascular clotting (disseminated intravascular coagulation) and pulmonary microembolism, resulting in pulmonary microvascular lesions[2–4] (Fig. 2–2). The pulmonary microvasculature has abundant collaterals that prevent pulmonary infarction, but clot in the microvasculature acts to increase pulmonary vascular resistance, which can increase cardiac work and result in decreased cardiac output. Additionally, endothelial and platelet factors released locally can cause bronchoconstriction and small airway closure, resulting in intrapulmonary shunting and hypoxemia.[3]

Finally, ventilation and perfusion must be reasonably matched. We have already discussed the problem that arises in a number of situations in which there is perfusion of nonventilated (or poorly ventilated) alveoli. This results in intrapulmonary shunting of venous blood causing hypoxemia.[5] Conversely, underperfusion of well ventilated alveoli also causes problems, because there is an effective or actual increase in dead space ventilation at the expense of perfused alveoli (assuming the same tidal volume). The effect is the same as a decrease in tidal volume already discussed with regard to chest wall injuries. There is a need for increased work of breathing. This problem is commonly present with severe hypovolemia, where the low cardiac output and pulmonary artery pressures preclude adequate perfusion of well ventilated midlung and apical segments. In addition, the

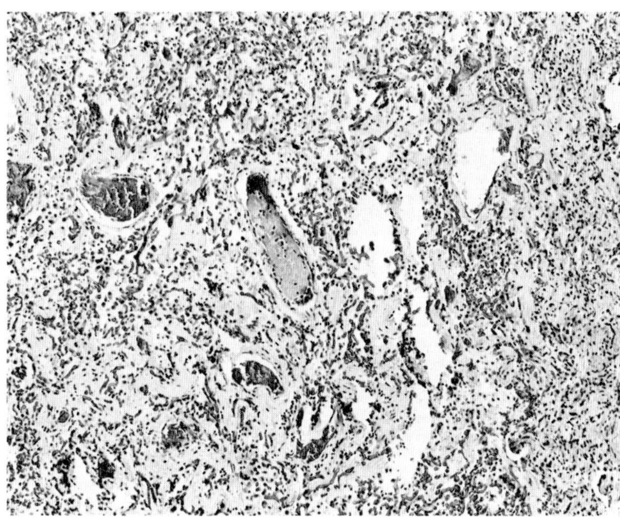

Figure 2–2.　Microscopic sections taken 24 hr after injury demonstrate pulmonary congestion and amorphous masses of material in pulmonary microvessels that take a positive stain for fibrin.

problem is compounded by the mixed venous desaturation that is associated with the low cardiac output.[4,5] Pulmonary emboli (both thrombotic and air) also are associated with the same pathophysiologic process, because ventilation generally continues in segments supplied by acutely occluded vessels.

CARDIOVASCULAR PATHOPHYSIOLOGY

The primary function of the cardiovascular system is to maintain flow of well oxygenated blood to vital organs at a rate appropriate for their metabolic demands.[10] This requires an adequate intravascular volume, unobstructed vessels, good cardiac filling and function, and peripheral vascular tone, although the interdependency of these various components also is obvious (Table 2–2). Hypovolemia or venous obstruction, which result in decreased cardiac filling, thereby decrease cardiac function, ultimately compromising flow. Similarly, decreases in peripheral tone produce increased microvascular sequestration of blood with central vascular volume depletion and decreased cardiac output. Blood pressure, per se, is a useful index of the adequacy of cardiovascular function because it is determined to some

Table 2–2.　**Causes of Impaired Cardiac Function**

Hypovolemia
Pulmonary/vascular obstruction
Cardiac compression
Cardiac dysfunction
Loss of vascular tone

extent by the function of these other components. However, an adequate blood pressure does not necessarily indicate normal cardiovascular function. For example, blood pressure may be grossly normal, due to compensatory mechanisms, in the presence of hypovolemia or cardiac failure when peripheral resistance is increased at the expense of severe maldistribution of blood flow.

The usual causes of cardiovascular compromise in traumatized patients are hypovolemia, myocardial contusion, pericardial tamponade, or tension pneumothorax. Occasionally, air or thrombotic emboli are the factors responsible. The effects on the cardiovascular system are indicated in Table 2–3. In patients with sepsis, alterations in vascular tone or permeability play a major role.[4] All of these abnormalities compromise flow in the cardiovascular system and may lead to impaired tissue and organ perfusion "shock." In many cases of chest trauma, multiple abnormalities coexist.

Hypovolemia

Most of the blood loss that follows an injury results primarily in depletion of the capacitance system, the systemic venules and small veins, which normally contain approximately 50% of the total body blood volume. Loss of blood from these vessels decreases filling of the right heart, resulting in a decrease in right heart output. Consequently, the pulmonary venous bed is depleted, left-sided filling pressures are decreased, and left heart output decreases, resulting in hypoperfusion of vascular beds.[9] Hypoxemia and hypercapnia may be present by the mechanisms already discussed and may contribute further to cardiovascular depression. Metabolic acidosis, although improving tissue oxygen delivery through the Bohr effect, may contribute further to cardiac depression and hypoxemia.

Myocardial Contusion

The right ventricle is more commonly damaged with chest injuries than the left. One of the more common injuries is a right ventricular myocardial contusion incurred when a patient's sternum strikes a steering wheel in an automobile accident (see Chapter 15). Patients who present to the emergency room alive with penetrating injuries of the heart also are more

Table 2–3. **Affect of Cardiopulmonary Pathology**

NORMAL PRESSURES	CENTRAL VENOUS AND RIGHT ATRIAL (5–7 mm Hg)	PULMONARY ARTERY (15 mm Hg)	LEFT ATRIAL (WEDGE) (7–10 mm Hg)
Hypovolemia	↓ ↓	↓	↓
Myocardial contusion			
Right	↑ ↑	↓	↓
Left	↑	↑	↑ ↑
Pericardial tamponade	↑ ↑	↓	↑
Tension pneumothorax	↑ ↑	↑	↓ ↑
Positive pressure ventilation	↑	↑	↑

likely to have injuries to the right rather than the left ventricle because of the anterior location of the former.

Right ventricular contusion leads to decreased contractility and decreased compliance of the ventricle. The right ventricle is thus unable to pump blood in adequate amounts, resulting in decreased filling of the left heart and thereby decreased left heart output. The result is decreased cardiac output with low left atrial (pulmonary wedge) pressures similar to that found with hypovolemia, but high right atrial pressures.[11]

A left ventricular contusion or injury also leads to low cardiac output and systemic arterial blood pressure, but left atrial pressures are high because the primary problem is a dysfunctioning left ventricle that is unable to pump blood efficiently into the systemic arterial circulation. The dysfunctioning left ventricle also leads to dysfunction of the right ventricle as the left ventricle enlarges and pushes the interventricular septum into the right ventricle. The thin-walled right ventricle is unable to expand because it is confined by the pericardial sac. The compressed right ventricle then is unable to pump adequate amounts into the pulmonary vasculature. The end result of severe dysfunction of the left ventricle is, again, low cardiac output with low systemic arterial pressures and high left and right atrial pressures. In addition to cardiac muscle dysfunction, arrhythmias that decrease effective cardiac output also are a significant problem with myocardial contusion.

Pericardial Tamponade

Pericardial tamponade exerts its adverse influence on the cardiovascular system by compressing the inferior and superior vena cava as they enter the right atrium and by compressing the right atrium, right ventricle, and left atrium. (The thicker walled left ventricle withstands the compression better than the other chambers of the heart.) Compression of the vena cava impairs filling of the right heart and thus impairs right ventricular output. Compression of the right atrium and right ventricle directly affects the function of these chambers and thus limits their capabilities for discharging blood into the pulmonary vasculature. Decreased filling of the pulmonary vasculature leads to decreased filling of the left heart. Left ventricular stroke volume decreases. The end result is low cardiac output, low systemic arterial blood pressure associated with extremely high right atrial pressure, and moderately elevated left atrial pressures.

Tension Pneumothorax

A tension pneumothorax has many adverse effects on the cardiovascular system. High pressure within one pleural cavity displaces the heart into the other. The high pressure displacement compresses or even kinks the inferior and superior vena cavae, decreasing filling of the right atrium and right ventricle. High pressures applied to the outside of the right atrium and right ventricle compress those chambers and further impair filling. Collapse of one lung and compression of the other increase pulmonary vascular resistance and further impair flow out of the ventricle. The end result of all of these adverse cardiovascular insults is to decrease right ventricular output. The resultant poor filling of the pulmonary vasculature compromises filling of the left side of the heart and is compounded by compression of the left atrium. As the cardiac output decreases, the systemic arterial blood pressure decreases. Right atrial pressure increases, sometimes to levels as high as 40 mm Hg.

Positive Pressure Ventilation

Positive pressure ventilation is not a primary abnormality that affects the cardiovascular system in patients with chest injuries, but it is frequently necessary to use positive pressure ventilation in such patients. Whereas positive pressure ventilation is used to support pulmonary function, all of the effects on the cardiovascular system are adverse.[10,12] Because so many patients with severe chest injuries require positive pressure ventilation, the cardiovascular effects of that ventilation must be considered.

Expansion of the lungs with positive pressure ventilation compresses the superior and inferior vena cavae as they enter the chest. This compression impairs right atrial and right ventricular filling, thus decreasing right ventricular output. Positive pressure expansion of the lungs also directly compresses the right atrium and the thin-walled right ventricle, further compromising their function. Inflation of the lungs by positive pressure compresses the pulmonary vasculature and increases the pulmonary vascular resistance. This further impedes flow from the right ventricle, which is poorly adapted to pumping against high pulmonary vascular resistance. All of these adverse effects—compression of the vena cavae, compression of the right heart, and compression of the pulmonary vasculature— impair right ventricular output. Low output from the right ventricle decreases filling of the pulmonary vasculature and thus decreases filling of the left heart. The results of all of these adverse effects on the cardiovascular system are a low systemic arterial blood pressure associated with high right-sided cardiac pressures and a low cardiac output.

These adverse cardiovascular effects are caused more by the mean airway pressure than peak airway pressures. The mean airway pressure, in turn, is determined primarily by the end-expiratory pressure.[13] In particular, those patients in shock who are unable to generate high filling pressures can have cardiovascular function compromised by even small increases in end-expiratory pressure.[13]

Compensatory Mechanisms

Several compensatory mechanisms come into play in response to cardiovascular dysfunction in patients with chest injuries. The three mechanisms that serve to compensate initially are discharge of the adrenergic nervous system, activation of the renin-angiotensin system, and release of vasopressin.

Adrenergic discharge constricts the venules and small veins, increases myocardial contractility, increases heart rate, and constricts the vascular sphincters in the skin, kidneys, and splanchnic viscera (the splanchnic viscera being the spleen, pancreas, liver, and gastrointestinal tract). Constriction of the systemic venules and small veins displaces blood to the right atrium and right ventricle. This increases right ventricular end-diastolic volume and right ventricular stroke volume. Increased myocardial contractility augments right ventricular stroke volume. An increased heart rate increases right ventricular output. This increased output distends the pulmonary vasculature and displaces blood into the left atrium and ventricle. Adrenergically mediated constriction of the pulmonary vasculature augments this displacement of blood into the left heart. Left atrial and left ventricular filling increases, and left ventricular stroke volume increases. Increased contractility and heart rate further increase the left ventricular output.

Adrenergic discharge successively constricts the vasculature of the skin, kidneys, and splanchnic viscera, ultimately limiting remaining blood flow to the coronary and cerebral arteries at the expense of all other vascular beds.[1]

Activation of the renin-angiotensin system also works to assist in compensation for the cardiovascular derangements associated with chest trauma. Low perfusion pressures and discharge of the adrenergic nerves to the kidneys lead to the release of renin from the juxtaglomerular apparatus. Renin generates angiotensin I that is converted, by the lungs, to angiotensin II, an extremely potent selective vasoconstrictor. Its vasoconstrictor effects are similar to those of discharge of the adrenergic nervous system. It selectively constricts the vasculature to the skin and splanchnic organs, but it does not constrict the vasculature to the kidneys. This selective vasoconstriction increases cardiac output and also diverts flow to the brain and heart.

Vasopressin also compensates for the cardiovascular derangements of chest trauma. In man, the cardiovascular stimulus for release of vasopressin is hypotension in the high pressure baroreceptors, such as those in the carotid bodies and aortic arch. Vasopressin probably is elevated after major trauma and shock and serves as a systemic vasoconstrictor. It constricts the vasculature to the skin and splanchnic organs. It then has the desirable effect of increasing cardiac output and of diverting flow to the brain and heart.

Thus, the compensatory mechanisms for low flow induced by hypovolemia, cardiac injury, or positive pressure ventilation include adrenergic discharge, activation of the renin-angiotensin system, and release of vasopressin. For unclear reasons, however, heart rate does not increase with institution of positive pressure ventilation.

ASSESSMENT OF CARDIOPULMONARY PATHOPHYSIOLOGY[1,11]

As noted in the previous chapter, the assessment of cardiopulmonary function starts in the emergency room. This involves observation of breathing and ventilation and the status of the circulation as denoted by peripheral perfusion and the presence or absence of neck vein distension. A persistent respiratory rate greater than 30 is an indication of serious respiratory trouble, requiring close observation of the patient, serial arterial blood gases, and chest radiographs. A respiratory rate greater than 35 that does not respond immediately to treatment of an underlying cause, such as pneumothorax, requires intubation regardless of the status of blood gases, because a respiratory rate at this level means that the patient is working hard to breathe and will fatigue unless mechanically supported. A decreasing level of consciousness with loss of vital reflexes, gag, cough, and swallowing is an indication for intubation, because the patient will be unable to protect the airway from aspiration. A carbon dioxide tension (P_{CO_2}) greater than 42 or 43 mm Hg when the patient is supported with supplemental oxygen is an indication for intubation.

With regard to circulatory function, assessment of presence or absence of the level of shock should be automatic (Table 2–4).

In most instances, the kidney is the guide to the adequacy of circulation. Urinary output above that necessary to excrete metabolic waste (0.5 ml/kg/hr) implies adequate

Table 2–4. Levels of Shock

	SIGNS AND SYMPTOMS	PRIMARY ORGAN AFFECTED
Mild	Cold, pale, vasoconstricted	Skin
Moderate	Urine <0.5 ml/kg/hr	Kidney-splanchnic bed
Severe	Restless, agitated, comatose electrocardiographic changes, cardiac arrest	Brain, heart

renal perfusion. This, when combined with warm, pink, well perfused extremities, provides assurance that circulation is adequate.

In the acute setting, the status of neck veins or central venous pressure should be repeatedly reviewed. Prominent neck veins in the presence of shock means either obstruction of venous return by a problem such as tension pneumothorax or compromise of cardiac function (Fig. 2–3).

In some instances in which there are large fluid requirements or an unstable cardiovascular system and urinary output is marginal or minimal, there may be reason to question the adequacy of the neck vein or central venous pressure assessment. This is particularly true in a setting of progressive pulmonary failure from contusion or the respiratory distress syndrome. Under these circumstances, pulmonary vascular resistance is increased and higher than normal right-sided filling pressures may be necessary to ensure adequate cardiac output. Moreover, most of these patients will have required endotracheal intubation and mechanical ventilation. At this point, a Swan-Ganz catheter is a useful guide for assessing cardiopulmonary function.[11] Central vein cannulation by a small needle permits the subsequent introduction of guides so that a balloon catheter can be floated into the pulmonary artery.

Because of problems in compliance of tubing, systolic and diastolic pressures as measured by central lines and Swan-Ganz catheters often are dampened and not reliable. However, mean pressure is consistent and should be reproducible. When mechanical ventilation is used, thoracic pressures are converted from negative to positive and increased filling pressures are necessary to preserve cardiac output. Thus, the higher the ventilatory pressure, the greater the intracardiac right- and left-sided pressures must be to maintain cardiac output.[14] In the supine position, with the patient spontaneously breathing, central

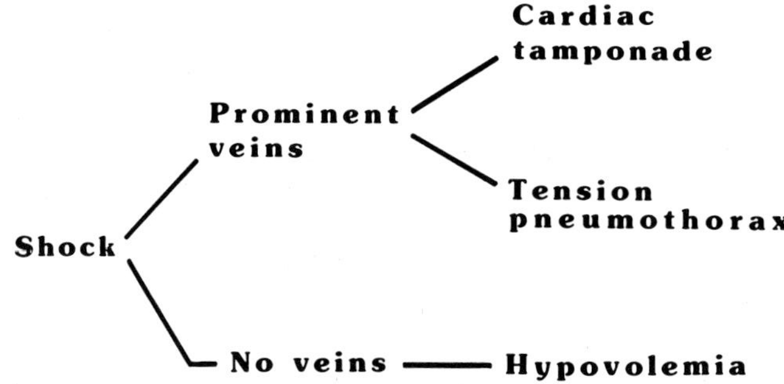

Figure 2–3. Observation of neck veins permits recognition of the basic causes of shock.

venous filling pressures of 5 to 10 cm of water or 8 to 12 mm Hg should be more than adequate. For patients on 10 or 15 cm of PEEP, right- and left-sided filling pressures of 20 to 25 mm Hg may be required to maintain adequate cardiac output.

Assessment of mixed venous oxygen tension (Po_2), assuming the arterial Po_2 is reasonably normal, provides information regarding adequacy of cardiac output. An arteriovenous oxygen difference of more than five volumes percent implies marginally adequate cardiac output, because oxygen extraction is being maximized. The oxygen difference of eight volumes percent is an absolute indication that cardiac output is inadequate, presumably due to impairment of cardiac function. Metabolic acidosis, as manifested by a normal to low Pco_2 and pH below 7.3, is another indication that the circulation is inadequate to ensure aerobic metabolism.

TECHNIQUES FOR CARDIOPULMONARY MONITORING[11]

Techniques required for cardiopulmonary monitoring include direct arterial puncture or cannulation, central venous cannulation, and pulmonary artery catheterization using a Swan-Ganz catheter.

Arterial Puncture

In the emergency room where arterial blood gas determinations are needed urgently, particularly in instances of shock, direct puncture of the femoral artery at the groin is the optimal method of obtaining blood samples. The artery is best punctured just below the inguinal ligament. This lies at a level 1 cm below the line between the pubic tubercle and anterior superior spine. The arterial pulse is trapped between two fingers of the nondominant hand, and using a 2- to 3-ml syringe, a #20 needle is advanced at right angles between the compressing fingers until arterial blood is obtained.

In a more elective setting, if the patient is not in shock, the radial or brachial puncture may be used for arterial blood sampling. The radial artery is most superficial over the distal radius, just lateral to the flexor carpi radialis tendon. A 1- or 2-ml syringe, combined with a #23 to #25 needle, is used to puncture the artery at right angles to the skin surface. Alternatively, the brachial artery can be palpated just medial to the biceps tendon in the antecubital area and punctured in similar fashion.

For continuous monitoring of patients in the operating room or critical care setting, arterial cannulation is optimal, the preferred choices being the radial, ulnar, and brachial arteries, in that order. The dorsalis pedis artery, posterior tibial artery, or even the femoral artery may be used if necessary. The groin is considered a relatively dirty area and contamination of arterial lines often occurs, so that femoral artery catheters may require changing or removal within a day or two of insertion, whereas the other catheters may retain their usefulness for weeks.

The technique of cannulation is similar to that for arterial puncture, except that the needle puncture is made at an oblique angle upward toward the proximal artery with the sharp end of the bevel down. This type of arterial puncture is more difficult, and an obliquity of more than 45° usually will result in the artery rolling away from the puncturing needle. A #18 to #20 needle is used for this puncture, and a guidewire is then advanced through the lumen of the needle into the artery once pulsatile flow is obtained. At this point, the needle is removed and a plastic catheter advanced over the flexible guidewire a variable distance into the artery. The stylet is then removed and the catheter securely fixed with suture or dressing. A stopcock is applied to the hub of the needle and a sterile protective dressing applied.

Central Venous Catheterization

Central veins appropriate for cannulation consist of subclavian, internal jugular, or common femoral. In the conscious patient, the subclavian vein is the one most commonly used for catheterization, because the procedure of introduction is better tolerated by the patient. Moreover, the infraclavicular area is relatively clean and not subject to trauma. The jugular vein is an acceptable alternative, particularly when the patient is under general anesthesia at the time of introduction. It requires a quiet or cooperative patient and preferably a hyperextended neck.

The subclavian vein passes upward from the axilla laterally, paralleling the course of the undersurface of the clavicle, from the junction of the inner third with the lateral two-thirds, and then passes downward into the mediastinum as it is joined by the jugular vein under the sternoclavicular joint to form the innominate vein. The exact location depends on whether the arm is adducted or abducted.

Usually, the cannulation is carried out with the arm at the side. The patient's upper body should be lowered so that the upper chest is dependent, the exploring needle entering the area corresponding to the middle of the clavicle and 1 or 2 cm below. A puncture is made with a 4-in, 18-gauge needle, and the needle is advanced toward the sternal notch, paralleling the immediate undersurface of the clavicle where the vein is in close contact with the bone. If the patient is on mechanical ventilation, the apex of the lung may rise and nearly surround the subclavian vein superiorly. As the needle is advanced under the clavicle, the stylet is removed repeatedly and syringe aspiration carried out. Failure to obtain blood requires repassage of the needle in a slightly cephalad or caudad direction. Once blood is aspirated from the needle, a flexible stylet is passed through the needle and the needle withdrawn. For central venous infusion or monitoring, a plastic catheter is passed over the stylet and the stylet removed.

Catheterization of the jugular vein is carried out in similar fashion. The patient's bed should be depressed and the feet elevated to raise and distend the cervical veins if possible. Needle puncture is carried out over the anterior edge of the midportion of the sterno-cleidomastoid muscle. A #18 needle is advanced downward and angled about 45°, with aspiration being carried out as the needle is advanced. The jugular vein is relatively superficial, lying just deep to the cervical fascia and lateral to the trachea. The needle should head toward the sternoclavicular joint. If initial puncture is not successful, another puncture site may be selected nearer to the clavicle, with angulation, as used previously. This gives a larger target, the jugular–subclavian junction, but carries a greater risk of complication. Once blood is aspirated, a catheter similar to that used for subclavian venous cannulation is passed over the stylet.

When a sample of venous blood is needed and the patient is in shock, the femoral vein just below the inguinal ligament is the venipuncture site of choice. A line should be drawn from the pubic tubercle to the anterior superior spine, because the groin crease may lie an inch or more below the actual inguinal ligament. The femoral pulse should be palpated just at the inguinal ligament. The femoral vein lies one fingerbreadth medial, and this site can be marked with a needle scratch. A #20 needle connected to a 3- to 10-ml syringe should be advanced at right angles to the skin surface. If blood is not aspirated, the needle is withdrawn and advanced medially or laterally until a specimen of blood is obtained.

The femoral vein is seldom cannulated because of the risk of thromboembolic complications, but, when necessary, it can be utilized temporarily, cannulation proceeding as with the subclavian and jugular vein.

Swan-Ganz Catheter Insertion

Swan-Ganz catheter insertion is initiated as described for subclavian and jugular vein cannulation. A flexible guidewire is passed through the needle or catheter if one is already in place. The needle or catheter is removed, the skin puncture site enlarged with a pointed scalpel blade, and a plastic sheath that will accommodate the Swan-Ganz catheter is passed over the guidewire and the stylet removed. The Swan-Ganz catheter is passed well into the vein and the balloon inflated with 2 ml of air. The catheter is then connected to a pressure monitor and advanced slowly. The venous stream usually will direct the catheter into the right atrium and subsequently into the right ventricle. The entrance into the right ventricle is noted by the characteristic ventricular pressure wave that normally is 30/0 mm Hg (Fig. 2–4). An additional 10 to 15 cm of catheter is advanced until a significant diastolic component is noted in the pressure tracing (Fig. 2–5). This denotes the entrance of the catheter into the pulmonary artery. The catheter is then advanced slowly to a total distance of about 45 cm in the average adult. Usually, the catheter will direct itself into the pulmonary zone of high flow (this corresponds to the midlung field as seen on lateral chest radiographs in the supine patient). When the catheter is in position in the lung field as noted by a dampening of the pressure tracing, the balloon is deflated (Fig. 2–6). This should give a normal pulmonary artery pressure curve. The balloon is slowly reinflated; a dampening of

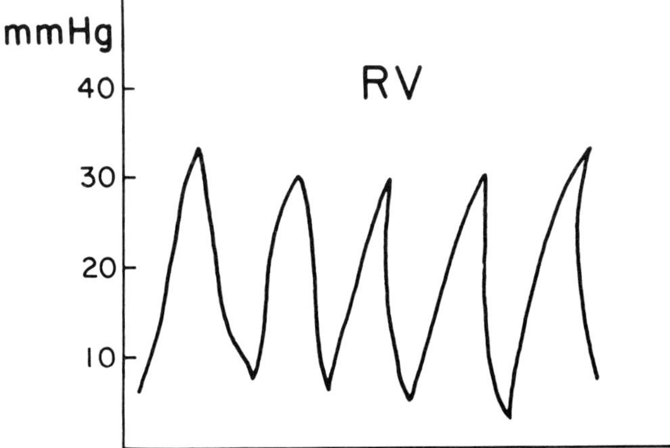

Figure 2–4. Ventricular pressure wave shows a spiking systolic component and diastolic pressure at zero.

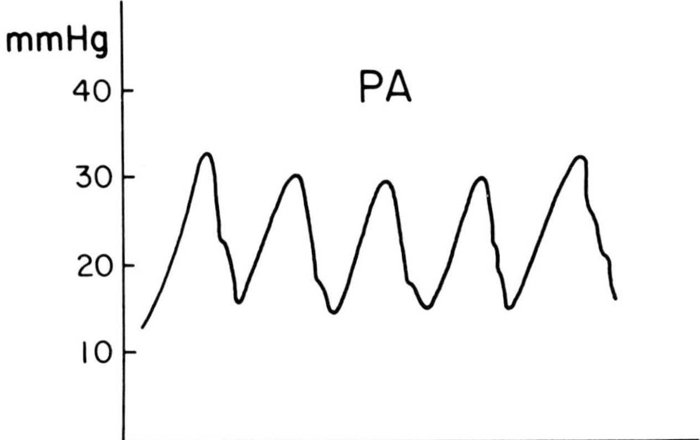

Figure 2–5. Pulmonary artery pressure tracing shows a similar systolic pressure to that of the right ventricle and, in addition, it shows a significant diastolic component.

the pressure tracing signifies a wedge position. An optimal location will be assured by adjusting the catheter position so that a 1-ml inflation dampens the pressure tracing. This dampened pressure tracing corresponds to the pulmonary wedge pressure, a reflection of the left atrial pressure.

The successful passage of a triple lumen Swan-Ganz catheter permits cardiac output assessment, assessment of mixed venous blood, and measurement of left-sided wedge pressures, all of which may be of value in monitoring the patient.

SUPPORT OF CARDIOPULMONARY FUNCTION[15]

With a combination of arterial and central venous lines, in particular a Swan-Ganz catheter, sophisticated monitoring of cardiopulmonary function is possible. This, combined with assessment of peripheral perfusion and urinary output, permits total continuous monitoring. Obviously, this type of monitoring is applicable only in an operating room or intensive

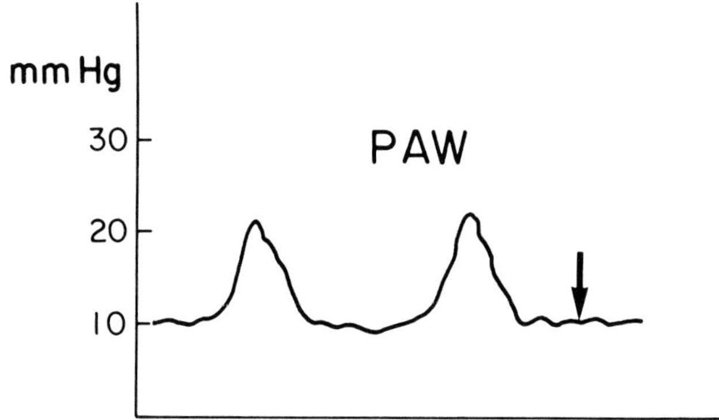

Figure 2–6. With the pulmonary artery obstructed by the balloon catheter, the wedge pressure (*PAW*) corresponds to the left atrial pressure.

care unit setting, but it is in one of these two environments that the critically injured patient should be found.

The most common cause of cardiopulmonary deterioration, 24 hr or more after injury, is the development of the respiratory distress syndrome of either trauma or sepsis. Both are caused by diffuse intravascular inflammation that results from a combination of shock with soft tissue injury or sepsis. The latter has, as its source, diffuse infection anywhere, including the lung. Both have in common diffuse compromise of vascular integrity with interstitial edema. Although interstitial edema is a generalized process, the impact is greatest on the lung and is reflected in alterations in pulmonary function. Loss of vascular integrity may result in hypovolemia, with corresponding circulatory breakdown.

Pulmonary Support

With an arterial cannula in place, serial monitoring of arterial blood gases is easily done, and such a catheter should be inserted in any unstable patient with respiratory failure, whether from chest wall or pulmonary injury or from indirect injury, such as that caused by the respiratory distress syndrome. The Po_2 should be sampled repeatedly and supplemental oxygen administered to maintain the Po_2 above 70 but below 100 mm Hg. A persistent respiratory rate greater than 35 with Po_2 less than 70 is an indication for mechanical ventilation, as is a Pco_2 above 42 mm Hg (Table 2–5). The patient on mechanical ventilation should have PEEP set at 2.5 cm of water. If the patient requires oxygen concentration above 30%, PEEP should be raised to 5 cm. At this point, failure to maintain a Po_2 of 70 mm Hg requires the oxygen concentration to be raised progressively to 50%. At this point, if the Po_2 is not adequate, rather than raise the fractional concentration of inspired oxygen (Fio_2), PEEP should be gradually increased to 10 to 15 cm of water before the decision is made to increase the Fio_2. Once 12 to 15 cm of PEEP has been reached, the Fio_2 should be increased as necessary to maintain the desired Po_2, even though, under some adverse circumstances, 100% oxygen may be required for short periods (Table 2–6).

When the ventilator is being used, the tidal volume should be set to maintain a tidal volume of 10 to 15 ml/kg. This should be adjusted to maintain the Pco_2 at approximately 40 mm Hg and within the range of 38 to 42 mm Hg.

Table 2–5. Ventilatory Function

	NORMAL RANGE	INDICATIONS FOR INTUBATION AND VENTILATION
Mechanics		
Respiratory rate	12–20 min	>35/min
Vital capacity	70 ml/kg	<15 ml/kg
Inspiratory pressure	−100 cm H_2O	>−25 cm H_2O
Oxygenation		
Pao_2	75–100 mm Hg	<70 mm Hg (on O_2)
Alveolar to arterial oxygen tension difference	50–75 mm Hg	<300 mm Hg (Fio_2 = 1.0)
Ventilation		
$Paco_2$	35–45 mm Hg	>45 mm Hg
V_d/V_t	0.3–0.4	>0.6

Table 2-6. Respiratory Failure Treatment

$Po_2 < 70 \rightarrow \uparrow$ Fio_2 as needed until $Fio_2 = 0.5$
$Po_2 < 70$ ($Fio_2 \rightarrow 0.5$ $\uparrow$ PEEP from 3 to 18 cm of H_2O as needed
$Po_2 < 70$ (PEEP 15) $\rightarrow \uparrow$ Fio_2 as needed to 1.0
Adjust dead space and tidal volume as necessary to maintain Pco_2 38–42 mm Hg

Support of Cardiac Function[15,16]

With regard to cardiac monitoring, the blood pressure and pulse should be recorded continuously. The critically injured patient should have an arterial line inserted and this connected to a monitor. Because of problems of compliance in the tubing, the mean arterial pressure, rather than systolic and diastolic pressure, should be used. This usually lies one-third of the way between diastolic and systolic pressure, or about 100 mm Hg in the patient with a blood pressure of 140/80 mm Hg. The primary gauge of the adequacy of circulation is the urinary output. A urinary output of 50 to 100 ml/hr indicates adequate renal perfusion and implies adequate cardiac output. In most instances in the trauma setting, a decrease in urinary output below these levels is an indication for increased increments of fluid or blood. In older patients or those with possible cardiac injury, this can be cross-checked by observing the status of neck veins or noting central venous pressure. If the former are not visible or the latter low, the need for fluids is confirmed (Table 2–7). When pulmonary dysfunction is developing simultaneously with problems of renal function, and there is doubt about the status of cardiac function, a Swan-Ganz catheter should be passed. Cardiac function can be assessed by measuring the cardiac index using a cold injectate. The cardiac filling pressure at the point at which the cardiac index and urinary outputs are optimized should be noted and fluids administered to maintain this filling pressure.

If pulmonary artery wedge pressure is low (<10 mm Hg) and cardiac index is low (<2 L/min), lactated Ringer's solution should be given sufficient to raise wedge pressure by 3 to 5 mm Hg. Cardiac index should be measured and, assuming cardiac index improves, additional fluid can be given as necessary to optimize cardiac index and urine output.

Should left-sided filling pressures be high, a diuretic may be tried and the cardiac index assessed before and after diuresis. Improvement in cardiac output with diuresis indicates that the Starling's curve will be optimized by lower filling pressures, and diuresis or fluid restriction should be used to optimize the cardiac output.

Should the patient fail to respond to fluid manipulation and should cardiac output and urine volume remain inadequate, cardiotonic drugs may prove useful.[16–20] At this point, pulmonary vascular resistance should be assessed. If vascular resistance is high and blood pressure is normal or high, afterload reduction should be tried. Sodium nitroprusside

Table 2-7. Optimizing Cardiac Index

FILLING PRESSURE	VASCULAR RESISTANCE	TREATMENT
Low (<10–15 mm Hg)	High or low	Fluid bolus
High (>15–20 mm Hg)	High or low	Restrict fluids; diuresis
Normal or high	High	Nitroprusside
Normal or high	Low or normal	Dobutamine
Normal or high	Normal or high	Amrinone

should be started at 0.5 μg/kg/min intravenously. This should be increased gradually as cardiac index and blood pressure are monitored. Blood pressure should be maintained above 80 as the infusion is increased to optimize cardiac output and organ perfusion.

If the patient's blood pressure is already low or afterload reduction has not optimized cardiac index or renal perfusion as manifest by diuresis, dobutamine may be useful to improve cardiac performance. This is administered at dosages of between 5 and 20 μg/kg/min.

Finally, if the response to the above measures is unsuccessful, amrinone should be tried. An initial loading dose of 5 to 10 μg/kg/min should be followed by maintenance infusion of 5 to 10 μg/kg/min. The initial loading dose should be omitted if the blood pressure is low. (See Chapter 7, Table 7–6.)

Impaired cardiac function is unusual in the young trauma patient in the absence of severe septic complications. In the absence of sepsis, poor cardiac function should lead to the suspicion that some treatable lesion may be present. Echocardiography has proved to be a valuable means of assessing the heart and permits recognition of fluid in the pericardium, impaired cardiac wall function, or internal cardiac derangement. Thus, if the patient does not respond promptly to the support just indicated, specific examination of the heart should be carried out. Pericardial fluid should be drained by needle, catheter, or operative means, depending on the acuteness and severity of the problem (Chapter 15). Internal cardiac derangements should be corrected if this is possible (Chapter 15).

Weaning Cardiopulmonary Support

Withdrawal of pulmonary support can be done by established criteria. In the absence of septic complications, most pulmonary lesions will improve progressively in a day or so after the initial injury.

An unstable patient who requires intubation and mechanical ventilation should be on full ventilatory support if paralyzed or requiring hyperventilation to treat a head injury (Table 2–8). If conscious and able to initiate ventilation, the patient should be on assist-

Table 2–8. Weaning from Ventilator

Full mechanical/ventilatory support
(Ventilator set so patient does not initiate breath)
↓
Assisted ventilation
(Patient takes no inhalations on his own, but initiates each breath)
↓
Intermittent mandatory ventilation
(Patient takes independent breaths on his own; ventilator assist for remainder)
↓
Continuous positive airway pressure
(Patient breathes on his own against fixed resistance)
↓
Patient breathes spontaneously/no resistance
(T piece provides humidified oxygen)
↓
Patient extubated/breathes on his own
(Humidified oxygen provided by mask)

Table 2–9. Ventilator Weaning F_{IO_2} and PEEP

$F_{IO_2}>0.5 \rightarrow \downarrow F_{IO_2}$ to maintain $PO_2>70$
$F_{IO_2}<0.5 \rightarrow \downarrow$ PEEP to maintain $PO_2>70$
PEEP<5 cm/$H_2O \rightarrow \downarrow F_{IO_2}$ to 0.3, $PO_2>70$

demand ventilation. In this mode, the ventilator fires in response to respiratory effort initiated by the patient.

Once the patient's condition has stabilized, and particularly when there are signs of improvement, progressive ventilator weaning should be instituted. This is accomplished by allowing the patient to take a certain number of breaths on his own; this is called intermittent mandatory ventilation (IMV). Ventilator settings are set a bit lower than necessary for total assist, perhaps 14 to 16 per minute initially, and the patient is allowed to take one or two unassisted ventilations each minute.

Usually, regardless of the state of pulmonary function, the patient will maintain reasonably normal blood gases. Requiring the patient to take at least a few breaths on his/her own each minute maintains strength in the respiratory musculature. At this point, an F_{IO_2} greater than 0.5 should be progressively cut back, provided the PO_2 can be maintained above 60 mm Hg (Table 2–9). This is done with variable degrees of rapidity, depending on the severity and acuteness of the patient's problem.

Once an F_{IO_2} of 0.5 is reached, any PEEP setting above 5 cm of water should be progressively cut back. Once a PEEP of 5 cm has been reached and once the patient is able to maintain adequate blood gases on that setting, the F_{IO_2} should be cut to 0.4. The IMV rate is then progressively decreased two points at a time, depending on the acuteness of the problem. Once an IMV rate of 4 is reached, the patient can be allowed to breathe spontaneously, ideally exhaling against a fixed resistance (known as CPAP). This is assuming that the patient tolerates the low IMV rate and CPAP satisfactorily with respiratory rates less than 24/min and with normal PO_2. The patient should be rested after 4 hr of spontaneous ventilation with CPAP, waiting for an optimal time for extubation. This should be early so that patients with severe respiratory problems can be observed closely during the course of the day. In the final stages of weaning, the patient is placed on a T piece for approximately 30 min and arterial blood gases obtained. If the PCO_2 is ≤40 mm Hg and the PO_2 is >70 mm Hg, with respiratory rate no higher than 24, extubation can be carried out.

After extubation, the patient is generally supported with humidified oxygen by mask or nasal prongs. This can be discontinued after 24 hr unless the patient has a tracheostomy in place, because the latter requires humidification until the tube is removed.

REFERENCES

1. Holcroft JW, Blaisdell FW. Shock: causes and management of circulatory collapse. In: Sabiston, ed. *Textbook of Surgery.* 14th ed. Philadelphia: Saunders; 1991:34–56.
2. Blaisdell FW. Traumatic shock. *Bull Am Coll Surg.* 1983;68:2.
3. Blaisdell FW, Lewis FR. *Respiratory Distress Syndrome of Shock and Trauma.* Philadelphia: Saunders; 1977.
4. Blaisdell FW, Holcroft JW. Septic shock. In: *Problems in General Surgery.* vol I. Philadelphia: Lippincott; 1984.
5. Cheney FW, Colley PS. The effect of cardiac output on arterial blood oxygenation. *Anesthesiology.* 1980;52:496.

6. Pepe PE, Hudson LD, Carrico CJ. Early application of positive and expiratory pressure in patients at risk for the adult respiratory distress syndrome. *N Engl J Med*. 1984;311:281.

7. Dantzker DR, et al. Ventilation-perfusion distribution in the adult respiratory distress syndrome. *Am Rev Respir Dis*. 1979;120:1039.

8. Rinaldo JE, Rogers RM. Adult respiratory distress syndrome: changing concepts of lung injury and repair. *N Engl J Med*. 1982;306:900.

9. Synder JV, et al. Mechanical ventilation: physiology and application. *Curr Prob Surg*. 1984;21:1.

10. Green JF. Determinants of systemic blood flow. In: Guyton AC, Young DB, eds. *International Review of Physiology, Vol 3: Cardiovascular Physiology*. Baltimore: University Park Press; 1979.

11. Abrams JH, Cerra F, Holcroft JW. Cardiopulmonary monitoring. In: *Care of the Surgical Patient*. New York: Scientific American; 1989:1–25.

12. Holcroft JW, Trunkey DD. Extravascular lung water following hemorrhagic shock in the baboon: comparison between resuscitation with Ringer's lactate and plasmanate. *Ann Surg*. 1974;180:408.

13. Nicotra MB, Stevens PM, Viroslav J. Physiological evaluation of positive end-expiratory pressure. *Chest*. 1973;64:10.

14. Rankin JS, et al. The effects of airway pressure on cardiac function in intact dogs and man. *Circulation*. 1982;66:108.

15. Rankin JS. Hemodynamic management. In: *Care of the Surgical Patient*. New York: Scientific American; 1988:1–12.

16. Rice CL. Pharmacologic support of the failing heart. In: *Care of the Surgical Patient*. New York: Scientific American; 1989:1–8.

17. Leier CV, Bambach D, Thompson MJ, et al. Central and regional hemodynamic effects of intravenous isosorbide dinitrate, nitroglycerin and nitroprusside in patients with congestive heart failure. *Am J Cardiol*. 1981;48:1115.

18. Leier CV. General overview and update of positive inotropic therapy. *Am J Med*. 1986;81(Suppl 4C):40.

19. Monrad ES, Baim DS, Smith HS, et al. Milrinone, dobutamine, and nitroprusside: comparative effects on hemodynamics and myocardial energetics in patients with severe congestive heart failure. *Circulation*. 1986;73:(Suppl 3):168.

20. Silke B, Verma SP, Midtbo KA, et al. Comparative hemodynamic dose-response effects of dobutamine and amrinone in left ventricular failure complicating acute myocardial infarction. *J Cardiovasc Pharmacol*. 1987;9:19.

3

Emergency Room Thoracotomy in the Management of Thoracic Trauma

DAVID H. WISNER, M.D.
BALAZS IMRE BODAI, M.D.

HISTORY: Injuries necessitating emergency thoracotomy, particularly penetrating cardiac injuries, have long been associated with a poor prognosis. The earliest description of penetrating chest wounds is found in the Edwin Smith papyrus written around 3000 BC.[1] Hippocrates called attention to the fatal nature of such injuries[2] and Boerhaave considered all cardiac wounds unsalvageable in the early 1700s.[3] Pericardiocentesis was suggested in 1649 by Riolanus,[4] but it was not attempted until 1826 when Dupuytren kept the French duc de Berry alive for several hours after a stab wound of the heart.[5] Three years later Baron Larrey, surgeon to Napoleon, successfully decompressed a cardiac tamponade by aspiration and demonstrated that dogs could survive cardiorrhaphy.[6]

In 1882, Bloc[7] sutured rabbit hearts, and a decade later DeVecchio[8] was successful in repairing stab wounds in the hearts of dogs. In the mid-1890s, two cases of successful pericardial repair after stab wounds were reported.[9,10] The first successful repair of a human heart laceration (the patient died 2 and a half days postoperatively) was reported in 1895 by Cappelen.[11] Despite these limited successes, Paget[12] concluded in 1896 that cardiac surgery had reached its limits and these wounds would forever be uniformly fatal. One year later, Rehn[13] successfully sutured a 1.5-cm laceration of the right ventricle in a patient who recovered fully.

Hill[14] in 1902 reported the first successful cardiorrhaphy in the United States. By 1906, 124 cases of cardiac injuries managed surgically were noted,[15] and in 1920 Tuffier[16] published a review of 305 cases. Cardiorrhaphy was well on its way to acceptance, and the role of thoracotomy was becoming established.

The last 50 years have seen a steady decline in the morbidity and mortality associated with thoracic injuries. Wide experience was gained as a result of wartime environments.[17–20] In 1943 Blalock and Ravitch[21] proposed pericardiocentesis as a method of conservative treatment for pericardial tamponade. This approach was employed with moderate success until cardiac surgery became widespread. Patients subjected to early thoracotomy appeared to fare better than those treated conservatively. Sugg and associates[22] reviewed 459 cardiac injuries in 1968 and found that 10 of 18 deaths occurred secondary to recurrent pericardial tamponade. No deaths were noted with the institution of early thoracotomy.[23–26] Repeated pericardiocentesis has now been largely abandoned in favor of a more aggressive approach using early thoracotomy. Some investigators still feel that pericardiocentesis may have a role as a diagnostic aid or prethoracotomy procedure to gain time for transport of the victim to the operating room.

Emergency thoracotomy was employed frequently in patients experiencing sudden cardiac arrest before 1960, before the advent of closed chest cardiac massage and defibrillators.[27] Few successes were reported outside the operating room and, despite the persistence of some enthusiasts for this procedure,[28–32] there remains little evidence of the success of emergency thoracotomy in cardiopulmonary arrests secondary to medical conditions.

Emergency thoracotomy has been applied to the increasing number of patients arriving at the hospital with some sign of life due to rapid transport capabilities. In the trauma center, left anterior thoracotomy was originally advocated for emergency room use in patients with penetrating cardiac injuries associated with pericardial tamponade as well as other hemorrhaging thoracic and abdominal injuries.[33–36]

Many centers have reported the successful repair of cardiac lesions in the emergency room.[37–41] These reports formed the basis for extension of the indications for emergency thoracotomy to include many other injuries.[15,42] Thoracotomy with aortic cross-clamping was first proposed by Sankaran and associates,[43] who demonstrated improved survival in animals using the technique before laparotomy. This concept was reinforced by Ledgerwood and co-workers,[44] who recommended thoracotomy and aortic occlusion in the operating room before laparotomy in patients with massive distention of the abdomen who were refractory to standard resuscitative measures.

Large series have been published reporting experiences with emergency room thoracotomy for a wide variety of injuries.[28,35,39,40,41,45–50] The technique also has been advocated for use in the surgical intensive care unit after open heart operations complicated by inadequate circulation in the postoperative period.[51]

INDICATIONS

The indications for emergency room thoracotomy have been the subject of controversy.[52] Suggested indications have included acute deterioration or uncontrolled hemorrhage in patients with penetrating wounds of the chest, intrapleural exsanguination, suspected hilar or great vessel injury, and arrest after blunt trauma.

The indications, cost, and benefits of resuscitative thoracotomy have been reviewed.[45,49,50,52,53] The mode of injury has been used as a criterion for performance of the procedure.[39,45,47,50,52,54–56] As experience with emergency room thoracotomy expanded, the indications for its performance in the trauma patient became more sound. The currently accepted indications for emergency room thoracotomy in the management of thoracic trauma are presented in Table 3–1. There is little debate as to the benefits of the procedure in penetrating cardiac and thoracic injuries; therefore, the indications in such injuries include acute deterioration, uncontrolled hemorrhage, or cardiac arrest in patients with presumed penetrating wounds of the heart as well as for patients with wounds suspected of penetrating the subclavian or great vessels who are threatened with exsanguination. Those patients who are suspected of having air embolism are likewise considered to be optimal candidates for emergency room thoracotomy. Thoracotomy should be performed in patients with blunt thoracoabdominal trauma only if there are signs of life or a normal sinus rhythm on the initial electrocardiogram. Patients with blunt trauma without signs of life or a sinus rhythm are not appropriate candidates.[39,50,57–60]

TECHNIQUE

Emergency room thoracotomy is optimally performed by a well trained trauma team. It should be done simultaneously with other resuscitative measures, including intubation, insertion of large-bore intravenous catheters, bladder catheterization, and blood sampling for typing and cross-matching. The procedure should be performed by the most experienced member present.

Successful thoracotomy in the emergency room depends largely on the rapidity with which it is performed. The entire chest is prepared, if possible, with an organic iodide solution. A left (or right, if the pathologic condition is presumed to lie in the right chest) anterolateral thoracotomy is best performed in the fifth intercostal space from the sternum to the midaxillary line (Fig. 3–1A). This is best accomplished by placing the incision in the pectoral or mammary crease, curving it upward medially, following the curvature of the rib. It is best to avoid slicing the internal mammary artery, but concern about this should not interfere with rapid and wide entry into the chest. The incision is carried through the pectoralis major, anterior serratus, and intercostal musculature. There is no need to control hemorrhage from the incision because these patients are hypotensive and bleeding is therefore minimal.

The incision should be tailored to the specific suspected injury. In patients with suspected injury to the left subclavian artery, incision at the third or fourth interspace may

**Table 3–1. Indications for Emergency Room
Thoracotomy in Thoracic Trauma**

Penetrating injuries
   Acute deterioration
   Uncontrolled hemorrhage
   Cardiac arrest
   Suspicion of major vessel injury
   Air embolism (hilar injuries)
Blunt injuries
   On-the-spot deterioration or arrest
   Vital signs present on scene or arrival

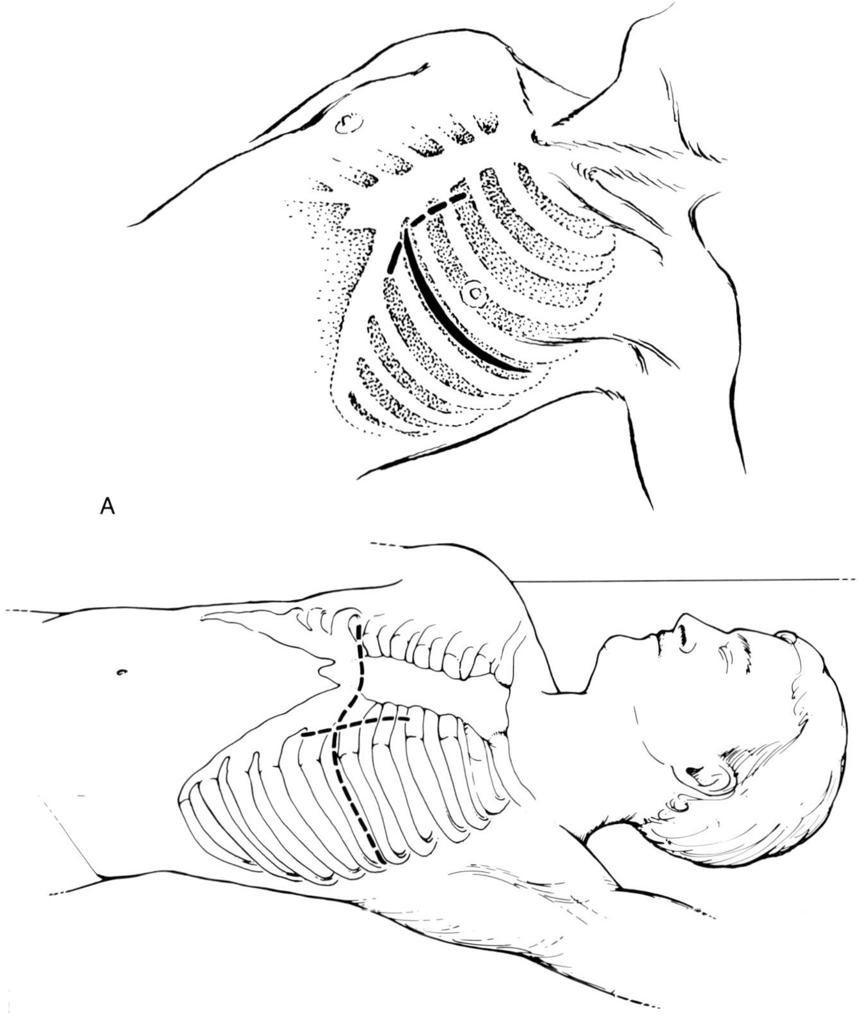

Figure 3–1.   **A:** Location of the incision. The pectoral or intramammary groove is the optimal location. **B:** The incision can be carried upward through costal cartilages as appropriate for exposure or across the sternum into the right chest to facilitate exposure of the right heart.

allow for easier clamping of the vessel. Alternatively, by curving the fifth or sixth intercostal space incision upward in the parasternal area, costal cartilages can be cut to permit exposure of the entire thoracic cavity or the incision can be extended across the sternum to expose the right heart (Fig. 3–1B). In those patients with right-sided injuries, thoracotomy should be performed first on the right side.

After the musculature has been divided, the pleura is incised sharply, bearing in mind that it is easy to damage the underlying lung. Once the incision is completed, a chest wall retractor is inserted and, if not already done so, the costal cartilages of the ribs immediately above and below the intercostal incision should be cut to facilitate exposure (Fig. 3–2). Clotted blood encountered in the thoracic cavity is rapidly evacuated.

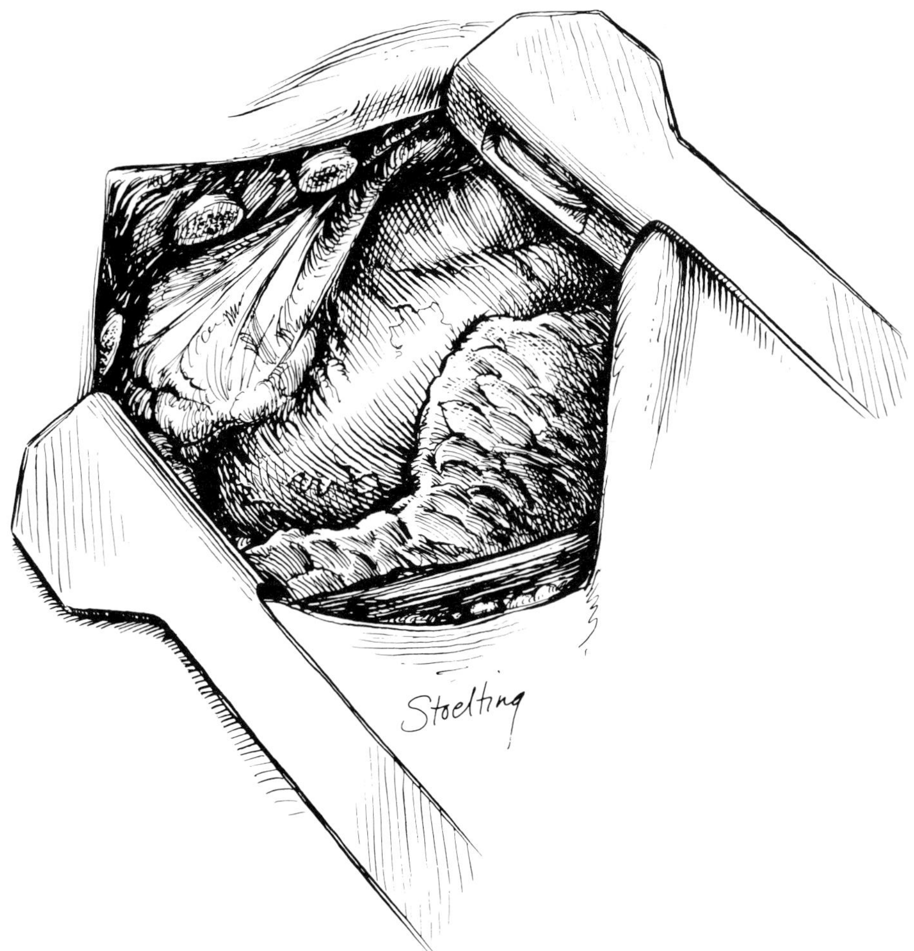

Figure 3–2.   Rib spreaders are inserted and spread to give exposure of the pericardium.

The pericardium should be immediately located and opened. A distended pericardium may be difficult to grasp. The pericardial incision can be begun with a knife and completed with scissors (Fig. 3–3). Pericardiotomy should be performed in a vertical manner to avoid injury to the phrenic nerve. When the pericardiotomy is completed, clots are rapidly evacuated and any spurting cardiac wounds are tamponaded with a gloved finger until definitive repair is accomplished. Stapling also has been described for temporary control of bleeding,[61] but has not been particularly effective in our experience. Definitive techniques of cardiac repair are discussed in another chapter.

The heart should be inspected to determine whether it is in asystole or fibrillation.[61] Fibrillation calls for application of internal defibrillating paddles. Defibrillation may have to be repeated several times. Asystole should be treated by cardiac massage until coarse fibrillations are obtained, then treated with defibrillation. In some instances, massage will be followed by spontaneous resumption of a heart beat. One critical aspect of cardiac

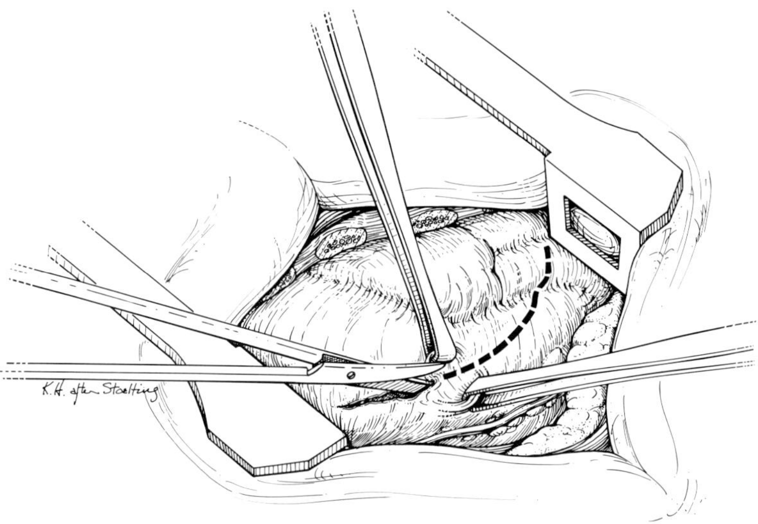

Figure 3–3. The pericardium is opened longitudinally to provide exposure of the heart as necessary.

massage is that the surgeon should monitor fluid administration during the period of arrest and immediately thereafter. The surgeon, with the heart in his/her hands, is in the best position to monitor cardiac filling. The collapsed, empty heart dictates rapid fluid infusion. On the other hand, overdistention of the heart may result in severe damage to cardiac muscle and may seriously compromise function. In the initial period after resumption of a heart beat, it is important to keep a hand around the heart to monitor distention and support the heart by manual compression for 10 to 15 min until a relative measure of stability is obtained.

Cardiac massage should be performed with two hands with pressure distributed over the palmar surface of both hands as opposed to the fingertips (Fig. 3–4), which may result in damage to the heart. The atria, which are quite thin, are particularly susceptible to iatrogenic injury. An alternative technique involves compressing the entire heart against the sternum using one hand with the thumb hooked over the sternum and the remaining four fingers compressing the heart upward (Fig 3–5). This is easiest to accomplish from the opposite side of the chest. It is important to avoid excess anterior displacement of the heart, which may result in decreased venous return.[62]

Once assessment of the heart is completed and resuscitation underway, the thoracic cavity should be inspected for sources of hemorrhage. The apex of the chest cavity and the hilar areas should be visualized. Pulmonary, vascular, and lung injury are assessed. Should there be massive air leaks or bleeding noted from the lung parenchyma itself, a large vascular clamp can be used across the hilum to occlude the entire lung. This is facilitated greatly by partial blunt division of the inferior pulmonary ligament. On occasion, it may be necessary to extend the thoracotomy across the sternum to the opposite side of the chest to allow exposure of the contralateral cardiac border.

Occasionally, patients with presumed arrest or persistent hypotension due to intraabdominal bleeding will require occlusion of the descending thoracic aorta. This can be done temporarily manually or with a sponge stick or an aortic occluder. Later, an arterial clamp

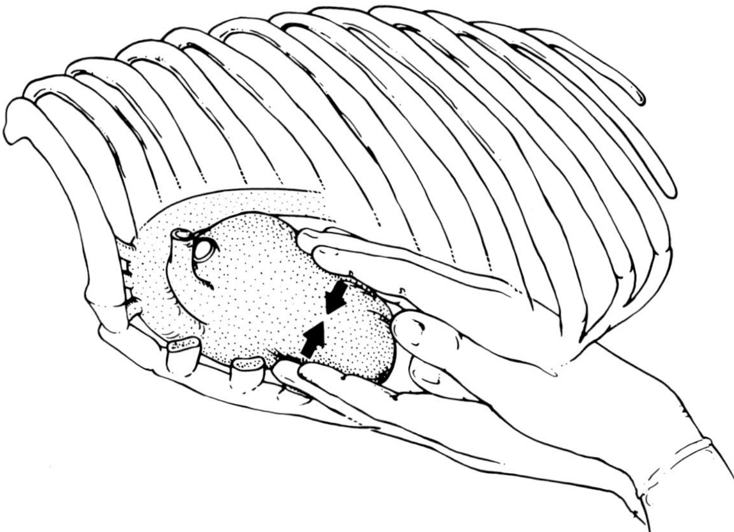

Figure 3–4. The ventricles are compressed with two hands. The fingers should exert uniform compression along the length of the digits to avoid rupturing the heart.

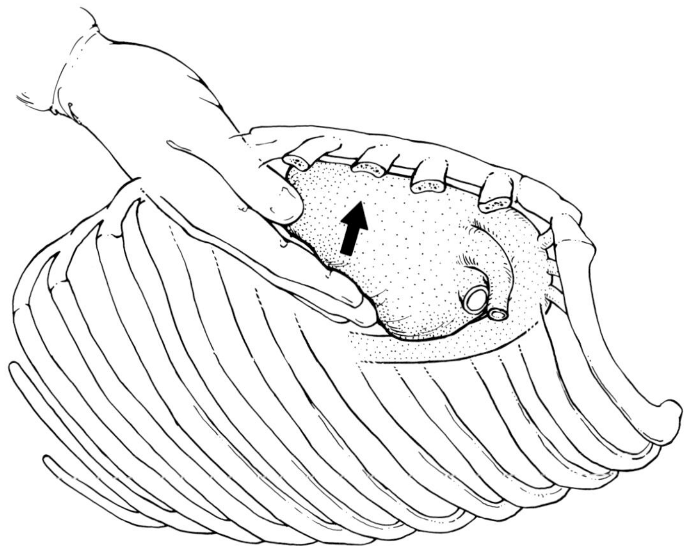

Figure 3–5. One-hand compression of the heart. This is best accomplished from the side of the table opposite the thoracic incision. The heart is compressed upward against the undersurface of the sternum with or without the thumb hooked over the top of the sternum.

such as a DeBakey aortic clamp can be substituted. This is best done with prior blunt or sharp dissection of the overlying pleura to fully mobilize the aorta. The diaphragm can be opened in its membranous portion to confirm intraabdominal bleeding, then laparotomy should be carried out immediately to control the source of hemorrhage.

RESULTS

Penetrating Trauma

Emergency thoracotomy often is more successful in penetrating trauma than it is in blunt trauma. The lung is the most frequently injured organ in penetrating trauma. The vast majority of lung parenchymal injuries respond well to conservative treatment with thoracostomy drainage alone. Thoracotomy is rarely required. In those who do ultimately require thoracotomy, only a small percentage have required that thoracotomy be performed in the emergency room. Thoracotomy performed in the emergency room can be lifesaving in instances of arrest; however, rare successful resuscitations have been reported after penetrating injury to the intrathoracic great vessels and to the lung hilum.[28,35,63,64] Baker and co-workers[28] salvaged 4 of 25 patients with injury to the great vessels and 5 of 15 patients with injury to the lung hilum. Mattox and co-workers[35] have reported success with 5 of 20 patients with hilar injuries and 3 of 10 patients with great vessel injuries. Only 1 of 31 patients with noncardiac penetrating injury who required emergency room thoracotomy survived in Ivatury et al.'s series.[65] It should be noted that in most series, patients with noncardiac penetrating chest trauma who arrived in the emergency room without vital signs could not be saved. Thoracotomy is rarely necessary before operating room transport in penetrating chest injury if the heart is not involved.[36,66–73] Major vessel hemorrhage and air embolism from pulmonary injury may be controlled by immediate thoracotomy with the appropriate hilar cross-clamping technique described previously in those few patients arriving in the emergency room in a moribund condition.

Repeated experience has shown that patients with penetrating cardiac injuries who decompensate on or just before arrival benefit most from emergency thoracotomy. The number of patients arriving at the hospital with penetrating cardiac wounds is small, since the prehospital mortality of such injuries has been estimated to be as high as 83%.[22,64,72,74–76] The best results of emergency room thoracotomy are obtained when used in patients with *pericardial tamponade*. As mentioned previously, multiple, repeated pericardiocentesis and observation have been abandoned as an acceptable treatment for pericardial tamponade. Thoracotomy in the emergency room for such injuries has resulted in a decrease in mortality[26,39,78] and the role of pericardiocentesis has been relegated to one of only transient application to stabilize the patient enough to allow surgical expertise to arrive or before transfer to the operating room.[38,79]

When one considers penetrating cardiac injuries as a group, the overall survival statistics associated with treatment begun in the emergency room by thoracotomy are encouraging (Table 3–2). Steichen and co-workers[25] were the first to report a significant series of moribund patients undergoing emergency thoracotomy; they had a salvage rate for the procedure of 34%. Several other reports have since appeared, also demonstrating excellent results with the resuscitation of these otherwise fatally injured patients.[33,38,80,81]

Mattox and co-workers[82] have presented convincing data supporting the effectiveness

**Table 3–2. Results of ER Thoracotomy
in Penetrating Cardiac Injuries**

| | | NUMBER OF | SURVIVAL | |
			NUMBER	PERCENT
AUTHOR	YEAR	PATIENTS		
Steichen[25]	1971	21	7	33
Beall[33]	1971	18	5	28
Mattox[35]	1974	44	24	55
Sherman[38]	1978	38	9	24
Breaux[79]	1979	41	5	12
Oparah[81]	1979	13	2	15
Baker[28]	1980	29	5	17
Ivatury[78]	1981	22	8	36
Rohman[64]	1983	73	24	33
Vij[88]	1983	24	4	17
Demetriades[86]	1984	11	1	9
Danne[59]	1984	33	?	40
Tavares[40]	1984	37	21	57
Roberge[94]	1986	31	6	20
Schwab[60]	1986	18	13	72
Ivatury[64]	1986	69	9	13

ER, emergency room.
Adapted with permission from Ivatury, et al.[39]

of emergency room thoracotomy for penetrating cardiac injuries. They report a better than 50% salvage rate in those patients who required thoracotomy in the emergency room if they presented with vital signs. It is interesting to note that no patient arriving without vital signs in the emergency room survived. Baker and co-workers[28] have reported 6 of 91 patients initially seen without vital signs who were successfully resuscitated. Five of the six patients had penetrating cardiac injuries and the sixth had sustained an isolated penetrating injury to the iliac artery. Ivatury and associates[39] have concluded that the only group deriving substantial benefit from emergency room thoracotomy are patients with penetrating thoracic injuries, particularly stab wounds. This experience has been confirmed by others[35,47,83] (Table 3–3).

Moore and associates[49] reported their experience with emergency room thoracotomy in 146 patients, of whom 12 left the hospital alive. They excluded those patients with pericardial penetration who were taken immediately to the operating room for treatment, thereby eliminating those most likely to benefit from the procedure. The results of that study indicate that survival is dependent on signs of life in the field and the prompt institution of resuscitative maneuvers, including transport to an emergency room. Those patients without a palpable pulse, reactive pupils, or at least agonal respiratory efforts uniformly fail to survive heroic measures. Cogbill and co-workers[46] expanded this experience. Of the 400 patients undergoing resuscitative thoracotomy, 294 (73%) died in the emergency department. Of the remaining 106 patients who reached the operating room, 28 (26%) survived the operation and were admitted to the intensive care unit, and 16 of these patients eventually were discharged from the hospital; however, four required institutional care secondary to irreversible neurologic damage. Overall, therefore, 12 (3%) of 400 patients undergoing thoracotomy for trauma survived with intact neurologic function. Harnar and associates[84] reported a 42% survival rate in patients when ventricular activity

Table 3–3. Results of ER Thoracotomy in Penetrating Noncardiac Thoracic Injuries

AUTHOR	YEAR	NUMBER OF PATIENTS	SURVIVAL	
			NUMBER	PERCENT
Mattox[35]	1974	30	8	27*
MacDonald[48]	1978	4	0	0
Moore[49]	1979	69	3	4
Baker[28]	1980	40	9	16*
Flynn[47]	1982	7	4	66
Vij[88]	1983	44	5	11†
Shimazu[58]	1983	17	2	12
Danne[59]	1984	?	?	40*
Washington[95]	1985	36	8	22‡
Adkins[63]	1985	25	?	12
Schwab[60]	1986	4	0	0
Ivatury[64]	1986	31	1	3*

ER, emergency room.
*Injuries to great vessels, pulmonary hilum.
†"Successful resuscitation" ? survival.
‡Injuries to chest, neck, or extremities.
Note: Except the reports marked *, others may have cardiac injuries included in the results.
Adapted with permission from Ivatury, et al.[39]

was present, but there were no survivors in those patients with asystole. This observation appears to be a consistent finding.[28,29,39–41,65,85,86]

Blunt Trauma

Patients sustaining blunt thoracoabdominal injury that is severe enough to require emergency room thoracotomy have a poor chance of survival (Table 3–4). The major series that have been reported in the literature have categorized all survivors of emergency thoracotomy into one group. This hides the fact that patients with blunt thoracoabdominal injuries only have a negligible chance for survival. The overall admirable survival rates reported for all injuries cannot be extrapolated to patients who have blunt trauma. Mattox and associates[35] have reported a 15% survival rate in patients with blunt trauma, but theirs was a small series (19 cases), and no patient without vital signs on admission survived. In an update of the original report, an additional 187 emergency thoracotomies were noted in which one patient with blunt trauma survived after cardiac arrest in the emergency department[87]; however, the total number of patients who had blunt injury was not stated. MacDonald and McDowell[48] had no success with two patients with blunt trauma. Baker et al.[28] were able to salvage only 1 of 60 patients admitted with a diagnosis of blunt trauma. In an early report, Moore and co-workers[49] salvaged 1 of 48 cases of blunt trauma. This patient, however, was noted to have a severe neurologic deficit after surgery. In an update of that report,[46] 195 patients with blunt trauma underwent emergency room thoracotomy. None of the 195 patients recovered fully after thoracotomy. The sole survivor in this group remained a neurologic invalid. Several recent series have confirmed the dismal prognosis in

**Table 3–4.   Results of ER Thoracotomy in Blunt
Thoracoabdominal Wounds**

AUTHOR	YEAR	NUMBER OF PATIENTS	PERCENT SURVIVAL
Mattox[35]	1974	19	15.7
MacDonald[48]	1978	2	0
Moore[49]	1979	48	2
Baker[28]	1980	60	1.6
Bodai[45]	1982	38	0
Flynn[47]	1982	20	0
Cogbill[46]	1983	195	0.5
Shimazu[58]	1983	217	2.2*
Vij[88]	1983	6	0
Danne[59]	1984	16	0
Schwab[60]	1986	15	0
Feliciano[96]	1986	53	3.8

ER, emergency room.
*Includes operating room thoracotomies.
Adapted with permission from Ivatury, et al.[39]

this group.[2,59,60,88] Resuscitative thoracotomy may be beneficial in patients with blunt trauma who present with deteriorating vital signs; it does not appear warranted, however, if the patient is admitted to the emergency room without some sign of life.

Bodai and co-workers[45] have analyzed 38 consecutive patients with blunt trauma requiring emergency room thoracotomy. There were no survivors in that series, and more than 85% of the patients had no obtainable vital signs or were agonal on admission. Most of these patients (60%) had multisystem organ damage, reflecting the massive nature of these injuries.

The report of Harnar and co-workers[84] appears to justify the performance of emergency room thoracotomy regardless of the findings at the scene or the mode of injury. They reported 8 of 65 patients with blunt injuries who survived; however, the report is unclear as to how many of these thoracotomies were actually performed in the operating room rather than the emergency room. Patients in whom closed cardiopulmonary resuscitation produced a palpable carotid pulse were transferred to the operating room for definitive care. Three-fourths of the survivors had thoracotomy performed in the operating room. It is apparent that if adequate volume is present to allow circulation with closed chest cardiopulmonary resuscitation, then hypovolemia is not severe enough to necessitate thoracotomy in the emergency room.

The reasons for the poor outcome in blunt trauma, as opposed to penetrating trauma, are speculative. A substantial portion of these patients die of brain injury.[45] This presumably is related either to direct cerebral injury or prolonged brain hypoxia before and during resuscitation. In addition, the incidence of multiple injuries is more extensive in blunt trauma, and surgical treatment therefore is lengthier and more complicated. Another contributing factor that may be responsible for difficult resuscitation and low salvage rates after blunt trauma is disseminated intravascular coagulation. Hemorrhagic shock alone in the absence of soft tissue injury is rarely associated with disseminated intravascular coagulation, whereas blunt trauma with soft tissue injury and shock is a potent activator of the process.[89] After blunt trauma, tissue fragments enter the bloodstream and in conjunction with circulatory stasis produce intravascular coagulation. With severe shock, protective mechanisms appear to be absent and unchecked intravascular utilization of clotting components results in a consumptive coagulopathy. This may have been a contributing factor in as many as 70% of the cases reported by Bodai and associates.[45] In those patients who survived an initial bleeding episode, subsequent multiple organ failure was almost universal, accounting for the high late mortality in that group.

COMPLICATIONS

Complications associated with emergency room thoracotomy are surprisingly rare and are mostly iatrogenic. These include laceration of the lung, injury to the phrenic nerve, laceration of the myocardium or coronary artery when opening the pericardium, and digital laceration of the heart during myocardial compression. Although generally performed in haste, attention should be paid to the proper placement of the thoracotomy incision. In males this usually corresponds to the interspace just below the left nipple. In females, manual upward retraction of the breast during thoracotomy will help prevent breast transection. In the latter instance, the dissection should be carried obliquely upward to the fifth interspace. The most common mistake is to enter the thorax too low.

During performance of pericardiotomy, it is important to avoid injury to the phrenic nerve, which lies on the pericardium. Therefore, we recommend that pericardiotomy incisions always be made in a vertical manner above and parallel to the nerve. In addition, on performance of pericardiotomy the underlying heart or coronary arteries may be injured. This is unlikely in the presence of tamponade because the pericardium is elevated away from the underlying heart.

During manual compression of the heart, the tension placed on the heart should be distributed over the palm or fingers of the hand. The atria are very thin, and cardiac rupture can occur with too vigorous attempts at cardiac massage and overvigorous fingertip compression.

Late complications include bleeding, infection, and neurologic injury. On termination of the procedure, closure should be accomplished in a meticulous manner. Attention should be paid to the internal mammary vessels, which may have been transected during the incision. They may cause considerable bleeding in the postoperative period, and this bleeding can be difficult to differentiate from bleeding from other sources. The pericardium is closed loosely if the pericardial contents are dry and the heart is not too distended. Failure to close the pericardium may, on occasion, lead to herniation of the heart into the left chest. Paricardial closure should be such that free drainage is permitted without compromising cardiac function.

Wound infections are remarkably uncommon in patients surviving emergency room thoracotomy.[51,90,91,94–96]

Ischemic brain damage has been noted as a complication of emergency room thoracotomy by some investigators,[46,91,92] although cross-clamping of the aorta does not seem to affect the brain adversely.[93] In addition, paraplegia secondary to spinal cord ischemia has been reported. These complications are presumably secondary to the low-flow state that these patients suffer as part of their injury.[44]

REFERENCES

1. Breasted JH. *The Edwin Smith Papyrus.* vol. 1. Chicago: University of Chicago Press; 1930.
2. Adams F. *Genuine Works of Hypocrites.* vol 2. New York: William Wood and Co; 1886.
3. Boerhaave H. Aphorismi de cognoscendis et curandis morbis (Aphorism 170). Vander Linden; 1709.
4. Riolanus J. En cheiridium anatomicum et pathologicum, in quo ex naturali constitutione partium, recessus a naturale statu demonstratur; ad usum theatri anatomici acornatum. Lugd. Bat., A. Wynjaerden; 1649.
5. Dupuytren. Cited by Cazan GM Jr. Multiple lacerations of the auricle. *Armed Forces Med J.* 1952;3:253.
6. Larrey DJ. *Clin Chir Paris.* 1829;2:284.
7. Bloc MH. Uber wunden des Herzen und der Herzbentelf. *Verh Dtsch Ges Chir.* 1882;11:108.
8. DeVecchio S. Sutura del cuore. *Riforma Med.* 1895;2:79.
9. Dalton HC. Report of a case of stab wounds of the pericardium. *Ann Surg.* 1895;21:147.
10. Williams DH. Stab wound of the heart and pericardium: suture of the pericardium—patient alive three years afterwards. *Med Rec.* 1897;51:437.
11. Cappelen A. Vulnus cordia, sutur of hjirtet. *Nord Mag Laegevidensk.* 1896;11:285.
12. Paget S. *The Surgery of the Chest.* London: Wright;1896.
13. Rehn L. Uber penetrirende Herzwanden and Herznaht. *Arch Klin Chir.* 1897;55:315.
14. Hill U. Report of case of successful suturing of heart and table of 37 other cases of suturing by different operators, with various terminations and conclusions drawn. *Med Rec.* 1902;62:846.
15. Phillips CV, Jacobensen DC, Braton DF, et al. Central vessel trauma. *Am Surg.* 1979;45:517.
16. Tuffier T. La chirurgie du coeur. Cinquieme Congres de la Societe Internationale de Chirurgie. Paris 1920. Extrait, Brussels, Hayez, 1920.
17. Blades B, Dugan DJ. War wounds of the chest observed at the thoracic center, Walter Reed General Hospital. *J Thorac Surg.* 1944;13:294.
18. Churchill ED. Trends and practices in thoracic surgery in the Mediterranean theater. *J Thorac Surg.* 1944;13:307.
19. Glass JL. Treatment of chest injuries in Viet Nam. *Am Surg.* 1969;35:227.
20. McNamara JJ, Messersmith JK, Dunn RA, et al. Thoracic injuries in combat casualties in Vietnam. *Ann Thorac Surg.* 1970;10:389.
21. Blalock A, Ravitch MM. Consideration of nonoperative treatment of cardiac tamponade resulting from wounds of the heart. *Surgery.* 1943;14:157.
22. Sugg WL, Rea WJ, Ecker RR, et al. Penetrating wounds of the heart. An analysis of 459 cases. *J Thorac Cardiovasc Surg.* 1968;56:531.
23. Beall AC, Patrick TA, Okies EJ, et al. Penetrating wounds of the heart: changing patterns of surgical management. *J Trauma.* 1972;12:468.
24. Botta AR, Lansing AM, Ransdell HT. Immediate operative treatment for stab wounds of the heart: experience with fifty-four consecutive cases. *J Thorac Cardiovasc Surg.* 1970;59:662.
25. Steichen FM, Dargan EL, Efron G, et al. A graded approach to the management of penetrating wounds to the heart. *Arch Surg.* 1971;103:574.
26. Pickard LR, Mattox KL. Thoracic trauma and indications for thoracotomy. In Mattox KL, Moore EE, Feliciano DV, eds. *Trauma.* Norwalk, CT: Appleton & Lange; 1988.
27. Stephenson HE Jr, Reid CL, Hintow JW, et al. Some common denominators in 1,200 cases of cardiac arrest. *Ann Surg.* 1953;137:731.
28. Baker CC, Thomas AN, Trunkey DD. The role of emergency room thoracotomy in trauma. *J Trauma.* 1980;20:848.
29. Hoffman J. Emergency department thoracotomy. *Ann Emerg Med.* 1981;10:275.
30. Jackimczyk K, Markovchick V, Rosen P. Traumatic cardiac arrest. In: Harwood AL, ed. *Cardiopulmonary Resuscitation.* Baltimore: Williams & Wilkins; 1982.
31. Stephenson HE. Artificial maintenance of circulation: open chest resuscitation. In: Stephenson HE, ed. *Cardiac Arrest and Resuscitation.* St. Louis: CV Mosby; 1969.
32. Stephenson HE. Present place of open chest cardiac resuscitation. In: Safar P, ed. *Advances in Cardiopulmonary Resuscitation.* New York: Springer-Verlag; 1977.
33. Beall AC Jr, Gastor RM, Bricher DL. Gunshot wound of the heart: changing patterns of surgical management. *Ann Thorac Surg.* 1971;11:523.
34. Kish G, Kozloff L, Joseph WL, et al. Indications for early thoracotomy in the management of chest trauma. *Ann Thorac Surg.* 1976;22:23.
35. Mattox KL, Espada R, Beall AC, et al. Performing thoracotomy in the emergency center. *JACEP.* 1974; 3:13.
36. Siemens R, Polk HC, Gray LA, et al. Indications for thoracotomy following penetrating thoracic injury. *J Trauma.* 1977;17:493.

37. Kaushik VS, Mankal AK, Awariefe OA, et al. Early thoracotomy for stab wounds of the heart. *J Cardiovasc Surg*. 1979;20:423.
38. Sherman MM, Saini VK, Yarnoz MD, et al. Management of penetrating heart wounds. *Am J Surg*. 1978;135:553.
39. Ivatury RR, Kazigo J, Rohman M, Gaudino J, Simon R, Stahl WM. "Directed" emergency room thoracotomy: a prognostic prerequisite for survival. *J Trauma*. 1991;31(8):1076.
40. Tavares S, Hankins JR, Moulton AL, et al. Management of penetrating cardiac injuries: the role of emergency room thoracotomy. *Ann Surg*. 1984;35:183.
41. Ivatury RR, Rohman M, Steichen FM, et al. Penetrating cardiac injuries: twenty year experience. *Am Surg*. 1987;53:319.
42. Mavroudis C, Roon AJ, Baker CC, et al. Management of acute cervicothoracic vascular injuries. *J Thorac Cardiovasc Surg*. 1980;80:342.
43. Sankaran S, Lucas C, Walt AJ. Thoracic aortic clamping for prophylaxis against sudden cardiac arrest during laparotomy for acute massive hemoperitoneum. *J Trauma*. 1975;15:290.
44. Ledgerwood AM, Kazmers M, Lucas CE. The role of thoracic aortic occlusion for massive hemoperitoneum. *J Trauma*. 1976;16:610.
45. Bodai BI, Smith JP, Blaisdell FW. The role of emergency room thoracotomy in blunt trauma. *J Trauma*. 1982;22:487.
46. Cogbill TH, Moore EE, Millikan JS, et al. Rationale for selective application of emergency department thoracotomy in trauma. *J Trauma*. 1983;23:453.
47. Flynn TC, Ward RE, Miller PW. Emergency room thoracotomy. *Ann Emerg Med*. 1982;11:413.
48. MacDonald JR, McDowell RM. Emergency department thoracotomies in a community hospital. *JACEP*. 1978;7:423.
49. Moore EE, Moore JB, Galloway AL, et al. Post-injury thoracotomy in the emergency department: a critical evaluation. *Surgery*. 1979;86:590.
50. Esposito TJ, Jurkovich GJ, Rice CL, Maier RV, Copass K, Ashbaugh DG. Reappraisal of emergency room thoracotomy in a changing environment. *J Trauma*. 1991;31(7):881.
51. Fairman RM, Edmunds LH. Emergency thoracotomy in the surgical intensive care unit after open cardiac operation. *Ann Thorac Surg*. 1981;32:386.
52. Bodai BI, Smith JP, Ward RE, et al. Emergency thoracotomy in the management of trauma: a review. *JAMA*. 1983;249:1891.
53. Moore EE. Prognostic factors in emergency department thoracotomy for trauma. *Curr Conc Trauma Care*. 1982;5:5.
54. Bodai BI, Smith JP, Blaisdell FW. Emergency center thoracotomy. *Surg Rounds*. 1982;5:105.
55. Baxter BT, Moore EE, Moore JB, et al. Emergency department thoracotomy following injury: critical determinants for patient salvage. *World J Surg*. 1988;12:671.
56. Clevenger FW, Yarbrough DR, Reines HD. Resuscitative thoracotomy: the effects of field time on outcome. *J Trauma* 1988;28:441
57. Cogbill TH, Moore EE, Millikan JS, et al. Rationale for selective application of emergency department thoracotomy in trauma. *J Trauma*. 1983;23:453.
58. Shimazu S, Shatney CH. Outcome of trauma patients with no vital signs of hospital admission. *J Trauma*. 1983;23:213.
59. Danne PD, Finelli F, Champion HR. Emergency bay thoracotomy. *J Trauma*. 1984;24:796.
60. Schwab CW, Adcock OT, Max MH. Emergency department thoracotomy (EDT): a 26-month experience using an "agonal" protocol. *Am Surg*. 1986;52:20.
61. Shamoun JM, Barraza KR, Jurkovich GJ, Salley RK. In extremis use of staples for cardiorrhaphy in penetrating cardiac trauma: case report. *J Trauma*. 1989;29(11):1589.
62. Gilston A, Resnekov L. *Cardio-Respiratory Resuscitation*. London: William Heinenan Medical Books; 1971.
63. Adkins RB Jr, Whiteneck JM, Woltering EA. Penetrating chest wall and thoracic injuries. *Am Surg*. 1985;51:140.
64. Ivatury RR, Rohman M. Emergency department thoracotomy for trauma: a collective review. *Resuscitation*. 1987;15:23.
65. Ivatury RR, Nallathambi M, Rohman M, et al. Penetrating thoracic injuries: in-field stabilization vs. immediate transport. *J Trauma*. 1987;27:1066.
66. Botta AR, Ransdell HT. Treatment of penetrating gunshot wounds of the chest: experience with 145 cases. *Am J Surg*. 1971;122:81.
67. Brutel de la Riviere A, Brummelkamp WH. Penetrating thoracic trauma. *Scand J Thorac Cardiovasc Surg*. 1980;14:123.
68. Graham JM, Mattox KL, Beall AC Jr. Penetrating trauma of the lung. *J Trauma*. 1979;19:665.

69. Levinsky L, Vidne B, Nudelman I, et al. Thoracic injuries in the Yom Kuppur War. *Isr J Med Sci*. 1975;11:275.
70. Mattila A, Laustela E, Tala P. Penetrating and perforating thoracic injuries. *Scand J Thorac Cardiovasc Surg*. 1981;15:105.
71. Oparah SS, Mandal AK. Penetrating stab wounds of the chest: experience with 200 consecutive cases. *J Trauma*. 1976;16:868.
72. Schwartz GR, Wagner DK. Emergency therapy: penetrating trauma to the chest, heart, and great vessels. *JACEP*. 1973;2:196.
73. Trinkle JK, Toon RS, Franz JL, et al. Affairs of the wounded heart: penetrating cardiac wounds. *J Trauma*. 1979;19:467.
74. Beall AC Jr, Ochsner JL, Morris GC Jr, et al. Penetrating wounds of the heart. *J Trauma*. 1961;1:195.
75. Boyd TS, Strender JW. Immediate surgery for traumatic heart disease. *J Thorac Cardiovasc Surg*. 1965;50:305.
76. Isaacs JP. 60 Penetrating wounds of the heart: clinical and experimental observations. *Surgery*. 1959;45:696.
77. Parmley LF, Mattingly TW, Manion WC. Penetrating wounds of the heart and aorta. *Circulation*. 1958;17:953.
78. Ivatury RR, Shah PM, Ito K, et al. Emergency room thoracotomy for the resuscitation of patients with "fatal" penetrating injuries of the heart. *Ann Thorac Surg*. 1981;32:377.
79. Breaux EP, Dupont JB Jr, Albert HM, et al. Cardiac tamponade following penetrating mediastinal injuries. Improved survival with early pericardiocentesis. *J Trauma*. 1979;19:461.
80. Carrasquilla C, Wilson RF, Walt AJ, et al. Gunshot wounds of the heart. *Ann Thorac Surg*. 1972;13:208.
81. Oparah SS, Mandal AK. Operative management of penetrating wounds of the chest in civilian practice; review of indications in 125 consecutive patients. *J Thorac Cardiovasc Surg*. 1979;77:162.
82. Mattox KL, Beall AC, Jordan GL, et al. Cardiorrhaphy in the emergency center. *J Thorac Cardiovasc Surg*. 1974;68:886.
83. DeGennaro VA, Bonfila-Robert EA, Ching N, et al. Aggressive management of potential penetrating cardiac injuries. *J Thorac Cardiovasc Surg*. 1980;79:883.
84. Harnar TRJ, Oreskovich MR, Copass MK, et al. Role of emergency thoracotomy in the resuscitation of moribund trauma victims: 100 consecutive cases. *Am J Surg*. 1981;142:96.
85. Bodai BI. Discussion of: Rohman M, Ivatury RR, Steichen I, et al. Emergency room thoracotomy for penetrating cardiac injury. *J Trauma*. 1983;23:570.
86. Demetriades D. Cardiac penetrating injuries: personal experience of 45 cases. *Br J Surg*. 1984;71:95.
87. Feliciano DV, Mattox KL. Indications, techniques, and pitfalls of emergency center thoracotomy. *Surg Rounds*. 1981;4:32.
88. Vij D, Simoni E, Smith E, et al. Resuscitative thoracotomy for patients with traumatic injury. *Surgery*. 1983;94:554.
89. Blaisdell FW, Lewis FR. Treatment of intravascular coagulation. In: Blaisdell FW, Lewis FR, eds. *Respiratory Distress Syndrome of Shock and Trauma*. Philadelphia: Saunders; 1977.
90. Evans J, Gray JS, Rayner A, et al. Principles for the management of penetrating cardiac wounds. *Ann Surg*. 1979;189:777.
91. Mattox KL, Von Koch L, et al. Logistic and technical considerations in the treatment of the wounded heart. *Circulation*. 1975;51-52(Suppl 1):210.
92. Baker CC, Caronna IT, Trunkey DD. Neurologic outcome after emergency room thoracotomy for trauma. *Am J Surg*. 1980;139:677.
93. Shackford SR, Walsh JC, Davis JW. The effects of aortic crossclamping and resuscitation on intracranial pressure, cerebral blood flow, and cerebral water content in a model of focal brain injury and hemorrhagic shock. *J Trauma*. 1990;30(7):768.
94. Roberge RJ, Ivatury RR, Stahl WM, et al. Emergency department thoracotomy for penetrating injuries: predictive value of patient classification. *Am J Emerg Med*. 1986;4:129.
95. Washington BW, Wilson RF, Steiger Z, et al. Emergency thoracotomy: a four-year review. *Ann Thorac Surg*. 1985;40:188.
96. Feliciano DV, Bitondo CG, Cruise PA, et al. Liberal use of emergency center thoracotomy. *Am J Surg*. 1986;152:654.

4

Radiologic Assessment of the Chest

RAYMOND E. PARKS, M.D.
JOHN P. LIVONI, M.D.

HISTORY: Radiology has made important contributions toward the advancement of thoracic trauma management during the past 100 years. X-rays were discovered in 1895 by William Conrad Roentgen. They were almost immediately utilized to visualize the thoracic contents, and the first scientific paper about chest radiographs was presented within a year of Roentgen's discovery. The first monograph, "The Roentgen Rays in the Diagnosis of Diseases of the Chest," made its appearance in 1906. The early radiographs of the chest were underpenetrated and were blurred by respiratory and cardiac motion. The early equipment required considerable time to produce a radiograph, often were accompanied by high voltage arcing and electromagnetism, and had unpredictable results. The radiographer, who usually was a nonmedical person with some skills or interest in photography and electricity, would fix the patient in a rigid position with straps and sandbags. The image was recorded on a glass plate that had silver bromide photographic emulsion rolled on its surface. A typical exposure would take several minutes and the finished product, if any image was obtained, would be blurred by respiratory and cardiac motion. All of the radiographs made before World War I were made on glass plates; the term "chest plate" has endured even to this day.

During World War I, several advances in diagnostic radiology took place. W.D. Coolidge invented the hot tungsten filament x-ray tube that provided a reliable production of a relatively large flux of radiation. At about the same time, x-ray film became available as a substitute for glass plates. The x-ray film had a double emulsion, one on each surface, and it was soon sandwiched between two fluorescent screens (intensifying screens), thereby reducing by 10 to 20 times the necessary dose required for a chest radiograph. These advances allowed instantaneous films of the thorax so that cardiac and respiratory motion did not interfere.

One of the most important advances of the past decade has been the expansion of basic knowledge and a keener appreciation of the anatomy and the pathophysiology of the plain chest radiograph. Although the frontal chest radiograph has been with us for more than 100 years, only in the past few years have improved concepts of interpretation become appreciated. Computed tomography (CT) has given a new dimension to the pathologic changes occurring within the thorax, and this information has led to a better understanding of the plain chest radiograph.

No attempt is made in this chapter to discuss the many and varied images of thoracic trauma, because this would be redundant in view of the detailed discussions elsewhere in this book. Thoracic trauma is a broad subject that includes penetrating and blunt injuries of the thorax from external sources, as well as internal trauma from inhalation, ingestion, foreign bodies, exertional, and iatrogenic. The imaging manifestations include the primary, secondary, and chronic effects of trauma that may occur during the emergent, progress, and convalescent periods of management.[1]

The purpose of this chapter is to discuss some of the principles used to obtain the maximum information from radiologic studies of the thorax injured by external trauma, either blunt or penetrating. Good radiologic diagnosis requires good images. Good images are the result of good positioning, correct exposure and data collection, and proper processing of the imaging information.[2] The worth of these diagnostic tools, whether it be a plain x-ray film, an angiogram, computed tomography (CT), ultrasound, or nuclear scan, is dependent on obtaining a satisfactory film for interpretation.

Good imaging results also depend on the interaction of the attending surgeon and the radiologist. Whenever possible, the thoracic surgeon should make his needs known by direct discussion with the radiologist performing and interpreting the study. If the radiologist understands the diagnostic problem, additional views or procedures often will supply the needed information. Requesting an examination with inadequate clinical information supplied to the radiologist often results in poor interpretation and an incomplete imaging study.

The logistics of radiologic examinations is dependent on the patient's whole status, and determination as to whether or not to perform a radiologic examination is the prerogative and responsibility of the attending trauma surgeon. Some critical, unstable patients may need life-saving surgery without delay, whereas others may be as seriously injured, but time may be taken to obtain a portable chest radiograph to help plan the surgery. Judgment on priorities is the essence of trauma management. Whether or not radiographic examinations are utilized is determined by available time for diagnosis, the potential benefit, and the additional risks of the radiologic procedure.

It is prudent to attempt to foresee the need for other radiologic examinations and to have a sequence plan in mind to save time and duplication. For example, the severe chest trauma patient who also has head trauma may need CT of the head. If iodinated contrast is to be administered, that contrast media also may serve to evaluate the kidneys if renal trauma is also suspected. If angiography is required for evaluation of the chest or abdomen, CT may be performed immediately before or after the angiogram and prevent the duplication of intravascular administration of the contrast media. An upper gastrointestinal study with barium or a barium enema for evaluation of a traumatic diaphragmatic herniation should not be performed if there is any need for urography, angiography, CT, ultrasound, or nuclear medicine investigation of the abdomen.

PLAIN CHEST RADIOGRAPH

A frontal chest radiograph is a required diagnostic aid in every case of thoracic trauma. An upright chest film made with fixed equipment is the ideal, but often only a recumbent chest film can be obtained because of the condition of the patient. A plain recumbent chest radiograph can be obtained on any injured patient, no matter how extreme the condition may be, and it can be made without moving the patient from the stretcher or treatment table. The determining factor is whether the few minutes necessary to obtain the radiograph should be taken if interruption of the emergency therapy of the patient is required. However, it usually is the case that the patient requiring resuscitation will benefit from radiologic assessment of the chest, and we make every effort in our environment to obtain a chest x-ray within 5 min of presentation of the patient. The only exception is the patient in extremis who requires open chest resuscitation.

Portable Versus Fixed X-Ray Equipment

The equipment used for obtaining a "portable" chest radiograph on the treatment table, operating room table, or intensive care bed requires an x-ray generator with a minimum capacity of 100 kw and 200 ma to permit the use of adequate tube-film distance with a reasonable short exposure time. Although a smaller portable unit with a capacity of 20 to 30 ma has been used successfully, especially for children and small adults, the modern portable unit has much greater capacity and will produce far superior results. The modern portable unit is usually battery operated and, when not in use, the batteries are recharged by plugging the unit into a standard 120 V current. These portable x-ray units produce radiation that has qualitative wave length characteristics similar to fixed radiographic units in the radiology department. Their capacity is about 20 to 30 kw, whereas fixed radiographic units are from 50 to 100 kw. A single portable chest x-ray requires an exposure of 2 to 4 ma, and the modern portable unit is capable of delivering several times that amount. These "cordless" x-ray generators are equipped with a rotating anode tube with a focal spot of 2 mm or less and compare favorably with fixed x-ray units in this respect.

The x-ray capability of portable and fixed generators is similar and more than adequate, but there are deficiencies of radiographs from portable x-ray units when compared with those from fixed equipment. The precise centering of the x-ray beam of fixed installation allows the use of a lead grid for the elimination of scattered radiation. With portable equipment, the x-ray beam cannot be aimed with precision at the center of the x-ray film. The x-ray film is hidden behind the subject's body, and it is difficult to position the x-ray so that the surface of the cassette holding the film is at right angles to the x-ray beam. Because of the difficulty of accurately aiming the x-ray beam, high-efficiency grids cannot be used and radiographs often are made with no grid or with a grid of low efficiency. With a fixed installation, the x-ray tube to film distance is precisely maintained, and, with most fixed units, it would be impossible to use the wrong distance. The tube-to-film distance of portable radiography is an unknown, unless one takes considerable time and effort to determine the distance. The tube-to-patient distance can be measured, but to this must be added the thickness of the chest. Another factor that allows fixed radiographic units to have an advantage over portable units is that, with their greater capacity, radiographic exposures are delivered in a shorter period of time, which decreases the likelihood of lack of clarity from motion.

Positioning

Positioning of the patient and film is most important. It is easy with a fixed unit and difficult with portable equipment. Usually the trauma patient's condition prevents cooperation. The placing of the film beneath the patient is usually best accomplished by inserting the cassette beneath a sheet underneath the patient because the sheet usually produces less friction than the patient's skin, prevents injury of the skin, and allows minor adjustment in the position of the cassette. The use of a tunnel built into the surface of the treatment or operating room table is very helpful, but the patient must be positioned over this tunnel for satisfactory results. Stainless steel tunnels work out quite well and do not produce any density in the final radiograph because they are uniform in absorption. The cassettes that hold the x-ray film contain intensifying screens, and the weight of the patient directly against the cassette may result in a warp of the cassette and poor contact of the intensifying screen with the x-ray film. Any warp or distortion of the cassette renders it useless because the image will not be sharp and will show artifactual densities.

The greater the distance from the x-ray tube to the film, the less the photographic magnification (Fig. 4–1). Generally, we prefer to make upright films of the chest with a distance of 2 m or more. In the recumbent patient, whether using a fixed or portable x-ray generator, it usually is not possible to obtain a distance greater than 1 m because of ceiling height limitation or tube support height limitation (Fig. 4–2). This shorter tube-to-film distance introduces magnification distortion, but it does have the technical advantage that a shorter exposure time is required because of the shorter distance. The tube-to-film distance should not be shorter than 36 in (90 cm) or intolerable geometric enlargement and lack of sharpness will result, particularly involving that anatomy not close to the film. The incident x-ray beam should be perpendicular to the center of the film, and the central axis of radiation should be directed at the center of the film. Any angulation results in a distortion of anatomy that may be confusing and may result in faulty conclusions. If the central ray is not in the center of the film, uneven density of the radiograph results, and this may suggest the presence of pleural fluid, consolidation, or other abnormality in areas where insufficient radiation is recorded and may suggest emphysema or pneumothorax of the portion of the chest that receives adequate radiation.

Other Views

Multiple views often are desirable, but in the critically injured patient usually only a frontal supine view is possible and practical. The examination can be enhanced by obtaining underexposed or overexposed film. In some departments, the cassette used in portable examinations is loaded with two pieces of film, and the cassette contains one pair of fast

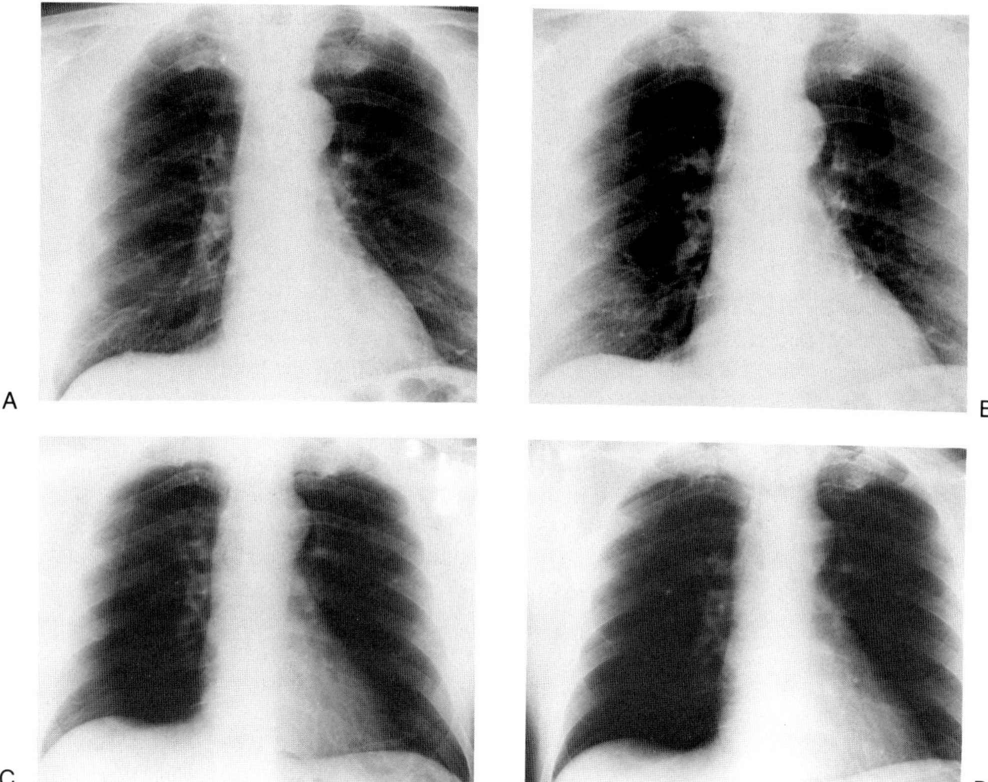

Figure 4–1. The effect of distance, position, and equipment on the appearance of the chest film. A normal volunteer was used for all four views and all were made within a few minutes' time. **A:** Upright anteroposterior chest radiograph made at 6 ft (180 cm) tube-object distance. **B:** Upright anteroposterior chest radiograph made at 40 in (100 cm) distance. The shorter distance caused magnification of structures that were not close to the film, which was behind the subject's posterior surface. The transverse diameter of the heart and of the thorax has increased. **C:** Supine anteroposterior chest radiograph made at 40 in (100 cm) distance. The recumbent chest film is similar to the upright film (B) in the degree of magnification. The diaphragm is not as high as the upright film because of visceral pressure on the diaphragm in the recumbent horizontal position. **D:** Supine anteroposterior chest radiograph made at 40 in (100 cm) with a portable x-ray unit. A, B, and C were made with a fixed x-ray generator in the radiology department. This illustrates that films made with portable equipment are no different from films made with fixed equipment if both are made under the same limitations. Portable films are often suboptimal because recumbent patients are sick and cooperation is difficult or impossible.

screens and one pair of slow screens so that with a single x-ray exposure, underexposed and overexposed films are obtained. The use of underexposed and overexposed films usually makes it easier to recognize the position of the endotracheal tube, intravascular catheters, and air leaks producing pneumothorax or pneumomediastinum. The overexposed film often will show details of the thoracic spine not visible on usual chest exposure (Fig. 4–2). A reduction of the x-ray beam to a coned-down small area results in an improved radiograph, and this technique will produce superior radiographs with maximum detail when interest is centered on a specific area. When making any radiographs, it is desirable to remove all overlying and underlying artifacts such as clothing, foreign bodies, tubes, dressing

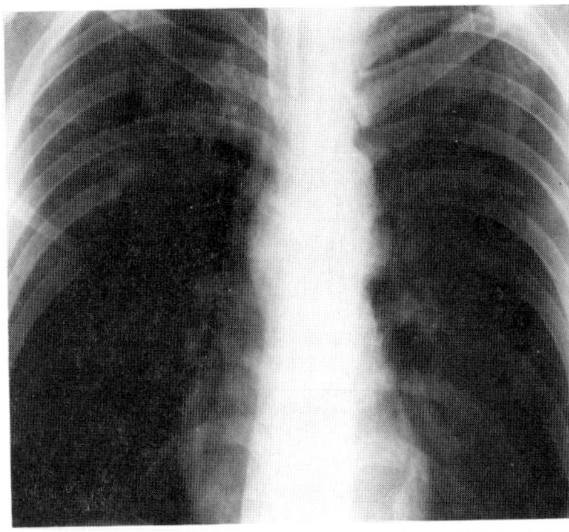

Figure 4–2.   Value of overpenetrated views. Supine chest film made in emergency room (*not shown*) showed fracture of posterior left seventh rib, but did not suggest the paravertebral hematoma seen on this overpenetrated film. The paravertebral hematoma was due to a compression fracture of the body of T7.

materials, and surgical appliances before exposing the film if these can be removed without disturbing the therapy of the patient. Any folds in the dependent skin of the thorax should be smoothed out to prevent skin fold densities (Fig. 4–3). Such artifactual densities cause considerable confusion in the interpretation of the radiograph and may result in false conclusions.

Inspiration Versus Expiration

The inspiratory phase of respiration provides more diagnostic information and is used whenever a chest radiograph is made. The densities that we see in the lung field, whether they be lung markings, atelectatic or consolidated lung, or any other density, are seen because they are contrasted with the surrounding air within the lung. Mediastinal structures, such as aortic knob and pericardial sac, are silhouettes seen only because the air in the lung field defines these non–air-containing densities. Therefore, an increase in the volume of air in the thorax should improve visualization and recognition of contrasted densities. Inspiration also lowers the level of the diaphragm and thus reveals a greater lung area for evaluation. If the patient is intubated, the radiograph can be obtained at full lung volume by stopping the ventilator at the height of its inspiratory phase. In the patient who is not on external ventilatory assistance, an inspiratory film requires the voluntary stopping of respiratory activity at full inspiration if the patient is conscious and can cooperate. Most acute emergent trauma patients cannot cooperate and, in these cases, the technician must anticipate when maximum inspiration will occur and hope that the radiographic exposure coincides. When patient cooperation is not available, the exposures should be as short as possible.

Films made in the expiratory phase often are adequate for evaluation of trauma effects, especially by an experienced radiologist or trauma surgeon. Expiratory phase films have been recommended for the detection of pneumothorax and pneumomediastinum (Fig. 4–4). Because the lungs have a reduced volume of air during the expiratory phase, pneumothorax air and mediastinal air should be visualized and recognized more easily. Our experience has indicated that expiratory films generally are better for the demonstration of pneumothorax,

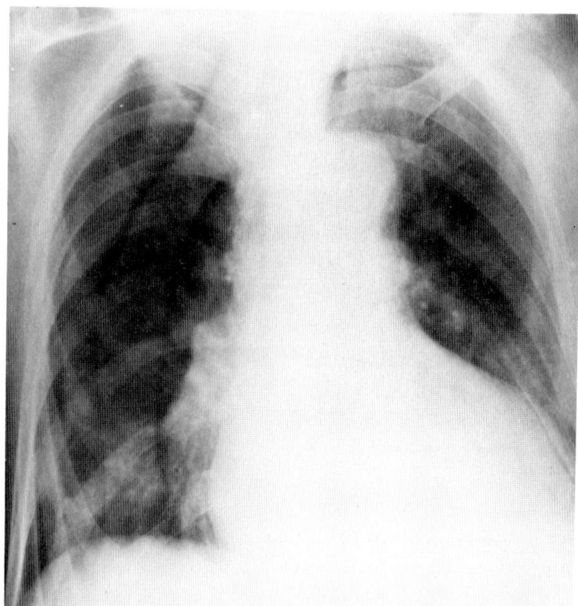

Figure 4–3. Skin folds. Chest radiographs made of a patient in a supine position often will show skin folds, especially if the skin is loose and redundant. Good technique includes prevention of these folds by inserting the radiographic cassette beneath the bed or table sheet and then smoothing out the folds that may occur in the skin or sheet. Skin folds often mimic pneumothorax, and thoracostomy tubes have been inserted to treat a pseudo-pneumothorax caused by skin folds.

but usually are not required, and usually are inferior for the demonstration of other radiographic findings. Expiratory films also have been recommended for demonstrating ischemic regions of the lung fields or large areas of air trapping. Emphysematous bullae, for example, may be recognized more easily in an expiratory film because the lucency of the large air-containing chambers becomes more apparent when the surrounding lung tissue becomes more dense. A portion of the lung that is deprived of pulmonary arterial perfusion due to embolus or thrombus may be visible on an expiratory phase film when compared with an inspiratory phase film. These considerations are not of importance during the acute emergent phase, but may be important considerations during the convalescent phase when the trauma patient is recovering in intensive care.

Lateral and Oblique Views

It is an axiom in radiology that more information can be obtained from additional views. The expense and inconvenience of obtaining additional views must be weighed against the potential benefit. In the acute traumatized patient, additional views often are not indicated because of the interruption of therapy and the movement of the body that may be required.

A lateral view of the chest often is desirable but usually not practical. In the emergency trauma patient, the lateral view of the chest has to be made recumbent using a horizontal

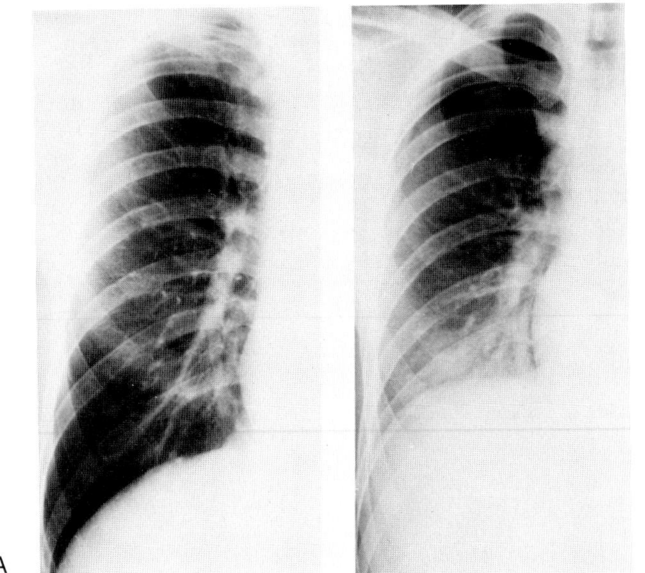

A   B

Figure 4–4.   Expiration film. Pneumothorax is seen at apex of the upright chest. **A:** The inspiration film shows the pneumothorax. The parietal pleura is separated from the visceral pleural by 15 mm. **B:** The expiration film made immediately before the inspiration film shows the pneumothorax to better advantage. The distance between the visceral and parietal pleura is 35 mm in this film. The edge of the lung (visceral pleura) is more distinct. A tiny bleb on the visceral pleural surface is best seen on the expiratory phase film. Expiration reduces the volume of the pleural cavity and the lung. The lung also becomes more dense because of the reduced volume of air. The pneumothorax remains essentially unchanged in volume and as a consequence is proportionately larger during the expiratory phase.

x-ray beam. This view often will demonstrate a pneumothorax or pleural fluid that might not be recognized on the frontal view, but the demonstration of the air, pleural fluid, or lung density cannot be localized to the right or left side unless it is recognized in the frontal view of the chest. Although the quality of the trans-table lateral view often is suboptimal, it usually answers the questions of whether or not a pneumothorax exists and if there is any large pleural fluid collection. The diagnostic value of the cross-table lateral view does not justify its routine use in trauma patients, but in selected cases it can be very helpful.

Oblique films can be made by using a vertical beam and rotating the patient in an oblique position. Oblique views also can be made with a horizontal beam, and the patient is rotated into an oblique position by bringing the side of interest upward. The oblique view made with a horizontal beam probably is the most reliable view for the demonstration of a small pneumothorax in a recumbent patient. When the patient is rotated with the involved side upward and an oblique film is obtained with a horizontal x-ray beam, even small collections of air are visible along the anterior axillary aspect of the elevated side of the chest. Fluid collections in the pleural space are well demonstrated in the dependent side of the chest by the horizontal lateral view. Oblique views of the chest are painful for the patient with rib fractures or chest tubes and usually are contraindicated if fractures of the spine or pelvis are present.

Decubitus Views

Decubitus views often are used to demonstrate small quantities of fluid or pneumothorax air in the trauma patient who is in relatively good condition and in whom there is no contraindication to assuming the decubitus position (Fig. 4–5). In the multitrauma patient, decubitus films usually are impractical or impossible. A decubitus view requires rotating the patient 90° so that the side of the body is dependent. If the patient has a fracture of the spine, pelvis, or multiple rib fractures, the decubitus position is contraindicated. The decubitus position may disrupt respiratory tubes, central lines, and peripheral intravenous lines unless care is taken to protect these. In some cases, respiratory and cardiac activity

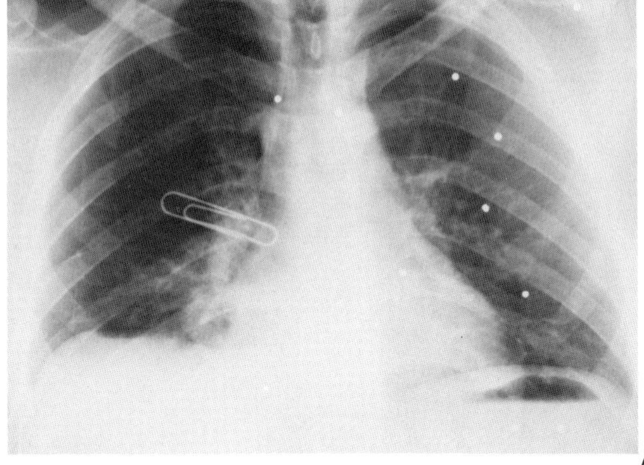

A

Figure 4–5.   Decubitus view. **A:** Upright film of chest of patient with a stab wound. Paper clip marks site of stab wound. Shotgun pellets are in chest wall from previous injury many years ago. The small air bubble at the dome of the right diaphragm suggests a tiny basilar pneumothorax because its upper border is not thick enough for the bubble to be subdiaphragmatic free air. A subpulmonary collection of blood with a tiny subpulmonary pneumothorax was suspected and a right decubitus view (**B**) showed approximately 300 ml of shifting fluid (blood), confirming the impression.

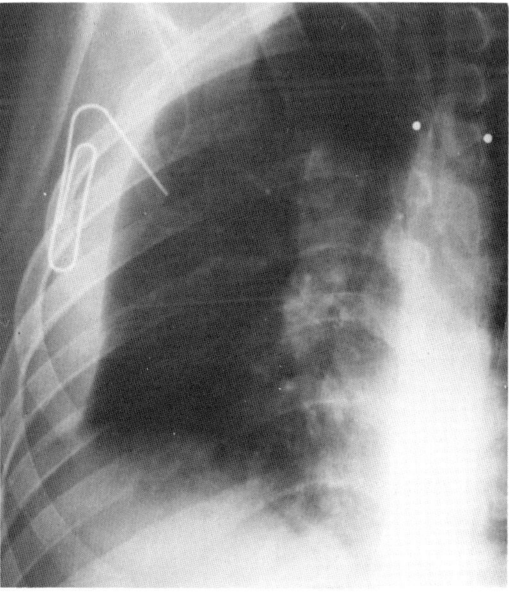

B

may be interfered with in the decubitus position. The information sought usually can be obtained with a shallow oblique view with a horizontal x-ray beam. In the convalescent patient or in the acute trauma patient who can assume the decubitus position, free-shifting fluid can be demonstrated and the amount estimated.

Rib, Sternum, Thoracic Spine, and Clavicle Films

During the acute, emergency phase of management, there is no special advantage of the radiographic demonstration of fractures of the ribs, sternum, or clavicle. These can be diagnosed clinically with good accuracy. The exception is first and second rib fractures, which are associated with a high incidence of underlying vascular injury. These should be looked for in parallel with apical capping.[3]

It is important to determine as early as possible whether a spinal fracture exists that might threaten the integrity of the spinal cord. This information can be detected by obtaining an overpenetrated frontal view of the thoracic spine and, if there is any suspicious finding, a trans-table lateral view of the thoracic spine of the patient will demonstrate the fracture. Any suggestion of disruption of an alignment of any of the thoracic vertebrae or any suggestion of a paravertebral hematoma or any rib fracture that involves the region of the head, neck, or angle of the posterior rib demands a lateral view of the thoracic spine. When the plain films suggest the probability of thoracic cord injury from fracture, dislocation, or penetrating foreign body, usually a more definitive examination is required, especially CT with a metrizamide myelogram.

Frequency of Plain Radiographs

The plain radiographs of the chest should be obtained as often as required, and the number of films and the views should be dictated by necessity. Financial cost and radiation exposure are limiting factors. Radiation exposure is more of a theoretical than a practical consideration as it applies to the trauma patient. The radiation risk involved, whether the patient be an infant, adult, or an unborn fetus, is so minimal that it is completely eclipsed by the actual or potential risk of the trauma effect. If the radiograph is required for the management of the patient, it should be obtained with no consideration of radiation risk. Harmful effects from diagnostic radiography levels of radiation have not been demonstrated, and the conclusion of probable hazard is extrapolated from larger doses of radiation that produce definite injury (Table 4–1).

Another concern for controlling radiation exposure to the acute trauma patient is the radiation exposure of the personnel. The attending personnel, unlike the patient, have repeated exposure risk because of their occupation and obtain no benefit from the radiation exposure. Whenever possible, personnel should withdraw from the area of radiation and, in all cases, should avoid the direct x-ray beam. When a chest x-ray is being made, a 2-m distance from the radiographic beam would be safe. Under certain circumstances, such as at the operating table or during active resuscitation, the surgeon or his assistants may be as little as 0.5 m away from the x-ray beam. When making a frontal portable chest x-ray, personnel located 0.5 m from the incident x-ray beam would receive approximately 0.004 mrem of radiation. This radiation dose is about the same as would be received during a 1-h

Table 4–1. Relative Radiation Dose

FRONTAL CHEST X-RAY (POSTEROANTERIOR, ANTEROPOSTERIOR, DECUBITUS)	×-UNITS
Lateral view, oblique, or overpenetrated chest films	2×
CT of chest	2000×
Fluoroscopy of chest	1000–5000×
Conventional tomogram of chest	1000×
Angiography	1000–5000×

travel in a jet airplane or a 24-h visit to a location of 6000 feet altitude. Although this exposure dose is extremely small, all personnel should withdraw during the moment of the actual x-ray exposure and under all circumstances should never be exposed to the direct x-ray beam.

How often should the chest trauma patient have a radiograph to determine progress? The answer, of course, is as often as required. Any patient who is intubated or on ventilation equipment cannot be evaluated reliably by auscultation. When an intravascular catheter is introduced or exchanged, especially by anyone with limited experience, it is best checked by radiography to detect complicating pneumothorax, hemorrhage, or faulty placement. The position of endotracheal and chest tubes deserves confirmation to avert complications (Fig. 4–6).

Review of the Chest Radiograph

In the chest trauma patient, frontal view of the chest is the most important and is the one view that is always obtained (Fig. 4–7). The frontal view usually will be obtained in the recumbent position and often there will be only partial inspiration.

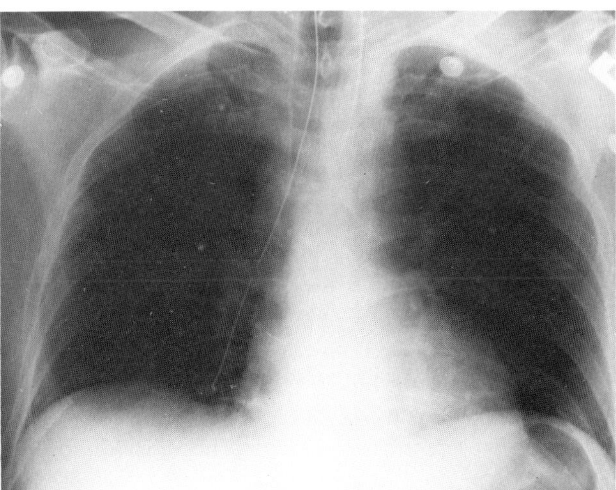

Figure 4–6.   Faulty tube placement. Portable recumbent chest film shows that the endotracheal tube entered the esophagus and the nasogastric tube entered the trachea. The endotracheal tube had its tip in a basilar bronchus of the lower lobe.

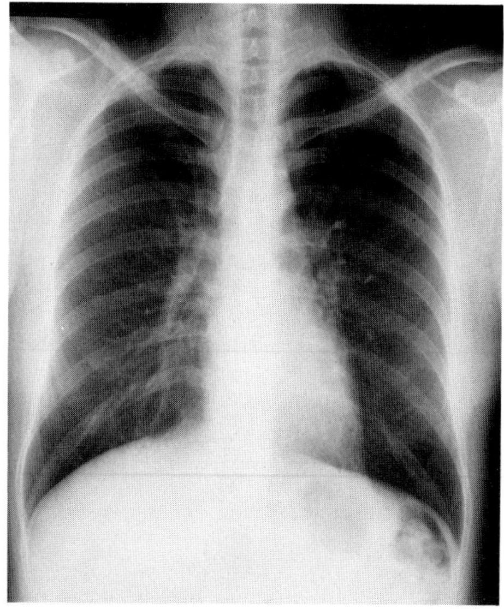

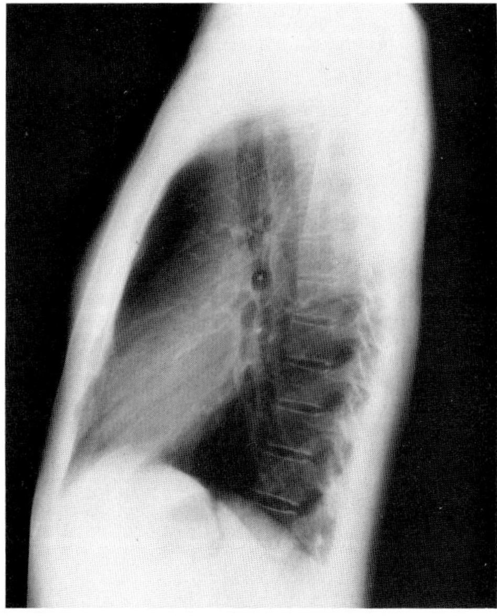

Figure 4–7. Radiologic anatomy. **A:** Posteroanterior view. **B:** Lateral view.

When reviewing the radiograph, it is best to display it on a good viewing box with uniform lighting, and it should not be studied by operating room light or lamps in the treatment area. A radiographic viewing box in a dimly lit room is best because extraneous room light does not make perception difficult due to reflections on the surface of the film. If previous films of the chest are available, they are always helpful and should be obtained and compared.

When looking at the initial chest radiograph of the thoracic trauma patient, a search should be made for evidence of air leaks, bleeding into the pleural space, lung contusion, hematoma, aspiration or atelectasis, widening of the mediastinal silhouette, bony injury, the position and location of tubes introduced into the body, and any clues suggesting injury to the diaphragm.[4] In other words, the possibility of any chest injuries that might result from severe thoracic trauma must be considered. Progress films of the chest made during the intermediate and convalescent phase would require other considerations.

Pneumothorax, if large, usually displaces the visceral pleura away from parietal pleura and is recognized along the lateral aspect of the lung. The presence of subcutaneous emphysema makes the recognition of pneumothorax more difficult because of the confusing overlying air shadows. A smaller pneumothorax will collect along the medial or lateral basilar aspects of the chest in the recumbent frontal view, and there may be no evidence of pneumothorax in the lateral or apical regions. Any localized area of radiolucency should be suspect for a pneumothorax, and this suspicion may be confirmed by additional views, usually best obtained by obtaining a shallow oblique view with a horizontal x-ray beam, if possible. Pneumothorax air may collect along the cardiac borders between the visceral and parietal pleura where it should not be confused with the pericardial air. Pericardial air in the recumbent chest produces a lucency above the diaphragmatic aspect of the pericardial cavity and this lucency crosses the midline.

Mediastinal air may be difficult to recognize, and a lateral film often is helpful. If the mediastinal air comes from the lung, it will be distributed throughout the mediastinum and may extend into the neck or into the subcutaneous spaces of the chest wall. Mediastinal air frequently collects along the cardiac contour within the mediastinal parietal pleura and, in this location, is identical with pneumothorax air that collects in the same location between the visceral and parietal pleura (Fig. 4–8). When mediastinal air is secondary to a torn

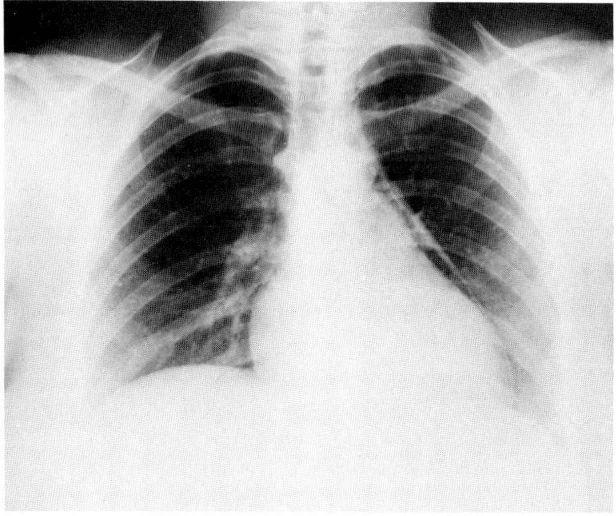

Figure 4–8. Mediastinal air. Air has collected along the left border of the anterior mediastinum defining the mediastinal parietal pleura. Pneumothorax air also may collect in the same location, but it would be located between the visceral and parietal pleura. The differentiation is easy in this case, because the lateral border of the air collection is wide, indicating that it is parietal mediastinal pleura with some fat and stromal tissue. If this were air in the pleural space, the lateral border of the air collection would be visceral pleura and would be very thin and continuous with the medial edge of the lung.

bronchus or trachea, it is usually copious. Mediastinal air caused by a torn esophagus usually is minimal and is rarely caused by external trauma.

Bleeding into the pleural space by pulmonary vessels or systemic arteries of the chest wall may be difficult to recognize on a radiograph of a recumbent patient. The blood collects along the posterior pleural space and does not appear along the lateral aspect of the pleural space until the fluid is sufficient in quantity to cause the lung to be displaced away from the chest wall. The fluid causes the lung to float anteriorly. The lung volume is reduced because of the encroachment on the available thoracic space by the pleural blood; this results in less air within the lung and therefore less blackness on the radiograph. Grayness of one lung compared with the other may be a sign of blood in the pleural spaces in the recumbent acute thoracically injured patient. Technical faults also can result in asymmetrical lung density. Slight rotation of the patient will cause one lung to be blacker than the other. If the central ray is not pointed at the center of the chest, one side of the chest may receive more radiation than the other, and this may account for a difference in the blackness of the lung fields. A recumbent oblique view made with a horizontal beam or a decubitus view usually will differentiate pleural fluid from these other technical faults. Extrapleural bleeding will cause inward displacement of the parietal pleura (the lung border), and this often is seen adjacent to rib fractures (Fig. 4–9). Extrapleural collections of blood at the apex of the lung cause the parietal pleura that forms the cap of the apex to be displaced downward, and this may be an indication of bleeding in the chest wall at the superior sulcus. This apical capping usually is a clue to venous or arterial bleeding from the aorta or brachiocephalic vessels, especially the proximal subclavian vessels. Venous bleeding usually produces only slight displacement of the apical pleural cap, whereas the arterial bleeding can produce considerably more displacement of the apical pleural cap. Displacement of the lung apex may be due to other causes, such as fibrosis from previous infection, radiation therapy, or neoplasm, and previous radiographs are helpful in determining if the displacement is due to bleeding. Increased density of the lung fields is not difficult to recognize, but it is difficult or impossible to differentiate between lung trauma effect (contusion, laceration, hematoma) and aspiration or atelectasis or a combination of these causes for lung density. Atelectasis is always a consideration with films taken of the acute emergency patient, especially if an endotracheal tube has been placed in the right or left bronchus.

Widening of the mediastinum or cardiac silhouette may be an indication of bleeding into the mediastinum or pericardial sac due to cardiac or great vessel injury. The optimal view, an upright posterior-anterior, is rarely obtainable.[4] Widening is difficult to evaluate on the recumbent frontal view during the acute emergency period; usually there are no previous films for comparison. A short-distance film tends to widen the mediastinal structures, and the detection of real widening is subjective and uncertain and should be cross-checked with a conventional posterior-anterior view as soon as the patient's condition permits.[5]

The changes in the lung fields should be inspected for infiltrates, areas of consolidation, or lucency that are consistent with lung contusion, hematomas, or air cysts. These are described in detail in Chapter 1. Infiltrates or consolidations that are apparent on the initial emergency room chest x-ray are diagnostic of intraparenchymal hemorrhage. Infiltrates related to aspiration, fat embolism, respiratory distress syndrome, or pulmonary embolism appear many hours to days later.

Enlargement of the cardiovascular silhouette is a manifestation of pericardial tamponade but is equally difficult to detect on the anteroposterior supine view. An upright anteroposterior view that demonstrates the "water bag sign" is the classic finding; the

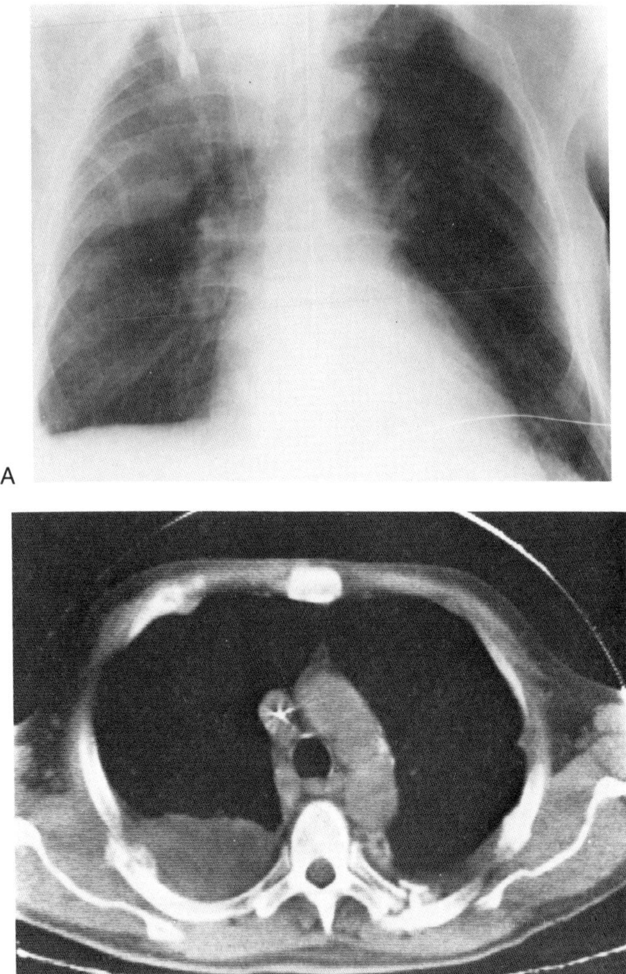

Figure 4–9.   Pleural fluid. **A:** Increased density of upper right chest is due to blood collected posterior to the upper right lung. The grayness of the right upper lung is because compressed lung has less air and the collected fluid is more dense than the air it displaced. Because the fluid is localized to the upper chest, it is probably a hematoma located in the subpleural space of the chest wall where there were several rib fractures. **B:** CT axial scan shows the posterior fluid decreasing the available space for the right lung. The posterior blood collection is well demonstrated and one of the several adjacent rib fractures is seen. (Figure continued on next page.)

diaphragmatic portion of the pericardium is widened by the blood collecting on the dependent surface of the diaphragm.

When the *diaphragm* has been injured (Fig. 4–10), it is usually obscured by fluid that has collected at the basilar region. The passage of a gastric tube may give a clue to a left diaphragmatic herniation.

Rib fractures often are not visualized when present, and a fracture of the *sternum* is not visualized on the frontal recumbent chest radiograph. The *thoracic spine* should be evaluated by obtaining an overpenetrated film and a later view if the frontal view is

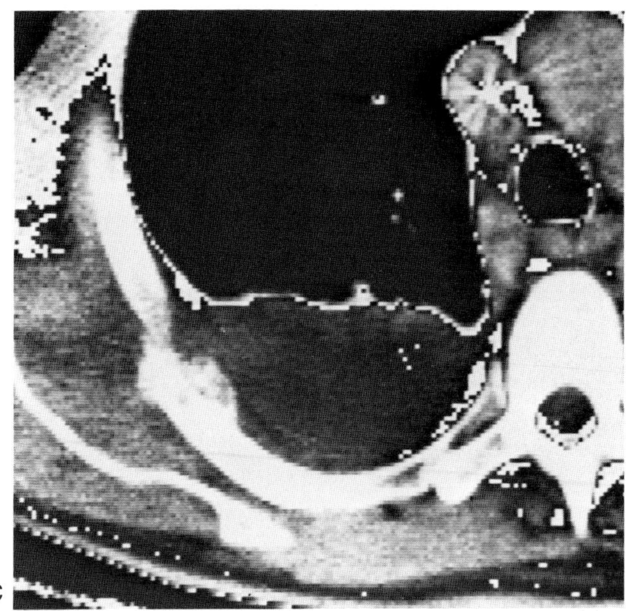

Figure 4–9, cont.   **C:** Window manipulation of the CT scan shows the pleural surface highlighted, confirming the impression that this was a subpleural chest wall hematoma.

suspicious. The clavicle and shoulder may be fractured, and these may not be evident on the recumbent frontal view of the chest.

Finally, chest tubes, central lines, endotracheal tubes, and gastric tubes should be evaluated for proper positioning. The recognition of an inappropriately positioned tube may be lifesaving when the chest tube is kinked or is located extrathoracically, the endotracheal tube is in the right main stem bronchus, or a central catheter tip is located in the pleural space.

Fluoroscopy

Fluoroscopy with television presentation of the image may be obtained by both fixed and portable fluoroscopic units. Portable fluoroscopic equipment with television has been available for the past 20 years, and most hospitals have such a unit that often is used in the operating room for orthopedic surgical procedures and for the placement of permanent transvenous pacemaker electrodes. The use of portable fluoroscopy does require that the patient be moved from the bed onto a radiolucent holder with space beneath it for the fluoroscopy unit.

Whenever dynamic information regarding motion is required, fluoroscopy is indispensable. Noncontrast fluoroscopy of the chest is no longer a common procedure. However, it still has some clinical usefulness. For instance, fluoroscopy can assist in localizing a radiopaque foreign body. Diaphragmatic motion can be assessed with fluoroscopy, and the dynamics of the respiratory cycle can be assessed with this technique.

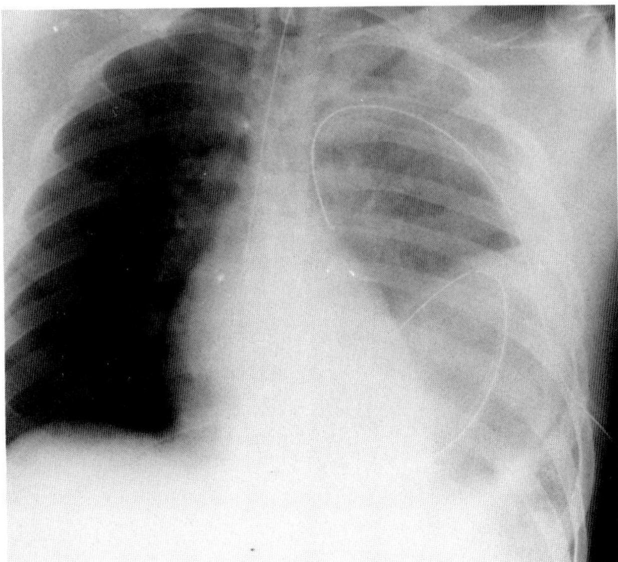

Figure 4–10.   Tube location. Film of chest made 10 min previously showed a left hemothorax. A chest tube was inserted into the left pleural space, and a nasogastric tube was passed into the stomach. A repeat film that was made to check the position of the chest tube reveals the nasogastric tube in the stomach fundus to be in a very high position, suggesting traumatic diaphragmatic herniation of the stomach. The stomach and spleen were found to have herniated through a large rent in the left diaphragm. There were fractures of the left 2 to 6 ribs (not visible on this film) and a fracture of the left clavicle.

Fluoroscopy of the esophagus is useful when penetrating or blunt damage to the esophagus is suspected. Initially, water-soluble contrast material such as meglumine diatrizaoate (Gastrografin) is swallowed under fluoroscopic observation. If there is no extravasation of contrast material, the esophagus can be studied with barium, which provides a much better contrast examination and provides better detection of mucosal and intramural abnormalities. A negative esophagram does not entirely exclude a tear because there are rare false negative studies.[6] Also, the rupture may be delayed due to esophageal wall ischemia.

Fluoroscopy of the more distal gastrointestinal tract is indicated if there is a clinical suspicion of diaphragmatic rupture.[7] These usually occur on the left, and any portion of the intestine may herniate into the left thoracic cavity. Rupture of the diaphragm may be silent, both clinically and radiographically. However, if there is herniation of the abdominal contents into the left hemithorax, barium examination of the colon or upper gastrointestinal tract will reveal the abnormally placed stomach, small intestine, or colon. Occasionally, the bowel will undergo strangulation, and this will be apparent radiographically.

REFERENCES

1.   Gling W. *Chest Trauma Diagnosis and Management*. Berlin: Springer-Verlag; 1981.
2.   Mintzer RA. *Chest Imaging: An Integrated Approach*. Baltimore: Williams & Wilkins; 1981.

3. Livoni JP, Barcia TC. Fracture of the first and second rib: incidence of vascular injury relative to type of fracture. *Radiology*. 1982;145:31–33.
4. Schwab CW, Larsen RB, Lind JF. Aortic injury. Comparison of the supine and upright portable chest films to evaluate the widened mediastinum. *Ann Emerg Med*. 1984;13:896.
5. Marnocha KE, Maglinte DDT. Plain film criteria for excluding aortic rupture in blunt chest trauma. *Am J Radiol*. 1985;144:19.
6. Love L, Berkow AE. Trauma to the esophagus. *Gastrointest Radiol*. 1978;2:305–321.
7. Wiot J. The radiologic manifestations of blunt chest trauma. *JAMA*. 1975;231:500–503.

5

Detection of Cervical Spine Injury in the Multitrauma Patient

VIRGINIA C. POIRIER, M.D.

HISTORY: Spinal injury with paralysis has been recorded throughout civilization. Ancient Greek and Egyptian medical records such as the 5000-year-old Edwin Smith surgical papyrus (dated at about 1600 BC) acknowledged a triage system for victims of traumatic spinal cord injuries.[1] The latter manuscript directed no treatment for those who were "unconscious of their arms and legs and in whom priapism and urinary incontinence were present." Accounts of historical figures such as Lord Nelson who suffered a spinal cord injury and tales from the battlefields of World War I consistently depicted the victims of spinal cord injury as doomed to death. Survivors were racked with infections, contractures, bedsores, and mental anguish. Until the discovery of antibiotics (concomitant with World War II) these patients died very quickly. In World War I, for instance, 98% died before they returned to the United States. Lack of effective treatment persisted until after World War II when Sir Ludwig Guttman, working at Stoke-Mandeville Hospital in England, virtually revolutionized the concept of health care for people with spinal cord injuries. He emphasized centralized comprehensive services as opposed to institutionalized custodial care. This development of a multidisciplinary approach to treatment of spinal cord injuries has been the most significant development in treatment of these patients and has now been adopted worldwide.

Nearly two-thirds of all spinal cord injuries occur in the cervical spine.[2] The early detection of cervical spine injury is essential in determining appropriate therapy and preventing neurologic injury or deterioration. Evaluation of the cervical spine in trauma victims with multiple injuries often presents a diagnostic challenge. Most of these patients have profound mechanisms of injury, altered mental status, and painful injuries to other organ systems. The risk of an overlooked cervical spine injury is substantial in these patients since the clinical exam is not reliable in this setting.

INDICATIONS FOR EVALUATION

Current trends in trauma care delivery have increased the number of patients seen in trauma centers for evaluation of possible cervical spine injury. There are now rigid protocols for emergency medical service personnel to protect the cervical spine in all accident victims. This is mandatory if we are to reduce iatrogenic cervical spinal cord injury secondary to extrication and transport. As a result of these protocols, virtually every accident victim presents to the emergency department on a backboard with the neck immobilized. Paradoxically, prolonged immobilization in a collar sometimes produces symptoms of neck pain that were not present when the collar was applied, and most patients so immobilized often do volunteer some degree of neck discomfort. Once such symptoms are elicited, it becomes difficult to omit an imaging evaluation of the cervical spine.

Referring clinicians are subject to many forces that favor liberal use of cervical spine radiographs, including the ever-present fear of misdiagnosis or mismanagement of these injuries. To accommodate this increasing demand and consider cost containment, a risk-tailored approach to cervical spine radiography is encouraged. Using four criteria, Kreipke et al.[3] were able to identify all patients with cervical spine injury. The criteria utilized were:

1. other severe injury
2. tenderness to direct spinous process palpation
3. altered mental status
4. focal neurological deficit.

Unfortunately, these four criteria carried a specificity of only 15%. Only 47% of patients with other severe injury proved to have cervical spine injury. Several other large series have found no evidence of cervical spine injury in any alert, mentally competent, nonintoxicated, neurologically intact patient who has no symptoms of neck discomfort or pain on palpation and has no other significantly painful injuries that might distract the patient's attention.[3–6]

Physical exam cannot be performed accurately unless the patient has a normal mental status, which implies absence of drugs, alcohol, or psychiatric disturbance. These are frequently present at the time of the accident and therefore invalidate accurate physical assessment of the cervical spine. Jacobs and Schwartz[7] found that the ability of clinicians to predict spinal injury on the basis of clinical history or physical exam is poor, with only half of cervical spine injuries identified prospectively. Zucker et al.[8] found a positive rate of cervical spine injury on cervical spine radiographs to be only 1.7% out of 1003 consecutive trauma exams. Several other large series[3,9] found a similar low yield (less than 3%) of fracture or subluxation in cervical spine radiographs from the emergency department.

Another reality of the emergency department is that, whether radiographs are indicated or not, the likelihood of the patients eventually undergoing cervical spine imaging is high. McNamara et al.[10] found that of patients who did not undergo cervical spine radiography at their initial emergency department visit, 52% subsequently had cervical spine radiographs taken within 6 months of their injury. In addition, 66% of patients were pursuing litigation. No doubt some trauma patients legitimately suffer from chronic posttraumatic cervical pain, accounting for a portion of these exams. However, recognizing the above, some experienced physicians feel that a baseline cervical spine series is justified.

Sensitivity of Cervical Spine Radiographs in Cervical Spine Trauma

With a complete trauma series of well positioned and optimally exposed radiographs of the cervical spine, recognition of significant injuries is quite high, with a sensitivity of 95% under ideal conditions. Unfortunately, a complete high quality exam frequently is impossible to obtain in the multitrauma patient due to time restraints imposed by other trauma priorities and lack of patient cooperation. Patients who are at highest risk for injury (Table 5–1) are most likely to have a technically compromised cervical spine exam.

The radiologist often is uncomfortable responding to the directive to clear the cervical spine. In its most common (but incorrect) usage, it is taken to mean that if no abnormality is identified on the cervical spine radiographs, then the patient is free of cervical spine injury. This definition is seriously flawed by its presumption of 100% sensitivity for cervical spine radiographs in the detection of cervical spine injury. Even if we assume an optimistic 95% sensitivity, most physicians would not be comfortable with a missed injury rate of 5%. Therefore, cervical spine radiographs cannot be considered the gold standard for cervical spine injury. Patients can have serious cervical spine injuries without obvious evidence of fracture or subluxation on the cervical spine radiographs. Inadequate radiographs are a common source of misdiagnosis in cervical spine trauma, especially in regard to visualization of the cervicothoracic and atlantoaxial regions. Ross et al.[11] reported that a single portable lateral view of the cervical spine was inadequate in visualizing the cervicothoracic junction in up to 25% of exams. Furthermore, the cross-table lateral cervical spine film alone was associated with a delayed diagnosis of unstable cervical spine injury in 15% of patients.

Precisely how many films constitute a complete cervical spine exam varies widely. A three-view series (lateral, anteroposterior, and odontoid views) is the minimum exam (Fig. 5–1). A "swimmer's" view of the cervicothoracic junction usually is necessary when examining the supine patient, since the cross-table lateral view rarely demonstrates the C7–T1 junction adequately (Fig. 5–2A). Five-view exams include supine oblique views, which are more likely to be of diagnostic quality and provide more information than the "swimmer's" lateral view and require only minimal motion of the patient's head[12,13] (Fig. 5–2B). Computed tomography (CT) is ideal for further evaluation of patients in whom complete visualization of the cervical spine cannot be accomplished with the initial trauma series radiographs.

Table 5–1. Clinical and Historical Characteristics of the High-Risk Patient[22]

High-velocity blunt trauma
Significant motor vehicle accident
Direct cervical region injury
Altered mental status at the time of trauma and/or during emergency
    department evaluation (includes alcohol, drugs, intoxicants, loss
    of consciousness, and mental illness)
Falls/diving injuries
Significant head/facial injury
Abnormal neurologic examination
Prominent neck pain or tenderness
Thoracic or lumbar spine fracture
Rigid spine (ankylosing spondylitis, etc.)

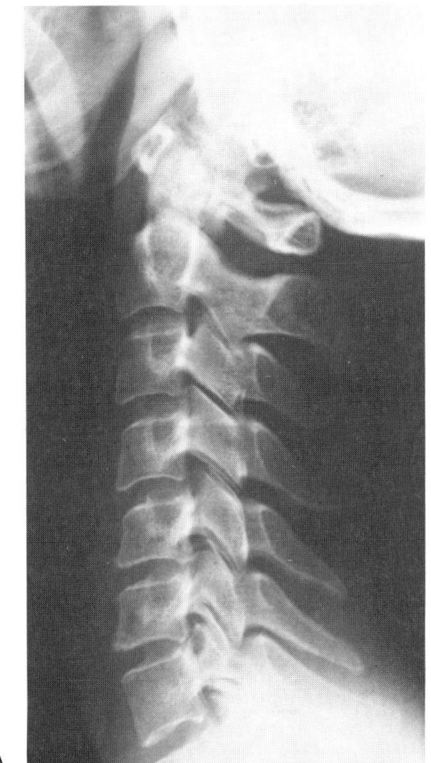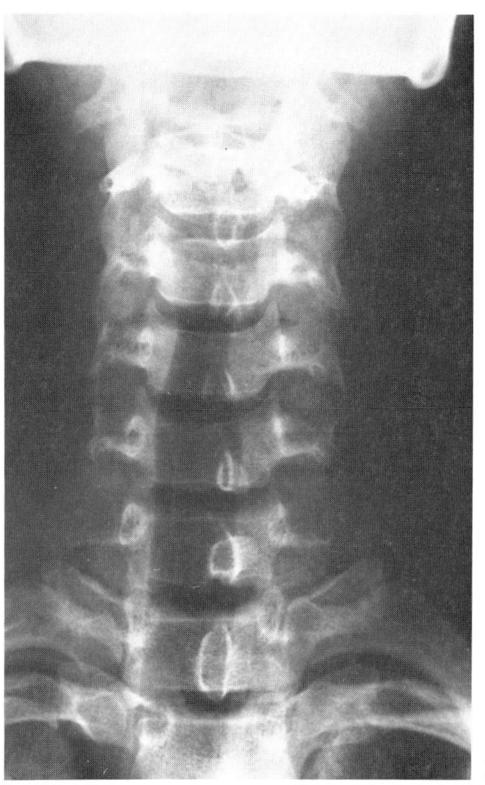

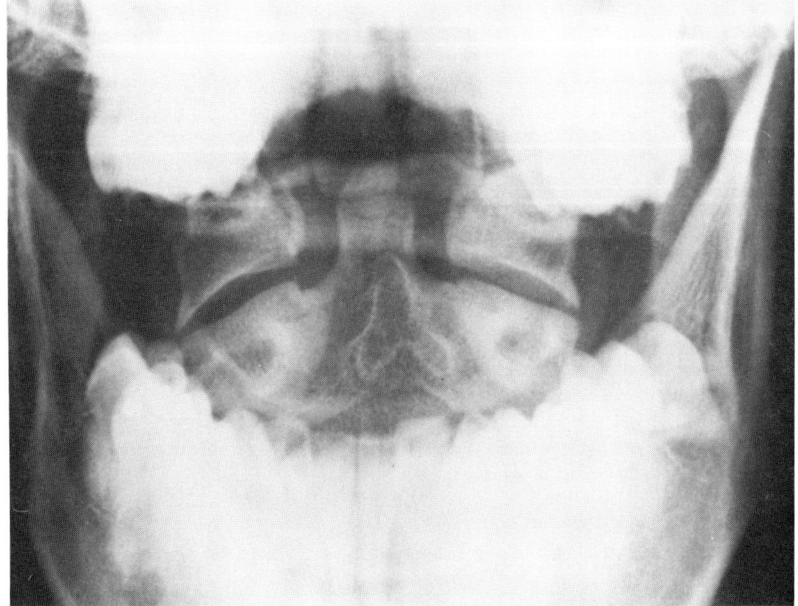

Figure 5–1.   Three-view cervical spine series: lateral (**A**), anteroposterior (**B**), and odontoid views (**C**).

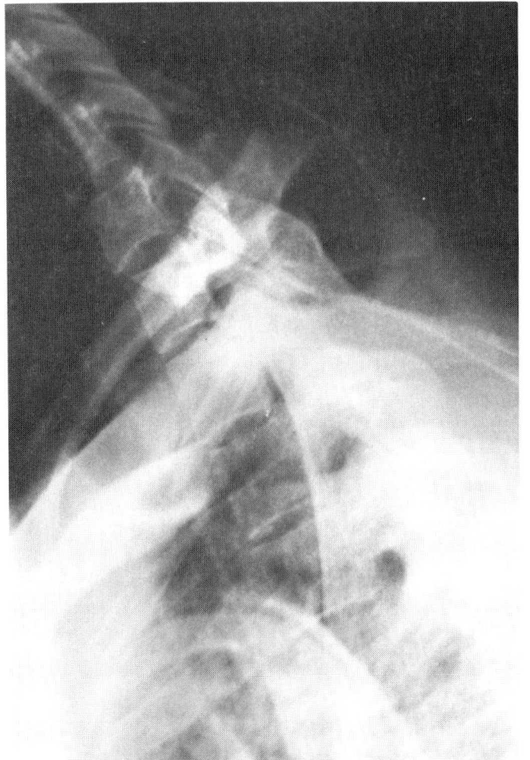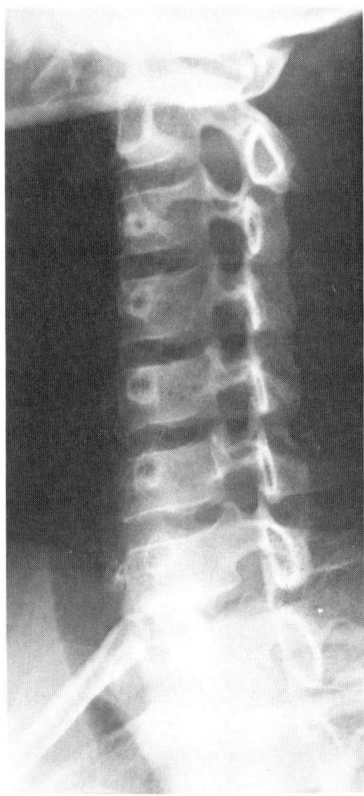

A   B

Figure 5–2. "Swimmer's" view (**A**) and supine oblique view (**B**). The latter two views often are required to obtain adequate visualization of the cervicothoracic junction.

Plain Film Evaluation of the Cervical Spine

Radiologic interpretation of cervical spine radiographs is a complex topic and several excellent texts have been written on this subject in recent years.[12–15] Additionally, the leading orthopedic treatise on fractures is Rockwood et al.'s multivolume text.[16]

The average number of cervical spine injuries per patient is 2.2,[14] so it is imperative to have a high index of suspicion even after identifying a single fracture. There is a significant incidence of combined upper and lower cervical spine injuries (15–25%) and of cervical injury associated with thoracolumbar fracture.[14]

The lateral view is the most important projection in the trauma series. Ninety percent of significant injuries potentially can be detected on this view.[17,18] When evaluating the lateral cervical radiograph, first make certain that the cervicothoracic junction can be adequately visualized. About 75% of adult injuries involve the lower cervical spine, whereas in children the upper cervical spine is more frequently injured.[13,17,18]

Measurement of the prevertebral soft tissues in the upper cervical spine is generally regarded as an important part of the cervical spine evaluation. However, there are many variables that may affect the presence of soft tissue swelling, including position of the cervical spine and phase of respiration in which the radiograph is acquired. If the prevertebral soft tissues measure above 7 mm at C3, there is a high probability of underlying injury.

Evaluation of Vertebral Alignment

Evaluation of vertebral alignment is established by evaluating four smooth uninterrupted lines (Fig. 5–3).

1. *Anterior vertebral line*. This line connects the anterior cortical margins of each contiguous vertebral body. Anterior osteophytes should be ignored in drawing this line.
2. *Posterior vertebral line*. This line connects the posterior cortical margin of the contiguous vertebral bodies.
3. *Spinolaminar line*. The junction of the spinous process with the lamina forms the point utilized for this line. This point delineates the posterior margin of the spinal canal. The spinal cord lies between the posterior vertebral and spinolaminar lines. Any offset of either of these lines could mean that a bony structure is impinging on the spinal cord.
4. *Spinous process line*. A line connecting the posterior tips of the spinous processes should form a smooth interrupted curve. An offset in this line usually indicates an underlying spinous process fracture.

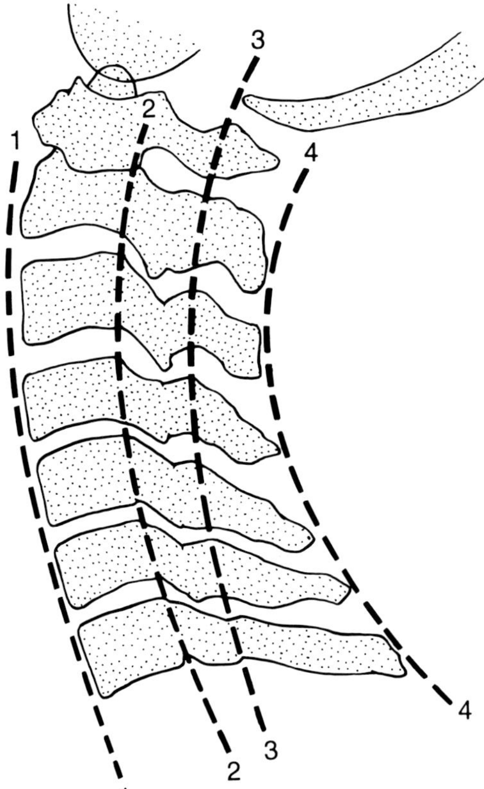

Figure 5–3.   Cervical vertebral alignment is evaluated using four smooth uninterrupted lines on the lateral radiographic view.

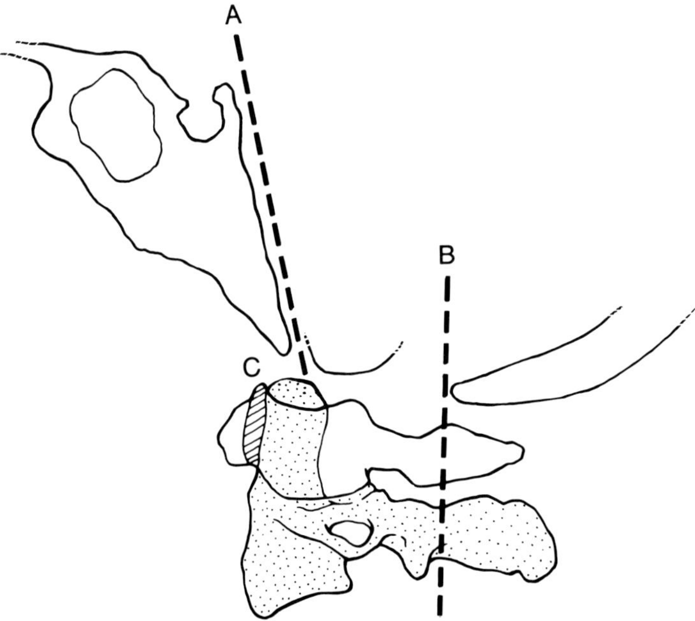

Figure 5–4.   Alignment of the craniocervical junction. **A:** Line on clivus of skull points to the tip of the odontoid; **B:** Spinolaminar line of C_1, extending to the posterior margin of the foramen magnum; **C:** Predental space should not exceed 2.55mm in adults and 5mm in children.

Evaluation of alignment in the upper cervical spine requires review of three areas (Fig. 5–4). Children and adolescents may demonstrate physiologic subluxation of C2 on C3 and of C3 on C4. The spinolaminar line will not be interrupted in these cases, however.

Determining Mechanism of Spinal Injury

Closed spinal trauma is generally classified according to the mechanism of injury: flexion, extension, axial loading (vertical compression), or rotation. Readers are referred to the excellent texts recommended at the beginning of this chapter for a more detailed discussion of this subject. Examples of cervical spine trauma based on mechanism of injury are listed in Table 5–2.

Flexion Injuries

A variety of injuries may be present after hyperflexion of the spine. There can be significant ligamentous damage even in the presence of normal radiographs, although widening of the interspinous distance frequently is observed. Progressive kyphosis and anterior subluxation may be present in the absence of bony involvement. Injuries resulting in facet subluxation have a high incidence of delayed instability.[18,19] Severe flexion forces can result in bilateral perched or locked facets (Fig. 5–5). This injury is associated with a high incidence of severe spinal cord damage. Disc herniation from a flexion injury also can result in spinal cord damage.

Table 5–2.   Cervical Spine Trauma—Mechanism of Injury[14]

Hyperflexion injuries
   Vertebral compression
   Anterior subluxation
   Bilateral locked facets
   Flexion teardrop fracture
   Spinous process (clay shoveler's) fracture
Hyperextension injuries
   Hyperextension sprain
   Fracture anterior arch C1
   Fracture posterior arch C1
   Hangman's fracture C2
   Anterior inferior vertebral chip fracture
   Extension teardrop fracture
   Laminar fracture
Axial compression
   Burst fracture
   Jefferson fracture C1

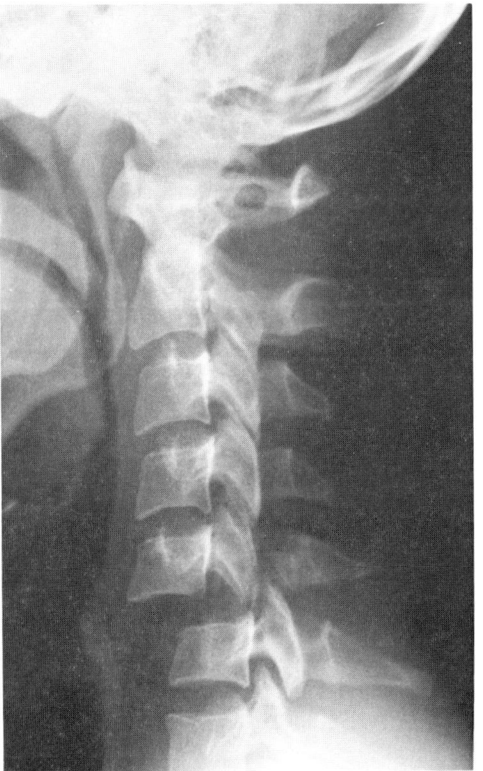

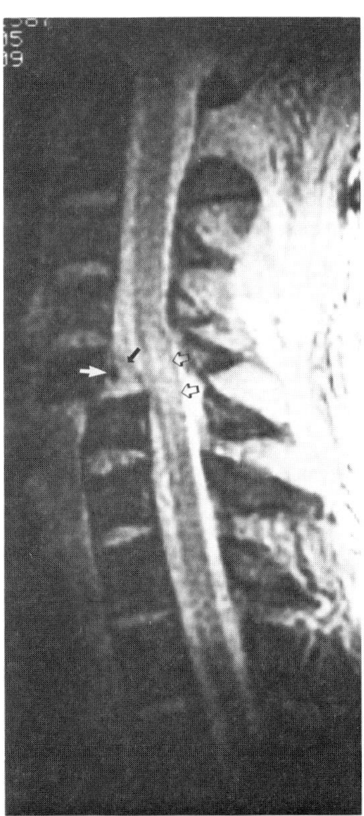

A   B

Figure 5–5. Flexion injury with bilateral locked facets on lateral plain film exam of the cervical spine (**A**). T_2-weighted MR exam (**B**) demonstrates an associated spinal cord contusion (*open arrows*), an intact posterior longitudinal ligament (*black arrow*), and a small epidural hematoma (*white arrow*).

Compression fractures of the vertebral bodies, typically involving the superior endplate at the anterior margin of the vertebral body, are the most common fracture associated with flexion. The most severe fracture associated with flexion is the "teardrop" fracture-dislocation of the cervical spine. The presence of this injury implies rupture of the entire posterior ligamentous complex and is associated with a high incidence of neurologic deficit.

Extension Injuries

Extension injuries to the cervical spine may disrupt the intervertebral disc, resulting in a widening of the anterior disc space and a separation of the adjacent vertebral bodies. In the presence of degenerative spondylosis, significant neurologic damage may occur because of impingement of the cord between the posterior osteophytes and the hypertrophied ligamentum flavum. A recent study using dynamic magnetic resonance (MR) imaging of the cervical spine in flexion and extension demonstrated spinal canal changes ranging from 1 to 5 mm, or 50% of the total canal diameter at a given level of stenosis.[20] If the force is sufficient, the anterior and posterior longitudinal ligaments may rupture, compromising the canal and injuring the spinal cord.

Axial Loading Injuries

Axial loading (vertical compression) of the spine results in burst fractures of the vertebral body. These fractures occur most commonly at the thoracolumbar junction and may be associated with retropulsion of bony fragments and/or fractures of the posterior elements. Burst fractures typically have a sagittal fracture line extending to the inferior endplate of the involved vertebra. The presence of posterior element fractures increases the potential for instability of these injuries. There may be significant compression of the spinal cord by retropulsion of bony fragments (Fig. 5–6). Most burst fractures have an intact posterior longitudinal ligament, and distraction typically reduces the retropulsed fragments.

Cervical Spinal Stenosis

Cervical spinal stenosis, either developmental or acquired, predisposes the spinal cord to injury. The anteroposterior (AP) diameter of the spinal canal should be evaluated on the lateral cervical spine radiograph using a method described by Pavlov et al.[21] Using a ratio of the AP diameter of the spinal canal divided by the AP diameter of the vertebral body, a normal ratio was found to be 1.00 (range 0.80–1.2). Patients with underlying spinal stenosis (ratio >0.80) often have transient bilateral motor and sensory symptoms after only mild to moderate injury. This ratio for evaluation of cervical spinal stenosis appears to be more accurate than previous direct measurements of the spinal canal on lateral spine radiographs. CT and MR can be used for more accurate overall assessment of spinal canal dimensions if further evaluation is required.

Diagnosis of Unstable Spinal Injury

For practical purposes, an unstable cervical spine is considered present if critical aspects of structural integrity of the spine have been compromised so that neurologic injury could

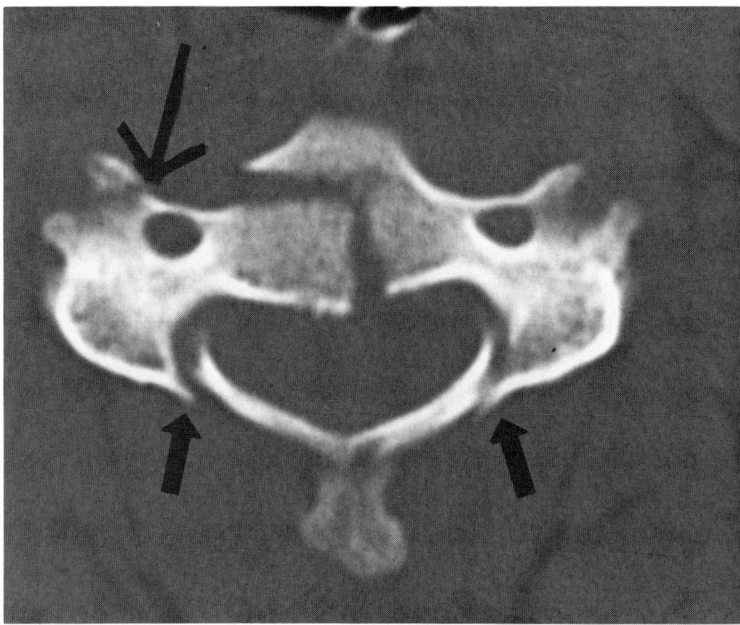

Figure 5–6. Axial CT image demonstrates a complex burst fracture of the cervical spine. There are both coronal and sagittal fracture lines through the vertebral body with a mildly retropulsed fragment. In addition, there are bilateral laminar fractures and a small corner fracture of the right transverse process (*arrows*).

occur if the cervical spine moved through a normal range of motion.[22] The ligamentous structures responsible for stability of the cervical spine are depicted in Figure 5–7. Traumatic loss of these binding elements may be difficult to assess on cervical spine radiographs. In the presence of a neurologic deficit, an unusual degree of neck pain, or marked prevertebral swelling, the radiologist should be alert to the possibility of an occult unstable injury such as a spontaneously reduced hyperextension dislocation. Findings suggestive of an unstable cervical spine injury are listed in Table 5–3.[13,23]

Denis popularized the three-column theory of spinal instability in which the integrity of two of the columns is required for stability[23] (Fig. 5–7A and B). Using this approach, the middle column is critical to maintaining stability. Acute instability is present when there is conclusive evidence of injury to the middle bony column or the middle ligamentous complex (Table 5–4).

Table 5–3. Findings Suggestive of an Unstable Cervical Spine Injury

Horizontal translation of a vertebral body greater than 3 mm
Abnormal widening or narrowing of a disc space
Widening of a facet joint
Widening of the interlaminar distance
Widening of the interspinous distance
Angular deformity of the spine greater than 11°
Vertebral compression fracture with greater than 25% loss in vertebral height

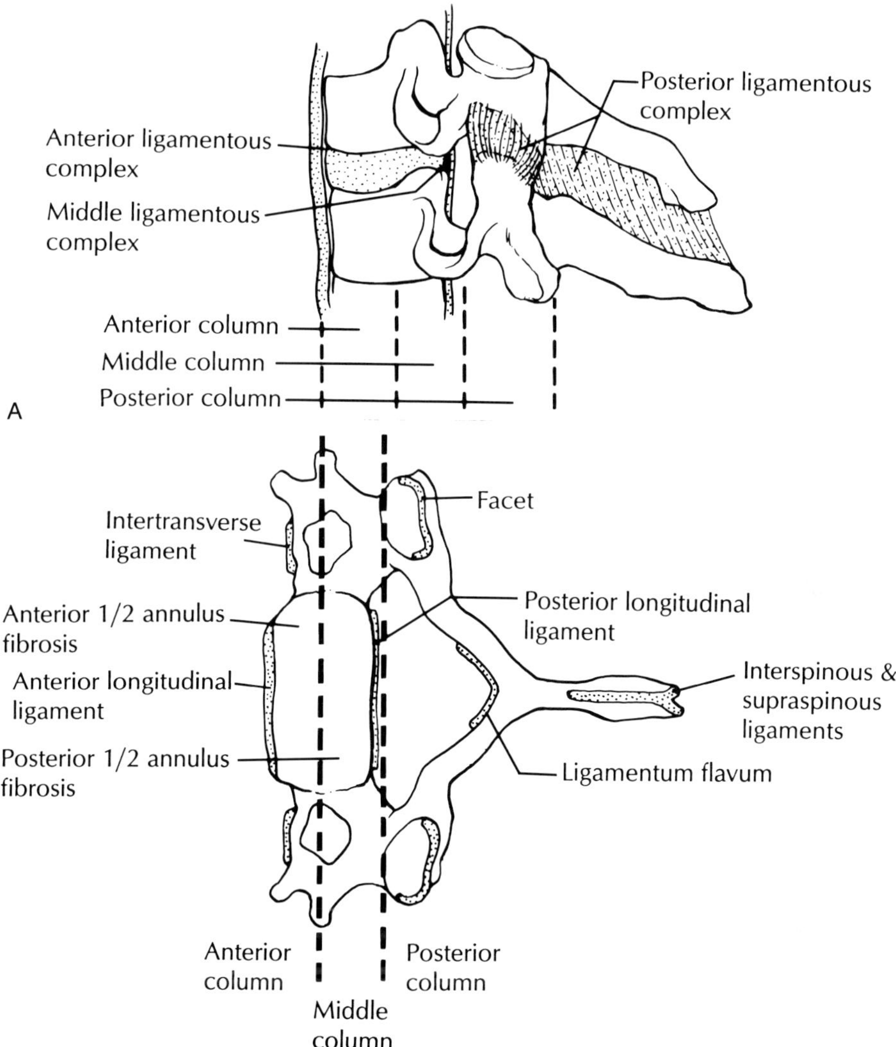

Figure 5–7.   Schematic representation of the structures and compartments responsible for spinal stability. **A:** Lateral view. **B:** Axial view.

Stating with confidence that the cervical spine is stable requires both static (erect lateral view) and dynamic testing (i.e., flexion and extension views). Supine lateral cervical films often will make the findings equivocal, whereas an erect lateral film will show the abnormal kyphotic angulation or subluxation. An erect flexion-extension series is almost always impossible or impractical to perform in multitrauma patients. Muscle spasm decreases cervical spine motion and makes detection of subtle injuries difficult. Thus, in this setting, patients should be immobilized in a rigid collar until muscle spasm diminishes so that the patient is able to execute the flexion and extension maneuvers satisfactorily. Some authors recommend waiting 10 to 14 days after injury. A White-Panjabi stretch test should be considered if one cannot obtain good flexion-extension views and cervical spine

**Table 5–4. Use of the Three-Column Theory to Predict the Stability
of Various Spinal Fractures[23]**

FRACTURE TYPE	COLUMN(S) DISRUPTED	PREDICTED STABILITY
Compression	Anterior	Stable
Burst	Anterior/middle	Unstable
Flexion-distraction	Middle/posterior	Unstable in flexion
Fracture-dislocaton	All	Highly unstable

instability is still suspected.[24,25] In patients with obvious cervical spine injury, it is better to treat patients with fractures in fixation and to perform motion studies after the fractures have healed.[13]

Delayed instability is commonly a complication of minor acute cervical spine injury (i.e., anterior subluxation or simple wedge fracture). The incidence of delayed instability after subluxation ranges from 21% to 50%.[26,27]

Use of Computed Tomography in Cervical Spine Trauma

In recent years, CT has assumed an increasingly important role in the evaluation of patients with spinal injury. Borock et al.[28] were able to clear the cervical spine in 93% of acutely injured blunt trauma patients within 24 hr using CT scanning as an adjunct to plain cervical spine radiographs. Indications for CT evaluation of cervical spine trauma as recommended by Mirvis and Young[15] are reviewed in Table 5–5.

One of the main advantages of CT is the cross-sectional view that provides visualization of the posterior vertebral arches and articulating processes. Axial CT imaging is especially accurate at assessing encroachment of the spinal canal or neural foramina. Most current CT scanners also provide the capacity for high quality two-dimensional reformations in virtually any plane as well as three-dimensional surface contour images. Some complex fractures may be better delineated utilizing nonaxial multiplanar reconstructions. Using thin section (1.5–2 mm) CT for the entire cervical spine is not practical, however, and most exams are confined to a small section of the spine. In general, it is wise to include one complete vertebral body above and below the suspected site of injury.

Table 5–5. Indications for CT Evaluation of Cervical Spine Trauma

Evaluation of patients with equivocal findings on cervical spine radiographs
Evaluation of patients with normal cervical spine radiographs and
    Focal neck pain
    Neurologic deficit(s) referrable to the cervical spine
Evaluation of patients with known cervical spine injury to determine details of fracture location, displacement, spinal canal compromise, and the presence of possible additional injuries unrecognized by plain radiographs
Evaluation of patients with known cervical spine injury as an aid in deciding on surgical or nonsurgical reduction and stabilization
Evaluation of the lower cervical spine in symptomatic patients unable to be "cleared" radiographically

Table 5–6.   Advantages of CT Imaging in Cervical Spine Injury

Axial display of spinal anatomy allows more accurate detection of complex spinal fractures, especially the posterior vertebral arch
Easy to perform in the trauma setting allowing rapid evaluation of combined craniocervical injuries
Accurately assess encroachment of the spinal canal and neural foramina
Less radiation dose than tomography
Improved contrast resolution compared with plain film radiography or tomography (excellent bone and soft tissue detail)
Two-dimensional reformatted image reconstruction in any plane

Despite the fact that CT is regarded by most authors as the gold standard for examination of spinal fractures, subtle, nondisplaced, axially oriented fractures can be missed by direct axial CT due to volume averaging, and high quality multidirectional tomography may prove more sensitive in such cases (e.g., fractures through the base of the odontoid).

Acheson et al.[2] found the three-view cervical spine radiographic series useful in detection of only 47% of fractures eventually discovered with CT imaging. Most of the occult fractures detected by CT imaging occurred in vertebrae immediately adjacent to ones that were initially identified as fractured on plain film radiography (20% of adjacent vertebrae were found to be fractured in this study). These authors also conclude that if cervical spine radiographs are normal, CT is unlikely to reveal a fracture. A summary of the advantages and disadvantages of CT imaging for cervical spine trauma is found in Tables 5–6 and 5–7.

Role of Magnetic Resonance Imaging in Cervical Spine Trauma

Although bone injury is well assessed with cervical spine radiographs and CT, ligamentous injury causing cervical instability or spinal cord impingement due to an associated herniated disc is best demonstrated and differentiated from intrinsic cord damage with MR imaging.[29–35] MR imaging has nearly completely replaced myelography in the evaluation of

Table 5–7.   Disadvantages of CT Imaging in Cervical Spine Trauma

Not practical as a survey exam for the entire cervical spine
Axial fractures may be missed (e.g., base of odontoid)
Subluxations may not be apparent without MPRs*
Pseudosubluxations may occur on MPRs* due to patient motion
Pseudofractures may be seen due to partial volume artifact
Artifacts may degrade CT image at the cervicothoracic junction, especially in large patients
Radiopaque materials (e.g., bullet fragments) produce streak artifact, which degrades the CT image
CT myelography is required to evaluate soft tissue pathology within the spinal canal (e.g., herniated disc or epidural hematoma)
Intramedullary spinal cord pathology cannot be assessed

*MPRs = multiplanar reconstructions.

Table 5–8.   Advantages of MR Imaging in Cervical Spine Injury

Evaluate noninvasively
    Occult vertebral compression fractures
    Intervertebral disc herniation
    Ligamentous injury
    Epidural hematoma
    Spinal cord injury
    Relationship of bone fragments to spinal cord
    Assess the cervicothoracic junction
Multiplanar imaging
No beam hardening artifacts like CT
No ionizing radiation

spinal cord injury. Advantages and disadvantages of MR imaging in cervical spine injury are summarized in Tables 5–8 and 5–9.

The role of MR imaging in the diagnostic workup of acute cervical spine injury is evolving. Current clinical indications for MR imaging in acute cervical trauma include patients with a progressive neurologic deficit, spinal cord injury in the absence of bone injury, or an unexpected level of neurologic signs above the level of radiographically identified injury. In addition, MR evaluation is useful to exclude a disc herniation, epidural hematoma, or spinal cord contusion before surgical intervention for a radiographically identified fracture-dislocation. The role of MR imaging in the absence of neurologic signs is more difficult to define at this point in time.

Cervical spine stabilization with MR-compatible devices are required for safe transport and successful imaging. Spinal immobilization may be accomplished using a Philadelphia collar or a cervical halo made of nonferrous materials. If necessary, in-line cervical traction can be achieved with MR-compatible graphite traction tongs and a series of nonferrous pulleys and water bags.[36] MR-compatible ventilatory support is now available as well. Devices that contain even small amounts of ferrous materials cast significant artifacts into the image and distort adjacent anatomic structures. Currently, graphite material has the advantage of great strength and compatibility with both MR and CT scanning.[37]

A discussion of the principles and physics of MR imaging is beyond the scope of this

Table 5–9.   Disadvantages of MR Imaging for Cervical Spine

Bone detail lacks the high resolution of CT
More difficult to perform on unstable patient due to inaccessibility of the patient
Contraindications:
    Cardiac pacemakers
    Cerebral aneurysm clips
    Claustrophobia
Need MR-compatible equipment (monitoring and ventilation equipment as well as cervical halo
    devices)
Exam time is currently longer than CT

chapter. The exact scanning parameters will vary from institution to institution and will depend on the type of machine used, the strength of the magnet, the type of coils used, and the patient's condition. Most MR imaging protocols include a combination of T_1- and T_2-weighted images. The latter produces "myelography-equivalent" images of the spine (Fig. 5–8).

T_1-weighted images are mostly useful for evaluation of vertebral anatomy and bony relationships of the spinal canal. Normal vertebral bodies have a hyperintense fatty marrow and a hypointense cortical margin on T_1-weighted imaging. T_2-weighted images are helpful for evaluation of extradural compression of the spinal canal and for differentiating cord contusion from hemorrhage. Gradient echo image sequences often are used in lieu of T_2-weighted images for MR trauma imaging because of their high sensitivity in detection of acute hemorrhage and the short acquisition time.

MR is quite sensitive in the detection of subtle vertebral fractures. Fractures are demonstrated as interruption of low signal from cortical bone or high signal from marrow fat (Fig. 5–9). MR is especially helpful in diagnosing horizontally oriented fractures that may be missed on CT scanning. MR also is excellent for demonstrating abnormalities of

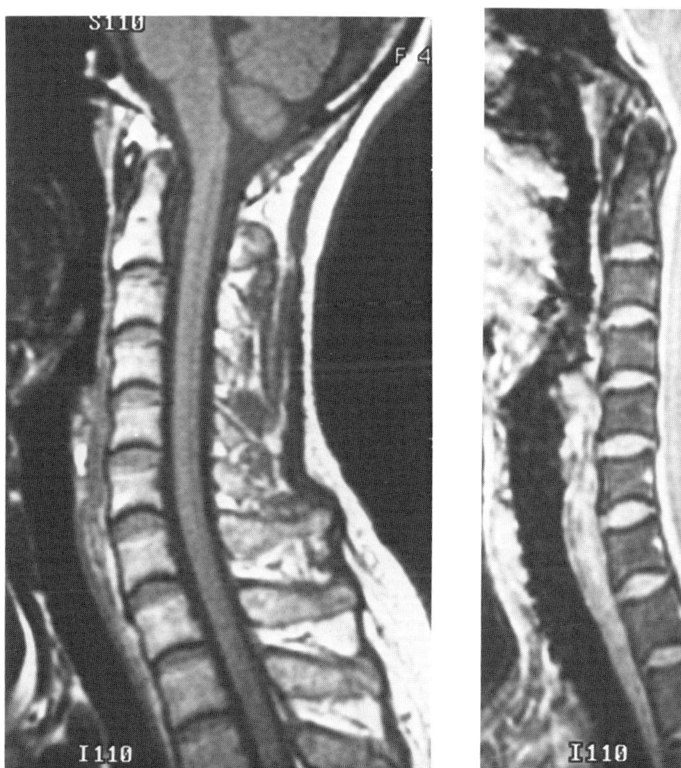
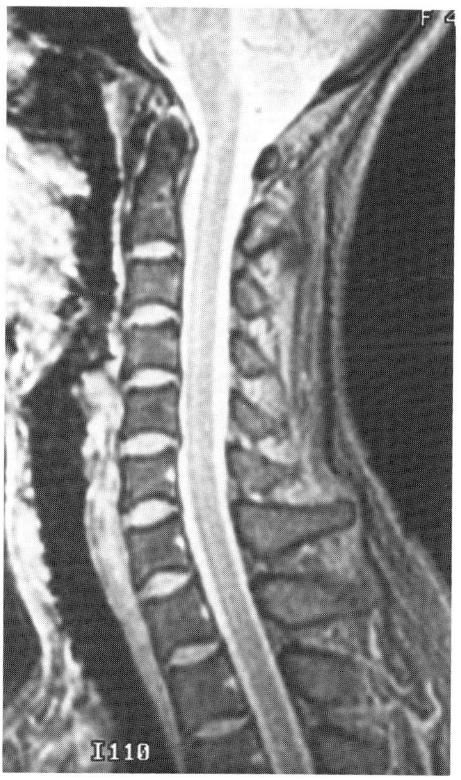

A   B

Figure 5–8.   Sagittal MRIs of the normal cervical spine. **A:** Normal T_1-weighted MR image. **B:** Normal T_2-weighted MR image.

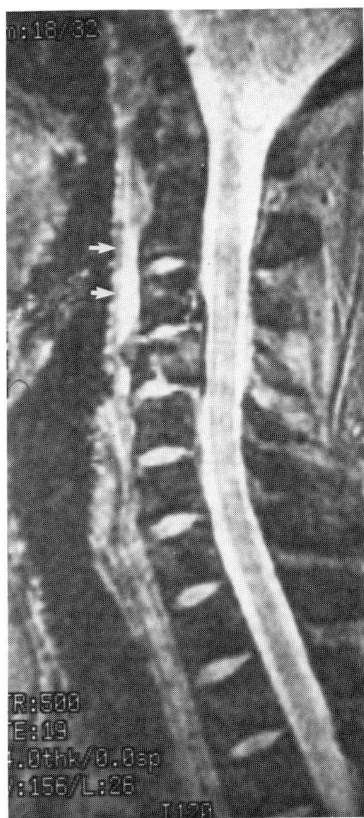

Figure 5–9. Gradient echo MRI demonstrates vertebral fractures at C3 and C4. There is increased signal through the fracture lines involving the posterior inferior corner of the C3 vertebral body and the sagittal fracture of C4. Also note increased signal in the prevertebral soft tissue swelling associated with these fractures (*white arrows*).

facet relationships due to its direct parasagittal imaging. MR is especially helpful in evaluating the cervicothoracic junction, which often is difficult to image adequately on trauma spine radiographs and occasionally with CT imaging as well. In a comparison of CT versus MR by Flanders et al.,[38] CT was found to be less sensitive for spinal cord injury, herniated disc, and prevertebral edema. CT failed to depict 40% of cases with obvious herniated discs on MR. Alteration of signal intensity of the vertebral marrow was a strong indicator of a significant compressive injury to the vertebral body even when a discrete fracture was not visible. When compared with CT, MR was poor in identification of smaller fractures such as those in the posterior elements.

MR evaluation of ligamentous injury to the cervical spine is evidenced by the following:

1. hyperintensity of the interspinous ligaments (secondary to tearing and hemorrhage) with or without splaying of the spinous processes
2. abrupt discontinuity of the linear signal void of the anterior or posterior longitudinal ligaments
3. hyperintensity and swelling of the prevertebral soft tissues on T_2-weighted imaging.

The ability of MR to demonstrate and characterize acute spinal cord injury exceeds that of other diagnostic techniques. Kulkarni et al.[30] noted three patterns of posttraumatic change within the spinal cord using MR imaging. Additionally, they found excellent correlation between MR patterns of cord injury and neurologic recovery. A type I signal pattern was consistent with acute hemorrhage, and these patients uniformly had a poor prognosis with no clinical improvement on follow-up exam. Type II injury was consistent with acute spinal cord edema and type III was a mixed signal appearance consistent with edema and punctate hemorrhages. Patients in the latter two categories experienced a significant functional neurologic improvement or recovery. Similar results have been substantiated by other authors.[34,38,39]

When significant hemorrhage is present within a spinal cord contusion, its appearance on MR imaging depends largely on the chemical state of the hemoglobin molecule and thus on the time from initial injury. Cord contusions are predominantly nonhemorrhagic and appear iso- or hypointense on T_1-weighted images and hyperintense on T_2-weighted images (Fig. 5–5B), whereas acute cord hemorrhage appears hypointense on T_2-weighted and gradient echo images.

Davis et al.[29] recently have shown the value of MR imaging in demonstrating both soft tissue and bony abnormalities of the spine secondary to hyperextension injuries. The plain film radiographic findings of hyperextension injury often are subtle, and fractures may be occult, even in unstable injuries. Anterior longitudinal ligament injuries give rise to hemorrhage and edema in the prevertebral space. Although prevertebral soft tissue swelling often is a clue to underlying cervical spine injury, measurements in normal subjects and those with cervical spine injury often overlap considerably. Its presence can be verified easily with T_2-weighted MR imaging, which can then further direct investigation of injuries such as spontaneously reduced hyperextension injury.

In summary, MR imaging is the most sensitive modality for detection of disc protrusions and spinal cord abnormalities in the acutely injured spine. Flanders et al.[38] believe that any center that treats spinal cord injuries must be required to provide quality MR images in an expeditious fashion. Continuing development of rapid imaging sequences, MR-compatible physiologic support and monitoring devices, and cervical traction and immobilization should foster increased use of this modality for imaging acute cervical spine injury.

Acknowledgment. I want to acknowledge my friend and colleague Carol S. Beatty, M.D., for all her encouragement, proofreading, and advisement during the evolution of this chapter. I also wish to thank my secretary, Ann Chamberlain, for her dedication and enthusiasm during the many rewrites required for completion of this chapter.

REFERENCES

1. Breasted JH. The Edwin Smith surgical papyrus. In: Wilkins RH, ed. *Neurosurgical Classics.* New York: Johnson Reprint Corporation; 1965:1–5.
2. Acheson MB, Livingston RR, Richardson ML, et al. High-resolution CT scanning in the evaluation of cervical spine fractures: comparison with plain film examinations. *AJR.* 1987;148:1179–1185.
3. Kreipke DL, Gillespie KR, McCarthy MC, et al. Reliability of indications for cervical spine films in trauma patients. *J Trauma.* 1989;29:1438–1439.

4. Roberge RJ, Wears RC, Kelly M, et al. Selective application of cervical spine radiography in alert victims of blunt trauma: a prospective study. *J Trauma*. 1988;28:784–788.

5. Bachulis BL, Long WB, Hynes GD, et al. Clinical indications for cervical spine radiographs in the traumatized patient. *Am J Surg*. 1987;153(5):473–478.

6. Ringenberg BJ, Fisher AK, Urdanela LF, et al. Rational ordering of cervical spine radiographs following trauma. *Ann Emerg Med*. 1988;17:792–796.

7. Jacobs LM, Schwartz R. Prospective analysis of acute cervical spine injury: a methodology to predict injury. *Ann Emerg Med*. 1986;15(1):44–48.

8. Zucker MI, Mower W, Hoffman JR, et al. Limiting utilization of cervical spine radiology by clinical parameters. *Am Soc Emerg Radiol*. 1991. Abstract.

9. Cadoux CG, White JD, Hedberg MC. High-yield roentgenographic criteria for cervical spine injuries. *Ann Emerg Med*. 1987;16(1):738–742.

10. McNamara RM, O'Brien MC, Davidheiser S. Post traumatic neck pain: a prospective and follow-up study. *Ann Emerg Med*. 1988;17:906–911.

11. Ross SE, Schwab CW, David ET, et al. Clearing the cervical spine: initial radiologic evaluation. *J Trauma*. 1987;27:1055–1060.

12. Daffner RH. *Imaging of Vertebral Trauma*. Rockville: Aspen Publications; 1988.

13. Harris JH Jr, Edeiken-Monroe B. *The Radiology of Acute Cervical Spine Trauma*. 2nd ed. Baltimore: Williams & Wilkins; 1987.

14. McCort JJ, Mindelzun RE. *Trauma Radiology*. New York: Churchill Livingstone; 1990.

15. Mirvis SE, Young JWR. *Imaging and Critical Care*. Baltimore: Williams and Wilkins; 1992.

16. Rockwood CA Jr, Green DP, Bucholz RW. *Fractures in Adults*. 3rd ed. Philadelphia: Lippincott; 1991.

17. Berquist TH. Imaging of adult cervical spine trauma. *Radiographics*. 1988;8:667–694.

18. Gehweiler JA Jr, Osborne RL Jr, Becker RF. *The Radiology of Vertebral Trauma*. Philadelphia: Saunders; 1980.

19. Streitwieser DR, Knopp R, Wales LR, et al. Accuracy of standard radiographic views in detecting cervical spine fractures. *Ann Emerg Med*. 1983;12:538–542.

20. Jordon J, Enzmann DR. Dynamic MR imaging of the cervical spine. Presented at the American Society of Neuroradiology June 1991, Washington D.C.

21. Pavlov H, Torg JS, Robie B, et al. Cervical spinal stenosis: determination with vertebral body ratio method. *Radiology*. 1987;164:771–775.

22. Vandemark RM. Radiology of the cervical spine in trauma patients: practice pitfalls and recommendations for improving efficiency and communication. *AJR*. 1990;155:465–472.

23. Denis F. The three column spine and its significance in the classification of acute thoracolumbar injuries. *Spine*. 1983;8:817–831.

24. White AA, Southwick WO, Panjabi MM. Clinical instability in the lower cervical spine: a review of past and current concepts. *Spine*. 1976;1:15–27.

25. White III AA, Panjabi MM. Update on the evaluation of instability of the lower cervical spine. Instructional course lectures—American Academy of Orthopedic Surgeons. 1987;513–520.

26. Harris JH Jr, Yeakley JS. *Current Problems in Diagnostic Radiology*. Chicago: Year Book Medical Publishers; 1989.

27. Cheshire DJ. The stability of the cervical spine following the conservative treatment of fractures and fracture dislocations. *Paraplegia*. 1969;7:193–203.

28. Borock EC, Gabram SGA, Jacobs LM, et al. A prospective analysis of a two-year experience using computed tomography as an adjunct for cervical spine clearance. *J Trauma* 1991;31(7):1001–1006.

29. Davis SJ, Teresi LM, Bradley WG Jr, et al. Cervical spine hyperextension injuries: MR findings. *Radiology*. 1991;180:245–251.

30. Kulkarni MV, McArdle CB, Kopanicky D, et al. Acute spinal cord injury: MR imaging at 1.5T. *Radiology*. 1987;164:837–843.

31. Mirvis SE, Geisler FH, Jelinek JJ, et al. Acute cervical spine trauma: evaluation with 1.5-T MR imaging. *Radiology*. 1988;166(3):807–816.

32. Kulkarni MV, Bondurant FJ, Rose SL, et al. 1.5 tesla magnetic resonance imaging of acute spinal trauma. *Radiographics*. 1988;8(6):1059–1079.

33. Beale SM, Pathria MN, Masaryk TJ. Magnetic resonance imaging of spinal trauma. *Top Magn Reson Imag*. 1988;1(1):53–62.

34. Schaefer DM, Flanders A, Northrup BE, et al. Magnetic resonance imaging of acute cervical spine trauma. Correlation with severity of neurologic injury. *Spine*. 1989;14:1090–1095.

35. Mirvis SE, Wolf A. Emerging MRI role: assessing cervical spine trauma. *MRI Decisions*. 1990;Jan/Feb. vol 4:21.

36. McArdle CB, Wright JW, Prevost WJ, et al. MR imaging of the acutely injured patient with cervical traction. *Radiology*. 1986;159:273–274.

37. Clayman DA, Murakami ME, Vines FS. Compatibility of cervical spine braces with MR imaging: a study of nine nonferrous devices. *AJNR*. 1990;11(2):385–390.
38. Flanders AE, Schaefer DM, Doan HT, et al. Acute cervical spine trauma: correlation of MR imaging findings with degree of neurologic deficit. *Radiology*. 1990;177:25–33.
39. Bondurant FJ, Cotler HB, Kulkarni MV, et al. Acute spinal cord injury: a study using physical examination and magnetic resonance imaging. *Spine*. 1990;15(3):161–168.

6

Angiography and Special Procedures: Computed Tomography, Duplex Scan, Ultrasound, and Magnetic Resonance Imaging

PAUL CAPEK, M.D.
WILLIAM R. FRY, M.D.

HISTORY: Angiography was conceptually considered soon after the discovery of x-rays.[1] The first angiogram performed on a living patient in 1923 is credited to Sicard and Forestier, who performed an arm venogram.[2] Direct arterial injection had been used to introduce salvarsan into the internal carotid arteries to treat syphilis, and in 1927 Moniz adapted this direct method to introduce sodium iodide and accomplished the first cerebral arteriogram.[3] The first cardiac catheterization is credited to Forssman, who blindly catheterized his own right heart and pulmonary artery through the antecubital vein in 1938. Having performed this procedure, he walked to the x-ray department to document his achievement.[4] Clinical applications of angiography slowly expanded, but it was not until 1953 when Seldinger introduced his technique for percutaneous insertion of catheters into blood vessels[5] that angiography enjoyed a marked increase in clinical use.

In the course of evaluating cervicothoracic trauma, the chest x-ray and cervical spine films are the primary initial screening modalities. Subsequently, evaluation of the soft tissues may be facilitated by certain specialized imaging procedures. The most urgent problem is to detect whether there is a major bleeding source. In this regard, angiography has represented the gold standard for the assessment of the integrity of major blood vessels. Computed tomography (CT) scanning has proved useful in similar circumstances, but the time required for the close serial cuts and the relative inaccessibility of the patient during the examination has resulted in relegating this examination to second choice as a screening procedure. Duplex scanning is currently proving to be an excellent screening technique for cervical vessel evaluation. It can be done quickly and is proving to be extremely accurate in diagnosing even minor vascular disruption. Magnetic resonance imaging (MRI) angiography is not a practical technique in the acute emergency situation, but it is proving to be of great value in spinal and neurological assessment.

ANGIOGRAPHY

Considerable refinements have occurred in imaging equipment, contrast agents, catheters, and catheterization techniques. The general trend is toward smaller, more controllable catheters and guidewires with which almost any blood vessel can now be identified and selectively imaged. Imaging equipment has become better with the advent of digital subtraction angiography (DSA). DSA allows the examinations to be performed considerably faster, with lower volumes of contrast and less patient discomfort. Even though translumbar aortography remains clinically useful, transfemoral catheterization is most commonly employed and has considerably increased the utility and safety of angiography.

Indications

Diagnostic angiography is the single best method to evaluate the vascular tree for occult injury. There are other promising, less invasive imaging techniques referred to above, but none yields a vascular evaluation that is as definitive as angiography. Future developments may alter this outlook, but currently an angiogram is still regarded as the "gold standard" (Fig. 6–1).

Penetrating and blunt trauma often injure blood vessels. Arterial vascular injury may be subtle but is catastrophic if missed. An angiogram taken during the silent period before major hemorrhage occurs may result in prompt intervention and cure, whereas a missed lesion can result in profound morbidity or death from exsanguination.

In certain cases such as vertebral artery injuries, endovascular occlusion therapy (embolotherapy) can be performed at the same time as the angiogram, further expanding the indications for this study.

Any penetrating trauma in proximity to a large artery may create a small pseudoaneurysm or intimal injury. The timing or urgency of arteriography after trauma can be controversial.[6-9] However, when dealing with possible injury to the aorta or brachiocephalic vessels, sudden deterioration of an apparently stable patient can occur when a temporarily contained hematoma ruptures into the pleural space or results in airway obstruction or stroke (Fig. 6–2). Only a strong clinical suspicion (based on the mechanism of injury) or an

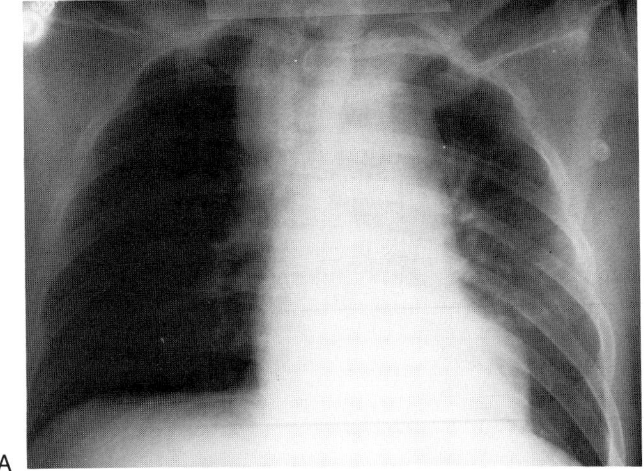

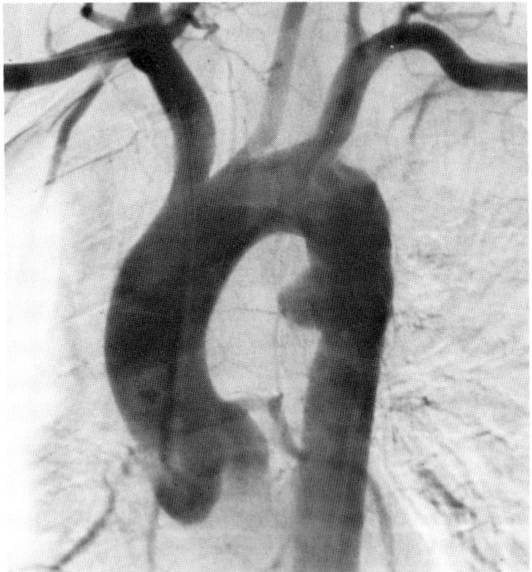

Figure 6–1. **A:** Blunt chest trauma was sustained in a motorcycle accident. There is widening of the mediastinum and indistinctness of the aortic knob. **B:** Thoracic aortogram demonstrates pseudoaneurysm of the aorta at the isthmus.

abnormal chest x-ray may prompt the decision to carry out angiography. Because chest x-ray findings are neither sensitive nor specific, the mechanism of injury often is the sole reason for evaluation.[10,11] If multiple findings are present on the chest film, the chance of aortic injury being present increases exponentially.

There are many other potential indications for angiographic evaluation and therapy in the traumatized patient (Table 6–1). If the patient is immobilized for a lengthy period (usually because of fractures or CNS injury), there is an increased incidence of pulmonary embolism. A pulmonary arteriogram is the single best examination to confirm or exclude this diagnosis.[12] A caval filter can be implanted immediately after the angiogram if a pulmonary embolism is present and there is a contraindication to systemic anticoagulation.

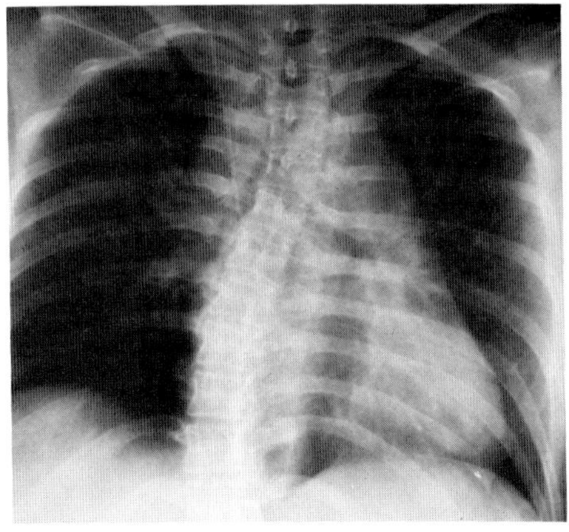

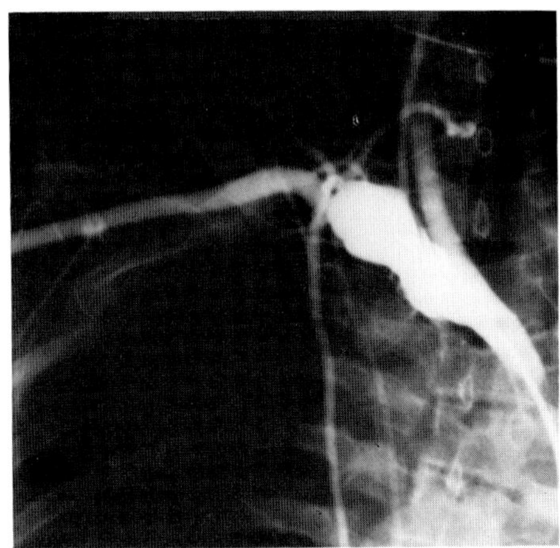

Figure 6–2. **A:** Blunt chest trauma with a non-displaced fracture of the first right rib and minimal right apical capping. **B:** Selective innominate arteriogram demonstrates a pseudoaneurysm of the right subclavian artery with an intimal tear.

Contraindications

Although an arteriogram can be performed in 30 min, in most instances the examination requires at least 2 hr. This period represents the primary problem: many personnel have to be assembled, and the patient must be transported and prepared. The main contraindication consists of *patients too unstable* to be removed safely for x-ray. Pressors, blood products, and fluids in marginally stable patients can all be administered during the angiogram, but this requires close collaboration between the clinical service and the angiography team.

Intracranial Hypertension

Intracranial hypertension is the second condition that must be controlled before angiography. Relative contraindications include a history of contrast allergy, cardiac or renal failure, and uncontrolled hemorrhage.

Table 6–1.   Radiographic Signs of Vascular Trauma*[11]

CHEST FILM FINDINGS	AORTIC RUPTURE (%)	NORMAL AORTA (%)
Mediastinal width (>8 cm) on upright CXR	93	50
Aortic knob alteration	93	50
Tracheal shift	53	40
Left mainstem bronchus depression	46	30
Left apical cap	40	10
Left hilar blurring	53	—
Obscured descending aorta	13	—
Displaced superior vena cava	13	10
Paratracheal stripe thickening	46	30
Right paraspinal line thickening	13	—
Left paraspinal line thickening	7	—
Pneumothorax or pneumomediastinum	—	10
Hemothorax	47	40
Pulmonary contusion	13	20
Bone fracture	67	90

$*p < .05.$
CXR, chest x-ray; SVC, superior vena cava

Known History of Contrast Allergy

Most contrast reactions are related to the osmotic load of the agent. True allergies are uncommon and may be avoided by preoperative oral or intravenous steroids as well as a nonionic contrast agent.[13–16] Most idiosyncratic contrast reactions are quite unpredictable and may not recur on reexposure. Interestingly, allergic reactions to intraarterially injected contrast are significantly less common than reactions to those administered intravenously.[17]

Cardiac Failure

The volume of contrast and fluid injected during an angiogram can precipitate cardiogenic shock from acute heart failure or an arrhythmia. A typical arch aortogram may give the patient a fluid bolus of 100 to 300 cc.

Impaired Renal Function

Diabetics and any patient with diminished renal function are at risk for acute contrast-aggravated renal failure. Adequate shock resuscitation including preangiogram hydration minimizes this risk, but some patients may require temporary or permanent hemodialysis.[18–21]

Uncontrolled Hemorrhage

Embolotherapy may achieve a definitive cure in the bleeding patient; however, if blood pressure cannot be sufficiently supported, the patient is at risk for death in the angiography suite.

Technique

Equipment

In general, a dedicated laboratory is required to perform all but the most basic types of angiography and vascular intervention. Dedicated x-ray generators and high quality image intensifying and recording systems are needed. Because trauma patients often are not completely evaluated for spinal injury, the ideal system allows the patient to be on a floating radiolucent table under a C-arm type of positioner. This allows full examination of any part of the patient. Less optimal is a fixed positioner. A rapid radiographic film recorder is needed to obtain optimal images; however, the newer DSA equipment obtains image quality that approaches that of film (Fig. 6–3). Biplane systems allow simultaneous filming in two projections at right angles to each other with a single injection of contrast. This significantly decreases the total amount of contrast needed. The room should be sufficiently sized to readily accommodate the patient, angiographers, technicians, all ancillary personnel, ventilators, beds, IV pumps, and any other necessary equipment.

Tools

There is a wide variety of needles, guidewires, and catheters available. With these tools it is possible to catheterize and treat practically any vessel in the body. The choice of tools is largely dictated by the experience and preference of the operator.

Contrast

The old ionic salts of tri-iodo benzoic acid are excellent contrast agents, but they induce an intense sensation of burning or pain while being injected. Their osmolarity is manyfold higher than blood, which may account for some of the induced hemodynamic changes, pain, and decreased hematocrit. The use of nonionic and ionic low-osmolarity agents has markedly lessened patient discomfort and has resulted in improved cooperation. A true anaphylactoid major reaction with cardiopulmonary collapse after contrast injection remains quite rare. The nonionics have lessened this risk further, although some risk

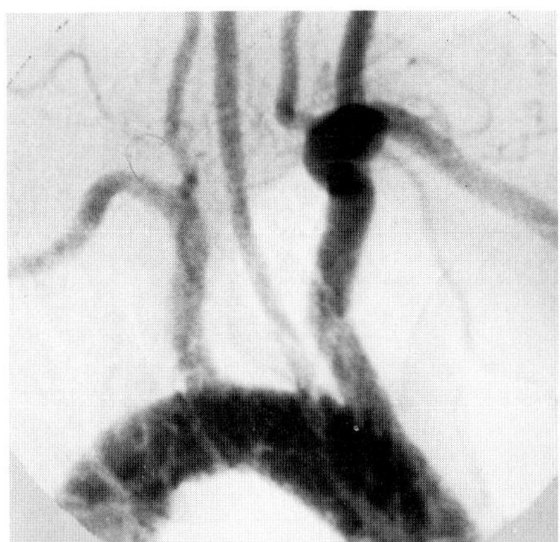

Figure 6–3. Digital subtraction angiography. This image was made after a superior vena cava injection of 40 ml of contrast material. The aortic arch and great vessels are well seen but subtle intimal damage could be missed.

remains. The presence of an anesthesiologist during the procedure is prudent if there is a history of significant allergic reaction.

Angiographer

Most radiologists are capable of performing simple diagnostic angiography and vascular intervention. Ideally, the procedure is performed by a radiologist with special training and interest in these procedures and patients (an interventional radiologist).

Vascular Access

Most vascular procedures are performed via puncture of the common femoral artery. This site is easily punctured, easily observed postprocedure, and readily controlled afterward if a problem arises. Alternate sites include axillary/brachial artery, although proximity of the brachial nerve harbors potential for permanent neurologic injury if a hematoma develops and goes unchecked. Unless promptly evacuated, an axillary sheath hematoma can result in a paralyzed and useless hand.

Complications

Overall, the transfemoral approach is probably the safest (0.7% complications) (Table 6–2). Potential complications include puncture site hematoma, thrombus formation and embolization, aneurysm rupture, subintimal passage of catheter/wire with subsequent vascular occlusion, wire/catheter break and embolization, cardiovascular derangements, drug reactions, and neurological complications of various types. All (except for groin hematomas) are rare but can yield devastating complications (e.g., cholesterol shower from an aortic aneurysm and subsequent myoglobinuria, renal failure, and eventual death).[22–24] This always must be weighed against the benefit of the study. Complication rates are higher in less experienced hands and centers that do fewer cases.

Preparation

If the patient's condition permits, he/she usually is sedated at the beginning of the procedure with a short-acting narcotic and benzodiazipine (fentanyl and midozalam). Ideally, the procedure is discussed at length with the patient and consent obtained preoperatively. Peripheral pulses are examined and charted.

Table 6–2.   Puncture Site Complications[24]

COMPLICATION	TRANSFEMORAL (%)	TRANSAXILLARY (%)	TRANSLUMBAR (%)
Hemorrhage	0.26	0.68	0.53
Arterial obstruction	0.14	0.76	0.00
Pseudoaneurysm	0.05	0.22	0.05
Arteriovenous fistula	0.01	0.02	0.00
Limb amputation	0.01	0.02	0.00
Total	0.47	1.7	0.58

Procedure

Local anesthetic (1–2% lidocaine) is infiltrated into the tissues around the puncture site. Neutralizing the lidocaine with bicarbonate decreases the pain of anesthesia. A hollow, 19–18-gauge needle is briskly advanced through both walls of the common femoral artery and slowly withdrawn. Pulsatile bleeding indicates that the needle is in the artery lumen and a guidewire is inserted. The needle is then removed and a catheter advanced over the wire into the vessel. Contrast is injected with a mechanical injector, with rapid filming of the vessel of interest. After completion, the catheter is withdrawn and compression applied to the puncture site. This usually is sufficient to achieve hemostasis within 10 min. Because the hemostatic plug is weak initially, the patients are kept at bed rest for the next 4 to 8 hr. The puncture site is frequently examined in the recovery area. If a hematoma starts to develop, it is readily controlled by simple local manual compression. Usually this is sufficient to control the bleeding; rarely a surgical groin exploration and suture closure of the arteriotomy are necessary. It is also possible for the patient to hemorrhage into the retroperitoneum without an appreciable hematoma in the groin. Puncture of the artery above the inguinal ligament increases this risk; therefore, careful attention should be given to any patient who complains of back or flank pain, especially if a high femoral puncture had been necessary.

Findings

Vascular injury takes the form of vessel laceration or division after penetrating trauma, avulsion, or obstruction after blunt trauma (Fig. 6–4). On angiography, these injuries may be manifest by frank extravasation, false aneurysm formation, arteriovenous fistula, spasm, dissection, partial or complete thrombosis, and distal embolism. All of these findings have a characteristic appearance. Occasionally the findings are quite subtle on arteriography, with only a small intimal flap or intimal irregularity. Rarely, it is possible to have a normal-appearing angiogram with significant injury to the vessel. This may be due to "blast" injury to the artery, which leaves the external layers damaged but a normal-appearing lumen. Small lacerations or false aneurysms may be missed if contrast is too heavy and the lesion not put in profile.

The presence of spasm may appear to be trivial, but it is always indicative of injury. Minor disruption of the intima may result subsequently in vascular thrombosis, so this is an indication at the very least for monitoring the distal circulation.

Embolotherapy

If frank extravasation or a pseudoaneurysm is seen in an end vessel of a well collateralized vascular bed, then the catheter can be directed into the injured vessel and be occluded by a catheter-delivered embolus. If temporary occlusion is desired, then particles of autologous clot or gelatin sponge (Gelfoam) can be injected. Clot recanalizes in 24 to 48 hr, Gelfoam in approximately 1 week.[25,26] If permanent occlusion is desired, then stainless steel coils[27,28] are deposited through the catheter or particles of polyvinyl alcohol foam are injected.[29,30] Liquid sclerosing agents such as ethyl alcohol or liquid glues such as isobutyl 2-cyanoacrylate (Crazy glue) cause too much tissue destruction to be of routine use in controlling bleeding traumatized vessels.[30] Embolotherapy has found application in controlling exter-

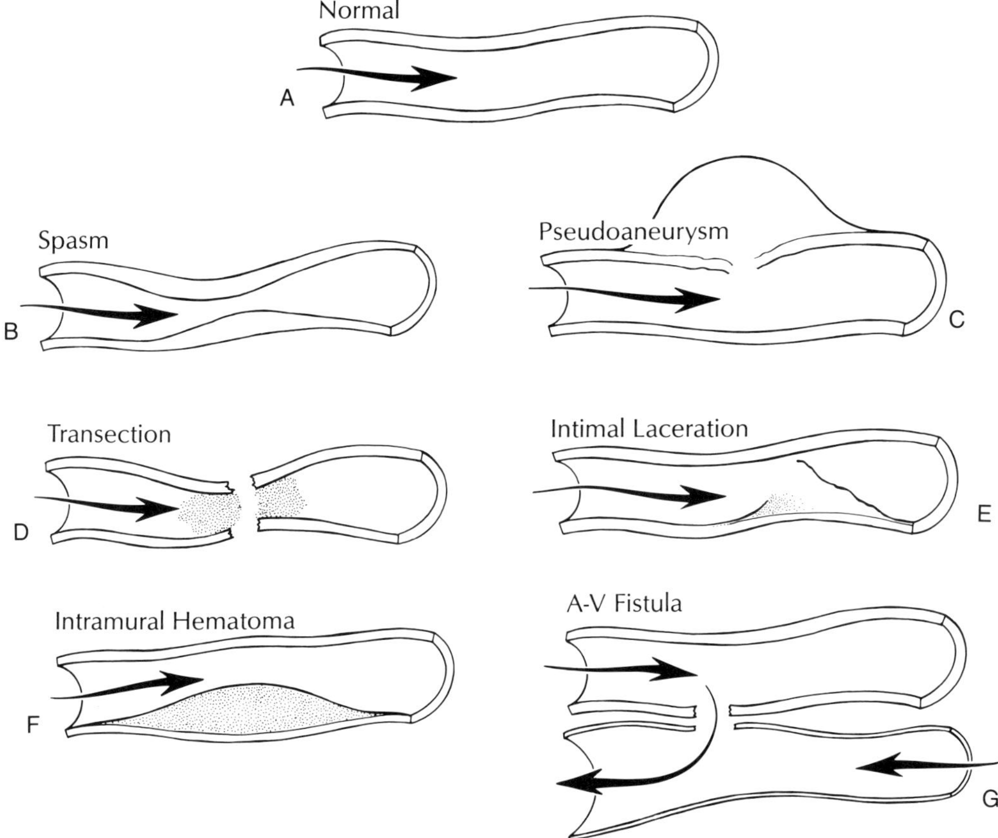

Figure 6–4. Nature of the injuries seen on angiography. **A:** Normal vessel. **B:** Vascular "spasm." **C:** False aneurysm. **D:** Disrupted vessel with thrombosis of the divided ends. **E:** Elevated intimal flap. **F:** Subintimal hemorrhage. **G:** Arteriovenous fistula.

nal carotid hemorrhage, vertebral bleeding, vertebral arteriovenous fistulae, and bleeding from bronchial and other small arteries.[30]

There is a wide variety of potential complications related to embolotherapy ranging from inadvertent embolization of nontarget tissues, to abscesses and sepsis, to inadequate or incomplete embolization and a return of symptoms.[31]

COMPUTED TOMOGRAPHY

CT is now a standard procedure available in all major American hospitals. It has proved to be extremely valuable in assessing central nervous system and abdominal trauma problems,[1] but its use in thoracic injuries has not been completely defined.[2,3] It has two primary disadvantages to that of simple radiological evaluation: the first is the expense and the second is that the procedure takes time to accomplish and removes the patient from direct contact with supporting personnel. As a result, its primary use has been under semielective circumstances or to assess secondary complications in the postoperative or postinjured patient.

Indications

Most thoracic injuries can be diagnosed quite well by a portable supine chest x-ray. Because the chest x-ray is readily available in the emergency room while the patient is undergoing resuscitation and only interrupts access to the patient for a minute or two at most, chest x-ray remains the standard method of initial assessment.

Abdominal and head CT often is carried out after initial stabilization of the patient. In some centers, whenever a patient has an abdominal or chest CT scan, 5 to 10 additional slices are taken through the chest; these slices add only 5 to 10 min to the procedure time.[4] Under certain circumstances, the CT may pick up additional important information, such as the occult pneumothorax, malposition of chest tubes, inadequately drained pleural collections, hemothorax, mediastinal hematoma, and pericardial fluid (Fig. 6–5).[5]

In the postoperative or postinjury period, CT may be of value to localize fluid or blood collections within the chest cavity that may be difficult to see or localize on routine chest x-ray. It is particularly important if the patient becomes septic and there is a question of adequacy of drainage of the chest. In patients who have persistent major air leaks, CT may provide information about the source of the leak, including location of pneumatoceles, or even bronchial tears, thus facilitating the decision for surgery.[6] It can be very helpful after lung contusions and provide information about the viability of lung tissue in the injured area. It also may facilitate the localization of empyema, which facilitates catheter drainage.

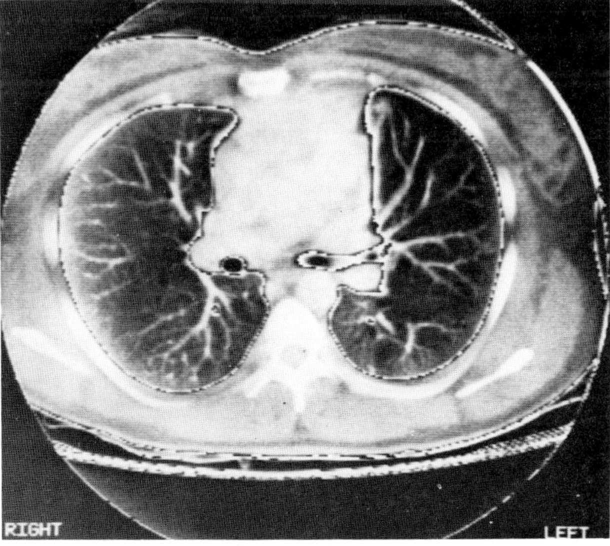

Figure 6–5.　CT examination of a middle-aged man who had sustained a parasternal stab wound. The anterior mediastinal hematoma is well shown with this technique.

Contraindications

Given the information that CT of the chest can provide, the primary contraindication to CT is the nonstable patient. When the patient has been stable from a cardiovascular respiratory standpoint for an hour or more, CT is appropriate if there is the need to assess head or abdominal injury and permits several cuts of the thorax when there is direct or indirect evidence of associated chest injury. It is rarely appropriate to use CT for primary assessment of the isolated chest injury.

Technique

Conventional third or fourth generation CT scanners have improved spatial resolution and short scan times of from 2 to 3 sec per slice. Depending on the urgency of the situation, slices can be taken 1 to 2 cm apart. If there are specific focal areas of interest, 2- to 3-mm slices may be appropriate, although this is rarely necessary. When the radiologist is familiar with the gross appearance of the vascular anatomy, the great vessels can be identified without the need for contrast. However, identification of specific vascular injury is facilitated by intravenous contrast administration.

Great Vessels

Although it is possible to diagnose rupture of the aorta or major vessels such as subclavian or innominate artery by CT, the study can be falsely positive as well as falsely negative (Fig. 6–6).[7] The greatest value of the CT is that it can distinguish a widened mediastinum caused by hemorrhage from widening caused by other etiologies.[8] Even more importantly, its superior sensitivity enables detection of occult hemorrhage when the mediastinum appears normal on conventional chest x-ray.[7] It also can identify anatomic variations and congenital abnormalities of mediastinal vessels that can produce abnormal mediastinal contours on the chest x-ray.[9] CT detection of any mediastinal hemorrhage mandates an aortogram, even though the aortic contour appears to be sharply preserved, because the last layer of the aortic wall to rupture is the adventitia. Hemorrhage associated with an intact adventitia and a gross rupture of the media and intima of the aorta usually represents bleeding from small vessels damaged by the shearing force of the trauma. The CT can demonstrate the traumatic aortic pseudoaneurysm associated with aortic rupture.[4,10,11]

Heiberg and colleagues have cautioned that false positive results in diagnosis of aortic tear may derive from the presence of streaking effects from catheters, motion, and arms within the gantry.[12] Thus, CT is useful to exclude the need for angiography when the patient has no evidence of mediastinal hemorrhage and to support the need to perform aortography in all patients with mediastinal hemorrhage or other evidence suggesting possible vascular injury.

Myocardial Contusion and Cardiac Rupture

In its ability to detect the presence of pericardial fluid, CT compares favorably with echocardiography.[5,10] A small amount of pericardial fluid is seen almost routinely on echo and is probably physiologic. On CT, physiologic pericardial fluid usually occupies the superior pericardial recesses and rarely extends inferiorly to surround the base of the heart.

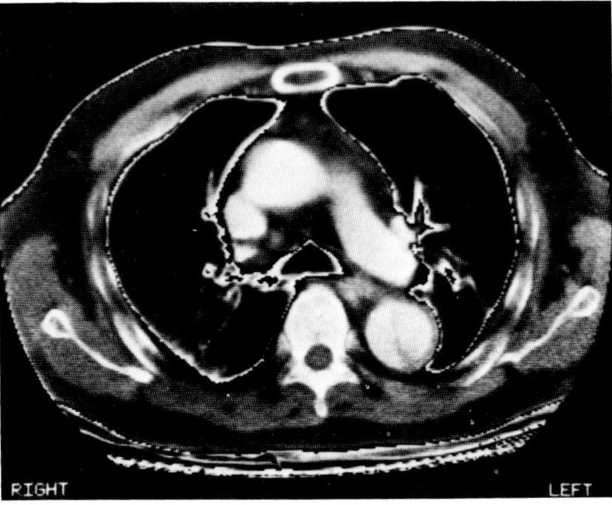

Figure 6–6. CT of the chest of an elderly man after administration of intravenous contrast material. True and false lumens are seen, confirming the clinical suspicion of aortic dissection. It is not known whether CT can demonstrate more subtle intimal damage.

The presence of fluid in this latter region should lead to suspicion of pericardial or cardiac injury. Major accumulations seen on CT are associated with tamponade and dictate immediate decompression in the patient not responding to resuscitation.

Pneumothorax

Pneumothorax is the most common intrathoracic complication of chest trauma. Plain chest x-ray can detect most pneumothoraces large enough to require immediate tube thoracostomy. However, CT identification of a small anterior, medial, or subpulmonic pneumothorax, which may be difficult to see on x-ray, may be of great value, particularly in the patient who requires or is about to require positive pressure ventilation.[5,10] Placement of a chest tube in such a patient with occult pneumothorax will avoid the subsequent risk of pulmonary deterioration from a tension pneumothorax. When patients are treated with a chest tube for pneumothorax, CT may reveal a large, unsuspected, residual pneumothorax in a region remote from the chest tube and dictate the placement of an additional drainage tube.

Hemothorax

A large hemothorax is readily detectable on routine chest x-ray. More than 500 to 1000 cc of blood can be present without being obvious on a marginal emergency room chest film. With a supine CT, fluid usually is recognized first in the apex of the hemothorax as an apical cap.[5,10]

Even though a hemothorax detectable only by CT is small and drainage may not be necessary, knowledge of its presence dictates further monitoring of that pleural space. It also may raise issues regarding associated injuries, such as ruptures of the diaphragm, aortic rupture, or pericardial rupture.

Bronchial and Tracheal Rupture

Rupture of the tracheobronchial tree usually results in obvious accumulations of air in the chest, mediastinum, or subcutaneous tissue. A small percentage of patients may fail to show obvious air on a routine chest x-ray. CT can permit recognition of small peribronchial or peritracheal accumulations of air that suggest the possibility of tracheobronchial rupture.[4] It can explicitly diagnose a tracheal tear in patients with indwelling endotracheal tubes when a herniating balloon is seen or when there is an abnormal dislocation of the endotracheal tube.[4]

Diaphragm Rupture

Gross laceration of diaphragm with major herniation of abdominal contents usually is readily diagnosed by conventional chest x-ray. However, the presence of chest wall injury, hemothorax, and pneumothorax may obscure the diagnosis. CT is useful in these circumstances to clarify the pathology.[12] Although CT almost never will show the laceration of the diaphragm itself, it will readily demonstrate even small visceral herniations and, in this regard, is more accurate than chest x-ray.

Parenchymal Injury

CT is not necessary or appropriate for the initial assessment of lung injury, but a subsequent consolidation may be assessed by CT and may demonstrate, by using contrast, a lack of viability of lung tissue, presence of air cysts, and localized areas of parenchymal disruption.[5,10]

Accuracy

McGonigal et al. compared of the efficacy of conventional chest x-ray with CT in 50 acutely injured patients.[5] They reviewed cases of hemo- and/or pneumothorax in 12 patients; only 5 were diagnosed by chest x-ray, whereas all 12 were seen on CT. CT identified pulmonary contusion in 10 patients; chest x-ray identified 4 and CT all 10. Three additional false positive diagnoses of pulmonary contusion were made by chest x-ray. The authors concluded that chest x-ray was less sensitive than CT in the detection of hemo- and pneumothorax (42% vs. 100%) and pulmonary contusion (40% vs. 100%).

McLean et al. determined the accuracy of CT scanning for diagnosing aortic rupture.[11] In 17 patients who underwent both CT scanning and aortography, five patients were found to have aortic rupture by aortography; CT scanning yielded three true positives and two false negatives. In 12 patients with a negative aortogram, CT scanning recorded four false positives and eight true negatives. The specificity was 23% and the sensitivity was 83% when compared with the aortography. The overall accuracy for CT scanning was 53%. Godwin and Tolentino agreed.[13] They also felt that CT lacked the spatial resolution to demonstrate significant injury reliably to the brachiocephalic arteries and was vulnerable to both false positive and false negative diagnoses in the assessment of aortic rupture.

DUPLEX SCAN AND ULTRASONOGRAPHY

Duplex Scan

Although angiography has been the standard method used for vascular examination, it is an invasive, expensive, time-consuming procedure, with risk of morbidity. When the indication for arteriography consists solely of wounds of proximity, the yield for angiography will be low for actual injury.[1-3] When dealing with the possibility of injury to the cervical blood vessels, the risk of missed injury may be catastrophic.

Alternative noninvasive techniques such as Doppler pressure assessment have been explored for screening for thrombotic destruction. However, it is difficult to measure carotid or vertebral artery pressures directly without risk of embolization. Measurement of carotid or ophthalmic artery pressures is technically even more difficult in the trauma setting. Moreover, these measurements do not take into account vascular injuries that produce arteriovenous fistula, pseudoaneurysm, or intimal flaps that may not reduce distal arterial pressures.

Only recently has noninvasive vascular imaging been applied in a systematic fashion to patients suffering cervical trauma.[4] Duplex scanning of the cervical vessels is ideally suited to the evaluation of potential traumatic injuries because both image and hemodynamic data are obtained. Additionally, vertebral artery injuries can be diagnosed with Duplex scanning, a capability other similar noninvasive techniques do not have.

We have used Duplex scanning in 52 patients suffering 56 traumatic cervical injuries.[5] The mechanism of injury included gunshot wounds (28 patients), stab wounds (20 patients), blunt injuries (2 patients), and shotgun wounds (2 patients). A normal cervical vasculature was demonstrated in 51 Duplex evaluations. Five studies revealed vascular injury. These injuries included a common carotid intimal flap, occluded internal and external carotid arteries, an occluded vertebral artery, and a stenotic vertebral artery. The accuracy of this Duplex scanning was confirmed in 11 patients by arteriography and in 6 patients by operative exploration. Of the remaining 30 patients with normal findings on Duplex screening, 10 returned for follow-up visits, and none of these patients developed vascular or neurological abnormalities. No patients returned with complications of a missed vascular injury.

Bynoe et al.[4] reported 59 carotid artery segments studied by Duplex scanning for potential vascular injury. In the group studied, only one patient had a false positive Duplex scan that suggested a carotid artery intimal flap. Arteriography showed only a shallow carotid plaque, and the patient was observed and no complications developed.[4]

These early experiences suggest that Duplex scanning may be the test of choice for the screening for cervical vascular injury. Currently, we screen all patients with cervical trauma for vascular injury by Duplex scan. Demonstration of a normal vasculature by this method obviates the need for further vascular studies. Due to the small experience with the diagnosis of arterial injury, cervical arteriography is used for final definitive evaluation before operative intervention in those patients stable enough to permit this latter technique.

Ultrasonography

Ultrasonography (US) as a diagnostic tool is used much less in the United States than in Europe and Japan. It is relatively inexpensive and can be readily available in the emergency room; it can be used to diagnose pneumothorax, pleural and pericardial effusion, cardiac function, and even aortic rupture.[6–8]

Its disadvantages are that it is operator dependent, the images can be difficult to interpret, and it does not have the global capability of a simple chest film or CT scan.

At UC Davis, US has been used primarily as 2-D echocardiography (ECHO).[8] It has proved to be extremely accurate in diagnosing and following pericardial effusions and in assessing myocardial wall motion and intracardiac injury. During a period of 3 years, 36 patients with possible cardiac penetrating injuries were evaluated by ECHO as part of their initial work-up (Fig. 6–7). In four instances, effusions were diagnosed and emergent treatment including cardiac repair was carried out. As a result, we consider that 2-D ECHO is a valuable tool in the triage of stable penetrating trauma patients when cardiac injury is suspected.[8]

Transesophageal Echocardiography

Transesophageal echocardiography (TEE) has been shown to be very accurate when dealing with nontraumatic dissections of the descending thoracic aorta.[10] This has resulted in enthusiastic application to trauma (Fig. 6–8). Unfortunately, adequate visualization of the arch and great vessels has been inconsistent.[9,10] Nevertheless, Shapiro expressed enthusiasm for this technique.[6] In addition to diagnosing myocardial injury in 63% of patients studied, aortic wall injuries were diagnosed in two patients, and the diagnoses were subsequently confirmed by angiography.

Intravascular Ultrasound

Intravascular ultrasound is a new diagnostic modality now becoming available in many centers.[11] It offers a high-resolution axial view of the aorta that is complementary to projected images obtained with conventional aortography.[12] Williams et al. supplemented a questionable aortogram with intravascular US and established the presence of significant thoracic aortic rupture by using a 6.5-F, 20-mHz transducer with a field of view approximately 30 mm.[12] The catheter was placed percutaneously in the groin and advanced, using fluoroscopic control, past the suspected injury, then slowly withdrawn while video recording the aortic lumen. This established that a laceration was present which, at surgery, involved one-fourth of the aortic circumference.

MAGNETIC RESONANCE IMAGING

MRI is becoming readily available for clinical imaging procedures in most medical centers in the United States. It has an *advantage* over conventional radiography in that it does not subject the patient to radiation. The spatial resolution of MRI approaches that of CT, and it has the ability to image nearly every pathologic entity visualized by CT scanning.[1] Solid masses can be differentiated from blood vessels without the use of intravenous contrast material, because the motion of blood in the vessel lumen results in it appearing lucent. It is an optimal technique for evaluating the spinal cord, vertebral column, and attaching ligaments (see previous chapter). Although rarely used except for the secondary assessment of trauma patients and their complications, there are theoretical and practical advantages that may well render it of much greater value in the future.

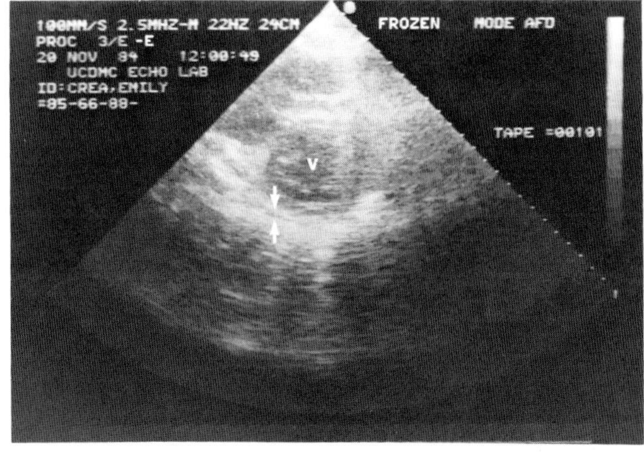

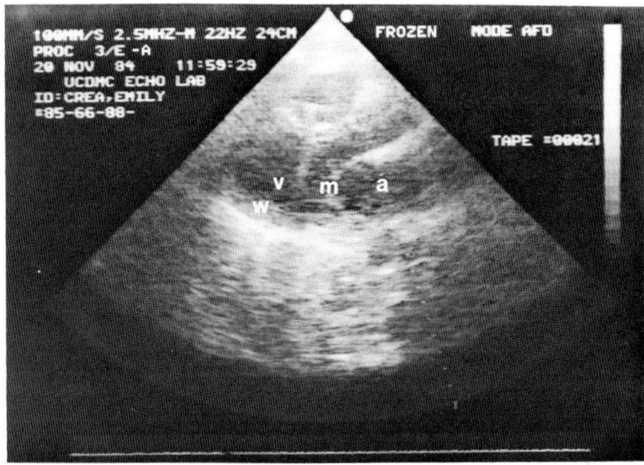

Figure 6 7. The echocardiogram has proved to be an extremely valuable tool in evaluating patients with cardiac injury. **A:** The transverse view. The left ventricle (*V*) is seen; behind the left ventricle fluid accumulation is noted in the pericardium (*arrows*). **B:** A longitudinal cardiac view. The left ventricular wall (*W*) did not move well and was compatible with the diagnosis of left ventricular contusion. M, mitral valve; A, left atrium.

The *disadvantages* at the present time are overwhelming when it is considered for acute trauma examination. The imaging times are longer than CT, metallic objects and other supportive monitoring devices produce imaging artifacts, and the patient is removed from the immediate proximity of the supporting personnel.

Great Vessel Evaluation

MRI is becoming increasingly reliable in the evaluation of vascular disease.[2–4] High spatial resolution can be obtained with MR angiography with the use of dedicated coils. Carotid arteries, in particular, have been studied with this technique with promising clinical results, as it has shown high sensitivity in the detection of lesions.[2] Pavone et al.[2] concluded that MRI and MR angiography performed at low-field strength had the same clinical value as

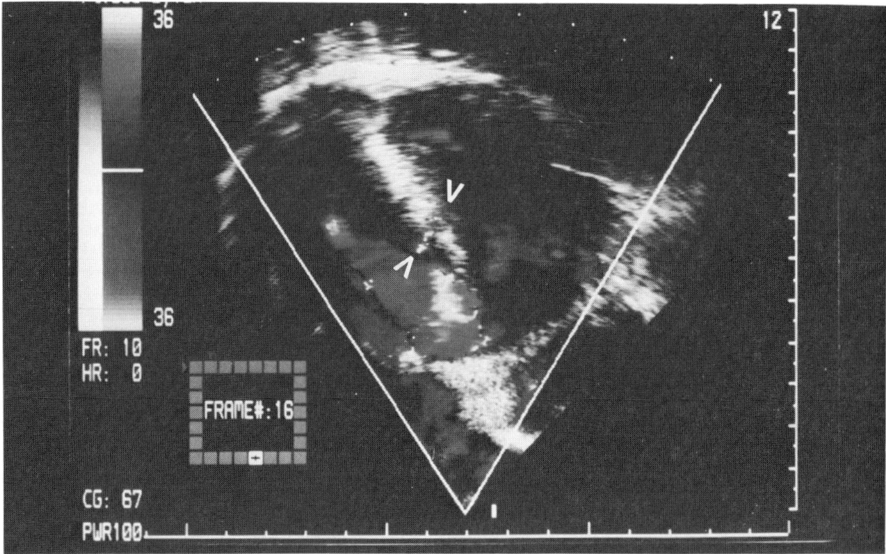

Figure 6–8. The transesophageal echocardiogram gives a more accurate assessment of valvular injuries and intracardiac shunts. Note the flow across the ventricular septum, indicating a traumatic VSD.

high-field strength MR angiography. They believe that clinical improvements as a result of the introduction of new techniques, such as three-dimensional time of flight and phase contrasting, will result in its accuracy being comparable to angiography.

Wielopolski et al.,[3] using three-dimensional MRI of the pulmonary vasculature, thought it was possible to obtain high resolution pulmonary vascular information with good image quality and little image degradation from moving blood and respiratory motion. In their hands, MRI generated excellent pulmonary vascular images in approximately 10 to 13 min. They concluded this technique was of great value in assessing the integrity of pulmonary vessels and in determining the presence of pulmonary emboli.

Axel et al.[5] obtained two-dimensional analysis of regional heart wall motion with MRI and concluded that MRI allowed noninvasive, regional analysis of within-wall motion. This included separation of components of rigid body motion and deformation, which permitted this analysis to be displayed as functional images. Webb and Sostman found that, in certain situations, MRI, at the present time, provides diagnostic information that is superior to that of CT.[1] They felt that, as a imaging modality, its value related to the ability to: a) image vessels, b) distinguish different tissues, c) image in nontransaxial planes, and d) obviate the administration of iodinated contrast material. This increased yield technically related to synchronizing imaging to the electrocardiogram. Webb and Sostman concluded that rapid technical developments in MRI are applicable to thoracic evaluation. They anticipate major advances in three areas: lung parenchymal imaging, pulmonary vascular imaging, and cardiac imaging. MRI of the lung parenchyma until now has been hindered by magnetic susceptibility artifacts, motion artifacts, and poor signal-to-noise ratio. The advent of shorter TE pulse sequences, better understanding of susceptibility variations, and faster imaging techniques should lead to new clinical applications in characterizing focal and diffuse pulmonary parenchymal disease.

Although MR now provides excellent anatomic and functional imaging of the heart, it has not provided enough unique information to achieve a major role in routine cardiac evaluation. The advent of fast imaging techniques, tagging methods, and greater understanding of contrast agents for the myocardium should lead to the emergence of the MR as the premier imaging modality.

REFERENCES

1. Haschek E, Lindenthal OT. A contribution to the practical use of the photography according to Roentgen. *Wien Klin Wochenschr.* 1896;9:63.
2. Sicard JA, Forestier G. Injections intravascularies d'huile iodee sous control radiologique. *CR Soc Biol (Paris).* 1923;88:1200.
3. Moniz E. L'encéphalographie artérielle son importance dans la localisation des tumeurs cérebrales. *Rev Neurol.* 1927;2:72.
4. Robb GP, Steinberg I. A practical method of visualization of chambers of the heart, the pulmonary circulation, and the great blood vessels in man. *J Clin Invest.* 1938;17:507.
5. Seldinger SI. Catheter replacement of needle in percutaneous arteriography: new technique. *Acta Radiol (Stock).* 1953;39:368.
6. Anderson RJ, Hobson RW, Bing CL, et al. Reduced dependency on arteriography for penetrating extremity trauma: influence of wound location and noninvasive vascular studies. *J Trauma.* 1990;30:1059–1065.
7. Weaver FA, Yellin AE, Bauer M, et al. Is arterial proximity a valid indication for arteriography in penetrating extremity trauma? *Arch Surg.* 1990;125:1256–1260.
8. Frykberg ER, Crump JM, Dennis JW, et al. Nonoperative observation of clinically occult arterial injuries: a prospective evaluation. *Surgery.* 1991;109:85–96.
9. Hartling RP, McGahan JP, Lindfors KK, et al. Stab wounds to the neck: role of angiography. *Radiology.* 1989;172:79–82.
10. Woodring JH, King JG. Determination of normal transverse mediastinal width and mediastinal-width to chest-width (M/C) ratio in control subjects: implications for subjects with aortic or brachiocephalic arterial injury. *J Trauma.* 1989;29:1268–1272.
11. Savastano S, Feltrin GP, Miotto D, et al. Value of plain chest film in predicting traumatic aortic rupture. *Ann Radiol.* 1989;32:196–200.
12. The PIOPED investigator group. Value of the ventilation/perfusion scan in acute pulmonary embolism. *JAMA.* 1990;263(20):2753–2759.
13. Kelly JF, Patterson R, Lieberman P, et al. Radiographic contrast media studies in high-risk patients. *J Allergy Clin Immunol.* 1978;62:181–184.
14. Lasser EC, Berry CC, Talner LB, et al. Pretreatment with corticosteroids to alleviate reactions to intravenous contrast material. *N Engl J Med.* 1987;317:845–849.
15. Katayma H, Yamaguchi K, Kozuka T, et al. Adverse reactions to ionic and nonionic contrast media: a report from the Japanese Committee on the Safety of Contrast Media. *Radiology.* 1990;175:621–628.
16. Wolf GL, Mishkin MM, Roux SG, et al. Comparison of the rates of adverse drug reactions: ionic contrast agents, ionic agents combined with steroids, and nonionic agents. *Invest Radiol.* 1991;26:404–410.
17. Shehadi W. Adverse reactions to intravenously administered contrast media. *Am J Roentgenol.* 1975;124:145–152.
18. Mason RA, Arbeit LA, Giron F. Renal dysfunction after arteriography. *JAMA.* 1985;253:1001–1004.
19. Gomes AS, Baker JD, Martin-Parederov, et al. Acute renal dysfunction after major arteriography. *Am J Roentgenol.* 1985;145:1249–1253.
20. Schwartz RD, Rubin JE, Leeming BW, et al. Renal failure following major angiography. *Am J Med.* 1978;65:31–37.
21. Kerstein MD, Puyau FA. Value of periangiography hydration. *Surgery.* 1984;96:919–922.
22. Ramirez G, O'Neill WM, Lambert R, et al. Cholesterol embolization: a complication of angiography. *Arch Intern Med.* 138:1430–1432.
23. Rosansky SJ. Multiple cholesterol emboli syndrome after angiography. *Am J Roentgenol.* 1984;143:683.
24. Hessel SJ, Adams DF, Abrams HL. Complications of angiography. *Radiology.* 1981;138:273–281.
25. Bookstein JJ, Chlodys RM, Foley D, et al. Transcatheter hemostasis of gastrointestinal bleeding using modified autogenous clot. *Radiology.* 1974;113:277.

26. Sniderman KW, Franklin J. Successful transcatheter Gelfoam embolization of a bleeding cecal vascular ectasia. *Am J Roentgenol.* 1978;131(1):157–159.
27. Gianturco C, Anderson JH, Wallace S. Mechanical devices for arterial occlusion. *Am J Roentgenol.* 1975;124:428.
28. Anderson JH, Wallace S, Gianturco C. Transcatheter intravascular coil occlusion of experimental arteriovenous fistulas. *Am J Roentgenol.* 1977;129:795.
29. Goldman ML. Bucrylate, silicones and ivalon as agents for intravascular embolization. In: Abrams HL, ed. *Angiography—Vascular and Interventional Radiology.* 3rd ed, vol 3. Boston: Little, Brown; 1983.
30. Sclafani SJ, Cooper R, Shaftan GW, et al. Arterial trauma: diagnostic and therapeutic angiography. *Radiology.* 1986;161:165–172.
31. Feldman L, Greenfield AJ, Waltman AC, et al. Transcatheter vessel occlusion: angiographic results versus clinical success. *Radiology.* 1983;147:1.

7

Anesthesia for Thoracic Trauma

AMIRA M. SAFWAT, M.D.

HISTORY: Although the use of anesthesia for chest surgery is of relatively recent origin, Plato originally used the term in a book that Timaeus published in the fourth century BC. He used it to mean the condition in which the impulse is not transmitted to the brain. Dioscorides, a Greek physician who served in Nero's army from AD 54 to 68, described the root of the mandrake (related to belladonna) as a sedative to bring sleep at night and to abolish pain during an operation "using a cyanthus of it for such as cannot sleep or are grievously pained and upon whom being cut or cauterized they wish to make no pain."[1]

The use of both ether and nitrous oxide to enliven parties brought these substances to the attention of Crawford Long, Horace Wells, and William T.G. Morton. In 1842, William E. Clarke, a medical student, administered ether to a friend for the extraction of a tooth, the dentist being Dr. Elijah Pope. Two months later, in March 1842, Crawford Long used ether for the removal of a small tumor from the neck of a friend. He apparently thought little of the experience and did not publish an account of it. On October 16, 1846, William T.G. Morton demonstrated the anesthetic properties of ether at the Massachusetts General Hospital when John Collins Warren removed a tumor from a man's neck.

In 1871, Trendelenburg, to facilitate operations on the upper air passages, did a tracheostomy and passed a tube with an inflatable cuff into the trachea. This was connected to an anesthetic cone for the administration of anesthesia. In 1878, endotracheal intubation as currently used was introduced by Macewin. He passed an oral endotracheal tube by the sense of touch for the relief of edema of the glottis and then employed this method for anesthesia in cases of extensive surgery within the mouth.

Subsequently Joseph O'Dwyer of New York and Rudolph Matas in 1900 expanded the utilization of endotracheal intubation and recommended its adaption for thoracic surgery. In 1928, Arthur E. Guedel described the inflatable cuff for the endotracheal tube that has since come into general use. In 1932, Ralph Waters and Gale introduced a cuffed tube that could be inserted into an individual bronchus permitting ventilation of a single lung.

Successfully managing patients with thoracic trauma requires a well coordinated team of emergency room physicians, surgeons, and anesthesiologists. The primary goals in such life-threatening situations are restoration of blood volume and cardiac output, protection of the airway, and control of ventilation. Anesthetic goals include successful resuscitation, safe analgesia and anesthesia, and creating optimum conditions for surgical intervention.

PREANESTHETIC CONSIDERATIONS

Resuscitation

The anesthesiologist can have an important role in the emergency room. When a severely traumatized patient arrives, an anesthesiologist should be available to assist with resuscitation and with initial evaluation. If possible, this anesthesiologist should remain in attendance if resuscitation and continuing treatment are required. Many of the complications that occur in emergency rooms could be avoided if an anesthesiologist were present to ensure proper placement of the endotracheal tube and adequate ventilation.

When intubation is required in the initial resuscitation, certain precautions must be observed. Cervical spinal injury requires stabilization of the neck during intubation, and fractures of the face and base of the skull are contraindications to nasal insertion of endotracheal and gastric tubes. Events that are important in anesthetic management sometimes are not documented during a crisis and can be appreciated only by personal observation. The anesthesiologist who remains in attendance will know the drugs and fluids that have been given, will be able to observe the patient's response to treatment, and will know the location and gauge of the intravenous catheters. Finally, in the event that a thoracotomy is performed in the emergency room, the anesthesiologist will be present to assist.

Preanesthetic Evaluation

The urgency of many thoracic injuries allows only a brief and sometimes incomplete evaluation. The primary concern is the effect of thoracic trauma on cardiopulmonary function. Information is needed regarding the nature of the thoracic injury, the patient's response to volume resuscitation, and the presence or absence of preexisting cardiopulmonary and vascular disease. Inspection and auscultation of the chest and, if the patient is intubated, appreciation of the total thoracic compliance are important parts of initial evaluation. Associated trauma to the central nervous system, the cervical spine, the abdominal area, and the lower extremities should be noted; pupil size, equality, and reactivity to light should be assessed as well as the level of consciousness because cerebral ischemia may result from shock or hypoxia. Evidence of occult blood loss into the abdomen and lower extremities should be sought. The possibility of hypothermia should be considered in all trauma patients. Resuscitation and surgical intervention usually are successful in healthy young patients after trauma, although some may be chronic drug or alcohol users. Unfortunately, the mortality in the elderly population is high because of the higher incidence of chronic diseases in this group.

Although paramedics in most big cities are capable of endotracheal intubation at the accident scene, aspiration pneumonitis remains a major cause of morbidity. Bleeding from the oral pharynx, whether due to airway injury or resulting from multiple attempts at laryngoscopy or nasotracheal intubation, can result in aspiration of blood or poor visualization of the larynx. Copious bleeding through the endotracheal tube usually results from pulmonary hemorrhage or tear and has to be attended to immediately in the operating room. A summary of the preanesthetic evaluation is shown in Table 7–1.

Transport to the Operating Room

When the injury is critical, the primary objectives during transportation are to continue resuscitation, to avoid deceleration-acceleration stress in a hypovolemic patient, and to prevent accidental loss of therapeutic channels (endotracheal tube, intravenous infusion line, chest tubes) during movement. Delays in transport should be minimized. Elevators should be under the direct control of the transporting team and the operating room should be ready. Clear directions to the proper operating room should be given and passage should be unobstructed by equipment or supplies. Operating room personnel should be available to continue transportation into the operating room area.

A common practice in major trauma centers is to designate a trauma operating room. Anesthetic machines can be set up in part in advance, as can administration sets for infusion of normal saline solution and blood. The room should be large enough for monitors and additional equipment that may be needed, such as cardiopulmonary bypass machines, autotransfuser, warming blanket, defibrillator, and x-ray machine.

The anesthesiologist is responsible for continuing resuscitation, administering the anesthetic, and monitoring the patient. The surgeon should be free to devote his attention to controlling the hemorrhage, administering open chest cardiac massage if needed, and restoring cardiopulmonary function, such as in relief of cardiac tamponade or tension pneumothorax. Extra personnel may be needed to assist with volume resuscitation, to bring

Table 7–1. Preanesthetic Evaluation

Airway and respiration
  Upper and lower airway patency; airway trauma, pulmonary aspiration?
Circulation
  Presence or absence of shock?
  Adequacy of volume resuscitation?
  Location and gauge of intravenous catheters?
  Amount of blood available or when it will be available?
Central nervous system
  Level of consciousness?
  Recent use of alcohol or other centrally active drugs?
  Pupils, size, equality, and reaction to light?
  Possibility of cervical spine injury?
Associated injuries to other systems
History (if available) of preexisting disease and medical treatment

samples to the clinical laboratory, or to bring blood and coagulation factors from the blood bank to the operating room.

Monitoring

Routine monitoring consists of an electrocardiogram, blood pressure cuff, precordial or esophageal stethoscope, pulse oximetry, and capnography. Invasive monitoring should be added only if resuscitation and surgical control of the bleeding can be effectively continued at the same time.

Transesophageal echocardiography (TEE) is a noninvasive tool for assessing cardiac function. It is considered the gold standard for myocardial ischemia detection.[2] Wall motion abnormalities could be the result of ischemic heart disease or newly diagnosed myocardial contusion. Left ventricular function can be determined by measurements of end-diastolic and end-systolic areas.[3] According to the following, fractional area change (FAC):

$$\text{FAC\%} = \frac{\text{End-diastolic area} = \text{End-systolic area}}{\text{End-diastolic area}} \times 100$$

The FAC provides a good estimate of the ejection fraction.

Preload or left ventricular filling usually is measured by pulmonary capillary wedge pressure; however, in patients with reduced ventricular compliance or mitral valve dysfunction, such measurements are grossly inaccurate and TEE can provide a better estimate of preload by measuring the left ventricular end-diastolic area. It is important to emphasize that in patients with reduced ventricular compliance, pulmonary capillary wedge pressure does not truly reflect preload.

TEE could also aid in the diagnosis of myocardial injury. It allows a complete examination of the mitral, tricuspid, and aortic valves, and color flow will allow the detection of ventricular septal defects. Pericardial effusion is detected easily and suggests the possibility of injury to the heart chambers or a periaortic leak from transection of the aorta.

There are several contraindications for the use of TEE; these are esophageal constrictions, the presence of tumor, or varices of the esophagus. Although placement is relatively easy, interpretation of TEE should not be attempted by an inexperienced anesthesiologist and should not detract that person from the anesthetic management or resuscitation measures. However, as anesthesiologists become more familiar with TEE, this probably will become standard monitoring especially during the anesthetic management of critical cases such as chest trauma. Table 7–2 lists the various monitored parameters and the conditions that may be recognized in patients with thoracic trauma.

ANESTHESIA PHASE

Anesthesia

The choice of induction agents depends on the adequacy of preinduction volume replacement and the possibility of ventricular dysfunction due to disease or trauma. Intravenous agents are generally preferred for rapid induction to reduce the risk of aspiration. Because

Table 7–2. Intraoperative Monitoring

MONITORING	PROBLEMS TO BE IDENTIFIED	INFORMATION OBTAINED
Routine		
Esophageal Stethoscope	Breath sounds	
Temperature probe (oral, rectal, or tympanic)	Hypothermia	
Electrocardiography	Hypothermia, arrhythmia, myocardial contusion, and hypocalcemia	
Capnogram	Inadequate ventilation	End-tidal CO_2
Pulse oximetry		
Hemodynamic	Oxygenation	O_2 saturation
Arterial catheter		Continuous systemic pressures, arterial blood gases, blood for cross-match, and other clinical laboratory studies
Central venous catheter		Right heart filling pressure, management of venous air embolism, infusion of cardiac and vasoactive drugs
Pulmonary artery catheter		Left heart filling pressure, cardiac output, core temperature, mixed venous blood samples
Transesophageal echocardiography		Wall motion abnormalities, ejection fraction, cardiac injury

of the myocardial depressant effects of thiopental, ketamine has been suggested as an alternative agent when the adequacy of blood volume is in question. Ketamine has sympathomimetic cardiovascular effects, but the effects are indirect. In the absence of additional sympathetic recruitment, ketamine may have a depressant effect. New intravenous induction agents have been lately introduced; these are propofol, etomidate, and midazolam, a short-acting benzodiazepine. These agents lack the myocardial depressant effect of thiopental but cause profound decreases in blood pressure in the hypovolemic patient. So far, ketamine in conjunction with a small dose of benzodiazepine is the agent of choice in such situations.

The new muscle relaxants vecuronium, pipecuronium, and doxycurium lack any cardiovascular effects; however, pipecuronium and doxycurium have not been tested in the trauma setting. Both are long-acting agents and seem to be attractive choices during long surgical procedures. However, the main concern usually is in the selection of the appropriate muscle relaxant during induction of anesthesia, especially during rapid sequence induction, for prevention of aspiration. So far, succinylcholine provides the best intubating conditions (i.e., vocal cord relaxation within 60 sec). Vecuronium 0.3 mg/kg will also result in excellent intubating conditions within 45 to 60 sec; however, this will lead to a longer duration of action at this dose. This may not be a major concern in chest trauma as the surgical procedure probably will outlast the duration of the drug. Anesthesia usually is maintained by using a balance of low-dose narcotic-inhalation agents (as tolerated by the patient) with muscle relaxants as adjuvants. Among the inhalation agents, nitrous oxide is avoided in the presence of hypoxemia, ventilation perfusion abnormalities, or gas cavities such as pneumothorax. Narcotics offer the advantage of causing very few circulatory disturbances. Amnesia can be provided by using scopolamine or diazepam. These recommendations are summarized in Table 7–3.

Airway Management

Trauma patients are presumed to be at high risk for aspiration of gastric contents. The most common method for immediately securing the airway is a rapid sequence of induction and intubation if the patient has not already been intubated in the emergency room. Endobronchial intubation is indicated when a major airway bleed occurs, overt bronchial injury with a major air leak occurs, pulmonary resection is anticipated, or repair of thoracic aortic transection is necessary (Table 7–4).

Endobronchial intubation should be performed only in the operating room. The use of the left-side tube is indicated in most instances as proper positioning of the right-side tube requires very careful positioning with fiberoptic confirmation. The main concern during right-side intubation is obstruction of the right upper lobe bronchus by the tip of the tube or the bronchial cuff, which could lead to severe hypoxemia if ventilation was mainly through that lung.

A serious anesthetic challenge is a difficult intubation in a hypoxemic patient. If the patient is already intubated, the orotracheal tube could be replaced by the endobronchial tube through the tube changer. Recent modifications of the tube changer permit insufflation of oxygen, and lengthening of the catheter allows safe replacement with the endobronchial tube.

The design of a new endobronchial blocker may facilitate endobronchial intubation and selective lung ventilation in an emergency setting. This new tube, Univent, is very

Table 7–3.   Anesthetic Induction

HEMODYNAMIC STATUS	SHOCK	HYPOTENSION	STABLE
Induction	Continue resuscitation	Ketamine	Barbiturate or diazepam and narcotics
Intubation	Usually has already been intubated	Rapid sequence induction and intubation with cricoid pressure	
Maintenance	Paralysis and oxygen initially; analgesia and anesthesia are added when the conditions are stable	Narcotics and low-dose inhalation agents with neuromuscular blockade	

Table 7–4.   Indications for Endobronchial Intubation

Major airway bleed
Bronchial injury with major air leak
Planned pulmonary resection
Thoracic aortic transection

similar to an endotracheal tube. Placement of that tube requires rotation of the tube toward the side to be isolated. Once the tube is placed, the endobronchial blocker is advanced and the cuff is inflated, after which selective lung ventilation can be performed (Fig. 7–1). In addition to its ease of insertion, this tube does not need replacement at the end of the procedure, as required with endobronchial tubes. A major disadvantage in the current tube design is that it has a low volume high pressure cuff, which is relatively contraindicated during prolonged ventilatory support.

In the presence of major bleeding, when blood floods the lumen of either the endobronchial or endotracheal tubes, the thoracic surgeon should be consulted and rigid bronchoscopy and endobronchial blocking of that segment is indicated to control the bleeding, allow safe ventilation of the patient, and prevent spillage in the normal lung.

In the patient with known or suspected cervical spine injuries, awake, blind, or fiberoptic assisted nasotracheal intubation can be attempted if the situation and time permit. In more urgent cases, the patient can be intubated without neck extension by retracting the tongue and using the epiglottis tip as a landmark for blind oral passage of an endotracheal tube that is appropriately curved with a stylet. Another person should assist in stabilizing the patient's head, since the anesthesiologist's attention is focused on endoscopy and intubation.

A patient who is already intubated on arrival in the operating room should have the endotracheal tube position rechecked and the length marking noted because displacement is possible during transport.

Ventilation

Proper endotracheal or endobronchial tube placement should always be verified by auscultation of the lungs, by monitoring pulse oximetry and end-tidal CO_2, and by fiberoptic bronchoscopy in the case of endobronchial intubation. Fiberoptic bronchoscopy can be performed safely by an experienced anesthesiologist. A fiberoptic bronchoscope swivel adapter is attached to the tracheal port of an endobronchial tube and the fiberoptic bronchoscope is passed through that. The patient should receive 100% oxygen at high flow rates to compensate for leakage around the scope. Proper positioning of the endobronchial tube is confirmed by visualization of the main carina, with the right main stem orifice to the right, and the proximal sleeve of the blue endobronchial cuff to the left, just beneath the orifice of the left main stem. The presence of bubbles around the blue cuff indicates an air leak and the cuff should be inflated until there is no air leak. Herniation above the carina can obstruct the right main bronchus and lead to inadequate ventilation (see Fig. 7–2 for proper tube confirmation).

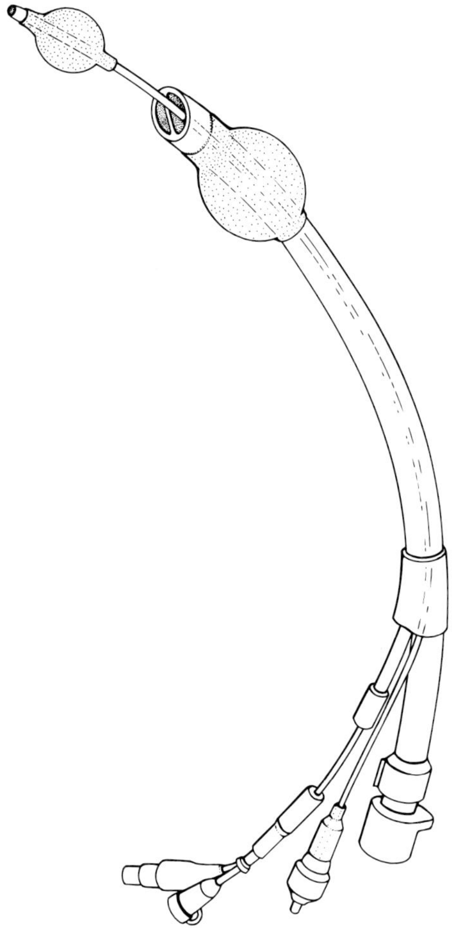

Figure 7–1. The Univent Inoue tube with the endobronchial blocker that is advanced toward the side to be isolated.

Ventilation for chest trauma and for one-lung ventilation should always be initiated using 100% inspired oxygen. The fraction of inspired oxygen could be decreased depending on the results of the arterial blood gases. A significant alveolar to arterial oxygen tension difference (fraction inspired oxygen = 1) indicates pulmonary shunting. The application of positive end-expiratory pressure (PEEP) should decrease the difference and improve oxygenation. It is important to remember that PEEP will decrease cardiac output in the presence of hypovolemia and this may increase venous admixture and decrease the arterial oxygen tension. PEEP may be required in patients with pulmonary edema, inhalation injury, pulmonary aspiration, and pulmonary contusion. Excessive airway pressures should be avoided in patients with pericardial tamponade and hypovolemia, since the cardiac output will be further compromised.

If oxygenation is inadequate during one-lung ventilation, then continuous positive airway pressure (CPAP) at 5 to 10 cm should be applied to the nonventilated lung.[4] This will allow differential perfusion to the ventilated lung and minimize shunting. If hypoxemia still

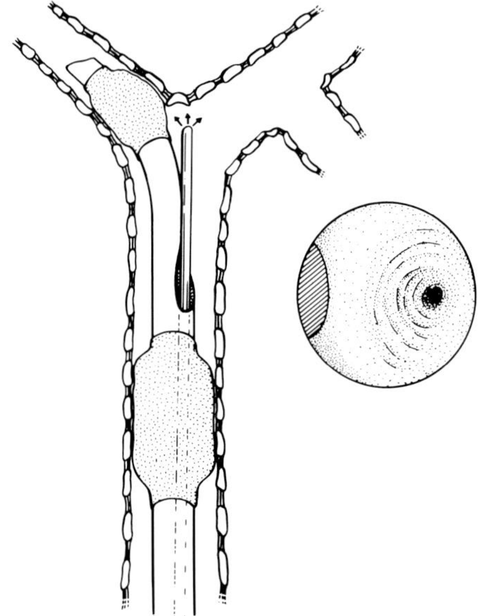

Figure 7–2.   An illustration of a clear view of the carina and right mainstem bronchial orifice with a rim of the blue endobronchial cuff just beneath the left main bronchial orifice, as seen through the fiberoptic bronchoscope.

persists as detected by the oxygen saturation monitor, then PEEP can be applied to the ventilated or dependent lung. If this does not correct the problem, then the deflated lung should be ventilated occasionally if the situation permits. Temporary occlusion of the pulmonary artery of the nonventilated lung may minimize shunting and improve oxygenation. Deflation of the lung usually results in hypoxic pulmonary vasoconstriction (HPVC) with redistribution of blood flow to the ventilated lung. Inhalation anesthetic agents do attenuate the HPVC response but this bears no clinical significance, as 100% inspired oxygen can be provided with these agents.[5] In severe hypoxemia, or patients with badly traumatized lungs with adult respiratory distress syndrome (ARDS), prostaglandin E_1 (PGE_1)[6] infusion usually results in improvement in oxygenation and ventilation. The use of an extracorporeal membrane[7] oxygenator is widely accepted and is applicable to those situations where there is an isolated lung pathology with no other injuries that could be adversely affected by systemic heparinization. The lungs are allowed to rest, and peak positive airway pressures are decreased; however, PEEP at 5 to 10 cm water should be applied to keep the alveoli open.[8] If there is respiratory failure with respiratory acidosis not responding to conventional pressure or volume ventilators, then high frequency jet ventilation should be instituted.

Pulmonary aspiration is a frequent complication of trauma and severely compromises the survival of the patient with thoracic injury. The severity of the pulmonary damage depends on the amount and type of material aspirated. Aspiration of gastric acid and food fibers usually is more severe than aspiration of blood or saliva. Intubation, mechanical ventilation, and high inspired oxygen concentration with addition of PEEP are indicated if hypoxia persists. Bronchoscopy is indicated only for aspiration of large particulate matter such as food or blood clots.

Circulatory Support

Advances in trauma resuscitation have finally put the crystalloids/colloids controversy to rest. Holcroft and associates[9,10] have shown convincing evidence of the successful use of hypertonic saline in dextran, in both the animal shock model and in trauma victims resuscitated in the field.

Appropriate hemodynamic monitoring is crucial for adequate cardiovascular control. Aggressive and invasive hemodynamic monitoring should be instituted immediately during the anesthetic management of major chest trauma. Swan-Ganz catheter placement is indicated under these situations: a) elderly victims of trauma, b) major pulmonary contusions, with ARDS pattern, c) patients with severe obstructive or restrictive pulmonary disease, and 4) myocardial contusions and emergency surgery (Table 7–5). It is important to note that TEE does not replace Swan-Ganz catheter monitoring, but information obtained from each is valuable and complementary and optimizes intraoperative management.

Emphasis has been placed on restoring blood volume to maintain circulatory stability. Adequate cardiac function is equally important since prolonged low cardiac output states will produce myocardial depression, renal failure, and pulmonary dysfunction. Figure 7–3 shows the pathophysiology of hemorrhagic shock and the points at which the anesthesiologist may attempt to intervene. When there is no improvement in mean arterial pressure (MAP) despite adequate volume replacement and control of hemorrhage, left ventricular dysfunction must be suspected and be confirmed by an elevated pulmonary artery wedge pressure. In this situation inotropic support using either dopamine or dobutamine (4–10 μg/kg/min) should be started. Dopamine improves ventricular function and is known to have selective renal vasodilatory effects. In equipotent doses both dopamine and dobutamine have the same effects on glomerular filtration rates and renal hemodynamics; however, dopamine has a direct tubular effect resulting in significant diuresis and natriuresis. If there is no response to either dopamine or dobutamine, then epinephrine could be administered starting at doses of 0.05 to 0.1 μg/kg/min.

A new group of drugs, phosphodiesterase type III inhibitors (PDI III), known as inodialators for their ability to improve contractility and increase cardiac output, are currently being used in conjunction with epinephrine or norepinephrine during cardiac surgery. These agents have vasodilatory effects, reduce pulmonary vascular resistance, and have little effect on the heart rate, thereby reducing myocardial oxygen consumption. There is potential use for these agents in patients with ischemic heart disease and depressed left ventricular function suffering from major trauma, in patients with severe right ventricular failure, and in patients who have blunted responses to the usual inotropic therapy (due to congestive heart failure and/or beta or calcium channel blockade).

Hypocalcemia due to citrate binding from massive transfusion should be corrected by

Table 7–5.   Indications for Pulmonary Artery Catheterization

Elderly victims of trauma
Major pulmonary contusions with ARDS
Severe obstructive or restrictive pulmonary disease
Myocardial contusion and emergency surgery

ARDS, adult respiratory distress syndrome.

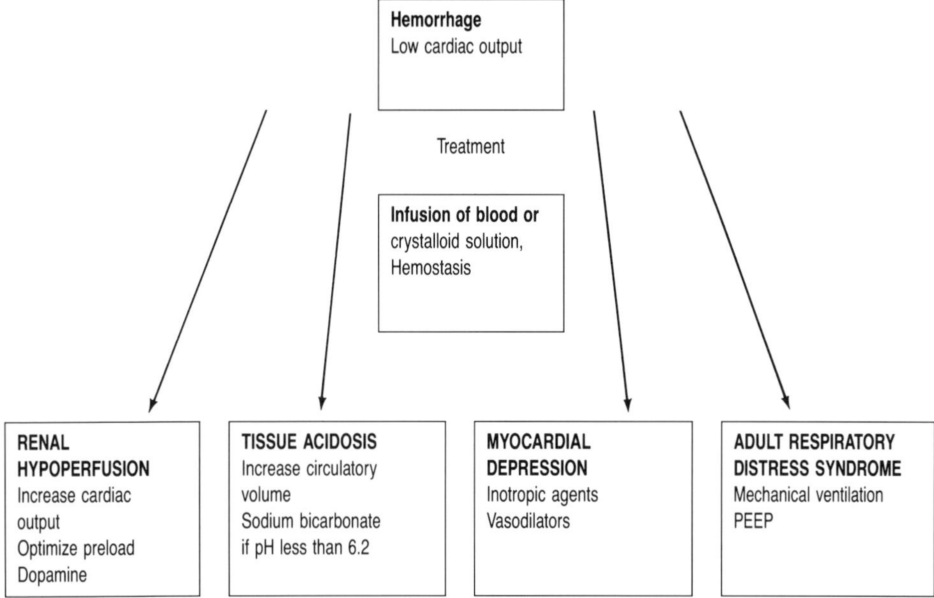

Figure 7–3.   Schematic diagram of the pathophysiology of hemorrhage and shock and therapeutic interventions.

infusions of calcium chloride. Such therapy is facilitated by analysis of serum ionic calcium levels. The lack of correlation between total serum calcium and ionic calcium has been demonstrated in patients receiving massive transfusion during hepatic transplantation.[11,12] Vasopressors generally are not used in the management of shock. They are occasionally a last resort when myocardial perfusion is jeopardized, and their use also has been suggested as a temporizing measure in neurogenic shock after spinal cord injury. Table 7–6 lists the commonly used inotropic agents.

Arrhythmias must be treated to optimize cardiac function. Sinus tachycardia due to left ventricular failure should be treated with digoxin for its vagotonic effect, but potent inotropic agents, such as dobutamine and dopamine, also should be given. Ventricular irritability, usually a result of hypoxia or acidosis, should be treated by correcting the cause; however, lidocaine bolus (1 mg/kg) may be given and an infusion started at 2 to 4 mg/min to maintain constant blood levels. Other antiarrhythmic drugs, such as procainamide, phenytoin, propranolol, and bretylium, can be used. Heart block secondary to penetrating injuries of the heart is best treated with transcutaneous pacemaker.

Acid-base Electrolyte Status

Serial determinations of arterial blood gases and electrolytes are mandatory and corrections should be made when such disturbances threaten to impair cardiac function. It is almost impossible to correct acidosis when there is uncontrollable hemorrhage and circulatory collapse, and repeated administration of sodium bicarbonate may cause an increased

Table 7–6.   List of Commonly Used Inotropic Agents

AGENT	DOSE RANGE	EFFECT	ADVANTAGES
Dopamine	1–2 μg/kg/min 2–10 μg/kg/min 10–15 μg/kg/min >15 μg/kg/min	DA_1, DA_2 β_1 DA β_1, α & DA α	Better renal perfusion through effect on dopaminergic receptors
Dobutamine	5–15 μg/kg/min	β_1 & β_2	Acts directly on beta-receptor, less tachy-arrhythmias: decreased pulmonary wedge pressure and systemic vascular resistance
Isoproterenol	0.015–0.1 μg/kg/min	β	Useful in presence of atrioventricular block and sinus bradycardia
Norepinephrine	High-dose 0.1 μg/kg/min	α on vessels β on heart	Used in combination with vasodilator therapy in cardiogenic shock or in sepsis
Epinephrine	Small doses Higher doses Recommended dose 0.04–0.01 μg/kg/min	β α	Useful during resuscitation for cardiac arrest or impending arrest
Digoxin	0.125–25 mg intravenously, repeat in 20 min	Vagotonic, very weak inotrope	Suppresses sinus tachycardia in congestive heart failure; decreases ventricular response in atrial fibrillation
CA^{2+}	10–20 mg/kg	+ + Inotropic	Enhances catecholamine effect, counteracts myocardial depression 2° to protamine or citrated blood
Amrinone	Loading dose: 1.25–2 mg/kg maintenance: 5–15 μg/kg/min	+ + Inotropic	Improves right ventricular function; increases cardiac output; effective in the presence of attenuated responses to adrenergic inotropes

osmotic load and brain cellular dehydration. Although hyperventilation may control acidemia, deleterious effects such as hypocapnia, decreased cerebral blood flow, and increased oxygen affinity to hemoglobin may occur.

Transfusion

The rapid infuser, or a Trauma Level I that has warming capabilities, is capable of delivering blood rapidly. If the patient has lower extremity fractures or injuries, then delivery of blood and fluids should be made through venous cannulations in the upper extremity.

In major chest trauma, blood volume should be replaced based on measurements of preload, cardiac output, and hematocrit concentration. The use of hypertonic saline in dextran for initial resuscitation minimizes the amount of crystalloid infusion, thereby decreasing hemodilution and interstitial fluid expansion.

In an era with fear of transmission of diseases such as autoimmune deficiency syndrome (AIDS), hepatitis, or cytomegalic virus (CMV), anesthesiologists and surgeons have been overtly conservative in using blood transfusion. For a young trauma victim, an acceptable hematocrit is 20% beyond which blood should be transfused, especially when more bleeding is anticipated. In the elderly patient with ischemic heart disease or pulmonary dysfunction, hematocrit should be maintained above 30%. Type O-negative blood usually is administered if there is no type-specific blood available.

Although there could be pro and con arguments for the use of blood filters, a great advantage in using them is the sparing of the IV administration set from blood clogging that would result in decreases in blood flow rate, necessitating replacement of such sets. It is preferable to avoid the infusion of Ringer's lactate through the blood line as the calcium in Ringer's lactate could stimulate coagulation of citrated blood.

Coagulation factors can be given according to estimated blood volume: 10 platelet packs and 2 U of fresh frozen plasma per 5 L of transfused blood in a patient weighing 70 kg. As noted above, calcium chloride may be required to counteract the effect of citrate after rapid infusion of stored blood. Prolongation of the corrected QT interval on the electrocardiogram indicates hypocalcemia; however, this will be a late finding and levels of serum ionic calcium should be continuously analyzed.

Summary

In summary, a number of problems can arise during the anesthetic management of trauma patients, the most important being hypotension, hypoxemia, and inability to ventilate. Immediate recognition of the problem and its management are mandatory. A brief summary of the differential diagnosis is shown in Table 7–7.

HOW TO DEAL WITH A DIFFICULT AIRWAY

Among the most dreaded and challenging airway situations facing an anesthesiologist are changing an endotracheal tube in a patient with a difficult airway or in a patient who has severe respiratory insufficiency with severe hypoxemia requiring high ventilatory pres-

Table 7–7.   Differential Diagnosis of Intraoperative Problems

Hypotension
Hypovolemia, cardiac tamponade, tension pneumothorax, air embolism, severe hypoxemia, hypocalcemia, transfusion of cold blood, surgical occlusion of venous return, transducer artifact, hypothermia
Hypoxemia
Pulmonary contusion, pulmonary edema, aspiration pneumonia, low cardiac output, main stem intubation, smoke inhalation
Inability to ventilate
Tension pneumothorax, bronchospasm, blood clot or foreign body in the airway, endobronchial intubation, overinflation of the endotracheal tube cuff, kinked endotracheal tube pulmonary congestion

sures, PEEP, and fraction of inspired oxygen. The tube changer with a ventilatory port is designed for use in these situations (see Fig. 7–4). When confronted with a difficult intubation, the tube changer is passed through the old endotracheal tube and oxygen is insufflated through the proximal port. The old tube is then pulled out and the new tube is slid over the changer. Once in place, the tube changer can be pulled out. In the patient with severe respiratory failure, interruption of ventilation could be costly. In such situations, it is preferable to visualize the larynx, then pass the tube changer alongside the orotracheal tube. An orotracheal tube is then slipped over the changer. Once it is in the oral pharynx, the old

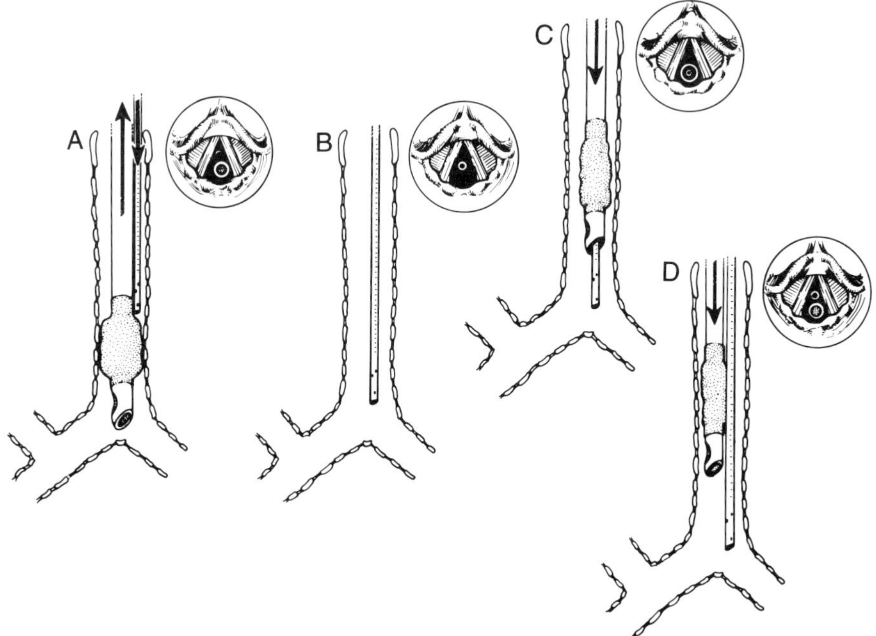

Figure 7–4.   Tube replacement utilizing the endotracheal tube changer (*TC*) with a ventilating port. **A:** The TC is introduced through the cords alongside the old endotracheal tube. **B:** Oxygenation is provided by the TC while the old tube is withdrawn. **C:** The new ETT could be advanced over the TC, or **D:** advanced alongside it if laryngoscopy is feasible.

tube can be pulled out and the new tube is advanced in the trachea and secured. This technique provides oxygenation during the brief period of pulling out the old tube. Another situation that is frowned on is changing an endobronchial tube after lengthy operations involving major fluid and blood losses. Facial edema and tongue and lip swelling make airway visualization almost impossible even though there was a normal anatomy previously. This can be dealt with after thoracic aortic tears by leaving the endobronchial tube in, using the tube changer, or using the bronchial blocker, Univent, which does not require replacement at the end of the case.

Airway and Ventilation Decisions

Because pulmonary gas exchange is likely to deteriorate in the first 24 hr postoperatively, a very conservative approach is justified in regard to extubation in high-risk cases. In addition, if the circulation is unstable, intubation and mechanical ventilation should be continued. Ventilator and oxygen settings can be initially identical to the settings that were used in the operating room, but since different ventilators may perform quite differently, arterial blood gas analysis should be done soon after arrival. Before leaving the patient, the position of the endotracheal tube should be checked.

Postoperative Analgesia

Epidural narcotics have significantly improved therapeutic modalities for pain relief and decreased morbidity and improved pulmonary function after thoracic surgery or trauma.[13–17] Contrary to former belief, thoracic epidural narcotics provide better relief for postthoracotomy surgery or rib fractures than lumbar epidural narcotics. In this author's experience, a smaller dose of epidural narcotic is required with thoracic epidural analgesia.

Epidural narcotics provide less respiratory depression than systemic narcotics, thus allowing early extubation and mobilization. They also do not produce sympathetic or motor blockade and thus have no deleterious effects on the cardiovascular system. The choice of the narcotic agent usually is predicated by the patient's response to the drug as well as the practice of the pain service and of the institution.

POSTANESTHESIA CONSIDERATIONS

Transfer from the Operating Room

The immediate postoperative objective is the safe physical transfer of the patient to the recovery room or intensive care unit, where physicians and nurses provide postoperative care. Although the details for accomplishing this objective are not particularly profound, they bear mentioning only because complications during transfer do occur. A prerequisite for physical transfer is the prior notification of the destination nursing unit so that a mechanical ventilator, electronic monitoring, and personnel will be immediately available to the patient on arrival. Prior notification can be facilitated by providing the nurses with a data sheet (see Table 7–8). The physical transfer should not be made if deterioration of

Table 7–8. Information for the Destination Nursing Unit
ICU Patient Information Sheet

(Addressograph)	
Admitting diagnosis:	
Surgical procedure:	
Ventilator: Volume: _______________________	Pressure: _______________________
Respiratory parameters:	
Tidal volume: _______________________	
Pressure: _______________________	
F_{IO_2}: _______________________	
PEEP: _______________________	
Rate:IMV: _______________________	
Patient's temperature: _______________________	
Arterial line: _______________________	RT LT
CVP/Swan-Ganz: _______________________	RT LT
IV: _______________________	RT LT
IV drips:	
Dopamine _______________________ µg/kg/min	
Dobutamine _______________________ µg/kg/min	
Nitroglycerine _______________________ µg/kg/min	
Nitroprusside _______________________ µg/kg/min	
Lidocaine _______________________ µg/kg/min	
Other _______________________ µg/kg/min	
Intraoperative complications:	
Comments:	
Estimated arrival time to ICU: _______________	

Anesthesiologist's Signature

---

cardiopulmonary function is likely to occur en route. A nonrebreathing system to deliver oxygen and high-pressure ventilation may be required as well as fluids, drugs, and even a portable defibrillator. Continuous monitoring by pulse oximetry, a portable monitor for electrocardiography, and arterial pressure are indicated in the patient whose condition remains critical.

Special care is required to avoid the complications of accidentally disconnecting, obstructing, or removing chest tubes, endotracheal tube, or intravenous tubing during movement of the patient. Infusions of drugs or fluid volume needed for cardiovascular support should be clearly labeled and running. Hallways should be unobstructed.

Transfer of the medical data on the patient is accomplished by a concise, accurate summary of essential information accumulated during the intraoperative course. This summary should be given verbally to the surgeon and entered into the patient's record as a postanesthetic note, which should include a statement of cardiovascular and pulmonary problems, a total of fluid volumes, an estimate of residual anesthetic and muscle relaxant effects, and a discussion of continuing therapy.

Patients undergoing thoracic surgery for major trauma usually will be admitted to an intensive care setting where there is intensive monitoring for several days. These patients will require ventilatory support and are least likely to develop respiratory depression resulting from rostral spread of epidural narcotics. However, those patients who do not undergo chest surgery but have numerous rib fractures are managed in a monitored area or telemetry unit. There are specific orders prescribed by the anesthesiologist or the pain service that deal with respiratory depression, infection, itching, or urinary retention—all potential problems of epidural narcotic administration (Table 7–9). The pain service provides continuous 24-hr coverage for in-house patients. Telemetry nurses participating in the care of such patients are educated and trained to take care of these patients.

CONSIDERATIONS FOR SPECIFIC AREAS OF INJURY

The pathophysiology and diagnosis of specific conditions are discussed in the chapters describing surgical management and will not be repeated here. The considerations to be discussed refer to anesthetic management.

Upper and Lower Airway

Rupture of the trachea or bronchus can lead to pneumothorax, pneumomediastinum, and subcutaneous emphysema. In the case of bronchial rupture, endobronchial intubation or

Table 7–9.　Acute Pain Service: Epidural Narcotic Standard Orders

1. Operating room dose: Drug _________ Mg _________ Time _________
2. Drug for continuing epidural analgesia:
   A.　PF morphine (1 mg/ml) _________ mg every 6–12 hr.
   B.　Fentanyl (10 μg/ml normal saline) infuse _________ μg (_________ ml)/per hr.
   C.　Other: Drug _________ Concentration _________ Dose _________ Interval _________
3. Fentanyl 50 μg (1.0 ml) into epidural catheter every 3 hr as needed for inadequate analgesia with prescribed dose above.
4. Maintain iv access (drip or heparin lock) for 24 hr after last dose of epidural narcotic.
5. Naloxone 0.4 mg at bedside.
6. No narcotics or other CNS depressants to be given except as ordered by the Acute Pain Service.
7. Monitoring: Respiratory rate and sedation scale every 1 hr for 1st 24 hr, and then every 4 hr.
8. Treatment of side effects:
   A.　Call Acute Pain Service if sedation scale = 3.
   B.　Call Acute Pain Service if respiratory rate is <8 breaths per min.
   C.　Naloxone 0.4 mg iv stat for sedation scale = 3 plus respiratory rate <8 breaths per min. Call Acute Pain Service.
   D.　Metoclopramide 10 mg iv q 6 h prn for nausea/vomiting. In addition, if age <60 yr, transdermal scopolamine patch to either mastoid area. Change every 72 hr as needed.
   E.　Diphenhydramine 25 mg iv every 6 hr as needed for severe itching.
   F.　For urinary retention, "in-and-out" bladder catheter as needed.
9. For inadequate analgesia or other problems related to epidural, call Acute Pain Service.
10. Triazolam 0.125 mg every 1 hr as needed. May repeat × 1.

Date _________________________　_________________________________ M.D.

Dr. _________________________ on the APS was notified about this patient at _________________ hr.

Appendix
Example of Bedside Sedation Scale

Sedation	Description
0 (none)	Alert
1 (mild)	Occasionally drowsy; easy to arouse
2 (moderate)	Frequently drowsy; easy to arouse
3 (severe)	Somnolent; difficult to arouse
S (sleeping)	Normal sleep; easy to arouse

insertion of a double lumen tube will permit ventilation during reanastomosis. In the patient who is already intubated with a conventional tube, bronchial intubation can be accomplished by advancing the tube while the surgeon guides the tip into the contralateral main stem bronchus. A double lumen tube should be changed to a conventional tube at the end of the procedure if postoperative ventilation will be required. The use of high-frequency positive pressure jet ventilation has been successful in the management of patients with bronchopleural fistulas, which provides adequate ventilation with little hemodynamic changes and lower mean peak airway pressures.

Chest Wall and Pleura

Pneumothorax is a potential complication in most thoracic injuries. When pneumothorax has not been recognized preoperatively and a chest tube inserted, tension pneumothorax may develop as a complication of positive pressure ventilation during anesthesia. In addition to positive pressure, the use of nitrous oxide to provide anesthesia can cause a gas cavity to expand rapidly. In dogs, the volume of experimentally induced pneumothorax increased by 100% after 10 min of exposure to 75% nitrous oxide. Although pleural gas may not be present on the initial evaluation, pneumothorax can be introduced iatrogenically by misdirected attempts at subclavian catheterization, pericardiocentesis, and external cardiac compression; it also could result from failure of chest tubes to provide the expected relief of accumulated gas. Therefore, tension pneumothorax always must be included in the differential diagnosis of low pulmonary compliance and cardiovascular collapse.

The Heart

Penetrating injuries to the heart and great vessels are such life-threatening emergencies that the patient should be transferred immediately to the operating room for control of hemorrhage. Compression of cardiac chambers by blood in the pericardial sac can be rapidly fatal as cardiac output is progressively compromised. The circulation can be supported by cautious blood volume expansion, by inotropic agents, and by correction of metabolic acidosis. Induction of anesthesia and positive pressure breathing may lead to decompensation. Sedation with ketamine and surgical decompression under local anesthesia have been recommended. Once the cardiac tamponade has been relieved, anesthesia may be induced. Since tachycardia is part of the physiologic compensatory response to the low cardiac output, attempts should not be made to lower the heart rate artificially.

Patients with anterior chest wall contusions, pain or tenderness of the chest, and/or sternum or anterior rib fractures may well suffer a myocardial contusion. Patients suffering severe myocardial injuries will manifest so at the time of the emergency room admission. Although the diagnosis of myocardial contusion is an autopsy diagnosis, a high index of suspicion should be raised when there is blunt chest trauma associated with ST segment changes or arrhythmias seen on the electrocardiogram. Routine admission of these patients to an intensive care setting for observation does appear to be costly and has been deemed unnecessary by some observers[18,19] (see Chapter 15). Numerous screening tests have been advocated. These are serial electrocardiographs, CPK levels with CPK-MB fractions, two-dimensional echocardiography, and recently, TEE.[20] TEE provides excellent images, can be performed easily at the patient's bedside, and has the advantage over the conventional transthoracic echocardiography in that it provides better imaging and is not subject to interference by lungs, chest tubes, and tape. It can be placed easily and abnormalities of cardiac structures and aortic transections can be identified easily. Recently, cardiac troponin T (TNT) has been considered more specific for myocardial injury than CK-MB measurements.

In one study, surgical procedures requiring general anesthesia were performed in patients diagnosed as having myocardial injury, and there was no apparent increase in morbidity and mortality and significant arrhythmias were absent.[21] However, optimizing the anesthetic management of such patients requires Swan-Ganz catheter placement and possibly intraoperative TEE. Those patients suffering from right or left ventricular dysfunction should receive the same medical management as patients suffering from an acute myocardial infarction (i.e., nitrates, inotropes, beta and calcium antagonists as necessary).

Thoracic Aorta

Blunt trauma resulting in tears of the thoracic aorta usually are a result of motor vehicle accidents. Victims of ascending aortic tears and disruptions usually die at the scene of the accident, but those who make it to the hospital have an 80% chance of survival after surgery.

Tears of the ascending aorta could involve the aortic valve annulus, leading to acute aortic regurgitation, or can extend into the arch. The usual site of tear is in the descending thoracic aorta at the level of the ligamentum arteriosum. Such tears could involve the entire aortic wall or part of the intima or media. Hematomas resulting from such tears usually are contained by the adventitia but dissection of the hematoma can result in occlusion of major vessels. The diagnosis and surgical management are described in Chapter 16; however, once a diagnosis is made, preparation for emergency surgery should be immediately initiated. Such patients should have large-bore intravenous catheters placed as well as an indwelling catheter in the upper extremity for arterial pressure monitoring.

The most important aspect in medical management of aortic disruption is prompt recognition and control of systolic blood pressure and heart rate so as to decrease the possibility of dissection or bursting of the hematoma with resultant exsanguination. The medical therapy usually consists of the use of short-acting vasodilators such as sodium nitroprusside and beta antagonists such as Esmolol or Labetalol. Esmolol is a short-acting beta 1 selective antagonist with a distribution $t_{1/2}$ of 2 min and elimination $t_{1/2}$ of 9 min, which can be easily titrated, whereas Labetalol is both a nonselective beta and alpha$_1$ antagonist that has a distribution $t_{1/2}$ of 6 min and elimination $t_{1/2}$ of 2.9 to 8.5 hr, when given intravenously. The use of Labetalol is particularly desirable when there is significant hypertension not readily controlled by sodium nitroprusside. Sodium nitroprusside should be used in conjunction with a beta antagonist. Sodium nitroprusside should not be used alone in aortic tears as the widening of the pulse pressure and tachycardia resulting from nitroprusside can result in more shearing force on the aortic wall and tear. The use of sodium trimethaphan was advocated as a hypotensive agent for these aortic injuries as it lowers both systolic and diastolic components of the blood pressure and has little effect on the heart rate. Sodium trimethaphan has been substituted by the new selective and nonselective beta and alpha$_1$ antagonists.

The use of vasodilator therapy is particularly indicated in the management of aortic regurgitation. Acute aortic regurgitation can lead to sudden ventricular decompensation and unlike chronic regurgitation, the left ventricular chamber is small and noncompliant and cannot cope with sudden volume overload. Vasodilators tend to lower the regurgitant fraction and improve hemodynamics.

Patients scheduled for ascending aortic repair will need to have such repair done using extracorporeal circulation with possibly profound hypothermia and circulatory arrest if the arch vessels are involved. The anesthetic management of such patients is similar to those patients undergoing open-heart surgery with the exception of rapid sequence induction and intubation, if indicated. If the patient is in shock or is hemodynamically unstable, then he should be brought promptly to the operating room to undergo resuscitation or restoration of blood volume while surgery is expedited by femoral cannulation and institution of cardiopulmonary bypass. Patients may benefit from the administration of steroids and barbiturates, in addition to profound hypothermia, for brain protection during circulatory arrest for arch repairs. Additional cooling of the brain may be accomplished by local application of ice packs around the patient's head. Upon weaning off cardiopulmonary bypass the main concern is to correct any coagulopathy and control of hypertension. As mentioned earlier, this could be readily achieved by using Labetolol and sodium nitroprusside. Labetolol can be given in increments up to 75 mg.[22,23]

Acceptable surgical techniques for repair of tears of the descending thoracic aorta are: a) clamp and repair, b) aortic bypass shunt, c) full cardiopulmonary bypass, and d) left heart bypass utilizing a centrifugal pump with or without heparinization. This is accomplished using the left atrial–femoral bypass or femoral vein–femoral artery bypass.

Proximal descending aortic rupture is the most common of all aortic injuries and it is interesting and challenging for the anesthesiologist because adequate cardiopulmonary function has to be maintained during the surgical procedure. Of utmost importance in the anesthetic management is the establishment of large-bore IVs and endobronchial intubation for selective lung ventilation, and the crucial aspects of medical management are maintaining heart rate and systolic blood pressure control.

Intraoperative monitoring for aortic injuries should consist of routine monitoring, invasive hemodynamic monitoring, cerebrospinal fluid pressure (CSF) monitoring, and somatosensory evoked potential (SSEP) monitoring. The latter two monitoring devices should be used only when it is safe to do so but have special value in predicting and possibly helping prevent paraplegia, a most devastating complication of descending aortic injury.

Hemodynamic monitoring will include the routine monitoring as well as arterial pressure monitoring proximal and distal to the aortic clamps, as well as Swan-Ganz catheter monitoring. As the proximal clamp often is placed above the left subclavian artery, the right upper extremity is the one that should be cannulated for direct arterial pressure measurements in the upper body. Perfusion pressure in the lower body (mainly kidneys and spinal cord) is monitored through intraarterial cannulation of the right posterior tibial, dorsalis pedis, or femoral artery. A Swan-Ganz catheter is useful in monitoring left atrial pressure as well as in guiding pump flow rates and volume.

The use of TEE is particularly condemned by this author. Rotation of the TEE probe could result in malrotation or malposition of the endobronchial tube and proper tube positioning is crucial for a successful anesthetic and surgical management of descending aortic tears.

Induction of anesthesia will be dictated by the patrient's hemodynamic situation. If the patient is hypovolemic or in shock, then small doses of ketamine, a benzodiazepine, and narcotics should be used as appropriate; however, if the patient is stable and receiving vasodilators for blood pressure control, then using a sufentanil anesthetic with low dose isoflurane is preferable. The heart rate and blood pressure control that a sufentanil anesthetic provides is particularly desirable in this situation.

Endobronchial intubation is indicated if the patient's condition is stable. This will offer several advantages: better surgical exposure, less trauma to the lung, and isolation of bleeding from the right lung, especially after heparinization. In an intubated patient, the orotracheal tube should be replaced by an endobronchial tube or by the new endobronchial blocker, Univent, which does not require tube replacement at the end of the case.

Hemodynamic control is of great value in ensuring an optimal outcome. Successful management of thoracic tears has been accomplished by simple cross-clamping of the aorta and oversewing. This sudden increase in afterload can result in an increase in myocardial wall tension, myocardial oxygen consumption, and left ventricle failure. Sodium nitro-prusside has been used effectively to decrease the MAP.[24] However, concern exists for patients who have an intracranial injury with increased intracranial pressure (ICP), since sodium nitroprusside can cause a further increase in ICP.[25] In such situations, the use of the centrifugal pump without heparinization using either left atrial–femoral cannulation or femoral vein–femoral artery cannulation is advocated. This technique delivers blood flow to the lower body of 1.5 to 2½ L flow and a distal arterial pressure can be maintained around 50 mm Hg. The pulmonary capillary wedge pressure (PAW) should be maintained between 12 and 15.

Renal protection is another major concern and although it is controversial, the administration of mannitol is preferable before cross-clamping if no bypass or shunt is to be used. Another major concern is the development of coagulopathy due either to dilution of thrombocytopenia or disseminated intravascular coagulation (DIC), which should be treated by blood component therapy and/or factors. Disseminated intravascular coagulation can follow shock and soft tissue injury, or can be secondary to a hemolytic transfusion reaction. Fibrinolysis also is activated and could result in secondary bleeding. Hypothermia also results in diffuse oozing; therefore, all attempts should be made to maintain normothermia. Hypocalcemia resulting from massive transfusion of citrated blood may result in myocar-dial depression as noted earlier, and should be corrected by administration of calcium chloride.

Another frequent complication associated with aortic tears is the presence of myocar-dial or pulmonary contusion, resulting in cardiac and/or pulmonary dysfunction, respec-tively. Inotropes, antiarrhythmics, and vasodilator agents often are used to treat myocardial dysfunction. Hypoxemia resulting from severe pulmonary contusion will require high levels of PEEP and inspired oxygen, precluding the use of one lung ventilation.

Spinal Cord Protection

There is no single approach or technique for prevention of spinal cord ischemia (see Chapter 16). CSF monitoring and aspiration, as well as SSEP monitoring, have been clinically effective and have possibly prevented spinal cord ischemia in some cases. Papaverine, in combination with CSF aspiration, steroid administration before clamping, and with CSF drainage, have been used successfully in preventing paraplegia in animals. Partial exsanguination before thoracic aortic occlusion is another alternative technique in controlling proximal hypertension and in preventing the use of sodium nitroprusside with its possible deleterious effects on SCPP. More sensitive tools are being developed for monitoring cord blood supply, ultimately leading to early identification and implantation of critical arteries and helping identify cases that need distal shunting.

At the completion of the surgical procedure, the patient should be kept sedated and intubated, and the endobronchial tube should be replaced with an oral tracheal tube if the situation permits. In the presence of a difficult airway or tissue swelling, the patient could be left with the endobronchial tube and that tube replaced when the swelling has subsided.

If a catheter was placed for CSF drainage and aspiration, then before the removal of the catheter, intrathecal morphine or duramorph is injected through that catheter. This allows approximately 24 hr of analgesia without the use of supplemental intravenous narcotic.

REFERENCES

1. Meade RH. *A History of Thoracic Surgery.* Springfield, IL: Charles C Thomas; 1961.
2. Van Daele MERM, Sutherland GR, Mitchell MM, et al. Do changes in pulmonary capillary wedge pressure adequately reflect myocardial ischemia during anesthesia? A correlative preoperative hemodynamic, electrocardiographic, and transesophageal echocardiographic study. *Circulation.* 1990;81:865–871.
3. Clements FM, Harpole D, Quill TJ, et al. Simultaneous measurement of cardiac volumes, areas and ejection fractions by transesophageal echocardiography and first pass radionuclide angiography. *Anesthesiology.* 1988;69:A4. Abstract.
4. Benumof JL. Conventional and differential lung management of one-lung ventilation. In: Benumof JL, ed. *Anesthesia for Thoracic Surgery.* Philadelphia: Saunders; 1987:271–287.
5. Benumof JL, Augustine DS, Gibbons JA. Halothane and isoflurane only slightly impair arterial oxygenation during one-lung ventilation in patients undergoing thoracotomy. *Anesthesiology.* 1987;67:910–915.
6. Vassar MJ, Fletcher MP, Perry CA, Holcroft JW. Evaluation of prostaglandin E_1, for prevention of respiratory failure in high risk trauma patients: a prospective clinical trial and correlation with plasma suppressive factors for neutrophil activation. *Prostaglandins Leukotrienes and Essential Fatty Acids.* 1991;44:223–231.
7. Pennington OG. Symposium-circulatory support. *Ann Thorac Surg.* 1989;47:75–178.
8. Keszler M, Ryckman FC, McDonald JV, Jr, et al. A prospective, multicenter, randomized study of high versus low positive end-expiratory pressure during extracorporeal membrane oxygenation. *J Pediatrics.* 1992;120:107–113.
9. Halvorsen L, Gunther RA, Dubick MA, Holcroft JW. Dose response characteristics of hypertonic saline. *J Trauma.* 1991;31(6):785–796.
10. Vassar MJ, Perry CA, Gannaway WL, Holcroft JW. 7.5% sodium chloride/dextran for resuscitation of trauma patients undergoing helicopter transport. *Arch Surg.* 1991;126:1065–1072.
11. Kost GJ, Jammal MA, Ward RE, Safwat AM. Monitoring of ionized calcium during human hepatic transplantation. Clinical values and their relevance to cardiac and hemodynamic management. *Am J Clin Pathol.* 1986;86:61–70.
12. Marquez J, Martin D, Vinji MA, et al. Cardiovascular depression secondary to ionic hypocalcemia during hepatic transplantation in humans. *Anesthesiology.* 1986;65:457–461.
13. Mackensie MC, Karagianes TG, Hoyt DB, Davis JW. Prospective evaluation of epidural fentanyl for pain control and restoration of ventilatory function following multiple rib fractures. *J Trauma.* 1991;31: 443–451.
14. Soliman IE, Safwat AM. Successful management of an elderly patient with multiple trauma. *J Trauma.* 1985;25:806–807.
15. Ullman DA, Fortune JB, Greenhouse BB, et al. The treatment of patients with multiple rib fractures using continuous thoracic epidural narcotic infusion. *Reg Anesth.* 1989;14:43–47.
16. Mackersie RC, Shackford SR, Hoyt DB, Karagianes TG. Continous epidural fentanyl analgesia: ventilatory function improvement with routine use in treatment of blunt chest injury. *J Trauma.* 1987;27:1207–1212.

17. Wisner DH. A stepwise logistic regression analysis of factors affecting morbidity and mortality after thoracic trauma: effect of epidural analgesia. *J Trauma*. 1990;30:799–805.
18. Baxter TB, Moore EE, Moore FA, et al. A plea for sensible management of myocardial contusion. *Am J Surg*. 1989;158:557–562.
19. Wisner DH, Reed WH, Riddick RS. Suspected myocardial contusion: triage and indications for monitoring. *Ann Surg*. 1990;212:82–86.
20. Shapiro MJ, Yanofsky SD, Trapp J, et al. Cardiovascular evaluation in blunt thoracic trauma using transesophageal echocardiography (TEE). *J Trauma*. 1991;31:835–840.
21. Hiatt JR, Yeatman LA, Child JS. The value of echocardiography in blunt chest trauma. *J Trauma*. 1988;28:914–922.
22. Sladen R, Klamerus KJ, Swafford MWG, et al. Labetolol for the control of elevated blood pressure following coronary artery bypass grafting. *J Cardiothorac Anesth*. 1990;4:210–221.
23. Goldberg ME, McNulty S, Levette A, Goldman S. Intravenous labetolol for induced hypotension in an adult patient undergoing coarctation repair. *J Cardiothorac Anesth*. 1988;2:673–677.
24. Shenaq SA, Chelly JE, Karlberg H, et al. Use of nitroprusside during surgery for thoracoabdominal aortic aneurysm. *Circulation*. 1984;70(Suppl I):1–7.
25. D'Ambra MN, Dewhirst W, Jacobs M, et al. Cross-clamping the thoracic aorta, effect on intracranial pressure. *Circulation*. 1988;78(Suppl III):198–202.

8
Cervical Injury

FELIX D. BATTISTELLA, M.D.
JAMES E. GOODNIGHT, M.D.

HISTORY: Earliest recorded history of cervical vascular injuries dates back to the 16th century when Ambroise Paré controlled bleeding originating from the carotid artery and jugular vein of a wounded patient who went on to survive with the development of hemiplegia and aphasia.[1]

Despite medical progress,[2] mortality rates for cervical vascular injuries remained high, with 15% mortality reported during the Civil War and 11% mortality as recent as World War I.[3] Management of neck wounds until this time was primarily expectant until World War II, when Bailey[4] and Beebe and DeBakey[5] stressed the principle of exploring all wounds penetrating the platysma. This procedure reduced mortality to 7%. In 1956, Fogelman and Stewart[3] published a large series of civilian injuries in which mandatory exploration was performed for wounds penetrating the platysma muscle. They also confirmed a major improvement in morbidity and mortality, and surgical exploration became the treatment of choice for neck wounds. With improvements in evaluation, prehospital care, surgical techniques, and postoperative care, a mortality of 6% was achieved during the Vietnam War.[6] Subsequent series in civilian populations have reported mortality rates of 2% to 10%.[7–15] Although mandatory exploration has been the established treatment choice for neck wounds, recent improvements in both quality and availability of diagnostic tests such as angiography, esophagography, and endoscopic evaluation of both the airway and the esophagus have led to controversy, with many surgeons advocating a selective approach to exploration of neck injuries in patients with low-risk wounds and no clinical evidence of additional injury.

Neck injuries requiring operative intervention are in large part the result of penetrating trauma. Cervical trauma is complicated by the high density of vital structures in the neck and, as expected, there are controversies in management of these injuries. Serious cervical injury may not be obvious initially, and the consequences of missed cervical injuries can be devastating. Failure to recognize a cervical spine fracture or the rare vascular injury after blunt trauma can lead to major neurologic complications. Bleeding in the neck can result in acute airway obstruction; unrecognized pharyngeal or esophageal injury can lead to deep cervical and mediastinal infection.

128

In recent years, the principle of mandatory exploration of all cervical wounds has been challenged by numerous centers.[7,8,10–12,14,16–20] The primary reason for controversy is that wounds penetrating the platysma muscle are not necessarily associated with significant underlying injury; when mandatory exploration is used, 40% to 70% of explorations do not require any specific treatment.[8,9,12,16,21,22]

The management of specific injuries to cervical structures are found in subsequent chapters. This chapter will offer an overview and assessment of cervical injury.

ANATOMY

For clinical purposes, the neck may be divided into three zones (Fig. 8–1). Zone 1 occupies the base of the neck below the cricoid cartilage; zone 2, the midneck between the cricoid cartilage and the hyoid bone or angle of the jaw; zone 3 extends from the suprahyoid region to the base of the skull. This section will deal with cross-sectional anatomy of the neck as might be perceived from a computed tomography (CT) scan.

Beneath the skin, there is a variable layer of subcutaneous fat, followed in the anterior two-thirds of the neck by the platysma muscle, which is readily identified as a discrete layer. An areolar plane lies under the platysma muscle, between it and the deep cervical fascia (fascia colli). The neck is conveniently divided into anterior and posterior portions by the palpable transverse processes of the midcervical vertebrae as shown in a cross-section of the midneck (Fig. 8–2). This division is enhanced by the prevertebral fascia. This fascial layer originates from the deep cervical fascia opposite the transverse processes and passes anterior to the scalenus anticus and longus colli muscles across the front of the body of the vertebrae behind the esophagus and pharynx. It sends out slips that encircle the scalenus medius and scalenus posterior in addition to the two aforementioned muscles. The deep cervical fascia provides the sheaths of the strap muscles, the sternohyoid, sternothyroid, and thyrohyoid, and encircles the sternocleidomastoid muscle. A slip extends deep to the sternocleidomastoid and encircles the jugular vein, the carotid arteries, and the vagus nerve as the carotid sheath. This division leaves a deep anterior space containing the trachea, esophagus, pharynx, and larynx surrounded by areolar fatty tissue that is in continuity with the mediastinum.

The posterior half of the neck contains no major vascular or nerve structures except for the individual nerves to specific muscles. The ligamentum nuchae fixes the deep cervical fascia to the spinous processes in the posterior midline of the neck, separating the posterior neck into two major compartments. Fascial slips from the deep cervical fascia and nuchal ligament encircle the muscles of the posterior neck.

The vertebral artery and vein at this level course in a canal that passes through the transverse processes that in the interprocess interval are encompassed by a dense layer of fascia.

The anatomy changes abruptly in zone 1, or the base of the neck, but the fascial layers remain essentially the same (Fig. 8–3). The deep cervical fascia inserts on the clavicle in front and the acromium, spine of the scapula, and the nuchal line posteriorly. The subclavian vessels usually do not rise to any appreciable degree above the clavicle. The subclavian vein is separated from the subclavian artery at the apex of their ascendence by the scalenus anticus muscle. The phrenic nerve lies on the anterior surface of this muscle under the deep fascia. The fatty, or areolar, space is broader at the base of the neck and

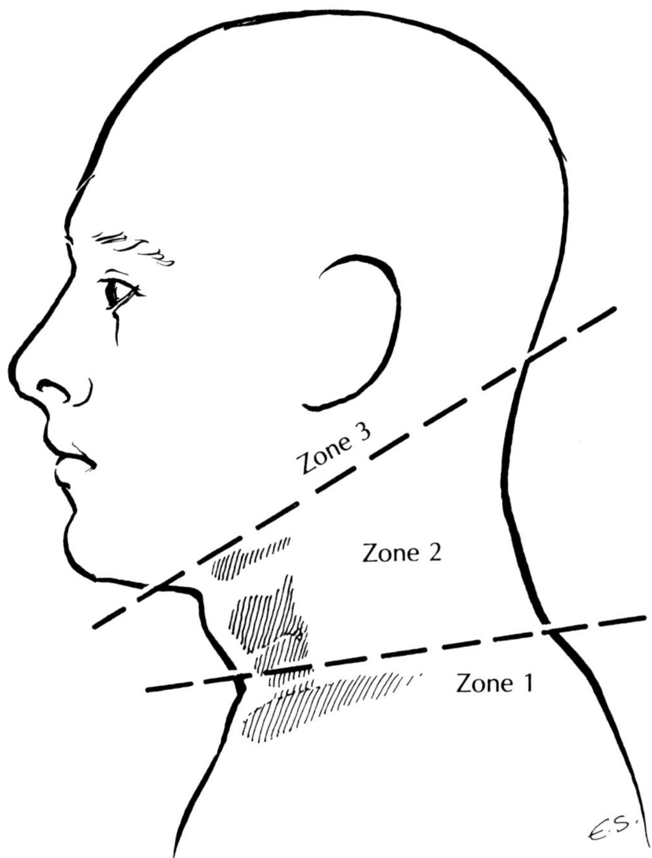

Figure 8–1.   Location of the three zones of the neck.

contains branches of the brachial plexus, which in this region still lie well posterior to the carotid sheath and vessels within. In this region, the vertebral artery passes from the posterior aspect of the subclavian artery toward the spinous process of the sixth cervical vertebra. The recurrent laryngeal nerve lies in a groove between the trachea and esophagus. The vagus nerve remains in its position between the jugular vein and carotid artery. The thyroid gland encircles the trachea at approximately the level of the first to the third tracheal cartilages and occupies the lateral side of the trachea.

The thoracic duct travels along the left margin of the esophagus to the base of the neck. It then passes behind the carotid sheath toward the medial border of the scalenus anterior muscle. Subsequently it turns inferiorly, paralleling the phrenic nerve, to drain into the left brachiocephatic vein, the left subclavian vein, or the left internal jugular vein.

Zone 3, in the anterior central portion of the neck, consists of the jaw and tongue muscles (Fig. 8–4). The most external of these originate from the hyoid bone as the hyoglossal and mylohyoid muscles. The pharynx assumes a funnel-like shape from above downward, lying just in front of the deep cervical fascia. At this level, the carotid artery has usually divided, with the external carotid artery generally lying immediately anterior to its

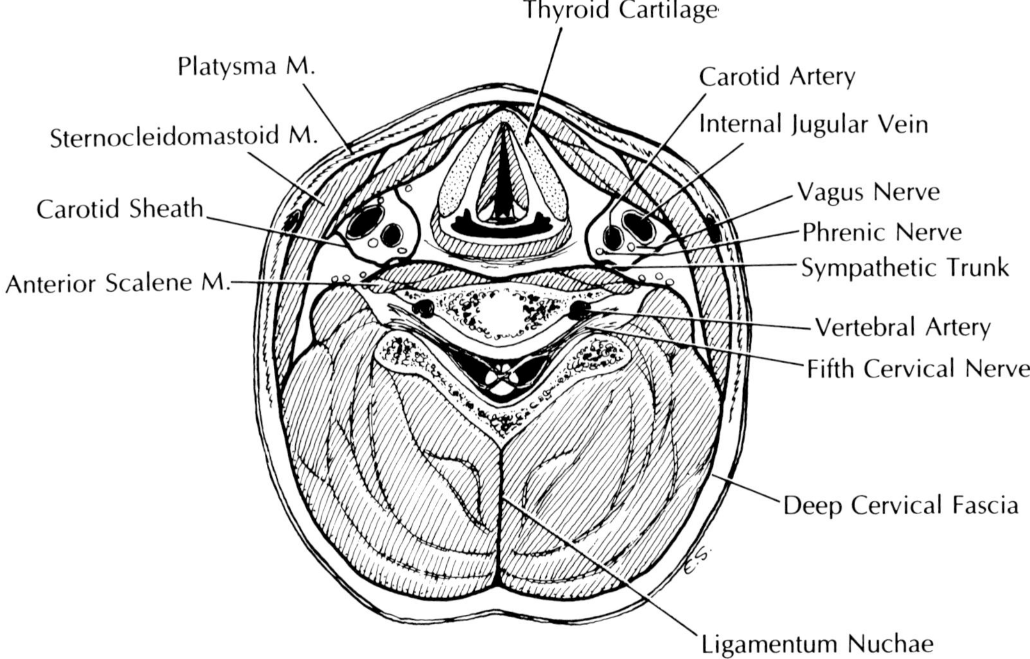

Figure 8–2.   Cross-section of the midneck (zone 2).

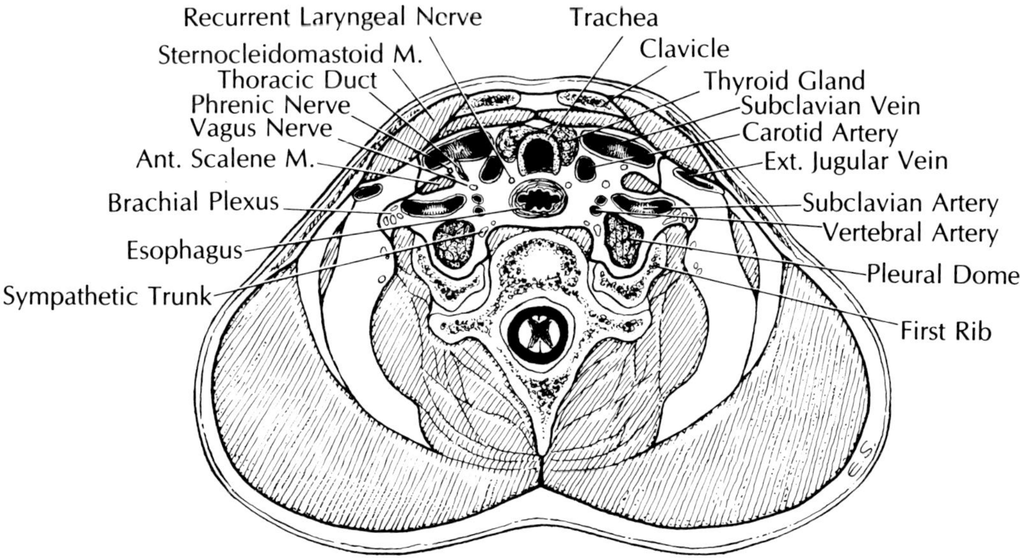

Figure 8–3.   Cross-section of the base of the neck (zone 1).

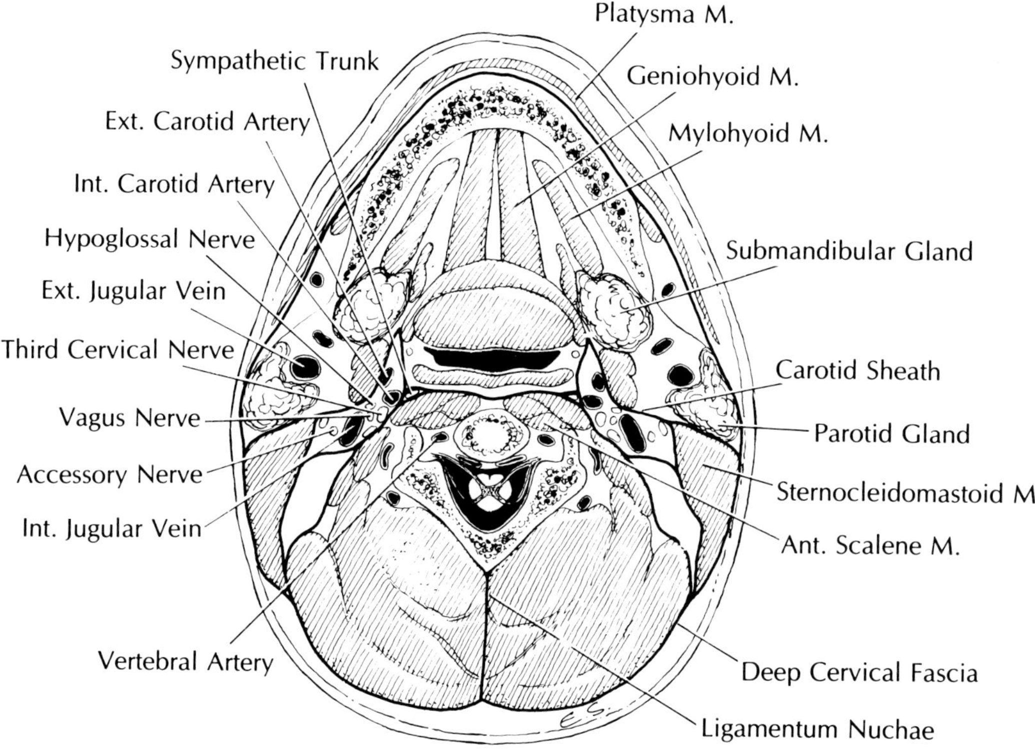

Figure 8–4. Cross-section of the upper neck (zone 3).

internal counterpart. The internal carotid artery ascends and runs progressively deeper into the neck and deep to the jugular vein. The 12th nerve crosses the internal carotid artery at approximately the tip of the mastoid process. The parotid gland is superficial to the vessels and occupies the space between the angle of the mandible and the mastoid process. The relationship of the nerves to deeper structures of the neck should be noted (Fig. 8–4). The sympathetic chain lies on top of the scalenus anticus and the longus colli muscles, the 11th nerve lies lateral to the jugular vein, and the tenth nerve is posterior to the internal carotid and between it and the jugular vein. The deep cervical nerves lie immediately posterior to the carotid artery.

The anatomy of the posterior half of the neck is not provided in detail, because no critical structures lie in this half of the cervical area, almost all of which is composed of muscle. It should be noted that as the nerve emerges from the sternocleidomastoid muscle posteriorly, the 11th nerve is superficial and relatively vulnerable in the posterior triangle of the neck before entering the trapezius muscle.

ASSESSMENT

The various types of *blunt cervical injuries* are presented in Table 8–1. Signs and symptoms of these blunt injuries are presented in Tables 8–2 and 8–3. Patients with blunt injury to the

Table 8–1. Cervical Injury

Blunt trauma
Vertebral fracture
  Stable
  Unstable
Spinal cord injury
Brachial plexus injury
Cranial nerve injury
Arterial injury
  Common, internal, external carotid, vertebral
Laryngotracheal
Pharyngoesophageal

neck should be handled carefully, because those with altered consciousness and those with complaints of cervical pain or with local neck findings should be presumed to have cervical fracture until proved otherwise. They should have the head and neck immobilized by a cervical collar or sandbags until all seven cervical vertebrae can be assessed radiologically.

Although the incidence of cervical spine injuries in fatal accidents is approximately 20%,[23] the incidence in polytrauma patients is less than 5%.[24] To improve the efficiency of the emergency radiology department and to minimize the economic impact of performing cervical spine x-rays on all blunt trauma victims, several investigators have concluded that asymptomatic patients who are alert and without alterations in level of consciousness by head injury, drugs, alcohol, or other painful injuries need not undergo radiologic evaluation of the spine.[25–28]

In the conscious patient without cervical discomfort or local findings, the probability of significant vascular injury is low. Nonetheless, stretch injuries of the carotid arteries do occur. If immediately available, Duplex scanning is an excellent screening tool for patients at risk for blunt carotid artery trauma.[29–31] Approximately half of the patients with carotid artery injury will not manifest external evidence of neck injury, and most will present with delayed focal cerebral ischemic symptoms.[32] If such injury is suspected, immediate arteriography or surgical exploration is indicated. Any neurological change, even a transient one, indicates possible arterial injury and should be evaluated with Duplex scan or arteriography (Chapter 6).

Airway evaluation is critical, because obstruction can develop rapidly from deep cervical hemorrhage. Palpable air in the neck or radiologic evidence of air may be associated with a laryngeal or tracheal injury. Hoarseness, laryngeal stridor, and intercostal or supraclavicular retraction are all manifestations of airway obstruction and demand

Table 8–2. Symptoms of Blunt Trauma

Cervical pain
Weakness
Numbness
Dyspnea
Swallowing difficulty

Table 8–3. Signs of Blunt Cervical Trauma

Deformity of neck
Paralysis or paresthesia
Air in neck
Hoarseness
Laryngeal stridor
Supraclavicular retraction
Hematomas
Bruits or thrills

immediate attention. Pain or difficulty with swallowing indicates pharyngeal or esophageal injury.

Injuries to cranial nerves are rare, but some branches are especially vulnerable. These branches are the marginal mandibular nerve (VII), which innervates the corner of the mouth and lower face, the main trunk of the vagus nerve (X), or the recurrent laryngeal branch that innervates the larynx. Injury to the vagus results in hoarseness or loss of volume of the voice. Injury to the spinal accessory nerve (XI) results in weakness of shoulder shrug; injury to the hypoglossal nerve (XII), tongue paralysis. Most of these nerve injuries occur in association with other cervical injuries. Avulsion-type injuries of the brachial plexus occur and are manifested by paresthesias and paralyses in the distribution of the involved segments.

When *penetrating injury* pierces the platysma muscle, the high density of critical structures in the anterior half of the neck results in high probability of significant injury. *Symptoms* of penetrating trauma consist of bleeding, hemoptysis, shortness of breath, hoarseness, difficulty swallowing, and weakness or paralysis (Table 8–4). The *signs* of penetrating trauma are shock, bleeding, hematoma, bruits or thrills, stridor, subcutaneous air, cervical air on radiographs or anterior displacement of the pharyngeal or tracheal shadow, and paralysis of anesthesia in the distribution of the cervical nerves (Table 8–5). Although these signs and symptoms typically are associated with significant injuries, as many as one-third of patients without signs and symptoms can harbor significant injuries.[33]

The relative incidence of injuries tabulated from 22 series is listed in Table 8–6. Venous injuries are the most common, with a superficial vein, such as the external jugular or the jugular itself, being the most often involved. Second in frequency are injuries to the common, internal, or external carotid arteries. Laryngeal and tracheal injuries follow and are similar in incidence to pharyngeal and esophageal injuries. Injuries to the brachial plexus and cranial nerves are relatively common, but injuries to the spinal cord are quite rare. The parotid gland may be injured in high cervical injuries and the thoracic duct in low cervical injuries; however, these injuries are rare.

Table 8–4. Symptoms of Penetrating Trauma

Hemoptysis
Shortness of breath
Hoarseness
Difficulty swallowing
Weakness, paralysis
Numbness

Table 8–5.   Signs of Penetrating Trauma

Shock
Bleeding
Hematoma
Bruits or thrills
Stridor
Cervical air
Displacement of traches or esophagus
Paralysis or anesthesia

In addition to a thorough history and physical examination, a chest x-ray should be obtained as a minimum in all patients with penetrating trauma to the neck to exclude intrathoracic injury.

INITIAL MANAGEMENT

Establishing an airway should be the first priority in any trauma victim; however, precautions should be taken not to aggravate any cervical spine injury that may by present. Although the incidence of cervical spine and cord injury after polytrauma is low, the consequences of a missed injury can be devastating. In the patient with respiratory distress, establishing an airway takes priority over obtaining x-rays to exclude injury to the cervical spine. The airway can be secured safely initially by employing the chin lift or jaw thrust maneuvers and, if needed, maintained by various means including nasotracheal intubation, orotracheal intubation with in-line manual cervical stabilization, or cricothyroidotomy

Table 8–6.   Penetrating Cervical Trauma*

INJURY	PERCENT
Arterial	16
Common, internal, external carotid	(9)
Vertebral	(1)
Subclavian, innominate	(3)
Other	(4)
Venous	21
Internal jugular	(9)
External jugular/superficial	(9)
Subclavian, innominate	(3)
Larynx and trachea	8
Pharynx and esophagus	8
Nerve	7
Cranial	(3)
Brachial plexus	(3)
Parotid gland	2
Thoracic duct	1
Thyroid gland	3

**Includes 4028 patients from combined referenced series.[7–9,11–22,37–40,51–53]*

when the above fail. The method chosen to establish an airway in an unstable patient should employ the technique with which the operator has had more experience and feels more comfortable with. Orotracheal intubation with proper precautions can be accomplished safely in the ER setting.[34]

Other urgent procedures and operations can and should be performed with proper spinal precautions. If a patient's condition permits, a lateral x-ray of the cervical spine can be taken in the resuscitation room. Although this view is the most useful, it is fraught with limitations and many injuries can remain undiagnosed (Chapter 5). It is often difficult to visualize the cervicothoracic junction, an area where unstable injuries can be missed. Thus, several views of the cervical spine are required to exclude injury, and patients with suspected spine injuries should be maintained in spinal precautions until cleared with roentgenographic studies. To permit early mobilization, these views should be obtained as soon as the patient has been stabilized.

With an airway secured, resuscitation of the patient is the next priority. External bleeding should be controlled by direct pressure, and aggressive fluid resuscitation should be instituted to reestablish adequate blood pressure. Resuscitation of moribund patients with penetrating neck trauma should include emergency room thoracotomy, as significant survival rates can be achieved even in these dire circumstances. In the patient with unexplained hypotension, neurogenic shock secondary to spinal cord injury should be considered.

INDICATIONS FOR SURGERY

The primary indication for cervical exploration after *blunt trauma* is airway obstruction. Impairment of ventilation may be due to crushing of the larynx, tracheal injury, or expanding hematoma. Emergency restoration of the airway may require cricothyroidotomy followed by tracheostomy. The second most common indication for surgery after blunt trauma is arterial injury.

After *penetrating trauma*, exploration is indicated whenever there is evidence of major injury. As already indicated, the neck is conveniently divided into three zones (Fig. 8–1). *Injuries to zone 1* should be evaluated by arteriography if the patient is stable, because, if major vessels in zone 1 are involved, thoracotomy is necessary to ensure adequate exposure and proximal control of arterial injury (Chapter 17).

For *arterial injuries* in zone 3, arteriography is indicated because high carotid and jugular venous injuries may be difficult to control. Arterial injuries may, on occasion, require ligation of the internal carotid artery. Recognition of the injury in advance is essential, because special procedures such as mandibular dislocation or fracture may be necessary to ensure adequate vascular exposure at the base of the skull for repair (Chapter 18).

Because *venous injuries* in zones 1 and 3 are difficult to expose, management should be nonoperative in the absence of evidence of arterial or other major injury unless bleeding is a problem. Immediate life-threatening problems related to sudden progression of arterial hematomas with compromise of the airway or rupture into the pleural space require prompt operation.

In the absence of airway obstruction or subcutaneous emphysema, the probability of *tracheal injury* is low, and the possibility of injury can be ignored in the absence of other evidence of injury. Occult *pharyngeal* or *esophageal injuries* are dangerous because they are the source of life-threatening infections of the deep cervical space and they rapidly and easily extend into the mediastinum. Wounds in proximity to these structures demand evaluation by barium swallow or exploration. One should be alert to tenderness, fever, or elevated white blood count as signs of injury.

If trauma is limited to the posterior half of the neck or if the line of penetration is clearly in a direction that does not involve the anterior neck (anterior to the vertebral transverse processes), observation is preferable to exploration. However, exploration should be performed for the slightest suspicion of injury. Patients treated by local exploration of a penetrating wound recover promptly with less morbidity than those whose injuries are missed.

Penetrating injuries to the *cervical spine* usually are the result of gunshot wounds, and, although devastating, these injuries are rare, accounting for less than 10% of all spine injuries.[35] Initial evaluation and treatment should focus on possible injuries to vital structures such as the carotid artery, trachea, and esophagus. Once these injuries have been ruled out or dealt with, attention can be directed toward the spine. Treatment of transpharyngeal cervical spine wounds requires adequate debridement of devitalized soft tissue and bone fragments followed by drainage to minimize the incidence of osteomyelitis. Other nongrossly contaminated injuries can be observed. Removal of retained intracanal bullet fragments in patients with partial cord lesions is appropriate; however, after complete lesions, surgical decompression and foreign body removal usually is not recommended.[36]

For *penetrating injuries in zone 2* of the anterior neck (penetration of the platysma), exploration is more expeditious than prolonged observation or arteriography and, for patients with shock, compromised airways, profuse bleeding, expanding hematoma, neurologic deficit, dysphagia, hematemesis or hemoptysis, subcutaneous emphysema, and recurrent laryngeal nerve injury, this approach is mandatory. Exploration in this group of patients will reveal significant injuries in 70% to 95% of cases.[10,11,13] However, in the stable patient without overt evidence of serious injury, there are an equal number of advocates for mandatory exploration[3,6,9,15,22,37–40] as those who recommend a selective exploration strategy.[7,8,10–12,14,16–20] Although some advocate observation alone, most agree that nonoperative evaluation should include evaluation with angiography, esophagography or esophagoscopy, and bronchoscopy. Advocates of the selective approach point not only to the elimination of morbidity associated with negative exploration but also claim a reduction in length of hospitalization. Those supporting mandatory exploration point to the significant increase in morbidity and mortality associated with missed injuries and minimal morbidity of negative exploration.

In a recent compilation of the current literature comparing the strategies of mandatory exploration with the selective approach, mortality rates for the two were found to be similar, with authors supporting mandatory exploration reporting a 5.9% mortality rate (11 series) and authors supporting the selective approach reporting a mortality rate of 3.8% (24 series).[41] In examining the clinical course of 4193 patients compiled from 26 series, a negative exploration rate of 46% was found in the mandatory group (10 series) as compared with 30% in the selective (16 series). Three of 16 patients (2%) required late exploration after initial observation in the mandatory group compared with 20 of 944 (2%) in the selective group.[41]

In centers where skilled radiologists and in-house surgical staff are immediately available, the selective approach to neck exploration in stable patients is efficacious. In facilities where staff are not readily available to evaluate and follow the patient closely and where a nonoperative management could lead to a delay in recognition of injury, a mandatory exploration policy should be followed. Mandatory exploration is associated with minimal morbidity; one-fourth to one-third of those explored will have clinically occult injuries.[9,33]

Although the approach to zone 2 injuries remains controversial, as just described, we favor an initial nonoperative evaluation for patients with an injury traversing the midneck and for patients in which the trajectory of the wounding object traverses two or more zones. Violation of more than one zone is common, with approximately 30% of injuries involving multiple zones.[37] In the stable patient, the wounding mechanism should be taken into account because wounds inflicted by high-velocity bullets or close-range shotguns are more likely to be associated with significant injuries and have a higher morbidity and mortality rate.[42] These types of injury undoubtedly are best dealt with by early exploration.

In summary, prospective studies looking at the selective approach have found equivalent morbidity and mortality rates. However, the selective approach mandates frequent reassessments of the patient to avoid complications related to progressive airway compromise during the diagnostic evaluation. As physical exam cannot exclude wounds to the carotid artery or the esophagus, evaluation should include arteriography as well as esophagography and, if these are equivocal, the injury should be explored. Most injuries to the trachea are apparent based on the patient's symptoms and physical findings. Should the possibility of an airway injury exist, laryngoscopy/bronchoscopy should be performed to evaluate the airway. Any abnormal findings mandate prompt surgical exploration. An algorithm for the management of patients with penetrating cervical trauma is outlined in Figure 8–5.

CERVICAL EXPLORATION

The routine incision for emergency exploration is along the anterior border of the sternocleidomastoid muscle. For those for whom cosmetics are extremely important, a transverse incision placed in a skin fold, with development of superior and inferior flaps, can be used. However, these flaps create delay under emergency circumstances. Moreover, the transverse incision is not easily extended to a sternotomy should chest exposure be necessary or cephalad extension if access to the upper neck is required. The incision along the sternocleidomastoid muscle permits all options and gives exposure of all structures of the anterior half of the neck.

Special consideration should be given to the possible need for proximal control of the carotid and subclavian arteries in patients with injuries at the base of the neck. The innominate artery can be controlled easily by extending the vertical neck incision onto the chest and performing a median sternotomy. Proximal control of the left subclavian is best achieved through a left anterolateral thoracotomy (Chapter 17). Exposure of the internal carotid at the base of the skull can be equally challenging. Adequate exposure of this area

Penetrating Cervical Trauma

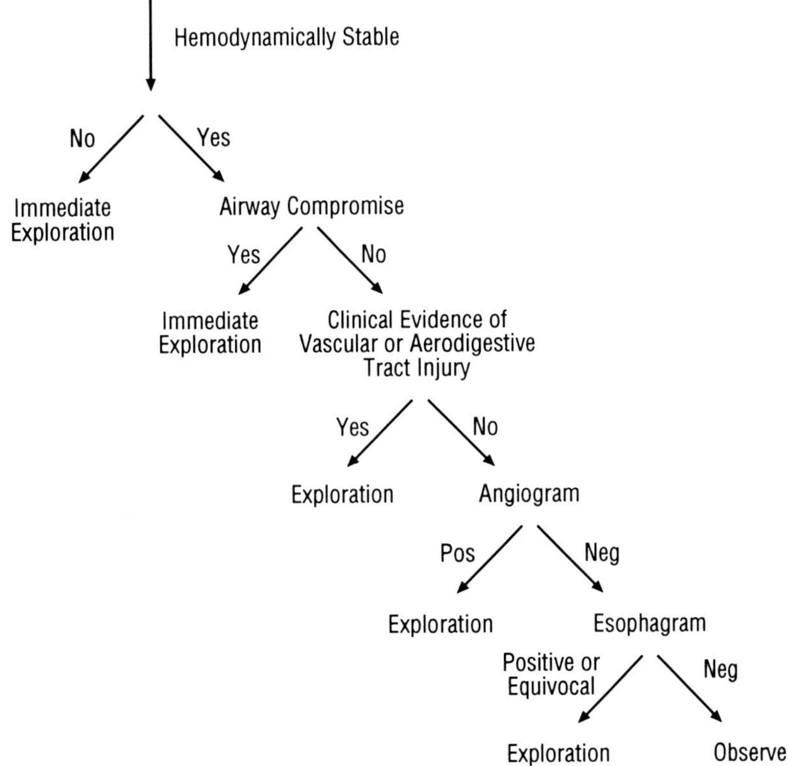

Figure 8–5.   Algorithm for management of penetrating neck injuries.

often will require either mandibular subluxation[43] or an osteotomy of the angle of the mandible[44] (Chapter 18).

The need for autogenous graft to be used in the repair of arterial injuries should be anticipated, and a groin or ankle should be prepared and draped for possible harvest of the saphenous vein.

The sternocleidomastoid incision can be limited if the trauma is penetrating, because the tract of injury can be picked up in the deeper portion of the neck and readily followed. Moreover, probing the site of penetration of knife or bullet provides a guide to the centering of the incision. This incision, placed along the anterior border of the muscle, avoids denervating the sternocleidomastoid and the trapezius muscles. It is carried down rapidly through skin, subcutaneous tissue, and platysma. As the neck is extremely vascular, bleeding points inevitably will require ligature or coagulation. The deep cervical fascia is best opened along the anterior border of the muscle itself and the muscle slightly rolled backward as the deeper portion of the neck is entered. Medial and deep to the sterno-cleidomastoid muscle, between it and the trachea, lies the carotid sheath containing the jugular vein anterolaterally, the vagus nerve just below the jugular vein, and the carotid artery deeper and slightly medial. In the absence of overt bleeding, the artery is the first structure to be explored, by carrying the dissection medial to the jugular vein. The vein is examined as it is mobilized and while the middle thyroid vein and the confluence of the common facial veins are divided. It is then retracted laterally, exposing the carotid artery. If high cervical exposure is required, the incision should be carried toward the mastoid process and the superior lobe of the parotid should be retracted medially as vessels running between the parotid and the sternocleidomastoid muscle are ligated.

For exploration of the trachea and esophagus, the carotid artery is retracted laterally, and the dissection carried medially down alongside the trachea to the scalene and longus colli muscles lying in front of the transverse processes. The esophagus is best exposed from behind, because in the upper half of the neck the pharyngeal musculature blends into the laryngeal musculature. The free areolar plane behind the pharynx or esophagus is entered and the lateral and posterior walls are inspected. The esophagus should be carefully encircled bluntly and then retracted or rolled to the right or left to facilitate examination. If there is doubt as regards an esophageal injury, a dilator passed orally to distend the esophagus will facilitate recognition of a laceration if one is present.

The trachea is easily seen and, at the level of the cricoid cartilage, it should be palpated carefully to delineate the larynx from the trachea. The strap muscles should be divided if necessary. Gentle blunt dissection will separate the trachea and esophagus. Sharp dissection should be avoided until the recurrent laryngeal nerve is identified. The thyroid vessels can be divided if need be and the gland mobilized as necessary to facilitate tracheal exposure.

Treatment of identified injuries will be discussed in detail in subsequent chapters.

Little controversy exists regarding the management of tracheal and esophageal injuries. These should be repaired primarily whenever possible. Venous injuries can be ligated with impunity; however, ligation of both internal jugular veins should be avoided if possible. The treatment of vertebral artery injuries is aimed at occluding the injured vessel, and this can be accomplished by either surgical ligation or embolization of the artery.[45–47] The treatment of carotid artery injuries remains controversial for patients presenting with neurological deficits. Much of this controversy stems from the early experience with revascularization of stroke victims resulting in increased mortality due to the conversion of an ischemic infarct to a hemorrhagic one. Repair of carotid injuries in patients with either a normal neurologic exam or with limited deficits is widely accepted and the repair of patients with profound neurologic deficits is generally recommended. The treatment of patients in coma remains controversial, with most surgeons advocating ligation rather than repair, especially if there is no retrograde flow through the vessel.[48–50]

CLOSURE

The cervical incision as described can be drained via a stab wound posterior to the sternocleidomastoid muscle (low to avoid injury to the 11th nerve). Drains for esophageal injuries should be brought out so that they do not cross over the carotid artery, especially in the presence of an ipsilateral carotid artery injury. No attempt should be made to close structures deep to the cervical fascia. If possible, the cervical fascia should be closed with running or interrupted absorbable sutures. The platysma muscle should be closed as well. The skin should be approximated carefully to avoid overlap of skin edges and sutures removed early to avoid cross-hatch marks.

COMPLICATIONS

The complications of cervical exploration are rare. They include hemorrhage and hematomas, with or without laryngeal edema and airway compromise. Infection is rare unless there has been gross wound contamination or a missed pharyngeal, esophageal, or tracheal injury. This latter type of contamination can produce a virulent cervicomediastinal infection, because the tissue planes of the neck and mediastinum are in free communication. Mortality after a negative neck exploration is zero, and morbidity is negligible, with most series reporting a few wound infections as the only complications.[22,37]

The most significant complications resulting from penetrating cervical trauma occur as the result of missed injuries. These can occur in patients after a thorough diagnostic evaluation as well as in those undergoing exploration. Missed injuries, especially those involving the carotid artery or the esophagus, result in both significant morbidity and a high mortality. Unexplained signs of systemic infection and increased local pain may be the only early manifestations of a missed injury to the pharynx or esophagus.

REFERENCES

1. Watson WL, Silverstone SM. Ligature of the common carotid artery in cancer of the head and neck. *Ann Surg*. 1939;109(1):1–27.
2. Fleming D. Case of rupture of the carotid artery and wounds of several of its branches successfully treated by tying the common trunk of the carotid itself. *Med Chir J Rev (Lond)*. 1817;3:2–4.
3. Fogelman MJ, Stewart RD. Penetrating wounds of the neck. *Am J Surg*. 1956;91:581–596.
4. Bailey H. Wounds of the neck. In: *Surgery of Modern Warfare*. 2nd ed, vol I. Baltimore: Williams & Wilkins; 1942:320–329.
5. Beebe GW, DeBakey ME. *Battle Casualties: Incidence, Mortality and Logistic Considerations*. Springfield, IL: Charles C Thomas; 1952.
6. Fitchett VH, Butsch DW, Eiseman B. Penetration wounds of the neck: a military and civilian experience. *Arch Surg*. 1969;99:307–314.
7. Belinkie SA, Russell IC, DaSilva J, Becker DR. Management of penetrating neck injuries. *J Trauma*. 1983;23(3):235–237.
8. Ayuyao AM, Kaledzi YL, Parsa MH, Freeman HP. Penetrating neck wounds: mandatory versus selective exploration. *Ann Surg*. 1985;202(5):563–567.
9. Bishara RA, Pasch AR, Douglas DD, Schuler JJ, Lim LT, Flanigan DP. The necessity of mandatory exploration of penetrating zone II neck injuries. *Surgery*. 1986;100(4):655–660.
10. Jurkovich GJ, Zingarelli W, Wallace J, Curreri PW. Penetrating neck trauma: diagnostic studies in the asymptomatic patient. *J Trauma*. 1985;25(9):819–822.
11. Noyes LD, McSwain NE, Markowitz IP. Panendoscopy with arteriography versus mandatory exploration of penetrating wounds of the neck. *Ann Surg*. 1986;204(1):21–31.
12. Golueke PJ, Goldstein AS, Sclafani SJA, Mitchell WG, Shaftan GW. Routine versus selective exploration of penetrating neck injuries: a randomized prospective study. *J Trauma*. 1984;24(12):1010–1014.
13. Wood F, Fabian TC, Mangiante EC. Penetrating neck injuries: recommendations for selective management. *J Trauma*. 1989;29(5):602–605.
14. Merion RM, Harness JK, Ramsburgh SR, Thompson NW. Selective management of penetrating neck trauma. *Arch Surg*. 1981;116:691–696.
15. Roon AJ, Christensen N. Evaluation and treatment of penetrating cervical injuries. *J Trauma*. 1979;19(6):391–397.
16. Rao PM, Bhatti FK, Gaudino J, et al. Penetrating injuries of the neck: criteria for exploration. *J Trauma*. 1983;23(1):47–49.
17. Bostwick J III, Schneider WJ, Jurkiewicz J, Stone HH. Penetrating injuries of the face and neck. *South Med J*. 1976;69(5):550–553.
18. Massac E Jr, Siram SM, Leffall LD Jr. Penetrating neck wounds. *Am J Surg*. 1983;145:263–265.
19. Sheely CH II, Mattox KL, Reul GJ Jr, Beall AC Jr, DeBakey ME. Current concepts in the management of penetrating neck trauma. *J Trauma*. 1975;15(10):895–900.
20. Cabasares HV. Selective surgical management of penetrating neck trauma: 15-year experience in a community hospital. *Am Surg*. 1982;48(7):355–358.
21. Narrod JA, Moore EE. Selective management of penetrating neck injuries. *Arch Surg*. 1984;119:574–578.

22. Saletta JD, Lowe RJ, Lim LT, Thornton J, Delk S, Moss GS. Penetrating trauma of the neck. *J Trauma*. 1976;16(7):579–587.

23. Alker GJ Jr, Oh YS, Leslie EV, Lehotay J, Panaro VA, Eschner EG. Postmortem radiology of head and neck injuries in fatal traffic accidents. *Neuroradiology*. 1975;114:611–617.

24. Soicher E, Demetriades D. Cervical spine injuries in patients with head injuries. *Br J Surg*. 1991;78:1013–1014.

25. Roberge RJ, Wears RC, Kelly M, et al. Selective application of cervical spine radiography in alert victims of blunt trauma: a prospective study. *J Trauma*. 1988;28(6):784–788.

26. Kreipke DL, Gillespie KR, McCarthy MC, Mail JT, Lappas JC, Broadie TA. Reliability of indications for cervical spine films in trauma patients. *J Trauma*. 1989;29(10):1438–1439.

27. Saddison D, Vanek VW, Racanelli JL. Clinical indications for cervical spine radiographs in alert trauma patients. *Am Surg*. 1991;57(6):366–369.

28. Fischer RP. Cervical radiographic evaluation of alert patients following blunt trauma. *Ann Emerg Med*. 1984;13(10):905–907.

29. Martin RF, Eldrup-Jorgensen J, Clark DE, Bredenberg CE. Blunt trauma to the carotid arteries. *J Vasc Surg*. 1991;14(6):789–795.

30. Fabian TC, George SM Jr, Croce MA, Mangiante EC, Voeller GR, Kudsk KA. Carotid artery trauma: management based on mechanism of injury. *J Trauma*. 1990;30(8):953–963.

31. Davis JW, Holbrook TL, Hoyt DB, Mackersie RC, Field TO Jr, Shackford SR. Blunt carotid artery dissection: incidence, associated injuries, screening, and treatment. *J Trauma*. 1990;30(12):1514–1517.

32. Mokri B, Piepgras DG, Houser OW. Traumatic dissections of the extracranial internal carotid artery. *J Neurosurg*. 1988;68:189–1097.

33. Ashworth C, Williams LF, Byrne JJ. Penetrating wounds of the neck: re-emphasis of the need for prompt exploration. *Am J Surg*. 1971;121:387–391.

34. Rhee KJ, Green W, Holcroft JW, Mangili JAA. Oral intubation in the multiply injured patient: the risk of exacerbating spinal cord damage. *Ann Emerg Med*. 1990;19(5):511–514.

35. Meyer PR Jr, Cybulski GR, Rusin JJ, Haak MH. Spinal cord injury. *Neurol Clin*. 1991;9(3):625–661.

36. Kupcha PC, An HS, Cotler JM. Gunshot wounds to the cervical spine. *Spine*. 1990;15(10):1058–1063.

37. Meyer JP, Barrett JA, Schuler JJ, Flanigan P. Mandatory vs selective exploration for penetrating neck trauma. *Arch Surg*. 1987;122:592–597.

38. Knightly JJ, Swaminathan AP, Rush BF. Management of penetrating wounds of the neck. *Am J Surg*. 1973;126:575–580.

39. McInnis WD, Cruz AB, Aust JB. Penetrating injuries to the neck: pitfalls in management. *Am J Surg*. 1975;130:416–420.

40. Markey JC Jr, Hines JL, Nance FC. Penetrating neck wounds: a review of 218 cases. *Am Surg*. 1975;vol II(41):77–83.

41. Asensio JA, Valenziano CP, Falcone RE, Grosh JD. Management of penetrating neck injuries: the controversy surrounding zone II injuries. *Surg Clin North Am*. 1991;71(2):267–296.

42. Ordog GJ. Penetrating neck trauma. *J Trauma*. 1987;27(5):543–554.

43. Fisher DF, Clagett GP, Parker JI, et al. Mandibular subluxation for high carotid exposure. *J Vasc Surg*. 1984;1(6):727–733.

44. Welsh P, Pradier R, Repetto R. Fibromuscular dysplasia of the distal cervical internal carotid artery. *J Cardiovasc Surg*. 1981;22:321–326.

45. Golueke P, Sclafani S, Phillips T, Goldstein A, Scalea T, Duncan A. Vertebral artery injury—diagnosis and management. *J Trauma*. 1987;27(8):856–865.

46. Hatzitheofilou C, Demetriades D, Melissas J, Stewart M, Franklin J. Surgical approaches to vertebral artery injuries. *Br J Surg*. 1988;75:234–237.

47. Reid JDS, Weigelt JA. Forty-three cases of vertebral artery trauma. *J Trauma*. 1988;28(7):1007–1012.

48. Richardson R, Obeid FN, Richardson JD, et al. Neurologic consequences of cerebrovascular injury. *J Trauma*. 1992;32(6):755–760.

49. Demetriades D, Skalkides J, Sofianos C, Melissas J, Franklin J. Carotid artery injuries: experience with 124 cases. *J Trauma*. 1989;29(1):91–94.

50. Liekweg WG Jr, Greenfield LJ. Management of penetrating carotid arterial injury. *Ann Surg*. 1978;188(5):587–592.

51. Elerding SC, Manart FD, Moore EE. A reappraisal of penetrating neck injury management. *J Trauma*. 1980;20(8):695–697.

52. Obeid FN, Haddad GS, Horst HM, Bivins BA. A critical reappraisal of a mandatory exploration policy for penetrating wounds of the neck. *Surg Gynecol Obstet*. 1985;160:517–522.

53. Shirkey AL, Beall AC Jr, DeBakey ME. Surgical management of penetrating wounds of the neck. *Arch Surg*. 1963;86:955–963.

9

Pharyngoesophageal Injury

MERVIN B. O'NEIL, JR., M.D.

HISTORY: The history of pharyngoesophageal surgery begins with an account in the Smith Surgical Papyrus from ancient Egypt. Case 28 of the 48 cases in this work represented anatomic, physiologic, clinical, and pathologic observations entitled "A Gaping Wound of the Throat Penetrating the Gullet."[1] The treatment at the time was medical therapy, although wound "stitching" was mentioned. Very little progress was made until the 17th and 18th centuries when Boerhaave published his classic description of rupture of the esophagus[2] and Verduc recommended surgical extraction of foreign bodies in the cervical esophagus that could not be removed by other means.[2] Open removal of a piece of bone was reported by Goursand and Roland in 1757.[2] By the 19th century, operation on the cervical esophagus for foreign bodies was considered safe. Cheever[3] in 1867 and Gross[1] in 1880 published a series of cases with few mortalities. This century also saw Kussmaul pass a lighted tube through the entire esophagus into the stomach, and Walter B. Cannon pioneered upper gastrointestinal x-ray in 1898 utilizing the esophagus of a goose.[2]

In the 20th century the introduction of endotracheal anesthesia and a better understanding of the open pneumothorax, combined with the introduction of antibiotics and improved gastrointestinal suture techniques, resulted in remarkable advances in esophageal surgery. Surgical experience during World War II led to the recognition of the importance of early exploration and repair on the slightest suspicion of esophageal injury, a principle that is still valid today. The first survivor of a spontaneous perforation was treated by drainage by Frink in 1941.[4] This was reported in 1947, the same year Barrett[5] reported the first successful esophageal closure of that injury. Since then, many reports of the successful treatment of spontaneous perforations have emerged.[6-9] Simultaneously, a growing literature on penetrating and blunt injuries to the neck and thorax warned about the importance of unsuspected esophageal injuries and the serious consequences of delays in treatment.[10-21] The principles of early recognition, administration of antibiotics, and early repair or drainage have been established and today are fundamental to the successful management of pharyngoesophageal lesions.[22-28]

The pharynx and esophagus are privileged to be in a rather protected position in the neck and chest. The benefit of this privilege is that injuries to these organs are infrequent. The price of this is that injuries to these organs frequently are missed, with disastrous consequences. Thus, to improve the results with these lesions, a high index of suspicion must be maintained, and aggressive efforts must be made to diagnose these injuries or to rule them out.

ANATOMY OF THE PHARYNX AND ESOPHAGUS

The first portion of the alimentary canal, the pharynx, is a musculomembranous tube, conical in form, with the base upward and the apex downward, extending from the undersurface of the skull to the level of the cricoid cartilage in front and the sixth cervical vertebra behind (Fig. 9–1). The pharynx averages about 12.5 cm in length, with its greatest

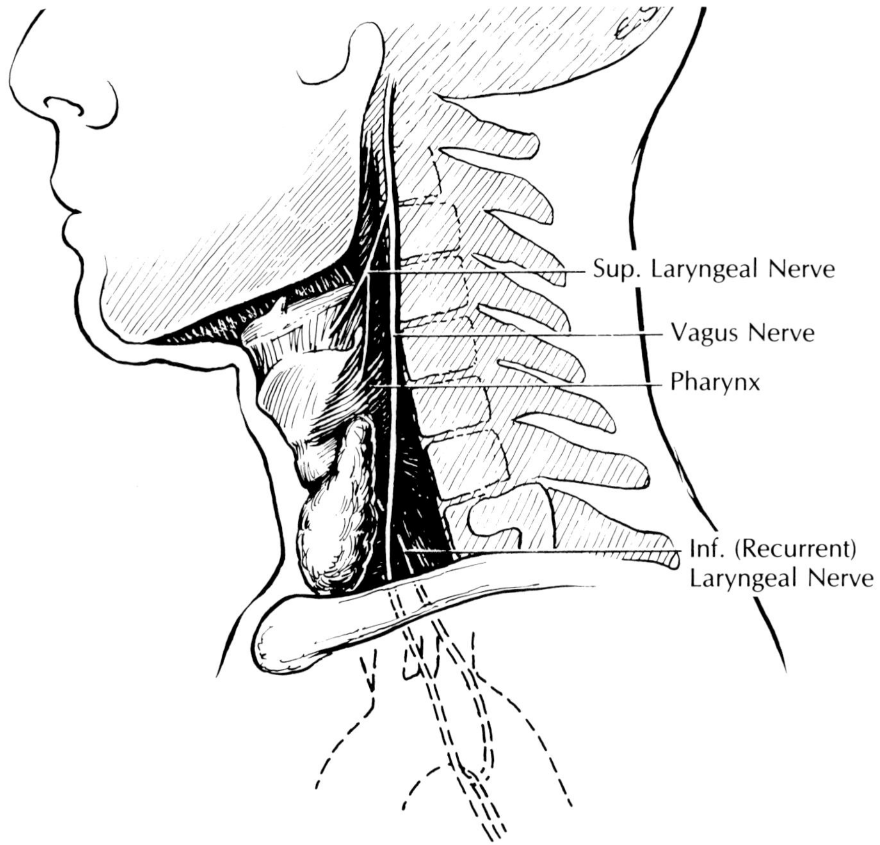

Figure 9–1. **A, B:** Lateral views of the neck showing the relative position of the pharynx and cervical esophagus lying just anterior to the vertebral column.

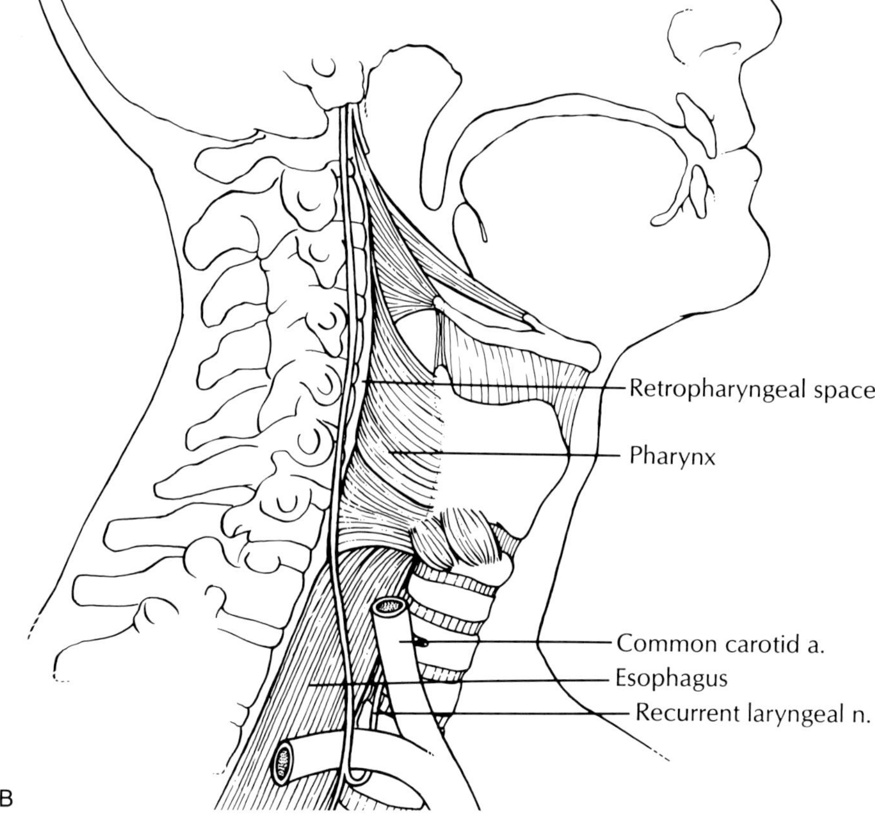

Figure 9–1, cont.

breadth lying immediately below the base of the skull where it projects on either side behind the orifice of the eustachian tube as a recess termed the "fossa of Rosenmüller." Its narrowest portion is at its termination in the esophagus. It is limited above by the body of the sphenoid as well as the basilar process of the occipital bone. Below it is continuous with the esophagus, and posteriorly it is connected by loose areolar tissue with the cervical portion of the vertebral column and the longus colli and rectus capitis anticus muscles. Areolar tissue is contained in what is called the retropharyngeal space. Anteriorly it is incomplete and is attached in succession to the eustachian tube, internal pterygoid plate, and the pterygomandibular ligament. The posterior termination consists of the mylohyoid ridge of the mandible, the mucous membrane of the mouth, the base of the tongue, the hyoid bone, the thyroid, and cricoid cartilages. Laterally it is connected to the styloid process and their muscles and is in contact with the common and internal carotid arteries, the internal jugular vein, and the glossopharyngeal, vagus, hypoglossal, and sympathetic nerves.

The pharyngeal musculature interdigitates with that of the esophagus. The latter averages approximately 25 cm in length, extending from the pharynx to the stomach. The muscular layers consist of an inner circular layer and an outer longitudinal layer that is striated in its cephalad portion and smooth in the distal two-thirds. It commences at the upper border of the cricoid cartilage opposite the sixth cervical vertebra and descends along the front of the vertebral column to the posterior mediastinum. It then passes through the diaphragm and enters the abdomen, terminating at the cardiac orifice of the stomach opposite the 11th thoracic vertebra about 2.5 cm to the left of the median plane. The general direction of the esophagus is vertical, but it takes two and sometimes three curves along its course. At its commencement it is placed in the median line, but it then inclines to the left side as far as the root of the neck, gradually passing to the midline again, and finally deviating to the left as it passes forward to the esophageal opening of the diaphragm. The esophagus also has anteroposterior flexures corresponding to the curvature of the cervical and thoracic portions of the vertebral column. The esophagus is the narrowest portion of the alimentary canal. It is constricted at its commencement at about the level of the third thoracic vertebra by the cricopharyngeas muscle and at the point where it passes through the diaphragm.

When empty, the esophagus is contracted so that the anterior and posterior walls come in contact; the lumen is stellate because of the longitudinal foldings of the inelastic mucous membrane. The caliber of the lumen varies from 1.5 to 2.5 cm, depending on the presence or absence of swallowed substances. The average distance for the origin of the esophagus from the upper incisor teeth is approximately 15 cm. The average distance from the incisor teeth to the cardiac opening of the stomach is approximately 40 cm.

The cervical portion of the esophagus lies behind the membranous portion of the trachea, with the thyroid gland folded over it laterally (Fig. 9–1). Posteriorly, it rests on the vertebral column and the longus colli muscles. The common carotid artery lies immediately lateral, and the recurrent laryngeal nerves ascend between it and the trachea.

The thoracic portion of the esophagus passes downward behind the aortic arch, separated from it by the trachea, and then descends in the posterior mediastinum just to the right of the descending aorta (Fig. 9–2). It enters the abdomen through the diaphragm at the level of the tenth thoracic vertebra anterior to the aorta. Its relationships are in front with the trachea, the left bronchus, the pericardium, and the diaphragm; behind, it rests on the vertebral column, the longus colli muscles, the right intercostal arteries, the thoracic duct, and the azygos minor vein. Just as it passes through the diaphragm, it passes somewhat anteriorly to lie immediately in front of the aorta. On the left side of the esophagus in the superior mediastinum are the terminal part of the arch of the aorta, the left subclavian artery, the thoracic duct, and the mediastinal pleura. On the right side, it is covered by the pleura and the azygos vein.

The right and left vagus nerves descend in close contact with the esophagus on its lateral aspects. The right nerve ultimately passes down behind the esophagus in the lower mediastinum, and the left nerve gradually descends to lie in front as the two nerves reach the diaphragm. In the lower part of the posterior mediastinum, the thoracic duct lies to the right of the esophagus.

The abdominal portion of the esophagus is approximately 1.5 cm long and is covered by peritoneum only on its ventral and lateral aspects.

The blood supply of the esophagus is segmental. The arteries supplying the esophagus are derived from the inferior thyroid branch of the subclavian artery, directly from the intercostal branches of the descending thoracic aorta, from the gastric branch of the celiac axis, and from the left inferior phrenic artery of the abdominal aorta. The veins are gathered

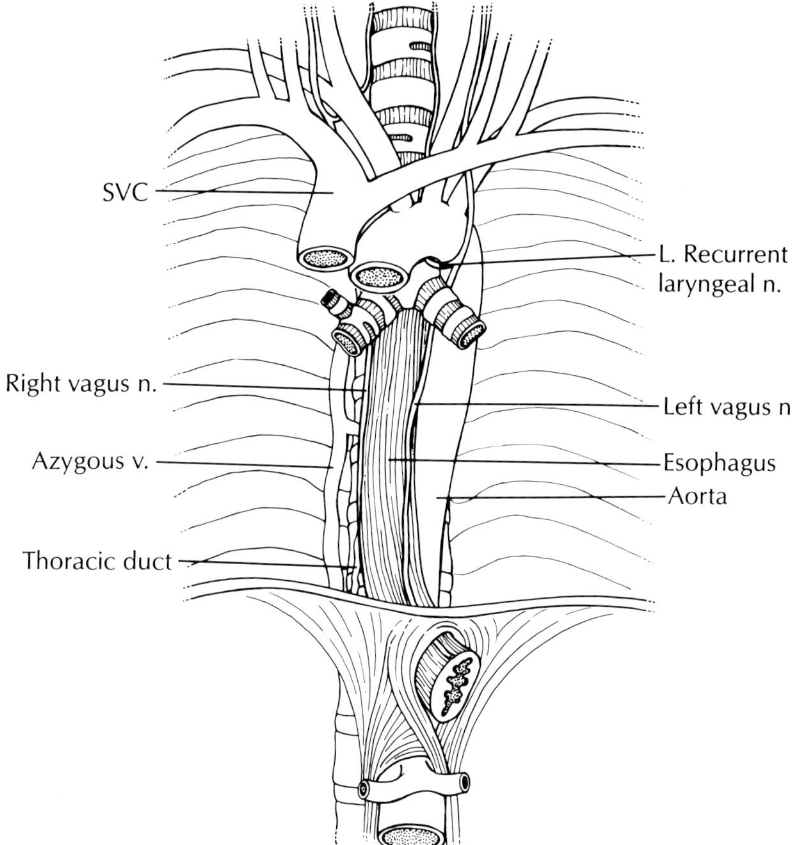

Figure 9–2. Anterior view showing the location of the thoracic esophagus behind the trachea and aortic arch above and medial and slightly anterior to the descending aorta below.

into a plexus that lies on the outer surface of the esophagus. The lower portion of the plexus communicates with the coronary vein of the stomach, the upper branches, and with the azygos and thyroid veins.

The entire cervical and thoracic portions of the esophagus lie in a loose areolar plane. As a result, the contents of the ruptured esophagus readily pass longitudinally in either direction, below upward or from upward downward. This lack of resistance results in devastating contamination of the huge cervical thoracic space, should pharyngeal or esophageal injury not be recognized and treated promptly.

ETIOLOGY AND MECHANISMS OF INJURY

A classification of esophageal injury is shown in Table 9–1. Intraluminal causes of injury are by far the most common and, of this group, iatrogenic perforations from instrumentation varies from 0.2% to 2%,[29] depending on the instrument used, the type of anesthesia, and the experience of the endoscopist. The fiberoptic esophagogastroscope is generally consid-

Table 9–1. Classification of Injury

Intraluminal causes of injury
   Endoscopy, dilations
   Foreign bodies
   Passage of tubes
   Caustic injury
   Miscellaneous
Extraluminal causes of injury
   Penetrating trauma
   Blunt injuries
   Operative injuries
Spontaneous perforation
   Increased intraluminal pressure
   Preexisting esophageal disease
   Neurogenic causes

ered to be safer than the rigid scope, although some report no difference in perforation rate between the two.[18] The 1974 survey by the American Society for Gastrointestinal Endoscopy reported an overall perforation rate of 0.13%, with a 0.09% perforation rate from endoscopy and 0.25% from esophageal dilation. The recent flurry of activity with the flexible transesophageal echocardiography probe also has resulted in very few perforations.

The most common site of perforation is at the pharyngoesophageal junction where the cricopharyngeus muscle produces an abrupt tapering at the esophageal inlet. Inadequate anesthesia, failure to appreciate the degrees of muscular narrowing in this area, large inflated endotracheal tube balloons, and inexperience contribute to these perforations. The second most common site of perforation is at the gastroesophageal junction where the esophagus passes through the narrowed diaphragmatic hiatus. Finally, perforation can occur where the esophagus bends around the aortic arch; this is especially true when rigid esophagoscopes are used.

Adding biopsy or dilations to endoscopy increases the risk of perforation.[15] Dilations are risky because they are performed to dilate strictures caused by such problems as reflux esophagitis, postoperative stenosis, and achalasia. The perforations in these cases usually are in the location of the diseased tissues. Poor visibility, false sense of security under direct vision, and excess perseverance leads to perforation, which often is unrecognized at the time.

Foreign bodies are another frequent cause of perforation. Coins and bones seem to be the leading offenders. Perforation can be caused by penetration of a sharp object; pressure necrosis can be caused by smooth objects and by well meaning endoscopists attempting to remove the foreign body. Whenever possible, a duplicate object should be studied to aid in selecting the appropriate instruments. This is particularly important with children. Attempting to push the foreign body into the stomach is especially hazardous. Occasionally, operative removal is necessary to prevent converting a relatively minor perforation into a major laceration.

Physicians have been inventing gastric and esophageal tubes for centuries, and every one of them at one time or another has caused an esophageal perforation. Celestin tubes and others for palliation of obstructing esophageal carcinomas can create perforation by erosion. Sengstaken-Blakemore and Linton tubes have caused perforation by necrosis; inadvertent inflation of the gastric balloon in the esophagus also will cause laceration or rupture. Endotracheal tubes and endotracheal tube obturators can lead to esophageal injury and perforation during difficult intubations.

Caustic injury is a well known cause of esophageal damage. Spontaneous perforation occurs with the more severe injuries. Other rare causes of intraluminal injury include perforation by sword swallowers, pneumatic blast injuries, and self-dilations.

Extraluminal causes of pharyngeal and esophageal trauma are far less common. The relative rarity of external injuries is accounted for by the protected position of the pharynx and esophagus in the neck and chest. A force sufficient to penetrate the thoracic esophagus often injures surrounding vital structures. Of 600 penetrating wounds that reach the esophagus, there were only three esophageal perforations in one series.[25] Of penetrating wounds that reach the esophagus, most were from gunshot wounds.[21] Sixty percent of these lesions were in the esophageal cervical region and two-thirds were associated with penetrating wounds to the trachea and great vessels. Any time a missile or object penetrates the neck or mediastinum, a pharyngeal or esophageal injury is a possibility. The greatest tragedy is to miss a major injury while dealing with the associated injuries.

Blunt trauma resulting in esophageal rupture or injury is rare. Most ruptures involve the cervical esophagus.[30,31] Beal et al.[30] recently reviewed the world experience with blunt esophageal injury in the 96 known reports since 1900, established an incidence of 0.001% of all blunt trauma admissions, and confirmed the variety of mechanisms leading to injury. In their review, the cervical esophageal injury occurred 70% of the time. Motor vehicle accidents were the most common causes, although something as apparently benign as the Heimlich maneuver was documented as the cause in two cases.[30] Blast injuries from compressed air and children biting inner tubes and soda bottles are rare but lethal injuries that require quick recognition and intervention.[32] Associated injuries are common in blunt esophageal injuries, and they can mask the esophageal injury, which contributes to the delay in diagnosis.

Injury to the esophagus can occur with various paraesophageal operations. Hiatal hernia repair, radical pneumonectomy, and vagotomy are responsible for esophageal injury. The incidence of esophageal perforation after abdominal vagotomy is about 0.5%.[33]

Spontaneous perforations of the esophagus are insidious and difficult to diagnose. They usually are not traumatic in origin. They are the result of a transient increase in intraluminal pressure from prolonged or forceful emesis. The tear usually is in the lower third of the esophagus on the posterolateral wall. Recently, these lesions have been further defined[19] into groups (Table 9–1). These are rarely the result of external trauma, but they represent a significant group of cases with high morbidity and mortality.

EVALUATION AND DIAGNOSIS

The most important part of the diagnosis of pharyngeal and esophageal injuries is a high index of suspicion. In iatrogenic injuries after endoscopy, the possibility that perforation has occurred is fairly obvious, but in other types of penetrating trauma the associated injuries may obscure that of the esophagus and delay its recognition. Multiple studies show that this delay in recognition and treatment contributes significantly to the morbidity and mortality of these injuries.[12,21,23] Successful management requires a high index of suspicion with prompt evaluation, diagnosis, and treatment.

The clinical manifestations of esophageal injuries vary with the site and magnitude of the injury. All the injuries are worsened by increased intraluminal pressure that pushes esophageal or gastric contents out into the cervicomediastinal space, creating a chemical and bacterial mediastinitis. During normal breathing, a negative mediastinal pressure is created, stimulating the movement of air and secretions into this relatively avascular space, further aggravating the situation. The extent that this process takes place and the length of time it rages unchecked will determine the severity of the damage, the treatment, and the ultimate prognosis.

The hallmarks of perforation are fever, leukocytosis, tachycardia, and general malaise. In the cervical region, pain, crepitation, tenderness, and swelling may be present as well. With intrathoracic perforations, severe pain usually is present, but other signs can be minimal. As time progresses, clinical signs of shock may develop.

Roentgenograms of the neck in cervical perforations may show subcutaneous emphysema or widening of the pretracheal space (Fig. 9–3). In thoracic perforations, mediastinal air is virtually diagnostic and may be accompanied by pleural effusion and mediastinal widening. If the perforation is in the intraabdominal portion of the esophagus, then the clinical picture will look like that of any perforated intraabdominal viscus with pain, tenderness, guarding, rebound, rigidity, splinting, and shock. In the acute injury, computed tomography (CT) and magnetic resonance (MR) scanning have not been helpful in diagnosis[30] but may be complementary in documenting effusions, mediastinal air, widening, etc. Both scans may lead to the recognition of the injury when diagnosis is delayed.

The definitive diagnosis is made by demonstrating the leak with a radiopaque soluble

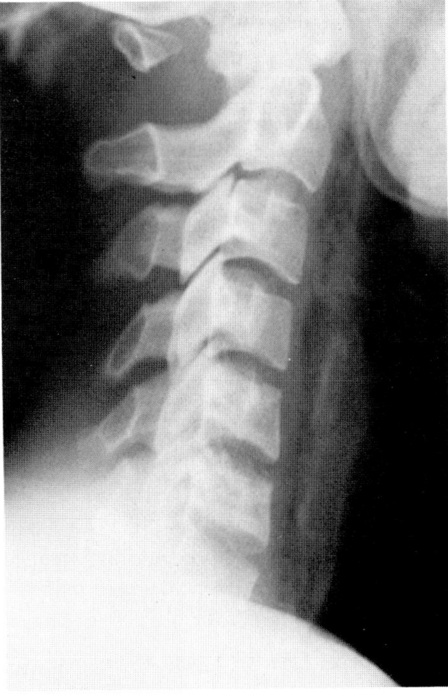

Figure 9–3.   Lateral radiograph of the neck demonstrates blood and air displacing the pharynx and esophagus anteriorly.

contrast swallow (Fig. 9–4).[29,34] This should be routine for all patients in whom it is suspected that a bullet or other penetrating object has traversed the anterior half of the neck or the posterior mediastinum. If an obvious leak cannot be seen and further detail is necessary, this can be followed with a barium swallow. Small amounts of barium are used at first to prevent a barium-contaminated mediastinum. False negative esophagograms do occur[30] and in the presence of other suggestive signs, clinical suspicion should persist. Esophagoscopy usually has been of minimal value in the past because the injury may be increased or missed altogether. Recently, however, Weigelt et al. have shown prospectively that esophagoscopy in the presence of a negative esophagogram can increase the accuracy of diagnosis to nearly 100%.[35] Clearly, if the esophagogram is positive, nothing further needs to be done to establish the diagnosis.

MANAGEMENT

Preoperative, Medical

The successful management of pharyngeal and esophageal perforations involves the application of several surgical principles. The first and most important is early diagnosis.

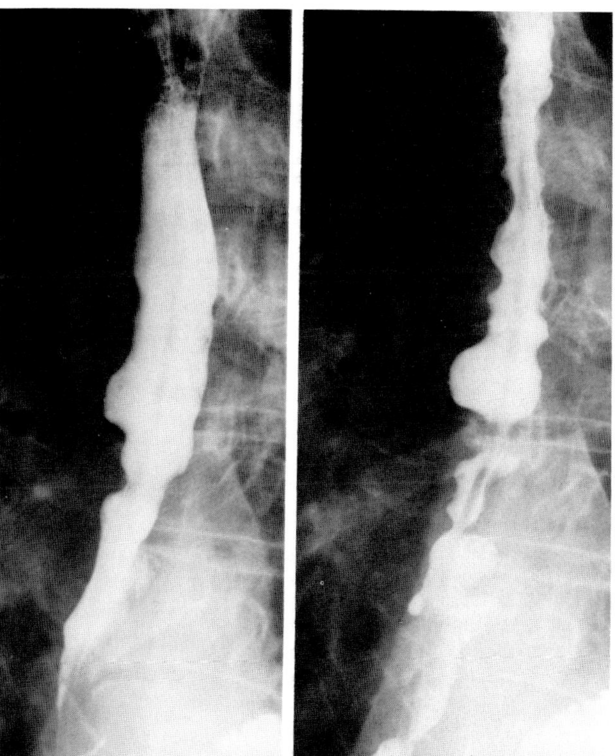

Figure 9–4.   Rupture of the distal supradiaphragmatic esophagus. Contrast media can be seen extravasating posteriorly over the body of the ninth thoracic vertebra.

Multiple studies have demonstrated that the best survival occurs in patients treated promptly (Table 9–2). First, identify the injuries promptly and operate within 12 hr of perforation.[10,15,21,34,36] Second, avoid the danger of continued contamination from the leak. In simple cases with minimal evidence of leak, the patient should be fasted. In severe intrathoracic perforations, esophageal exclusion may be necessary. Third, begin broad-spectrum antibiotics immediately when the injury is suspected. Fourth, institute adequate nutritional support early, because the advent of total parenteral nutrition has significantly reduced the morbidity and mortality associated with severe injuries. Fifth, initiate early and adequate drainage in any case not repairable surgically or that develops as a complication of surgical repair. The application of these steps will vary with the severity of the systemic response and the location of the injury.

Cervical pharyngeal and esophageal injuries present with varying degrees of contamination and systemic response so their management is best individualized.[37] Patients with minimal symptoms and minimal evidence of clinical sepsis can be treated by stopping oral intake and by the use of antibiotics, intravenous hydration, and observation. Success in this setting results from drainage of localized contamination back into the esophagus or the spontaneous sealing of an associated leak in which there has been minimal contamination. The patient needs to be observed carefully, and any sign of sepsis should lead to prompt surgical intervention to secure adequate drainage.

Although some investigators have recently advocated the same approach for iatrogenic injuries,[11,18] the standard of care for intrathoracic injuries remains adequate surgical drainage. Those who advocate primary medical therapy for esophageal perforations are in the minority.[29] In selected cases, medical nonoperative treatment as already outlined can be used. This approach can be used for patients with small tears with little contamination, as manifest by minimal symptoms and minimal clinical evidence of sepsis, who show no signs of progression over the initial 24 hr of observation. In addition, patients with delayed diagnosed injuries who are handling the process well can be considered for nonoperative management. It must be recognized, however, that the signs of mediastinal sepsis initially can be very subtle and that delay in intervening surgically can be catastrophic. Thus, these patients need to be observed very closely and at the first sign of deterioration they should undergo surgical drainage. In general, patients with pneumothorax, pneumoperitoneum, mediastinal emphysema, systemic sepsis, shock, and respiratory failure will die if treated nonoperatively, and all of these patients should be promptly explored. Spontaneous perforation of the distal esophagus (Boerhaave's syndrome) presents initially with pain and rapidly progresses to hypotension and shock. Unrecognized and untreated, the mortality

Table 9–2.   Principles of Management

Operative repair within 12 hr
Stop continuing contamination
Fasting
Esophageal exclusion
Broad-spectrum antibiotics
Good nutritional support
Prompt drainage of secondary leaks

approaches 100%, because these ruptures are inevitably extensive tears. With aggressive surgical therapy within 12 hr of onset, the mortality can be reduced to 20%.

Surgical

Cervical perforations are approached by an incision along the anterior border of the sternocleidomastoid muscle on the suspected side of perforation (Fig. 9–5) (Chapter 7). The pharynx or esophagus is visualized and, if the tear can be seen, it is closed with absorbable suture material and the area widely drained. If the site of a presumed esophageal injury is not obvious, a large-bore (32–40F) catheter or dilator should be passed by the area of presumed injury. Distention of the esophagus in this fashion usually will reveal the site of injury. If this is not successful, using the tube to distend the esophagus with air while the wound is filled with saline will demonstrate the site of the leak. Occasionally, the injury cannot be identified and, in those cases, wide drainage should be used. The patient is given nothing orally for 5 to 7 days and a meglumine diatrizoate swallow is repeated. In the absence of obstruction or significant leak, oral feeding can resume. Occasionally, a small fistula persists, but usually it is sealed off from the neck structures and without distal obstruction will soon close.

In patients with multiple injuries, the approach to the cervical portion of the injury will depend on the priority relative to the other injuries. In cases in which exploration for life-threatening conditions does not allow time for diagnosis of the esophageal lesion, air can be instilled into the esophagus to assess the presence of cervical emphysema. In case of doubt, open surgical drainage should be employed.

Intrathoracic perforations can be managed in several ways, depending on the severity of the injury and the delay in diagnosis before institution of therapy.[38] Generally, the hemithorax into which overt injury or greatest potential contamination has occurred is the side that should be approached, and most often this will be the left pleural space. However, upper thoracic lesions may be more optimally exposed from the right chest, because the aortic arch partially obscures the esophagus when the mediastinum is exposed from the left.

Early injuries that are recognized and treated promptly in which there is minimal mediastinal soilage and reaction can be closed in a single layer with synthetic absorbable suture material. The closure should be bolstered with a local tissue flap to prevent recurrent leakage. These flaps include pleura, pericardium, diaphragm, intercostal muscle, or stomach wall and depends on the location. These flaps are especially important if the tissue reaction has prevented a technically satisfactory closure. In some situations, a partial closure of the friable esophagus can be achieved over a large T tube.[39] The mediastinum should be left open and the chest drained with large-bore thoracostomy tubes. Gastrostomy drainage and feeding jejunostomy are necessary adjuvants.

In high-velocity injuries with gross disruption of the esophagus, an attempt should be made to ascertain the amount of viable esophagus. If possible, the esophagus should be repaired with a single-layer suture technique bolstered with local tissue. When there is extensive tissue loss and the other injuries preclude any extensive primary reconstructive efforts, esophageal exclusion with drainage should be performed. Reconstruction is then accomplished later.

In wounds more than 12 hr old, closure of the leak usually is not possible. The wound edges are often friable and indurated, unsuitable for closure. In these cases, buttressing the

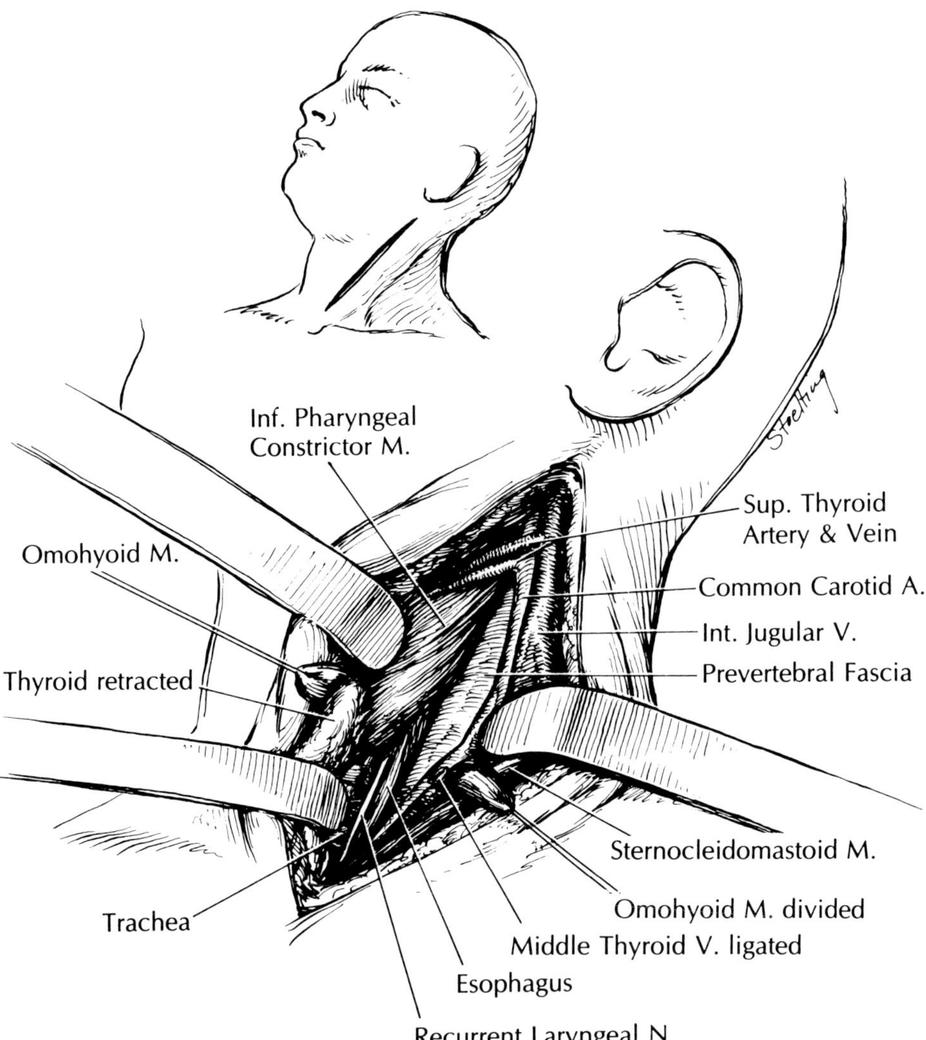

Figure 9–5. The approach to the pharynx and esophagus by an incision placed anterior to the sterno-cleidomastoid muscle. **A:** Left-sided approach.

leak with a pleural flap, cleansing the thorax, decorticating the lung, and draining the area may be all that is possible. In severe cases with major systemic sepsis, esophageal exclusion may be justified. Recently, successful esophageal exclusion has been reported with a Sengstaken-Blakemore balloon tube, but we favor a surgical approach such as that advocated by Urschel and co-workers.[28] An umbilical tape or Silastic band can be tied around the distal esophagus under the vagus nerves. Diverting cervical esophagostomy completes the exclusion (Fig. 9–6). Later, after resolution of the acute process, the distal band can be removed and esophageal continuity restored. Rarely, in situations in which the perforation is accompanied by a distal obstruction (such as a carcinoma), primary resection and anastomosis may be possible, but only if it can be accomplished within a few hours of

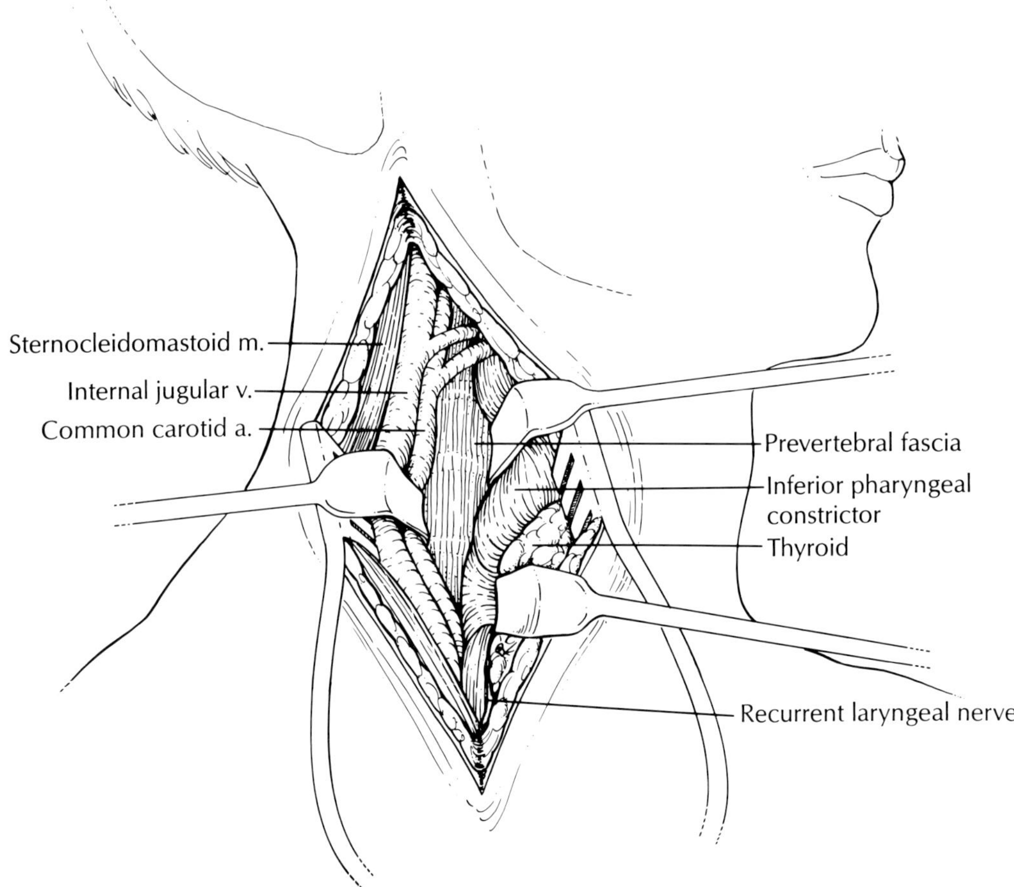

Figure 9–5, cont.   **B:** Right-sided approach.

perforation. In cases of prolonged delay before diagnosis, in the absence of toxemia, where the systemic signs of infection have been controlled by antibiotics and by natural defense mechanisms, transesophageal sump drainage of the abscess cavity in the mediastinum has been successful.[40]

POSTOPERATIVE MANAGEMENT

Postoperative management consists of minimizing the contamination by eliminating all oral intake. Adequate intravenous fluids must be provided, especially in those cases with severe contamination and resulting mediastinitis. Fluid requirements can be very large in these patients with established mediastinitis and sepsis. If there is any uncertainty about the adequacy of fluid replacement, the insertion of a Swan-Ganz catheter and measurement of hemodynamic parameters, including cardiac output and wedge pressure, are of value to guide replacement therapy. Broad-spectrum antibiotics are continued into the postoperative

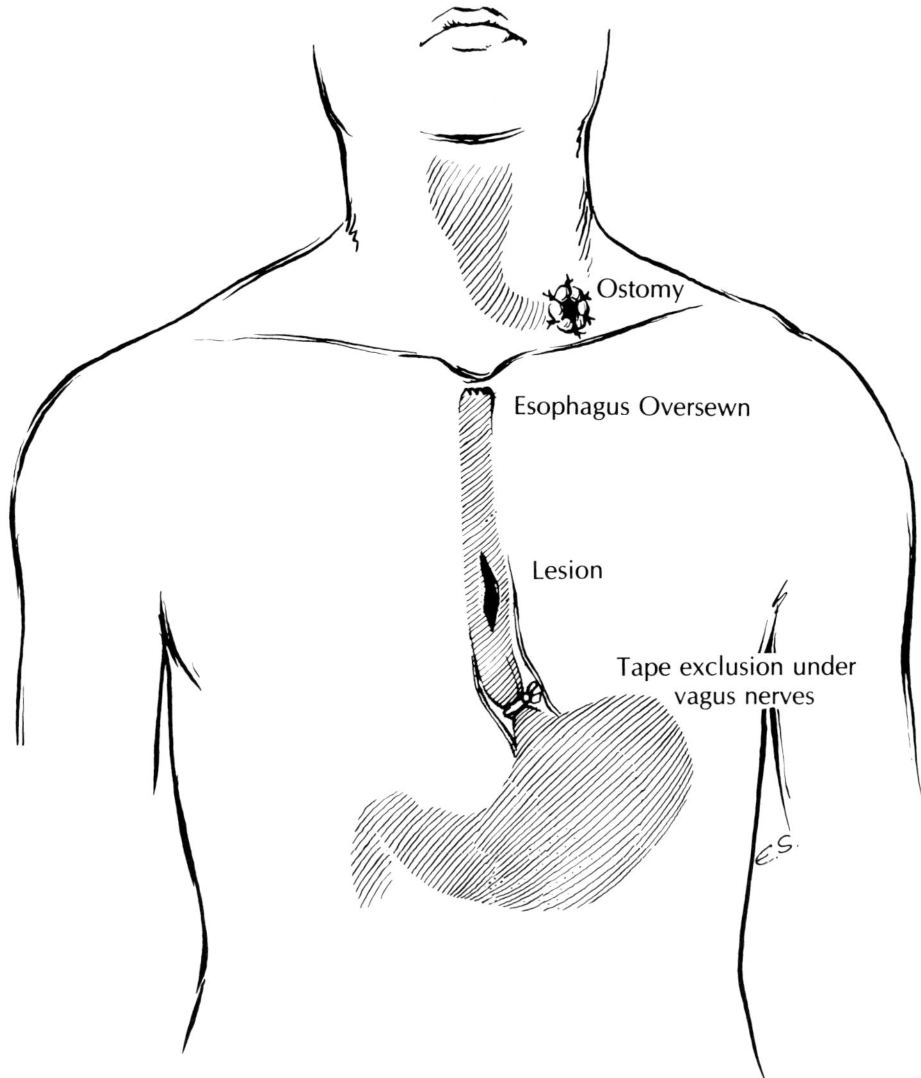

Figure 9–6. Technique of esophageal exclusion. A proximal cervical esophogostomy is followed by oversewing the distal esophagus. Transabdominal ligation of the distal esophagus is carried out by a tape placed under the vagus nerves. A feeding gastrostomy completes the procedure.

period. In general, with adequate drainage and control of continued contamination, a 7- to 10-day course suffices.

Attention to nutrition is critical. At the first sign of a complicated course or in those already nutritionally deficient, total parenteral nutrition should be instituted. In those patients in whom the abdomen was entered for other reasons, such as trauma, a feeding jejunostomy placed at the time of operation can be used.

If the postoperative course is benign, the esophageal leak can be assessed in 7 to 10 days with another meglumine diatrizoate swallow. If no leak is detected, barium can be used to be certain, and then oral feeding can resume. Drainage tubes should be left another 24 to 48 hr after eating to be sure a fistula does not develop. In cases of persistent fistula, total parenteral nutrition should be instituted and oral feeding withheld. In the absence of distal obstruction, most of these fistulas will close.

COMPLICATIONS

The postoperative complications of esophageal injuries are dependent on whether closure has been done, the presence or absence of leak of the closure, the amount of mediastinal and pleural contamination, and the presence of other injuries and their complications. These consist of esophageal leak or fistula, empyema and sepsis, and esophageal obstruction.

Esophageal leak from an anastomosis will occur in many cases and is related to the adequacy of the tissue and repair. It can be reduced by buttressing the repair with local tissue flaps. Adequate drainage of the chest and mediastinum with large-bore thoracostomy tubes should control this fairly common complication. Most persistent leaks or fistulas will close in time in the absence of distal obstruction. Often the patience of the surgeon and patient is severely tested waiting for these leaks to close. Nutrition and attention to the patient's overall condition is critical at this time. Total parenteral nutrition should be initiated early to support the patient's nutritional needs.

An occasional patient will demonstrate signs of continuing progressive sepsis despite what seems to be adequate drainage. Both the ipsilateral and the opposite chest should be assessed carefully for the development of an empyema. Open surgical drainage or tube thoracostomy should be used as appropriate. If sepsis is not promptly controlled by these means, the patient should be reoperated on and a formal esophageal exclusion performed by tying off or dividing the distal esophagus and diverting the cervical esophagus in the neck. Esophageal continuity can be restored at a later time if the patient survives.

Even more rarely, an esophagorespiratory fistula can develop. This usually occurs between the membranous portion of the distal trachea or proximal main stem bronchi and the adjacent esophagus. If recognized early (within 24–48 hr), these fistulas should be treated surgically by dividing the fistula, debriding the wound edges, closing the openings primarily, and interposing a flap of healthy tissue such as sternocleidomastoid muscle between the two structures. A direct surgical attack on those fistulas that are recognized late (more than 48 hr) will be doomed to failure. Instead, drainage of the area must be done, the distal esophagus ligated, and proximal esophagostomy done. Endotracheal intubation should be used if necessary to control respiratory failure. Great attention must be paid to pulmonary toilet and keeping the airway clear; often a tracheostomy may be necessary to accomplish this. Patience is required because it may take 1 or 2 months for these fistulas to close. After 2 to 3 months, if there is not further progression of healing and all sepsis under control, then an attempt should be made to close the fistula surgically. This may require esophagectomy with subsequent gastrointestinal esophageal substitution.

Esophageal stricture and obstruction are the last major complications, particularly after ingestion of caustic material. The first esophagogram after the repair may give an early indication of impending stricture, but often the obstruction may not be apparent for several months. Each patient should have a routine esophagogram at 1 and 3 months after repair. In addition, if any symptoms develop, radiologic evaluation should be done. Most strictures so discovered will respond to periodic dilations. The first dilations should be under direct vision with the rigid esophagoscope; subsequent dilations can be by the patient with mercury-weighted bougies. They will be required frequently at first, with gradually decreasing intervals. It may take as long as 1 yr for the stricture tendency to be overcome. In particularly severe cases of caustic ingestion, esophagectomy may be necessary. Interval feeding is recommended, either by gastrostomy or jejunostomy. After healing has taken place, reconstruction can be undertaken with gastropharyngostomy, jejunopharyngostomy, or right colon bypass. Rarely, the pharynx also may have to be reconstructed using myocutaneous flaps.

RESULTS

The mortality in esophageal injuries is influenced by age, general health, location and size of injury, cause of injury, interval between injury and treatment, the type of treatment, and presence of preexisting esophageal disease. The mortality in most series ranges from 10% to 30%.[10,41] Intrathoracic perforations seem to be twice as lethal as cervical perforations. Delay in therapy increases the mortality significantly. Similarly, old age and preexisting esophageal disease increases the morbidity and mortality.

REFERENCES

1. Brewer LA. History of surgery of the esophagus. *Am J Surg*. 1980;139:730.
2. Meade RH. *A History of Thoracic Surgery*. Springfield, IL: Charles C Thomas; 1961.
3. Cheever DW. *Two Cases of Esophagotomy for Removal of Foreign Bodies with a History of the Operation*. 2nd ed. Boston: James Campbell; 1868.
4. Frink WW. Spontaneous rupture of esophagus: report of a case with recovery. *J Thorac Surg*. 1947;16:291.
5. Barrett NR. Report of a case of spontaneous perforation of the esophagus successfully treated by operation. *Br J Surg*. 1947;35:216.
6. Lyons WS, Seremetis MG, deGuzman VC, et al. Ruptures and perforations of the esophagus. *Ann Thorac Surg*. 1978;25:346.
7. Burnet CM, Rosemurgy AS, Pfeiffer EA. Life-threatening acute posterior mediastinitis due to esophageal perforation. *Ann Thorac Surg*. 1990;49:979.
8. Postlewaithe RW. *Perforation and Rupture in Surgery of the Esophagus*. New York: Appleton-Century-Crofts; 1979.
9. Symbas PN, Hatcher CR, Harlaftis N. Spontaneous rupture of the esophagus. *Ann Surg*. 1978;187:634.
10. Barry BE, Ochsner JL. Perforation of the esophagus. *J Thorac Cardiovasc Surg*. 1973;65:1.
11. Cameron JL, Kieffer RF, Hendrix TR, et al. Selective non-operative management of contained intrathoracic esophageal disruptions. *Ann Thorac Surg*. 1979;27:404.
12. Dubost C, Kaswin D, Duranteau A, et al. Esophageal perforation during attempted endotracheal intubation. *J Thorac Cardiovasc Surg*. 1979;78:33.
13. Faerber N, Schwartz AM, Pinch LW, Leonidas JC. Unusual manifestations of neonatal pharyngeal perforation. *Radiology*. 1980;31:581.
14. Gelfand ET, Risk R, Callaghan JC. Accidental pneumatic rupture of the esophagus. *J Thorac Cardiovasc Surg*. 1977;74:132.
15. Flynn AE, Verrier ED, Way LW, et al. Esophageal perforation. *Arch Surg*. 1989;124:1211.
16. Hirsch M, Abramowitz HB, Shapira S, Barki Y. Hypopharyngeal injury as a result of attempted endotracheal intubation. *Diagn Radiol*. 1978;129:37.
17. Talbert JL, Rodgers BM, Felman AH, Moazam F, et al. Traumatic perforation of the hypopharynx in infants. *J Thorac Cardiovasc Surg*. 1977;74:152.
18. Katz D. Morbidity and mortality in standard and flexible gastrointestinal endoscopy. *Gastrointest Endosc*. 1969;15:134.
19. Michel L, Grillo HC, Malt RA. Esophageal perforation. *Ann Thorac Surg*. 1981;33:203.

20. Rao KVS, Mir M, Cogbill CL. Management of perforations of the thoracic esophagus. *Am J Surg.* 1974;127:609.
21. Symbas PN, Tyrus DH, Hatcher CR Jr. Penetrating wounds of the esophagus. *Ann Thorac Surg.* 1972;13:552.
22. Barringer M, Meredith J. Distal esophageal perforation esophageal exclusion using a modified Sengstaken-Blakemore tube. *Am Surg.* 1982;48:518.
23. Defore WW, Mattox KL, Hansen HA, et al. Surgical management of penetrating injuries of the esophagus. *Am J Surg.* 1977;134:734.
24. Finley RJ, Pearson FG, Weisel RD, et al. The management of nonmalignant intra-thoracic esophageal perforations. *Ann Thorac Surg.* 1980;30:575.
25. Oparah SS, Mandal AK. Operative management of penetrating wounds of the chest in civilian practice. *J Thorac Cardiovasc Surg.* 1979;77:162.
26. Schaefer SD, Bucholz RW, Jones RE, et al. The management of transpharyngeal gunshot wounds to the cervical spine. *Surg Gynecol Obstet.* 1981;152:27.
27. Symbas PN, Hatcher CR, Vlasis PA. Esophageal gunshot injuries. *Ann Surg.* 1980;191:703.
28. Urschel HC, Razzuk MA, Wood RE, et al. Improved management of esophageal perforation; exclusion and diversion in continuity. *Ann Surg.* 1974;179:587.
29. Jones RJ, Samson PC. Esophageal injury. *Ann Thorac Surg.* 1975;19:216.
30. Beal SL, Pottmeyer EW, Spisso JM. Esophageal perforation following external blunt trauma. *J Trauma.* 1988;28:1425.
31. Micon L, Geis L, Siderys H, et al. Rupture of the distal thoracic esophagus following blunt trauma: case report. *J Trauma.* 1990;30:214.
32. Guth AA, Gouge TH, Depan HJ. Blast injury to the thoracic esophagus. *Ann Thorac Surg.* 1991;51:837.
33. Wirthlin LS, Malt RA. Accidents of vagotomy. *Surg Gynecol Obstet.* 1972;125:913.
34. Foley MJ, Ghahremani CG, Rogers LF. Reappraisal of contrast media used to detect upper gastrointestinal perforations: comparison of ionic water-soluble media with barium sulfate. *Radiology.* 1982;144:231.
35. Weigelt JA, Thal ER, Snyder WH III, et al. Diagnosis of penetration cervical esophageal injuries. *Am J Surg.* 1987;154:619.
36. Cheadle W, Richardson JD. Options in management of trauma to the esophagus. *Surg Gynecol Obstet.* 1982;155:380.
37. Lundy LJ, Mandal AK, Lou MA, Alexander JL. Experience in selective operations in the management of penetrating wounds of the neck. *Surg Gynecol Obstet.* 1978;147:845.
38. Attar S, Hankins JR, Suter CM, et al. Esophageal perforation: a therapeutic challenge. *Ann Thorac Surg.* 1990;50:45.
39. Mulder DS, Barkum JS. Injury to the trachea, bronchus, and esophagus. In: Mattox KL, Moore EE, Feliciano DV, eds. *Trauma.* Norwalk, CT: Appleton & Lange; 1988:335–347.
40. McNamee CJ, Meyns B, Pagliero KM. New method for dealing with last-presenting spontaneous esophageal ruptures. *Ann Thorac Surg.* 1991;52:151.
41. Keszler P, Buzna E. Surgical and conservative management of esophageal perforation. *Chest.* 1981;80:158.

10

Laryngeal Trauma

CRAIG W. SENDERS, M.D.

HISTORY: Descriptions of laryngeal trauma are available only in relatively recent times, presumably because injuries to the larynx were either immediately fatal or trivial. Habicot,[1] a Parisian surgeon, did a tracheostomy in 1620 on a boy whose airway was obstructed. The boy, apparently to avoid being robbed, attempted to swallow a small bag of money, which resulted in acute laryngeal obstruction. Habicot performed a tracheostomy and through this was able to push the bag down the esophagus into the stomach.

Intubation of the larynx for acute obstruction by croup was introduced by Eugéne Bouchut in 1856 to 1858.[2] Pierre Bretonneau performed the first tracheotomy (successful) for croup in 1825.[3] The technique of tracheotomy was subsequently perfected in 1885 by the conscientious labors of Joseph P. O'Dwyer of New York.[4] In 1945, traumatic laryngectomy with survival was reported by Jackson and Jackson.[5] The entire larynx of a quarryman in this instance was torn away by a premature blast.

Laryngeal trauma may be divided into two categories, external and internal. Internal laryngeal trauma is caused by intubation and endoscopic and other surgical procedures and will not be discussed in this chapter. External laryngeal trauma includes direct blunt and penetrating injuries to the larynx.

After the introduction of the lap seat belt, the incidence of laryngeal trauma appeared to increase.[6] The "padded dash syndrome" and "seat belt syndrome" referred to a constellation of injuries that included laryngeal trauma.[7,8] After a sudden deceleration, the torso of a person wearing a lap belt is thrown forward so that the forehead or face strikes the windshield (Fig. 10–1). This hyperextends the neck, causing the exposed larynx to strike the dashboard. Frequently, these individuals suffer multiple facial lacerations, with or without facial fractures, and blunt laryngeal trauma. Because of the extreme hyperextension of the neck, some victims may also suffer fracture of the second cervical vertebrae, the so-called hangman's fracture.[8] With the use of the shoulder harness, however, these types of injuries have decreased in frequency.[9,10]

The reason external laryngeal injuries are not as common as might be expected, despite its seemingly obvious vulnerability, is because the larynx is quite well protected by bony and cartilaginous structures. The vertebrae obviously protect it posteriorly. The mandible protects the laryngeal structures from above as well as below and the sternum

160

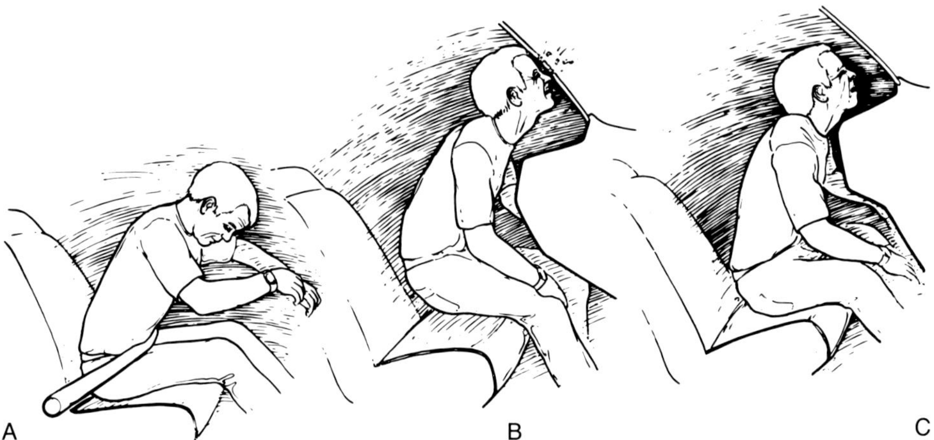

Figure 10–1.   Padded dash syndrome. **A:** Thrown forward, mandible protects anterior neck. **B:** Face strikes windshield hyperextending neck and exposing anterior neck. Cervical spine fracture may occur. **C:** Larynx strikes dash.

affords protection inferiorly.[11] When a potential victim is thrown forward, the neck flexes, which provides protection by the mandible. The flexibility of the larynx and trachea and the presence beside them of the sternocleidomastoid muscle give some protection from lateral injury.[12] Last, the compliance of the laryngeal cartilages provides the larynx with some resistance to trauma, although progressive calcification of these cartilages with age causes the larynx to become increasingly susceptible to trauma.[13]

ANATOMY

The larynx consists of a rigid cartilaginous framework, united in a dynamic mechanism by intrinsic and extrinsic muscles and ligaments, and lined by mucous membrane (Fig. 10–2). The larynx lies anterior to the fourth, fifth, and sixth cervical vertebrae. The laryngeal cartilages consist of the epiglottic, thyroid, cricoid, and arytenoid cartilages and two small accessory cartilages, the corniculate and cuneiform. The corniculate and cuneiform cartilages are small, nonfunctional accessory cartilages lying above the arytenoids in the aryepiglottic folds.

The thyroid cartilage is suspended from the hyoid by the thyrohyoid ligament. The inferior cornu of the thyroid cartilage articulates with the cricoid cartilage in a pair of true synovial joints.

The cricoid cartilage is fixed to the thyroid cartilage by the cricothyroid ligament. The cricoid is the only intact circumferential ring of cartilage in the laryngotracheal bronchial tree and it is therefore rigid and nonexpansile. The posterosuperior aspect of the cricoid expands to support the two arytenoid cartilages. Inferiorly, the cricoid attaches to the first trachea ring by an intercartilaginous ligament.

The arytenoid cartilages sit on the posterosuperior cricoid cartilage. The vocal cord reaches from the vocal process of the arytenoid cartilage to the thyroid cartilage. The arytenoids articulate with the cricoid cartilage at the synovial cricoarytenoid joints,

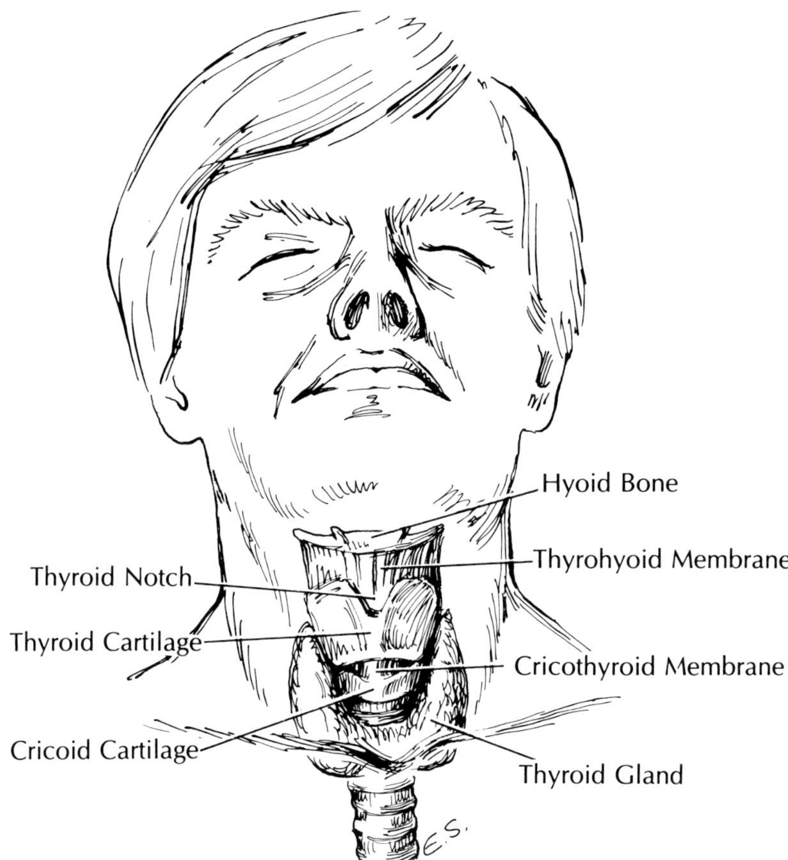

Figure 10–2.   Anterior thoracic anatomy of the trachea. The great veins and aortic arch pass anterior to the trachea.

permitting three-dimensional movements and changes in vocal cord position, thus modifying voice and airway.

The epiglottis is a single, leaf-shaped cartilage attached to the upper thyroid cartilage by the thyroepiglottic ligament. The aryepiglottic folds are folds of mucous membrane that sweep from the epiglottis to the arytenoid cartilages. The aryepiglottic folds separate the pyriform sinuses from the larynx.

The intrinsic and extrinsic laryngeal muscles and ligaments function to provide vocal cord movement for voice and airway function.

The nerve supply to the larynx consists of two branches of the vagus nerve, the superior and recurrent laryngeal nerves. The superior laryngeal nerve supplies sensation to the larynx above the vocal cords and motor innervation to an extrinsic muscle, the cricothyroid. The recurrent laryngeal nerve innervates all of the other intrinsic muscles and provides sensation below the vocal cords.

The superior laryngeal nerve, a fourth bronchial arch derivative, courses to the neck behind the internal carotid artery and divides into the external and internal laryngeal nerves. The external laryngeal nerve supplies the cricothyroid muscle; the interior laryngeal nerve passes through the thyrohyoid membrane to supply the mucous membrane of the larynx.

The recurrent laryngeal nerve, a sixth bronchial arch derivative, has a different course on the right and left. On the right side it passes from front to back around the subclavian artery just distal to the artery's origin from the innominate. After passing around the artery, it then courses upward in the groove between the esophagus and the trachea. It enters the larynx between the cricoid and thyroid gland and behind the superior thyroid artery. If the subclavian artery has an aberrant origin, the recurrent laryngeal nerve may not be recurrent at all and enters the larynx directly at the level of the cricoid cartilage. On the left side, the recurrent nerve takes origin from the vagus as it passes anterior to the aortic arch and then courses under the arch just lateral to the ligamentum arteriosum, a remnant of the sixth bronchial arch. It then passes upward medially between the esophagus and trachea in similar fashion to the nerve on the right.

MECHANISM OF INJURY

Penetrating Laryngeal Injuries

The most common cause of penetrating injuries of the upper airway has been military combat situations. The experience in Vietnam was such that Miller reported 35 cases of penetrating laryngeal trauma during a 2-yr period.[14] Twenty-five of the injuries were caused by moderate-velocity metallic fragments, and 10 were associated with high-velocity bullets. In the civilian sector, the most common cause of penetrating laryngeal trauma is the knife, although bullets also are responsible.[15,16]

When *bullet wounds* penetrate the larynx, there is a high fatality rate due to loss of the airway. The dramatic tissue destruction caused by high-velocity missiles is described well by Owen-Smith.[17] Because of the delicate nature of the larynx, any bullet wound to this area causes severe damage; these victims frequently never survive to reach a hospital but die of respiratory obstruction in the field. With a large laryngeal wound, therefore, it is often judicious to establish the airway with an endotracheal tube through the wound. Later, under more controlled circumstances, a tracheotomy may be performed. In addition, there may be damage to the great vessels of the neck that will require immediate attention. After the victim has been stabilized, attempts to repair the laryngeal defect may be made. Because the defect can be very extensive, some patients eventually may require a laryngectomy, although the decision to do this should very rarely be made initially. In a series of six patients with bullet wounds to the larynx, Harrison reported that three ultimately required a laryngectomy.[18]

Knife wounds are the most common cause of penetrating injury to the larynx in the civilian sector.[15] Suicide attempts typically produce a slash-type wound across the anterior neck.[16] Laryngeal and vascular injuries are quite common and the need for intervention is obvious. The extent of injury from a stab wound requires a careful evaluation as the extent of injury is not obvious. In one study, 65% of patients with anterior neck stab wounds had associated thyroid cartilage injury.[16] Fiberoptic laryngoscopy can determine the likelihood of significant laryngeal or pharyngeal injury. For patients with a normal fiberoptic exam and radiographic swallow study without voice changes, observation is appropriate.

Blunt Laryngeal Trauma

The most common cause of blunt laryngeal trauma is motor vehicle accidents.[15,19–22] Pennington[6] showed that a vertical midline or paramedian laryngeal fracture was the most common type of injury after automobile accidents. Due to the calcification of the laryngeal cartilages, the amount of horizontal fracturing, or comminution, increased with the age of the patient.

Clothesline-type trauma also can cause serious injury to the larynx and to the cervical spine (Fig. 10–3). The incidence appears to be increasing with the more common use of recreational vehicles.[23] Typically, young adults are involved in riding motorized bikes, snowmobiles, or water skiing, and therefore are the most susceptible age group to this type of injury. The strung-out wire or cable may strike the neck directly or it may hit the anterior chest wall and slide to the neck (Fig. 10–3). If the cable strikes the larynx directly, it will cause laryngeal injury in a similar manner to blunt laryngeal trauma. In the latter situation, where the cable strikes the anterior chest wall and slides to the neck, the larynx is suddenly tugged superiorly, which may result in complete laryngotracheal separation, often with associated cricoid fractures.[23] In any clothesline-type injury, an associated cervical spine fracture must be looked for.

Attempted strangulation also can be responsible for laryngeal fractures. Harm and Rajs studied 37 such victims.[13] Of the 14 who were older than 40 years of age, 11 sustained fractures of the hyoid bone or thyroid cartilage, whereas of the 23 who were under 40 years of age, only 9 sustained fractures. Increased calcification, which occurs naturally with aging, makes the larynx much more susceptible to this type of injury. Temporary vocal cord paralysis also may occur; Peppard reported five cases of vocal cord paralysis after attempted strangulation.[24] As may be anticipated, all had attained normal vocal cord function within 3 months.

External laryngeal injury in children is rare and easily overlooked.[25] Holinger and Schild reported on 159 patients with internal or external laryngeal trauma.[26] Of these, 42

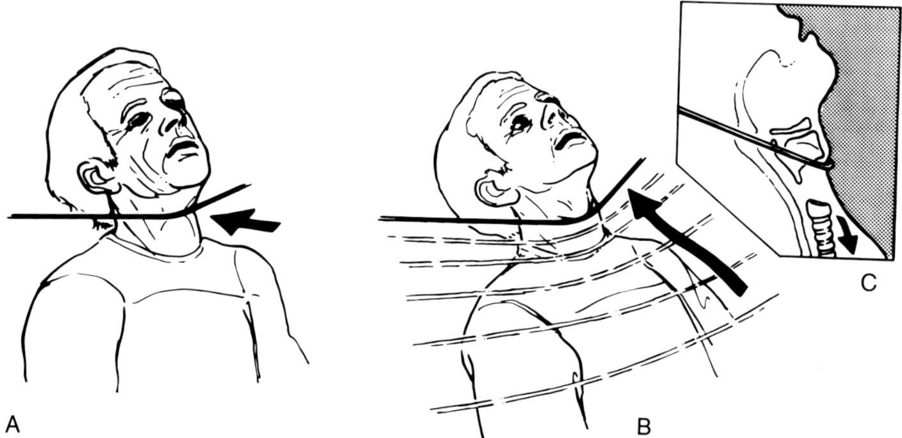

Figure 10–3. Clothesline injury. **A:** Cable striking larynx directly, resulting in localized blunt laryngeal trauma. **B:** Cable strikes anterior chest and slides up to neck. **C:** This pulls larynx superiorly causing laryngotracheal separation.

were in children less than 18 months of age and, of these, only one was due to external laryngeal trauma. By contrast, there were 29 patients with laryngeal trauma in the 19- to 25-yr age group and, of these, 27 had external laryngeal trauma. Meyer et al.[25] reported only 30% of the blunt laryngeal trauma in children was caused by motor vehicle accidents, whereas 50% was caused by accidents of other types. The incidence of soft tissue injury without cartilaginous injury was more frequent than in adults.

There are several factors that make children less susceptible to external laryngeal injury. First, the laryngeal cartilages are not calcified and are extremely flexible.[25,27] In addition, the ligaments surrounding the larynx are very pliable and allow for greater mobility of the larynx when traumatized. The larynx rests at a different level in the child than in the adult[25,28] (Fig. 10–4). At birth the cricoid is at approximately the level of C4; it progresses to C7 in the adult. The higher position of the larynx in the infant gives it greater protection by the mandible and makes it less susceptible to external trauma.

PATHOPHYSIOLOGY

Mild laryngeal injury typically occurs in a younger person with compliant laryngeal cartilages (Fig. 10-5). In this situation the larynx is compressed against the cervical vertebrae but snaps back to its appropriate position without sustaining a fracture. The snap-back causes stretching and pulling on the intralaryngeal structures, resulting in minor hematoma formation of the true vocal cords. Occasionally, the vocal cords may tear. In addition, the anterior vocal ligament may become detached with this manipulation.[6] Vocal

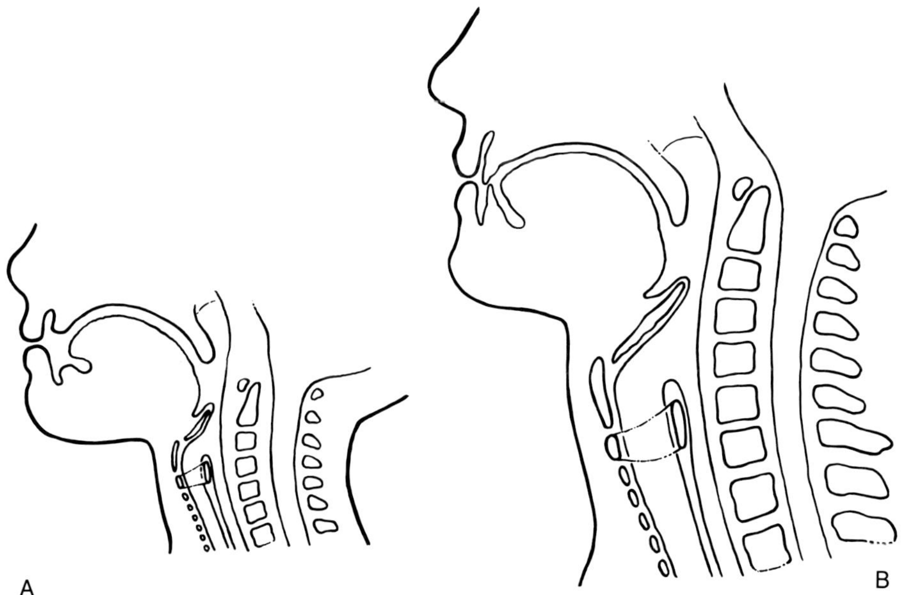

Figure 10–4.   **A:** Infantile larynx rests at a higher position with a posterior tilt. The cricoid is approximately at the level of C4. **B:** In the adult larynx the cricoid rests at C7. Because the posterior tilt of the larynx is less, the epiglottis does not visually obstruct the larynx.

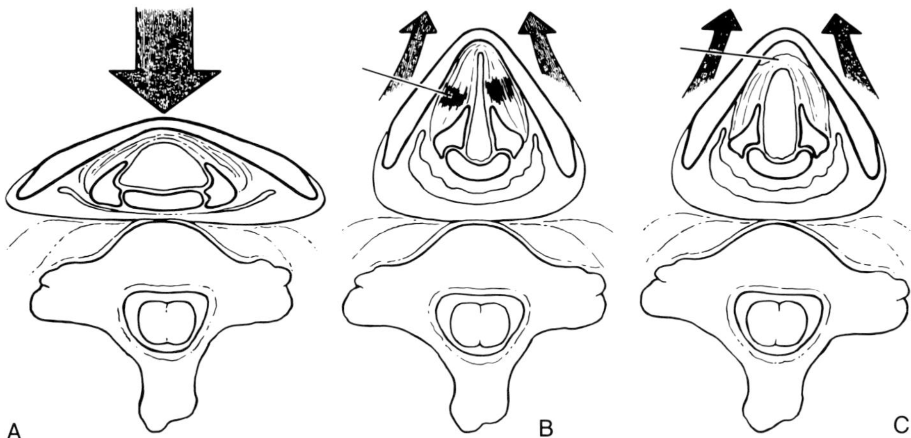

Figure 10–5. Laryngeal injury without fractures. **A:** Compression against vertebrae. **B:** In the minimally calcified larynx, the snap-back may result in hematoma formation of TVC. **C:** Rarely the anterior vocal ligament can become detached.

ligament detachment may occur with or without a fracture and results in foreshortening of the glottic aperture. The main symptoms are dysphonia and odynophonia, but the diagnosis often can be difficult to make clinically as a change in the cord length of 2 mm may not be noticed by the examiner. Unfortunately, a small change in cord length can result in lifelong hoarseness, especially in a woman. A computerized tomography (CT) may show this deformity, however.

In the calcified larynx of a victim over 40 years of age, compression of the thyroid cartilage may cause a vertical fracture, often with comminution and associated numerous horizontal fractures (Fig. 10–6).[6,29] Fractures of the cricoid are produced in a similar manner as fractures of the thyroid but can be much more devastating. With any fracture of the thyroid cartilage, rupture of the thyroepiglottic ligament may occur and is associated with a mucosal tear and herniation of the preepiglottic fat pad into the laryngeal space (Fig. 10–7).[6]

Cricotracheal separation can occur from a clothesline injury (Fig. 10–3) or from lateral laryngeal trauma. Lateral trauma also can result in a hinge-like action on the cricotracheal attachment that may produce partial or complete separation (Fig. 10–8). Anatomical features are presented in Table 10–1.

ASSESSMENT OF LARYNGEAL DAMAGE

Symptoms and Signs (Tables 10–2 and 10–3)

Patients with isolated laryngeal trauma often present with dysphonia or aphonia, varying degrees of dysphagia, subcutaneous emphysema, respiratory distress, and occasionally with hemoptysis. The amount of airway distress may be minimal or severe. Initially, mild respiratory distress may progress rapidly to severe respiratory distress. Therefore, most cases of significant laryngeal trauma require a tracheotomy, either expectantly or pro-

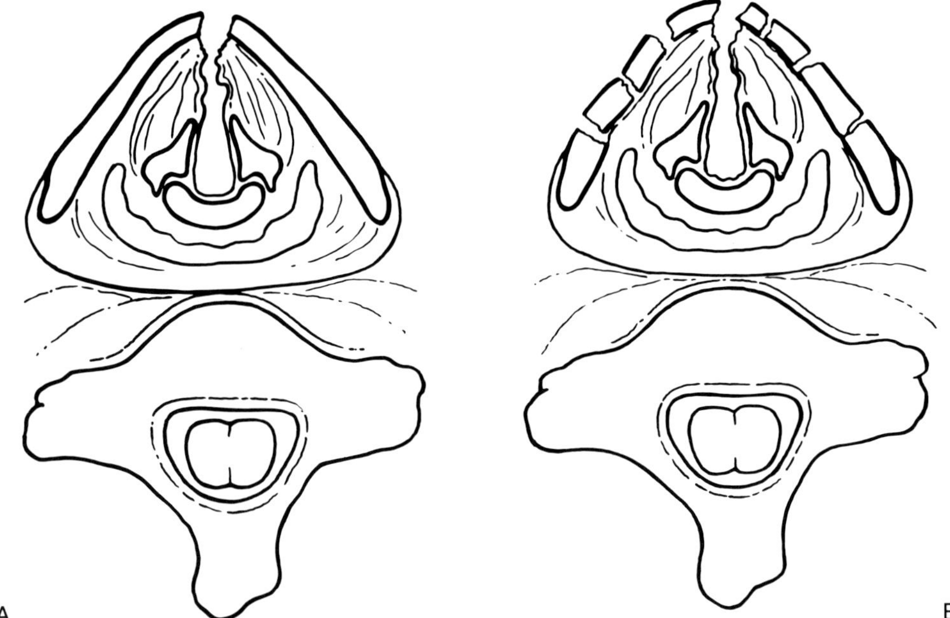

Figure 10–6. Laryngeal fracture. **A:** Compression with vertical fracture is most common. **B:** In a highly calcified larynx, multiple vertical and horizontal fractures may occur. The snap-back injury is reduced.

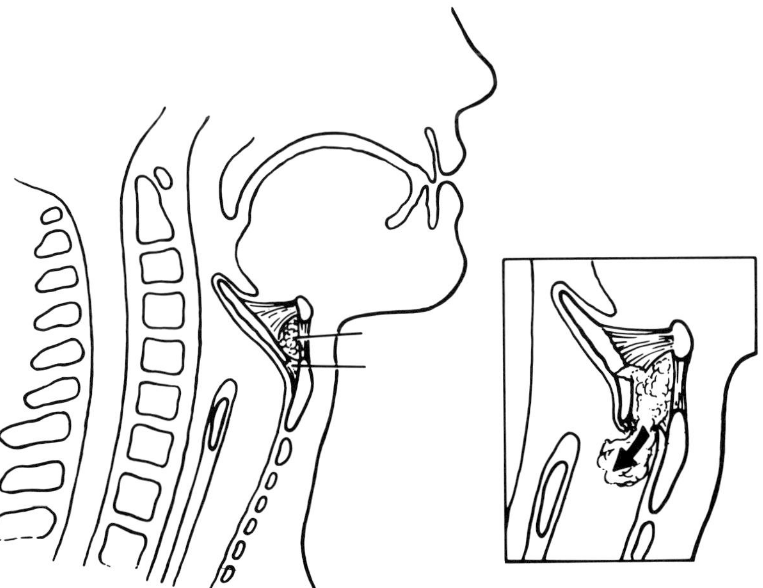

Figure 10–7. Rupture of thyroepiglottic ligament may obstruct airway and indirect view of the larynx.

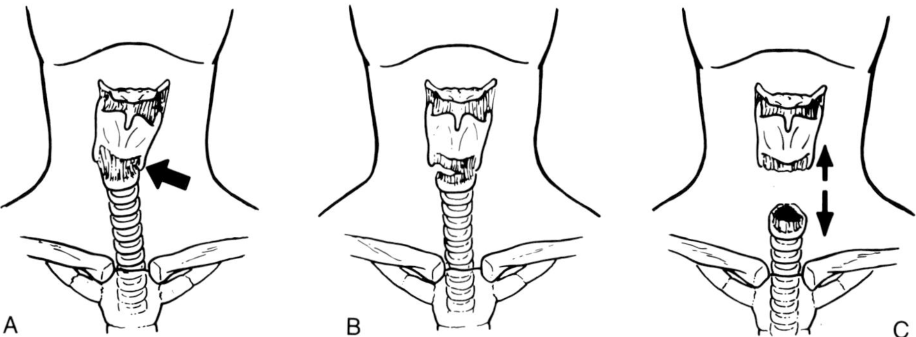

Figure 10–8. Cricotracheal separation from lateral trauma. **A:** Lateral trauma. **B:** Parietal cricotracheal separation. **C:** Complete cricotracheal separation with tracheal retraction into the mediastinum.

phylactically. These patients should not be intubated unless the laryngeal exam indicates only minimal trauma for fear of intubating a false passage.

External examination may reveal subcutaneous emphysema, although this may be a normal finding after a tracheotomy, particularly if the patient was ventilated by a mask during the tracheotomy. There often is a loss of the thyroid prominence, although in many women the prominence is normally recessive. Also, in many patients with excessive edema and hematoma formation, along with subcutaneous emphysema of the neck, this flattening may be difficult to appreciate. The larynx often is tender, and there may be a loss of the normal laryngeal crepitus.

Whenever feasible, all patients with laryngeal trauma should undergo an indirect or fiberoptic laryngeal examination to establish vocal cord mobility and to look for lacerations, edema, and hematoma formation. In patients with rupture of the thyroepiglottic ligament and herniation of the preepiglottic fat pad into the laryngeal lumen, the indirect examination may be nonfruitful. Here, only the direct examination can ascertain the degree of laryngeal injury.

Despite all of these signs and symptoms, this injury may go undiagnosed in an intubated patient when the diagnosis was not suspected at the time of intubation or when the airway distress is mild and is blamed on facial, neurological, or chest injuries. In this

Table 10–1. Laryngotracheal Injury: Anatomic Features

Cartilaginous fracture may range from a simple nondisplaced thyroid fracture to a severe comminution of both thyroid and cricoid cartilages

Mucosal lacerations and hematoma can lead to extensive stenosis of the laryngeal airway

Thyrotracheal or laryngotracheal separation results in marked subcutaneous emphysema and airway compromise

Ligamentous tears with avulsion of the thyroepiglottic ligament leads to anterior commissure blunting, hoarseness, and posterior displacement of the epiglottis with airway compromise

Injury to recurrent laryngeal nerve will result in vocal cord paralysis; with bilateral cord paralysis, airway obstruction is likely

Cricoarytenoid joint rupture leads to ankylosis, vocal cord immobility, and voice and airway compromise

Table 10–2.   Symptoms of Laryngotracheal Injury

Airway obstruction; stridor and intercostal and supraclavicular retraction may not be present initially
  but may rapidly develop
Dysphonia or aphonia, depending on the degree of vocal cord injury and surrounding edema
Cough secondary to aspiration, endobronchial bleeding, or vagal stimulation
Hemoptysis due to mucosal laceration
Neck pain aggravated by coughing or swallowing, especially with hyoid fracture
Dysphagia or odynophagia, primarily due to associated esophageal laceration or bruising

situation, the laryngeal trauma may be discovered when the patient is extubated when the airway deteriorates unexpectedly. Sometimes, laryngeal trauma is not diagnosed until many hours later when the patient develops persistent dysphonia or progressive airway problems.

After the airway is secured or judged to be stable in a very mild injury a search for other injuries must be undertaken. These patients often have a cervical spine injury that may be missed during initial concern over patency of the airway with potentially devastating results.[30,31] Pneumothorax is a common associated finding, and routine chest x-ray is indicated.[31]

In addition to a complete examination of the head and neck vocal cord motion, an endolaryngeal injury should be evaluated by indirect laryngoscopy or fiberoptic laryngoscopy. Vocal cord paralysis may be temporary, as from edema. Unilateral vocal cord paralysis should be managed conservatively.

Radiographic Evaluation

As neck trauma usually requires standard cervical films, the initial recognition of laryngeal injury may be on the lateral cervical film (Fig. 10–9).

CT scans should be obtained in all cases with dysphonia where the planned management is conservative to help identify cases where surgical intervention is recommended, such as anterior vocal cord ligament detachments and nondisplaced cricoid fractures. A CT scan also is of benefit in the patient with severe laryngeal trauma where the indication to explore the larynx may be unclear. The CT scan may help avoid an unnecessary exploration on those patients in whom the internal derangement is due to edema and hematoma rather than displacement of the laryngeal cartilages (Fig. 10–10).[29,32] Magnetic resonance (MR) scans are of little benefit in assessing cartilage displacement.

An esophagram with water-soluble dye can alleviate concern about a hypopharyngeal or esophageal tear when there is no other reason to explore the patient.[33]

Table 10–3.   Signs of Laryngotracheal Injury

Deformity of the neck: flat thyroid contour
Subcutaneous emphysema—air crepitation
Laryngeal or tracheal tenderness
Crepitation over the laryngeal framework

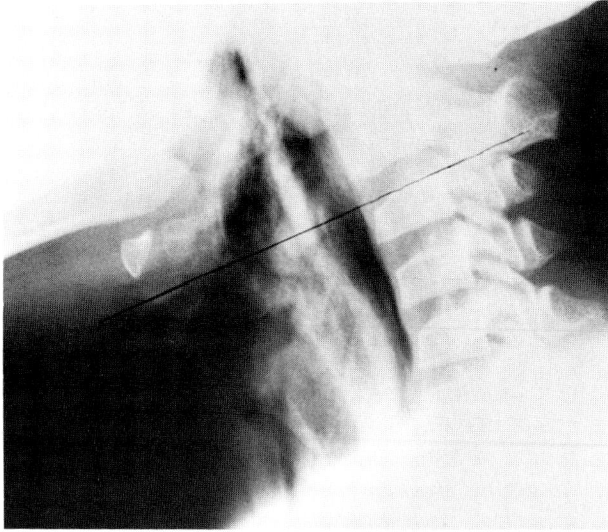

Figure 10–9. The lateral neck film shows extensive, subcutaneous air and an elevated hyoid bone. Normally, the hyoid bone is below a line drawn along and parallel to the superior surface of the C3 vertebral body. Operative findings confirmed laryngeal fracture and elevated hyoid.

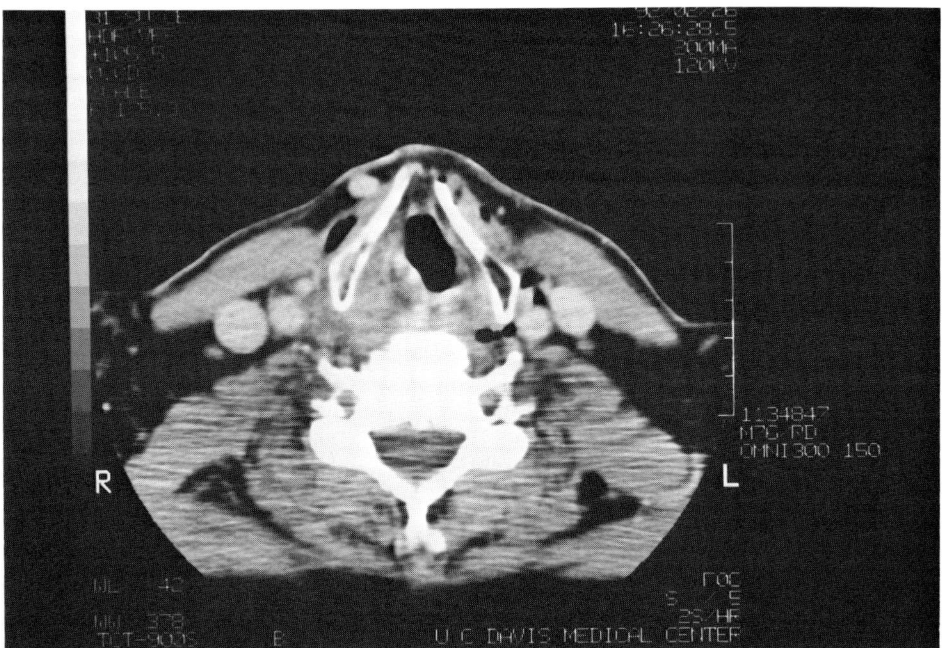

Figure 10–10. CT scan showing edema and hematoma formation of right true vocal cord. Subcutaneous emphysema is prevalent, but cartilage fractures are not demonstrated.

Endoscopy

Direct laryngoscopy, bronchoscopy, and esophagoscopy should be performed on all patients if they have undergone a tracheotomy and in all cases where an open exploration is planned.

MANAGEMENT

Emergency Treatment

The first concern in managing blunt laryngeal trauma is preservation of the airway. One must also keep in mind that the patient may have cervical spine injuries. Intubation should be avoided if at all possible because of the danger of manipulation of the neck in the presence of a possible cervical spine injury and because a false passage may be created when inserting the tube, which may induce a respiratory crisis. Moreover, patients with laryngeal trauma should not be sedated as this may aggravate their respiratory problems.

In an emergency situation, the patient may be ventilated with a mask while an emergency tracheotomy is performed. Mask ventilation will greatly increase the subcutaneous emphysema, however. The emergency tracheotomy should be done through a vertical incision so as to give better exposure in the presence of traumatized anatomy and to provide rapid entry into the airway with minimal bleeding[31] (see Chapter 21).

Cricothyrotomy should be discouraged, as the cricoid itself may be fractured, making the procedure difficult or even impossible to perform.[22] Furthermore, attempting the cricothyrotomy may greatly increase the damage to the area, making the ultimate treatment much more difficult. Oxygenation through a 14-gauge angiocatheter inserted into the trachea may buy additional time while a tracheotomy is performed.

Definitive Treatment

Principles of Laryngeal Healing

In the management of laryngeal trauma, the primary goal is to maintain an adequate airway and a normal voice. By understanding laryngeal physiology and the unique healing properties of the larynx, one may be able to facilitate normal laryngeal healing with the correct medical and surgical management.

The larynx is quite unique in its ability and manner of healing.[34] Exposed cartilage, which has no blood supply, depends on its nourishment from the perichondrium and has a strong susceptibility to infection, which produces an extensive inflammatory reaction. In the healing process, granulation tissue formation is replaced by collagen deposition. Small amounts of scarring in key locations may produce drastic changes in respiratory and vocal functions.

Because of the adverse effect of scarring within the lumen on function of the larynx, healing by secondary intention should be prevented, especially in critical areas. The subglottis, the anterior commissure, and, to a lesser degree, the posterior commissure, are naturally prone to detrimental scarring. For this reason, in these areas it is particularly important to reapproximate torn mucosa with 4-0 or 5-0 chromic sutures. In the area of the cricoid, if mucosa is missing, a free graft of mucosa usually works well. It is very important to initiate early repair, preferably within the first 24 hr, to avoid secondary healing with its prolific granulation tissue formation. If the repair must be delayed for any medical reasons, steroids and antibiotics may decrease this response.

It is generally considered that stenting actually may be detrimental.[34] Because of the constant laryngeal motion, there is a tendency for frictional epithelial loss from the stent. Secondary healing with granulation tissue followed by collagen deposition is the invariable result. In addition, the constant pressure of the stent on the cartilage of the arytenoids can cause permanent changes. Peacock, in his book *Wound Repair* states: "the surgeon, from time immemorial, has had the uncontrollable urge to put a tube through every aperture or circular structure he operates upon . . . from a general standpoint . . . the biological foundations of wound repair strongly suggest that a great number of such tubes exert deleterious influences on healing and that considerable damage has been produced on tubular organs because of such practice . . . there is no question that such a tube is deleterious to the basic mechanisms of wound healing."[34,35]

Undoubtedly, stenting is beneficial to the healing of the larynx in some situations, but it is not without a cost. Therefore, the benefits versus the detriments must be weighed carefully before use. Stents and keels should be used only when specific indications for their use are met.

Classification of Injuries Based on Their Management

Schaefer and Close devised several forms of treatment that were based on the clinical findings and the principles of laryngeal healing.[22] Below is a modified classification based on the optimal treatments (Table 10–4).

Group 1: Conservative Management Without Tracheotomy

A form of conservative management without a tracheotomy is recommended for those patients who have no airway compromise and minor laryngeal injury. This implies that there is only minor edema, hematoma formation, or lacerations of the endolarynx. Further, there is no exposed cartilage or herniation of the preepiglottic fat. The vocal cords are not foreshortened—indicating an intact anterior vocal ligament—and the arytenoids are not dislocated. A CT scan is recommended, which may show nondisplaced fractures of the larynx but no evidence of detachment of the anterior vocal ligament.

Table 10–4.   Classification Based on Treatment

Group 1:	Conservative management without tracheotomy	
Group 2:	Conservative management with tracheotomy	
Group 3:	Operative management	
Type A:	Open exploration without splinting	
Type B:	Open exploration with keel	
Type C:	Open exploration with stent	

Adapted with permission from Schaefer.[22]

This treatment includes inhospital close observation of the airway, voice rest, cool humidification, and elevation of the head of the bed. Steroids are of benefit to decrease edema if given early. Antibiotics are recommended if there are lacerations. One should be cautioned that, with the use of steroids and antibiotics, mediastinitis from a hypopharyngeal or esophageal tear may be masked.

Group 2: Conservative Management with Tracheotomy

A form of conservative management with a tracheotomy is recommended for those patients with significant airway compromise or pending airway compromise with minor laryngeal injury. Although lacerations may be present, there should be no exposed cartilage or herniation of the preepiglottic fat pad. The CT scan may show nondisplaced fractures of the larynx or cricoid but no evidence of detachment of the anterior vocal ligament.

The management includes a low tracheotomy, direct laryngoscopy, bronchoscopy, and esophagoscopy. When indicated, the dislocated arytenoid is relocated endoscopically.[36] Although arytenoid dislocation can occur without significant airway compromise necessitating a tracheotomy, it is unlikely to occur in patients with mild to moderate external laryngeal trauma.

Postoperatively, the patient should be placed on voice rest with cool humidification and elevation of the head of the bed. Antibiotics are recommended for lacerations, but steroids are not, as the airway is secure and they will decrease wound healing. For patients with nondisplaced cricoid fractures, repeat direct laryngoscopies with laser excision of granulation tissue are recommended at 2- to 4-week intervals or when symptomatic.

Group 3: Open Exploration

Group 3A: Open Exploration Without Splinting.   An open exploration with a tracheotomy is recommended with severe laryngeal injury. Any of the following criteria necessitate an open exploration: a) exposed laryngeal cartilage, b) herniated preepiglottic fat pad, c) displaced laryngeal or cricoid cartilages on CT scan or clinical exam, and d) evidence of detachment of vocal ligament on CT scan.

The treatment for this type of injury involves a low tracheotomy, followed by direct laryngoscopy, bronchoscopy, and esophagoscopy. An open exploration is done through a horizontal neck incision. A standard laryngofissure is performed. However, often there is a midline or paramedian vertical fracture that may be used for entering the laryngeal lumen. The subglottis is entered through the cricothyroid membrane. Care is taken to ensure that the mucosal incision passes through the anterior commissure and then extends laterally in the thyrohyoid membrane to avoid the epiglottis. It is rare that there is absent or missing mucosa and, with care, all mucosal lacerations may be closed with 4-0 or 5-0 chromic sutures. Occasionally, mucosal flaps may need to be developed to cover small defects. If the thyroepiglottic ligament is ruptured, this should be repaired and the excessive herniated preepiglottic fat should be trimmed. Rarely, an epiglottectomy may be required. If the perichondrium of the endolarynx is detached, it may be reattached with quilting sutures that pass through the laryngeal cartilage. Quilting sutures should not be placed at the level of the true vocal cord. The laryngeal fissure or fractures of the thyroid cartilage can be repaired with nylon suture or wire. If the framework remains unstable, microplates or miniplates should allow stabilization and avoid the need for a stent.[37]

A suprahyoid laryngeal release will decrease the tension on the repaired lacerations and fractures. The wound is closed in a standard manner and a Penrose drain is inserted into the overlying soft tissues.

Group 3B: Open Exploration with Keel Insertion.   The need for a keel is determined by the presence of lacerations near the anterior commissure. The keel is left in place for 4 weeks, after which it is removed. Otherwise, the treatment is the same as for Group 3A, open exploration.

Group 3C: Open Exploration with Stent.   In the following situations, the use of a stent is recommended because the benefits outweigh the disadvantages: a) unstable thyroid cartilage fractures after repair, b) displaced or multiple cricoid cartilage fractures, and c) laryngotracheal separation.[11,22,31]

In cases of laryngotracheal separation, a low tracheotomy is mandatory to preserve the blood supply to the tracheal segment but can be quite difficult when the trachea has retracted into the mediastinum. Rather than grabbing blindly with hemostats into the mediastinum for the trachea, Sofferman describes locating the detached tracheal segment with one's finger and then carefully using hemostats to bring it up into the neck.[38] This greatly reduces the chances of an inadvertent laceration of the brachycephalic vein, which most certainly would lead to a morbid outcome.

Various stents have been recommended, from polyvinyl chloride endotracheal tubes, to Montgomery stents, to finger cots packed with sponge. Any of the above will work for laryngeal or subglottic stents, but we recommend a finger cot filled with sponge that has been oversewn, as this is soft and not as likely to cause epithelial loss. The stent should be sewn into position with translaryngeal or transtracheal sutures over buried buttons. Normally, 4 weeks is an adequate amount of time for stenting. In cases where the cricoid cartilage has been left denuded, a free mucosal graft should be used. This may be sewn directly into position or wrapped around the finger cot. The routine use of split thickness skin or dermis grafts is not recommended with stent use.

POSTOPERATIVE CARE AFTER OPEN EXPLORATION

Postoperatively, the head of the bed should be elevated and the patient should be maintained on voice rest with cool humidified oxygen or air. In addition, nasogastric feedings and antacids are recommended for 10 days to help rest the larynx. Antibiotics are given, but steroids serve no purpose after a tracheotomy, although they may be given preoperatively if there is a delay in exploration due to other injuries. If a keel or stent was not used, the tracheotomy is removed usually 2 to 3 weeks postoperatively after the patient tolerates full corking for 24 hr. Otherwise, the tracheotomy is removed 2 to 4 weeks after the keel or stent has been removed and the airway demonstrates its adequacy by allowing full corking for 24 to 48 hr.

COMPLICATIONS

Delay in diagnosing and definitively treating these injuries is the factor most commonly responsible for complications, and these can be devastating. Apart from the immediate danger of sudden airway obstruction, the untreated laryngeal injury may cause long-term deformities within the larynx whose correction would challenge even the most skilled otolaryngologist and require a prolonged period of rehabilitation. Secondary healing that results in granulation tissue formation and scarring may produce irreversible damage to the larynx and subglottis. Glottic webs and laryngeal or subglottic stenosis not only result in a very poor voice but may result in the need for a permanent tracheostomy. The results are clearly most optimal if the repair of the laryngeal trauma is instigated within 24 hr after injury.[20,22] If there is an unavoidable delay, as may occur because of other associated injuries, steroids and antibiotics should be given to decrease the granulation tissue formation and the inflammatory response of the damaged tissues.

Additional postoperative complications consist of airway obstruction, recurrent laryngeal nerve injury, airway obstruction, or hemorrhage. Should the inlying airway be dislodged prematurely, acute respiratory obstruction may be manifested. Other complications include temporary or permanent loss of laryngeal function and voice and laryngeal or tracheal stenosis. Hemorrhage is a relatively rare complication in the absence of a coagulopathy. Therefore, if bleeding persists, both coagulation and platelet function should be assessed. Because platelet dysfunction is more common than a coagulopathy, platelet transfusions may be arbitrarily used if there is a persistent ooze. The tracheostomy or endotracheal tube balloon cuff usually prevents aspiration of blood.

Postoperative atelectasis or major airway obstruction should be treated by endoscopy, aspiration of mucous plugs, and clotted blood from the main or secondary bronchi.

The management of injury to the recurrent laryngeal nerve is controversial. In a patient with a unilateral vocal cord paralysis without a displaced cricoid fracture, open exploration is not recommended because further injury to the nerve is possible. Often this type of paralysis may resolve as the edema within the nerve itself resolves. If it does not return after 6 months or longer, Teflon paste injection, hydroplasty, or nerve-muscle transfers may give excellent results.[38,40] If the cricoid has displaced fractures, it is possible that they may be impinging on the recurrent laryngeal nerve. Careful removal of these fragments may aid recovery with or without exposure of the nerve.

Bilateral vocal cord paralysis is common after laryngotracheal separation. The outcome of nerve reanastomosis is poor due to synkinesis.[41] However, if the nerve is avulsed from the posterior cricoarytenoid muscle, it should be reimplanted.[39,42] In situations where both recurrent laryngeal nerves are severed, unilateral reanastomosis can be considered in the hope that adequate function may be regained.

The management of subglottic stenosis is complex. The reader is referred to the listed references. After major injuries prophylactic endoscopy should be considered at 4 to 6 weeks. Subglottic stenosis that has no vocal fold involvement can be successfully treated with laryngotracheal resection.[43] Symptomatic stenosis that involves the immediate subglottic space are best treated with cricoid division and cartilage grafting.[44–46] Most grafting techniques will require the placement of a laryngeal/subglottic stent for 3 to 12 weeks.

REFERENCES

1. Habicot N. Question chirurgicale sur l'operation de la bronchotomic. In: Meade RH, ed. *A History of Thoracic Surgery.* Springfield, IL: Charles C Thomas; 1961.

2. Bouchat JA. Sur la nouvelle methode de traitement du croup per la tubage du larynx. *CR Acad Sci.* 1858;47:476.
3. Garrison FH. *History of Medicine.* Philadelphia: Saunders; 1929.
4. O'Dwyer F. Intubation of the larynx. *NY Med J.* 1885;17:145.
5. Jackson C, Jackson CC. *Disease of the Nose Throat Ear.* Philadelphia: Saunders; 1945.
6. Pennington CL. External trauma of the larynx and trachea. *Ann Otol Rhinol Laryngol.* 1972;81:546.
7. Butler RM, Moser FH. The padded dash syndrome: blunt trauma to the larynx and trachea. *Laryngoscope.* 1968;78:1172.
8. Rogers LF. Injuries* peculiar to traffic accidents: seat belt syndrome, laryngeal fracture, hangman's fracture. *Tex Med.* 1974;70(1):77.
9. Guertler AT. Blunt laryngeal trauma associated with shoulder harness use. *Ann Emerg Med.* 1988;17(8);838.
10. Huelke DF. Shoulder belts and laryngeal trauma (letter). 1989;18(11):1257.
11. Gussack GS, Jurkovich GJ. Treatment dilemmas in laryngotracheal trauma. *J Trauma.* 1988;28(10):1439.
12. Close DM. Traumatic avulsion of the larynx. *J Laryngol Otol.* 1981;95:1157.
13. Harm T, Rajs J. Types of injuries and interrelated conditions of victims and assailants in attempted and homicidal strangulation. *Forensic Sci Int.* 1981;18:101.
14. Miller LH. Laryngotracheal trauma in combat casualties. *Ann Otol Rhinol Laryngol.* 1970;79(6):1088.
15. Gluckman JL. Laryngeal trauma: surgical therapy in the adult. *Ear Nose Throat J.* 1981;60:366.
16. Stanley RB Jr, Crockett DM, Persky M. Knife wounds into the airspaces of the laryngeal trapezium. *J Trauma.* 1988;28(1):101.
17. Owen-Smith MS. Wound ballistics. In: *High Velocity Missile Wounds.* London: Edward Arnold; 1981:15–33.
18. Harrison DF. Bullet wounds of the larynx and trachea. *Arch Otolaryngol.* 1984;110:203.
19. Camnitz PS, Shepherd SM, Henderson RA. Acute blunt laryngeal and tracheal trauma. *Am J Emerg Med.* 1987;5(2):156.
20. Fuhrman GM, Stieg FH, Burek CA. Blunt laryngeal trauma: classification and management protocol. *J Trauma.* 1990;30(1):87.
21. Myers EM, Iko BO. The management of acute laryngeal trauma. *J Trauma.* 1987;27(4):448.
22. Schaefer SD, Close LG. Acute management of laryngeal trauma: update. *Ann Otol Rhinol Laryngol.* 1989;98(2):98.
23. LeJeune FE Jr. Laryngotracheal separation. *Laryngoscope.* 1978;88:1956.
24. Peppard SB. Transient vocal paralysis following strangulation injury. *Laryngoscope.* 1982;92:31.
25. Myer CM III, Orobello P, Cotton RT, Bratcher GO. Blunt laryngeal trauma in children. *Laryngoscope.* 1987;97(9):1043.
26. Holinger PH, Schild JA. Pharyngeal, laryngeal, and tracheal injuries in the pediatric age group. *Ann Otol Rhinol Laryngol.* 1972;81:538.
27. Dunbar JS, Kramer SS. Radiology of trauma to the pediatric larynx. *Ear Nose Throat J.* 1981;60:356.
28. Richardson MA. Laryngeal anatomy and mechanisms of trauma. *Ear Nose Throat J.* 1981;60:346.
29. Schaefer SD. Use of CT scanning in the management of the acutely injured larynx. *Otolaryngol Clin North Am.* 1991;24(1):31.
30. Alonso WA. Surgical management and complications of acute laryngotracheal disruption. *Otolaryngol Clin North Am.* 1979;12(4):753.
31. Alonso WA, Pratt LL, Zollinger WK, Ogura JH. Complications of laryngotracheal disruption. *Laryngoscope.* 1974;84:1276.
32. Meglin AJ, Biedlingmaier JF, Mirvis SE. Three-dimensional computerized tomography in the evaluation of laryngeal injury. *Laryngoscope.* 1991;101(2):202.
33. Dolgin SR, Kumar NR, Wyoff TW, Maniglia AJ. Conservative medical management of traumatic pharyngoesophageal perforations. *Ann Otol Rhinol Laryngol.* 1992;101:209.
34. Olson NR. Wound healing by primary intention in the larynx. *Otolaryngol Clin North Am.* 1979;12(4):735.
35. Peacock EE. Healing and repair of viscera. In: *Wound Repair.* Philadelphia: Saunders; 1984.
36. Casiano RR, Goodwin WJ. Restoring function to the injured larynx. *Otolaryngol Clin North Am.* 1991;24(5):1215.
37. Woo P. Laryngeal framework reconstruction with miniplates. *Ann Otol Rhinol Laryngol.* 1990;99(10 Pt 1):772.
38. Sofferman RA. Management of laryngotracheal trauma. *Am J Surg.* 1981;141:412.
39. Crumley RL. Teflon versus thyroplasty versus nerve transfer: a comparison. *Ann Otol Rhinol Laryngol.* 1990;99(10 Pt 1):759.
40. Dedo HH. Injection and removal of Teflon for unilateral vocal cord paralysis. *Ann Otol Rhinol Laryngol.* 1992;101(1):81.
41. Crumley RL. Laryngeal synkinesis: its significance to the laryngologist. *Ann Otol Rhinol Laryngol.* 1989;98(2):87.
42. Miglets AW. Functional laryngeal abduction following reimplantation of the recurrent laryngeal nerves. *Laryngoscope.* 1974;84:1996.

43. Grillo HC, Mathisen DJ, Wain JC. Laryngotracheal resection and reconstruction for subglottic stenosis. *Ann Thorac Surg*. 1992;53(1):54.
44. Cotton RT. The problem of pediatric laryngotracheal stenosis: a clinical and experimental study on the efficacy of autogenous cartilaginous grafts placed between the vertically divided halves of the posterior lamina of the cricoid cartilage. *Laryngoscope*. 1991;101(12 Pt 2, Suppl 56):1.
45. Healy GB. Subglottic stenosis. *Otolaryngol Clin North Am*. 1989;22(3):599.
46. McCaffrey TV. Management of subglottic stenosis in the adult. *Ann Otol Rhinol Laryngol*. 1991;100(2):90.

11

Tracheal and Bronchial Injury

RUSSELL W. SAWYER, M.D.
JOHN R. BENFIELD, M.D.

HISTORY: In 1792, Hugh Munroe of Scotland alluded to the treatment of tracheal injury by discussing the need for suture of a transverse tracheal wound.[1] Initial observations of tracheobronchial injury were made by W.H. Winslow in 1874, when he described a bifurcation injury to a canvas back duck that had been healing a previous left bronchial rupture, when its life was interrupted by a sportsman.[2] Seuvre, in 1873, reported the first case of a traumatic bronchial rupture, and expressed the opinion that bronchial rupture was inevitably fatal.[3] It became apparent, however, that severe bronchial injury was not necessarily fatal when, in 1927, Krinitzki described a patient who had survived 20 years after a traumatic rupture of his right main stem bronchus.[4]

Successful operations to treat the bronchus probably began around 1907, when Goeltz did a bronchotomy and closure for removal of a foreign body. An operation to treat the delayed sequelae of trauma to the tracheobronchial tract initially was described by Nissen, who did a successful pneumonectomy to treat a stricture secondary to a complete bronchial rupture in 1931.[5] Acute surgical therapy for tracheobronchial trauma was first described by Sanger, in 1945, who reported the successful suture of a bronchial laceration.[6] Four years later the first suture of a complete bronchial rupture was reported by Griffith, and in 1957, Beskin described successful closure of a tracheal rupture.[7,8] Sophisticated tracheobronchial repairs are now routinely done.

It has been estimated that about 25% of traumatic deaths result from chest injuries.[9] In the United States such injuries are mostly from blunt trauma secondary to motor vehicle accidents, but there also is an increasing incidence of penetrating thoracic trauma.[10]

The true incidence of blunt tracheobronchial injury is difficult to establish, because many patients who sustain such injuries die before reaching the hospital.[11,12] There is, however, evidence that the incidence of tracheobronchial injuries that present for treatment may be increasing because of improvements in prehospital care of trauma victims.[13] Major

178

tracheobronchial injuries remain uncommon, but they are of great significance, because they can result in death or substantial functional compromise. Most tracheobronchial injuries can be repaired, with a successful outcome, if they are recognized in a timely manner and managed appropriately.

ANATOMY

The trachea, proximally, originates from the larynx at the lower border of the cricoid cartilage, at about the level of the sixth cervical vertebra; it terminates at the carina, at the level of the upper border of the fifth thoracic vertebra where it divides into right and left main stem bronchi.

The relationships of the trachea and main stem bronchi to adjacent structures are shown in Figure 11–1. In the neck, the trachea lies in the midline, behind the infrahyoid muscles and the thyroid gland, and anterior to the cervical portion of the esophagus. The course of the trachea is progressively posterior with an angle of 30° in the supine position. It passes under the sternum deep to the innominate vein, which overlaps the trachea just below the sternal notch. Caudad to this, it passes under the aortic arch, at the point of origin of the innominate and left common carotid arteries. The carina lies behind the aortic arch. In the neck and thoracic inlet, over most of its course, the jugular veins are lateral and anterior to

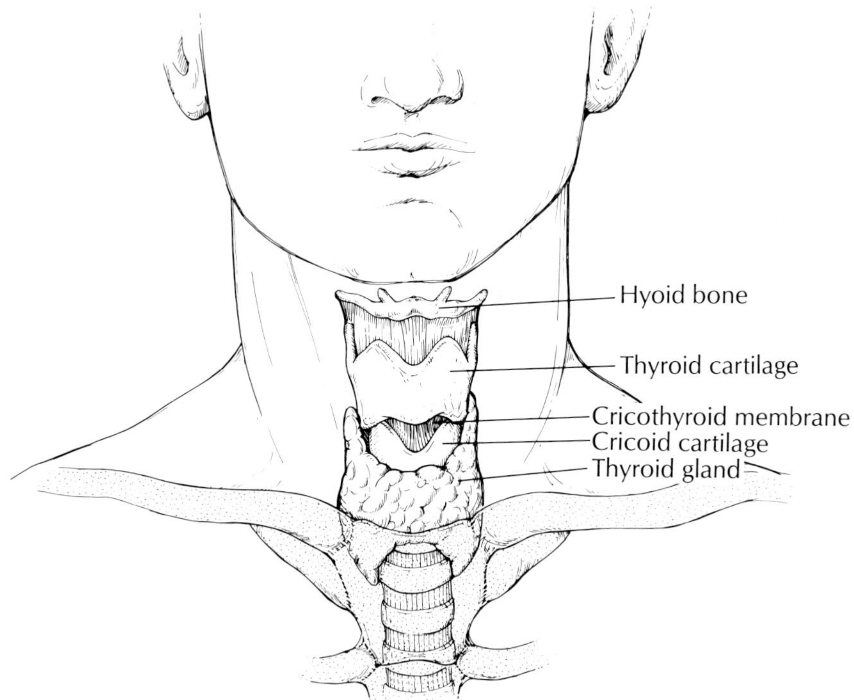

Figure 11–1. Anterior thoracic anatomy of the trachea. The great veins and aortic arch pass anterior to the trachea.

the trachea. The common carotid arteries run behind the trachea, and the vagus nerves lie between these and the jugular veins. The recurrent laryngeal nerves ascend at the posterolateral borders of the trachea in the tracheoesophageal groove.

A patent lumen of the trachea is maintained against fluctuations in pressure by 16 to 20 cartilaginous rings that encircle approximately two-thirds of the tracheal circumference. The submucosal trachealis muscle forms the wall of the posterior one-third of the trachea where it is commonly called the membranous portion of the trachea.

The right main stem bronchus is shorter, straighter, and at a smaller angle with the trachea than the left bronchus (Fig. 11–2). It lies just below the azygous–vena cava junction, and behind the right pulmonary artery. In adults, the right upper lobe bronchus is about 1 cm long before it trifurcates into the apical, anterior, and posterior segmental bronchi. Just distal to the upper lobe bronchus is the 2-cm bronchus intermedius, which divides into the middle lobe bronchus anteriorly and the lower lobe bronchus behind. The middle lobe bronchus varies in length, between 1 and 2 cm, in adults, before bifurcating into medial and lateral segments. Directly posterior and slightly more distal to the anterior origin of the middle

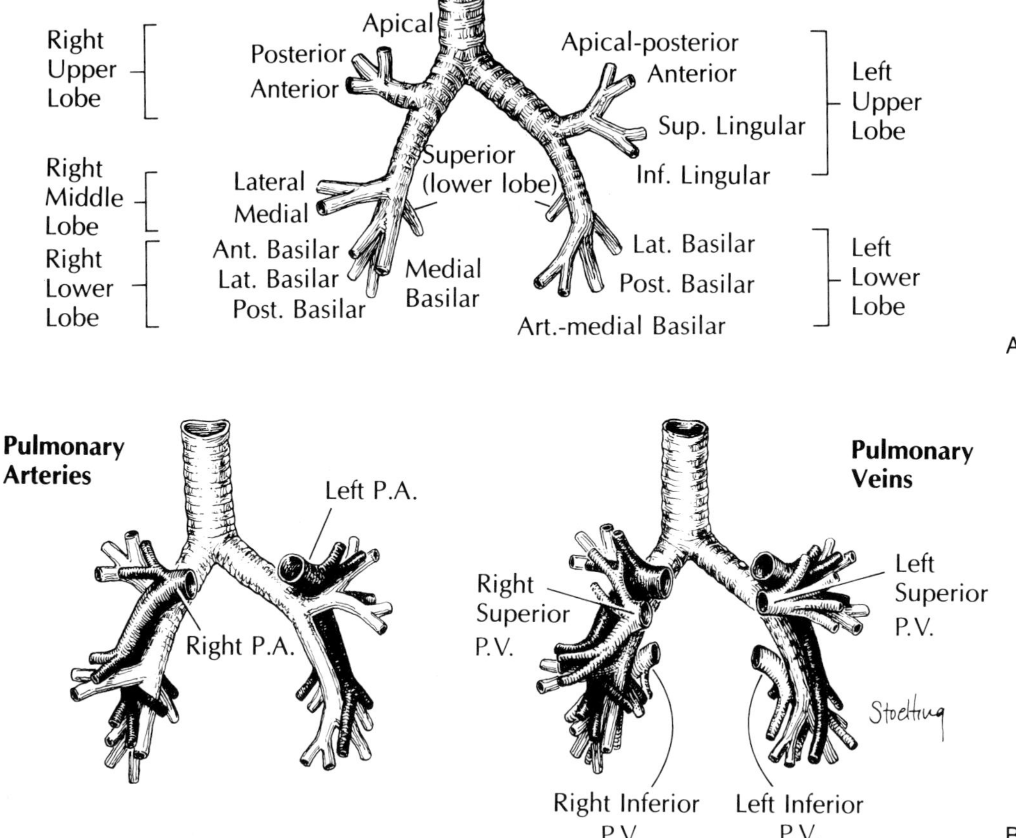

Figure 11–2.   **A:** The anatomy of the trachea and bronchi are depicted (see text). **B:** The pulmonary arterial and venous anatomy in relationship to the bronchi (see text).

lobe bronchus is the superior segmental bronchus to the lower lobe. Distal to the superior segmental bronchus, the lower lobe bronchus gives off the bronchi to the anterior, medial, lateral, and posterior-basal segmental bronchi.

The left main stem bronchus is smaller in diameter than the right (Fig. 11–2). It is about 3 cm long in adults and it passes under the arch of the aorta; this relationship explains why depression of this bronchus is a cardinal finding in thoracic aortic rupture or aneurysm. Medially and anteriorly the left main bronchus abuts the pericardium and the left atrium. The upper lobe bronchus arises anteriorly and laterally, and it is approximately 1 to 1.5 cm long before it divides into its superior and inferior division. The superior division extends upward, and it divides into the apical posterior and anterior bronchi. The inferior division supplies the lingula, which has superior and inferior lingular segmental bronchi. Approximately 0.5 cm distal to the upper lobe bronchus, the lower lobe bronchus gives off its first branch, the superior segmental bronchus. The lower lobe bronchus continues for an additional 0.5 cm before bifurcating into the anteromedial basal segmental bronchus and a common bronchus, which subsequently divides into lateral and posterior basal bronchi.[14,15]

MECHANISM AND PATHOGENESIS

Blunt trauma affects the cervical trachea more frequently than the thoracic trachea. There are three postulated mechanisms for blunt trauma to the trachea other than a direct blow to the hyperextended neck: a) a sudden forceful compression in the anteroposterior dimension of the chest that results in a simultaneous increase in the lateral diameter of the chest. As the lungs remain in contact with the parietal pleura secondary to negative intrapleural pressure, the increased lateral dimension results in traction on the carina causing a laceration or transection of the trachea or main stem bronchus; b) a sudden increase in intratracheal pressure against a closed glottis that results in a linear rupture of the tracheobronchial tree. This occurs because the greatest wall tension is generated in the large diameter airways (Law of LaPlace); and c) an acceleration or deceleration type of injury that produces a shearing force on the tracheobronchial tree between the relatively stationary areas of the cricoid cartilage and the carina[16] (see Chapter 10).

Penetrating trauma to the trachea depends primarily on the wounding agent and its trajectory. The intimate anatomic relationship of the trachea to the heart, lungs, great vessels, and esophagus explain the high incidence of serious associated injuries in both blunt and penetrating trauma of the thorax.

Most, but not all, individuals with a major airway injury die at the scene of the accident as a result of asphyxia or aspiration of blood and intrapulmonary hemorrhage.[11] However, even a complete bronchial transection may be compatible with survival if the open bronchus is sealed by adjacent soft tissues. An incomplete airway injury may result in subsequent granuloma formation, stenosis of the bronchus, and recurrent sepsis in the involved lung segment. Complete bronchial disruption results in total atelectasis usually without sepsis. Right to left shunting initially is severe (>30%), but it rapidly decreases because chronic atelectasis usually is associated with a shunt of less than 5% of the cardiac output[17,18] (Fig. 11–3).

Most patients with chest injuries (particularly blunt trauma) have an array of associated injuries. For example, Shorr et al. reported 515 thoracic trauma victims among whom only 84, or 16%, had isolated trauma; 84% had associated extrathoracic injuries, including

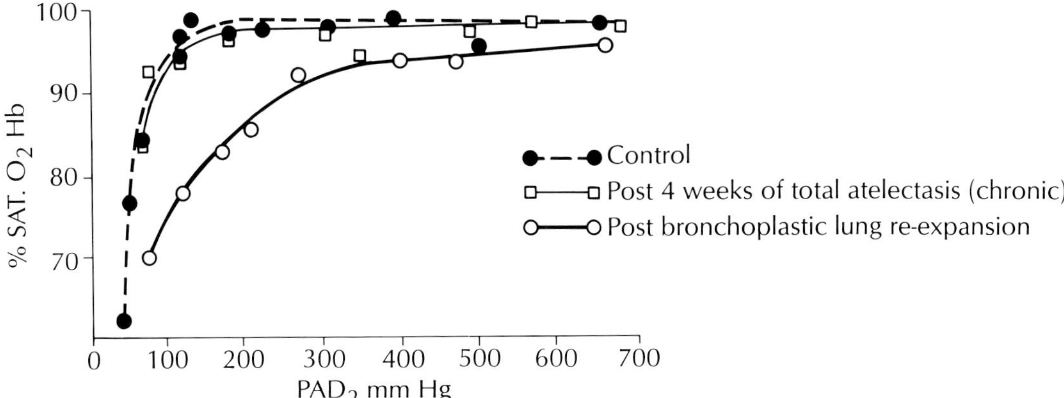

Figure 11–3.   After bronchial occlusion left to right shunting rapidly decreases. Chronic atelectasis usually is associated with a shunt of <5%. Successful reinflation eliminates shunt, but retains abnormally high pulmonary vascular resistance.

43% with head injury, 40% with intraabdominal injury, and 29% with additional bony or significant soft tissue injury.[19] Therefore, in considering the anatomy of tracheobronchial trauma, one also must consider the potential injury to the remainder of the body.

DIAGNOSIS

The key to prompt and accurate diagnosis of tracheobronchial injuries is to have a high index of suspicion. This point cannot be overemphasized because more than two-thirds of patients have stable vital signs when they are first seen.[19] Therefore, one must look for other signs, some of which may be subtle or difficult to recognize, if tracheobronchial injuries are to be discovered in a timely fashion. Table 11–1 summarizes the common findings associated with tracheobronchial injury.

Signs that should arouse suspicion of a tracheobronchial injury are based on a knowledge of the anatomy and the mechanism of injury. Fractures of ribs, sternum, clavicle, and scapulae reflect the fact that large amounts of energy have been imparted to the chest wall and thoracic viscera. Fracture of the first rib is associated with a 14% incidence of underlying vascular injury, and may be associated with injury to adjacent nerves that also

Table 11–1.   Findings in Tracheobronchial Injury

Cough
Dyspnea
Hemoptysis
Subcutaneous emphysema
Fracture of the bony thorax (ribs, scapula, clavicle, and sternum)
Pneumothorax
Pneumomediastinum
Pneumopericardium

occupy the narrow thoracic inlet.[20] However, the absence of bony injury does not exclude the possibility of tracheobronchial injury (about 25% of patients with significant tracheobronchial trauma can be expected to be without bony thoracic injury).[19]

Subcutaneous emphysema and dyspnea frequently are noted on initial evaluation.[21–24] Other physical findings consistent with a tracheobronchial disruption include hemoptysis, cough, and the rapid development of pneumothorax after endotracheal intubation and institution of positive pressure ventilation.[23] The presence of acute respiratory distress in association with absent breath sounds and mediastinal shift is evidence that a tension pneumothorax is present. These findings dictate immediate chest tube placement without waiting for a chest radiograph. In contrast, pneumothorax without hypotension, hypoxia, or mediastinal deviation usually should be treated by chest tube insertion, after a chest radiograph has been obtained. In trauma victims, we strongly advise against expectant treatment of minimal pneumothorax.

Pneumomediastinum or pneumopericardium may occur separately or together. Each of these findings also can be a sign of a ruptured bronchus, with its attending grave prognosis[19] (Fig. 11–4). Hemothorax to some degree occurs in almost every patient with

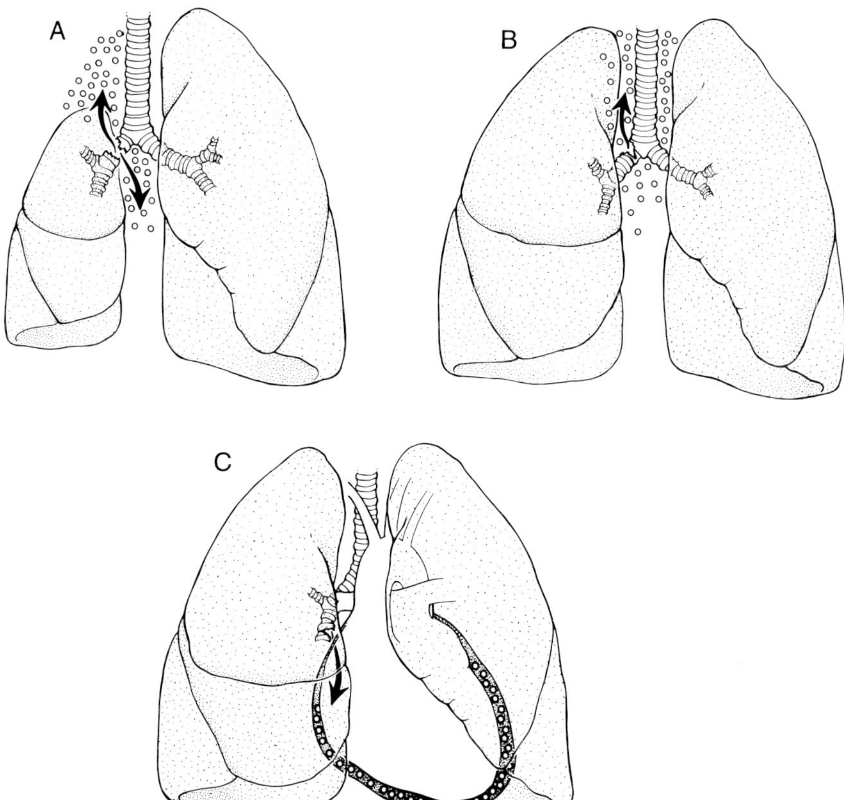

Figure 11–4.   Bronchial disruption causing pneumothorax and pneumomediastinum (**A**), pneumomediastinum (**B**), and pneumopericardium (**C**). Pneumomediastinum may be obvious or subtle, e.g., associated only with accentuation of the heart border on plain chest radiograph.

major chest trauma. Most often hemothorax results from chest wall or parenchymal injury; it also may be present in patients with tracheobronchial injuries.[22]

Diagnostic studies should include radiography and endoscopy. Conventional chest radiography is frequently helpful and it is often the first available study (Fig. 11–5). Rib fractures, particularly of ribs 1–5, other bony thoracic fractures, as well as pleural, mediastinal, pericardial, and subcutaneous air generally are easily detectable on a standard chest radiograph. However, one-fourth of patients with tracheobronchial injury have initial chest radiographs that appear completely normal.[12,24] Bronchography (Fig. 11–6) is helpful in evaluating chronic sequelae of tracheobronchial injury but it rarely, if ever, is indicated in the acute setting.

The diagnostic modality of choice to evaluate tracheobronchial injury remains tracheobronchoscopy.[12,19] Primary indications for bronchoscopy are hemoptysis, subcutaneous emphysema, unresolving air leak, persistent pneumothorax, or pneumomediastinum.[23] Both flexible fiberoptic and rigid bronchoscopy remain useful modalities in acute tracheobronchial injury. The examination is best performed in the operating room under general anesthesia by experienced endoscopists; in such a setting accurate diagnosis usually can be expected.[12]

However, bronchoscopic findings may be difficult to interpret.[25] Figure 11–7 shows the types of injuries that may be found. Blood in the airway or inability to visualize the distal bronchial tree should alert the bronchoscopist to the possibility of underlying tracheobronchial injury.[23] In some cases, repeated bronchoscopy may be indicated, if only to ensure a clear airway.[12,24]

Penetrating trauma presents a set of challenges that are slightly different from blunt injury. In level I trauma centers where surgeons have chosen to explore all zone II neck wounds that penetrate the platysma, preoperative endoscopy often is advisable because

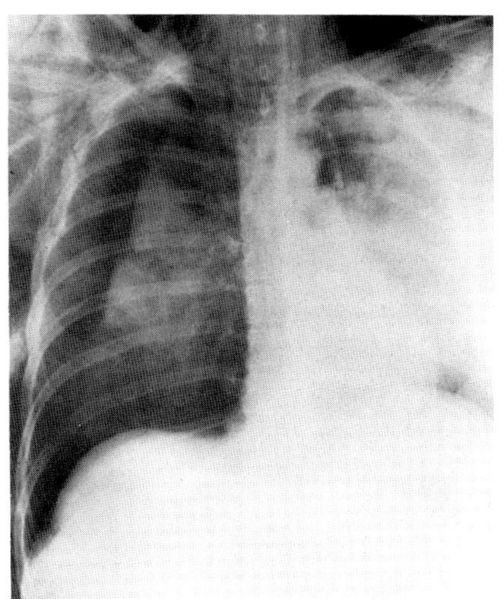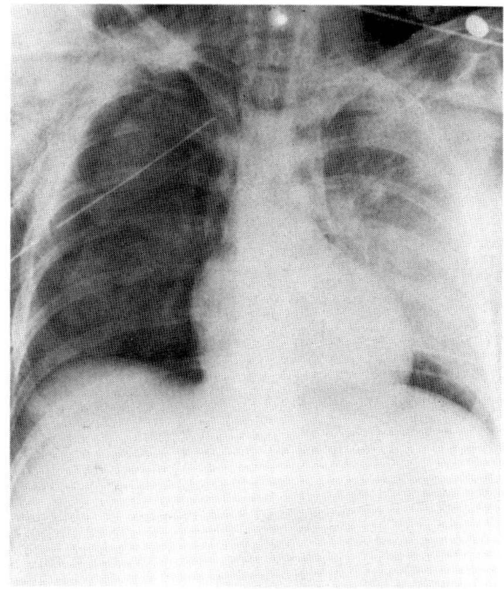

A
B

Figure 11–5. The initial chest radiograph (**A**) shows extensive subcutaneous air, a right pneumothorax and left hemothorax, and pulmonary contusion. After bilateral chest tube placement, the subsequent chest radiograph (**B**) shows a persistent right pneumothorax that required thoracotomy and repair of a tracheobronchial tear.

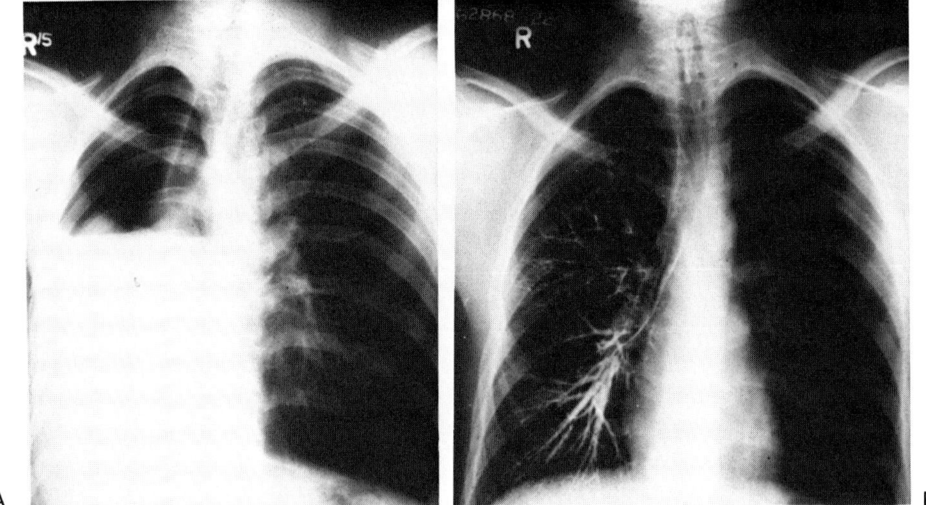

Figure 11–6. **A:** Preoperative chest radiograph. Note hemopneumothorax and mediastinal shift that result from complete right main stem bronchial transection. **B:** Bronchogram revealing fully patent bronchus after bronchoplastic repair.

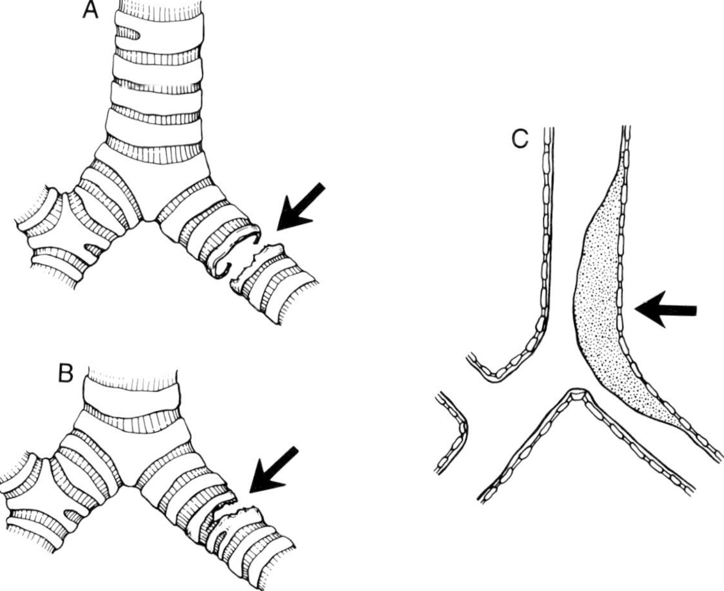

Figure 11–7. Major types of bronchial injury. **A:** complete disruption, **B:** partial tear, and **C:** submucosal hematoma. Such injuries may be difficult to assess during initial bronchoscopy.

intraoperative evaluation of the trachea and esophagus may be difficult. If the patient's condition remains stable and there is time to complete the work-up, expectant management may be acceptable. We recommend an aggressive diagnostic approach, most often to include definitive surgical exploration.[24,26]

TREATMENT

Most patients with a tracheobronchial injury will have other associated injuries, and therefore management priorities need to be established. The usual principles of first ensuring a patent airway with adequate ventilation and ensuring adequacy of circulation apply. Cervicothoracic airway control always takes priority.[21] After airway control, bleeding injuries should be treated first, whether they are located in the chest or in the abdomen. Attention then can be turned to repair of the tracheobronchial injury.

Specific treatment for tracheobronchial injuries requires proper positioning of the patient, choice of the proper incision, and a fundamental knowledge of cervicothoracic anatomy. Most penetrating injuries to the cervical region can be approached through a transverse collar incision or by incision overlying the border of the sternocleidomastoid muscle. After penetrating injuries the skin wound often can be extended and debrided. When the injury is to the left side of the trachea or on the left main stem bronchus within 2 to 3 cm from the carina, a left posterolateral thoracotomy provides satisfactory exposure. This permits mobilization of the distal tracheobronchial tree from under the aortic arch. Sternotomy occasionally may be advisable to treat tracheal injuries. Other tracheal injuries are easily visible through a right posterolateral thoracotomy. Occasionally a partial or complete mediansternotomy is needed, particularly when associated mediastinal injuries must be ruled out or treated.

Closure of tracheal lacerations are performed with one layer of interrupted simple sutures (Fig. 11–8). We prefer to use synthetic collagen absorbable suture, usually of 4-0 diameter. Large devitalizing disruptions of the tracheobronchial tree should be repaired after adequate debridement to vital tissue. Although rarely necessary in the traumatic setting, up to 6 cm of trachea can be resected. This requires mobilization of the trachea, division of the inferior pulmonary ligament, and hilar-mediastinal dissection, sometimes with incision of the pericardium. Further relief of tension may be facilitated with a laryngeal release procedure.[29–31] Sutures must be placed precisely, and suture knots should be on the external surface of the trachea when possible. Peribronchial and peritracheal tissues should be retained so as to keep the tracheobronchial collateral blood supply. The importance of the liberal use of a muscle or pleural flap to buttress the trachea and separate it from the esophagus when there have been simultaneous injuries of both has been properly stressed.[27] This valuable technique decreases the incidence of tracheoesophageal fistula and postoperative leak.[24,28]

Single or double selective intubation of the trachea may be necessary to ensure airway control during the repair (see Chapter 7). Patients are extubated as soon postoperatively as possible. Prolonged intubation stresses the repair and increases the incidence of anastomotic disruption and stenosis.

Selected patients with small tracheobronchial tears may be managed nonoperatively. This approach should be reserved for those patients who remain hemodynamically stable and have no other associated intrathoracic injuries. All nonoperatively managed patients should be treated with prophylactic antibiotics and should be watched closely for signs of airway obstruction and pulmonary or mediastinal sepsis.[24] In general, nonoperative treatment is avoided.

The need for tracheostomy is rare unless there is an associated laryngeal injury.[29] Crush injuries of the trachea with obstruction are best treated with a cricothyroidotomy or tracheostomy tube passed beyond the area of injury. The tube generally can be removed within a week, depending on the severity of the injury and/or associated injuries.

POSTOPERATIVE CARE

Principles of postoperative care are the same as for all trauma victims. It is first necessary to ensure effective ventilation and provide adequate volume replacement. A short period of nasogastric intubation usually is indicated to minimize the risk of aspiration. Aspirated blood, bronchorrhea, and excessive secretions require vigorous pulmonary hygiene. Repeated therapeutic bronchoscopy may be necessary in the first few days to ensure a clear airway and nonatelectatic lung segments. These patients have painful incisions, often with associated rib fractures, and they must be able to ventilate adequately and clear their secretions. Epidural analgesia has constituted a major advance in the management of postoperative or postinjury pain control. Early and prophylactic use of epidural analgesia in thoracic trauma patients is advisable.

COMPLICATIONS

Possible morbidities may include acute and chronic atelectasis, pneumonia from aspiration of blood or gastric content, adult respiratory distress syndrome (ARDS), and recurrent or

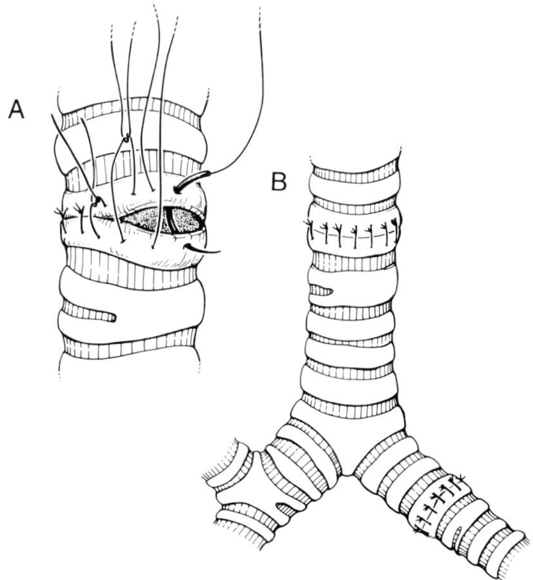

Figure 11–8. **A:** Closure of tracheal laceration with reapproximation of proximal and distal segments. **B:** Suture knots should be placed on the external surface of the trachea. Absorbable suture material is preferred.

persistent pneumothorax or empyema. The most common cause of prolonged air leaks or empyema is anastomotic leak. There also is a risk of wound infection.[19]

Complications are best prevented, if possible. The nature of bronchial secretions should be monitored by gram stain, and bacterial cultures with sensitivity testing. Purulent secretions should be treated promptly with specific antibiotics. Compulsive pulmonary hygiene, including therapeutic bronchoscopies, may be necessary. Early intervention and drainage should be utilized when septic complications develop from ongoing leaks.

Progressive stenosis of the airway (Fig. 11–9) is always a possibility after a major injury. Tracheal injuries with stenosis may go undetected. Unrecognized injuries (1 week to 22 years) still can be repaired with good return of function to the reexpanded chronically atelectatic lung segment[17,32] (Fig. 11–3). The involved bronchus is opened and suctioned free of bronchial secretions. Bronchoplastic repair should be undertaken if the chronically atelectatic lung or segment can be easily inflated and deflated (i.e., there is evidence of compliance and elasticity). If repair is not feasible, secondary to infection or fibrosis, then resection of the involved lung should be accomplished to avoid chronic infection and pulmonary hypertension.[33]

RESULTS

Morbidity is fairly common after tracheobronchial injury. The largest series of patients reported to our knowledge described a 7% incidence of atelectasis, pneumonia, and ARDS, respectively; about 5% of patients had persistent air leak or empyema.[19] Mortality rates vary among reports largely because of differing incidences of associated injuries. The life expectancy of patients who survive the first 24 to 72 hr of their hospital admission has been about 75% to 80%. The remaining mortalities after injury most often are from ARDS, sepsis, and multisystem organ failure.[19,21,23]

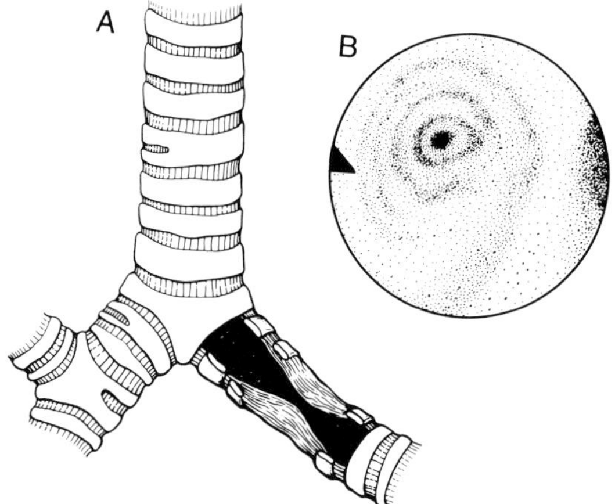

Figure 11–9.   Posttraumatic left main stem bronchial stricture, shown schematically (**A**) and as seen at bronchoscopy (**B**).

REFERENCES

1. Meade RH. *A History of Thoracic Surgery.* Springfield, IL: Charles C Thomas; 1961:206, 777–778.
2. Winslow WH. Rupture of bronchus from wild duck. *Phila Med Times.* 1874;255:April 15.
3. Seuvre M. Crushing injury from wheel of omnibus: rupture of right bronchus. *Bull Soc Anat Paris.* 1873;48:680.
4. Krinitzki SI. Zur Kasuistik einer vollstandingen Zerreibung des rechten luftrohrenastes. *Virch Arch.* 1927;266:815.
5. Nissen R. Total pneumonectomy. *Ann Thorac Surg.* 1980;29:390.
6. Sanger PW. Evacuation hospital experience with war wounds and injuries of the chest. *Ann Surg.* 1945;122:147.
7. Griffith JL. Fracture of the bronchus. *Thorax.* 1949;4:105.
8. Beskin CA. Rupture-separation of the cervical trachea following a closed chest injury. *J Thorac Surg.* 1957;34:392.
9. National Safety Council (1991). *Accident Facts.* 1991 ed. Chicago, IL.
10. Wilson RF, Murray C, Antonenko DR. Nonpenetrating thoracic injuries. *Surg Clin North Am.* 1977;57:17–36.
11. Bertelsen S, Howitz P. Injuries of the trachea and bronchi. *Thorax.* 1972;27:188.
12. Baumgartner F, Sheppard B, DeVirgilio C, et al. Tracheal and main bronchial disruptions after blunt chest trauma. *Ann Thorac Surg.* 1990;50:569–574.
13. De La Rocha AG, Kayler D. Traumatic rupture of the tracheobronchial tree. *Can J Surg.* 1985;28:68.
14. Woodburne RT. *Essentials of Human Anatomy.* New York: Oxford University Press; 1983;348:9.
15. Scannel JG. *Pulmonary Resection—Anatomy and Techniques in Thoracic and Cardiovascular Surgery.* Norwalk, CT: Appleton-Century-Crofts; 1983.
16. Kirsh MM, Orringer MB, Behrendt DM, et al. Management of tracheobronchial disruption secondary to nonpenetrating trauma. *Ann Thorac Surg.* 1976;22:93.
17. Benfield JR, Harrison RW, Perkins JF, Long ET, Herman GP, Adams WE. The reversibility of chronic atelectasis. *Surg Forum.* 1958;8:473–478.
18. Long ET, Adams WE, Benfield JR, Mikouchi T, Reimann AF, Nigro SL. Altered hemodynamics in the pulmonary circulation following reaeration of an atelectatic lung. *J Thorac Cardiovasc Surg.* 1960;40:640–652.
19. Shorr RM, Crittenden M, Indeck M, et al. Blunt thoracic trauma—analysis of 515 patients. *Ann Surg.* 1987;206:200–205.
20. Phillips EH, Rogers WF, Gaspar MR. First rib fractures: incidence of vascular injury and indications for angiography. *Surgery.* 1981;89:42.
21. Ramzy AI, Rodriguez A, Turney SZ. Management of major tracheobronchial ruptures in patients with multiple system trauma. *J Trauma.* 1988;28(9):1353–1357.
22. Jurkovich GJ, Moore EE. Hemothorax. In: Edlich RF, ed. *Emergency Medical Therapy.* Norwalk, CT: Appleton-Century-Crofts; 1984.
23. Jones WS, Mavroudis C, Richardson JD, et al. Management of tracheobronchial disruption resulting from blunt trauma. *Surgery.* 1984;95:49–58.
24. Flynn AE, Thomas AN, Shecter WP. Acute tracheobronchial injury. *J Trauma.* 1989;29(10):1326–1330.
25. Benfield JR. Traumatic bronchial rupture and other major thoracic injuries (editorial). *Ann Thorac Surg.* 1990;50:523.
26. Scientific American Medicine. Care of the Surgical Patient. Committee on pre and postoperative care, American College of Surgeons. New York, New York. Chapter 4, pp 31–33.
27. Mathisen DJ, Grillo H. Laryngotracheal trauma. *Ann Thorac Surg.* 1987;43:254.
28. Symbas PN, Hatcher CR, Vlais SE. Bullet wounds of the trachea. *J Thorac Cardiovasc Surg.* 1982;83:235–238.
29. Couraud L, Velly JF, Martigne C. Post-traumatic disruption of the laryngotracheal junction. *Eur J Cardiothorac Surg.* 1989;3(5):441–444.
30. Dedo H, Fishman N. Laryngeal release and sleeve resection for tracheal stenosis. *Ann Otol Rhinol Laryngol.* 1969;78(2):285–296.
31. Montgomery WW. Suprahyoid release for tracheal anastomosis. *Arch Otolaryngol.* 1974;99(4):255–260.
32. Eastridge CE, Hughes FA, Pate JW, et al. Tracheobronchial injury caused by blunt trauma. *Ann Rev Respir Dis.* 1970;101:230.
33. Kelly JP, Webb WR, Moulder PV, et al. Management of airway trauma I: tracheobronchial injuries. *Ann Thorac Surg.* 1985;40:551.

12

Chest Wall Injuries

DONALD D. TRUNKEY, M.D.

HISTORY: Wounds of the chest are recorded in the first medical writings, the Edwin Smith Papyrus.[1] This papyrus probably originated during the time of Imhotep (3000 BC) and recorded 58 cases, of which 3 were concerned with chest wounds. One of these cases, number 28, involved the neck with a penetrating wound to the esophagus. Case number 40 involved a wound of the anterior thorax penetrating the sternum at the manubrium. Treatment was advised and consisted of binding it with fresh meat the first day and subsequently with grease, honey, and lint. The third and final case involved a compound fracture of the ribs over the breast. This was thought to represent a fatal wound and treatment was not advised.

During Greek and Roman times, open wounds of the chest were universally fatal. At the battle of Mantinea in 362 BC, Epaminondas was pierced by a spear in the chest. Upon hearing of the victory of the Thebans, he removed the spear knowing that he would die from a fatal open pneumothorax.

Galen cared for gladiators with chest wounds, but what treatment was rendered consisted primarily of a poultice and leaving the wound open. This did not change until the time of Theodoric, who advised closing chest wounds. This advice was not universally accepted, and even the master military surgeon Paré treated open chest wounds for 2 or 3 days to allow the blood to escape and after this had ceased the wound was closed. It was not until 1767 that Hewson made the observation that a patient with an open wound to the chest might not be able to breathe but could do so easily when it was closed.

It was an additional 40 years, however, before Baron Larrey, another great French military surgeon, confirmed that observation in a wounded soldier.[2] He noted in his memoirs:

A soldier was brought to the hospital at the Fortress of Ibrahym Bey, immediately after a wound penetrated the thorax between the 5th and 6th true ribs. It was about 8 cm in extent. A large quantity of frothy and vermillion blood escaped from it with a hissing noise at each inspiration. His extremities were cold, pulse scarcely perceptible, countenance discolored, and respiration short and laborious: In short he was every moment threatened with a fatal suffocation. After having examined the wound, the divided edges of the part, I immediately approximated the two lips of the wound and retained them by means of adhesive plaster, and a suitable bandage around the body. In adopting this plan I intended only to hide from the sight of the patient and his comrades, the distressing spectacle of a hemorrhage, which would soon prove fatal; and I therefore thought that the effusional blood into the cavity of the thorax could not increase the danger. But the wound was scarcely closed, when he breathed more freely, and felt easier. The heat of the body soon returned, and the pulse rose. In a few hours he became quite calm, and to my great surprise, grew better. He was cured in a very few days, and without difficulty.

There are few descriptions of open pneumothorax, air hunger, and shock that are more lucid than this by Larrey during the Napoleonic wars.

One of the most famous open chest wounds was that of Alexis St. Martin, who was shot in the lower chest in 1822. William Beaumont recorded his treatment in 1825.[3] The gunshot wound was caused by a short-range blast within a yard of St. Martin's chest "fracturing and carrying away the anterior half of the sixth rib, fracturing the fifth, lacerating the lower portion of the left lobe of the lung, the diaphragm, and perforating the stomach. The whole mass of materials forced from the musket, together with fragments of clothing and pieces of fractured ribs, were driven into the muscles and cavity of the chest." Beaumont attended St. Martin within a half hour of the accident and found that his patient had lung and stomach herniating through the wound. "After cleaning the wound from the discharges and other extraneous matter, and replacing the stomach, and lung as far as practicable, I applied the carbonated fermenting poultice and kept the surrounding parts constantly wet with a lotion of muriate of ammonia and vinegar." Beaumont returned within an hour expecting to find the patient dead. To his surprise, he was not only alive but improved. Closing the wound had saved the patient's life. Unfortunately for St. Martin, but fortunately for gastric physiology, the wound did not heal completely and there was a gastric fistula that led Beaumont to make his famous observations.

The principle of closing an open pneumothorax did not become universal until after the first year of World War I.[1] However, in order for these wounds to be closed, it was necessary to understand the physiology of negative intrathoracic pressure. In 1875, a German internist, Buelau, introduced closed underwater drainage of an empyema. In 1889, T. Holmes, consulting surgeon to St. George's Hospital in London, introduced intercostal drainage for large chest wounds but did not advocate an underwater seal. Positive pressure ventilation was introduced in the early 1900s, and surgical techniques were improved during World Wars I and II with a subsequent decrease in mortality (Table 12–1). The most significant recent treatment advance has been the introduction of ventilators by the Scandinavians in the early 1950s.

Injuries to the chest wall far and away constitute the most common thoracic injury. Following automobile accidents, one-third of hospital admissions have severe chest wall injuries.[4] In elderly patients, isolated rib fractures may be responsible for mortality. In all patients, rib fractures are associated with life-threatening, underlying injuries. For those involving the upper six ribs, the consequences are usually intrathoracic; those that involve the lower six ribs have a high incidence of associated spleen, liver, and/or renal damage. Every trauma surgeon must be knowledgeable in assessing these injuries and dealing with their management.

Table 12–1. Mortality from Chest Wounds

CONFLICT	%
Crimean War	79.0
Civil War	62.5
Franco-Prussian	55.7
World War I	24.6
World War II	12.0
Recent civilian experience	4.0–7.0

ANATOMY

Conceptually, the bony thorax is a parabaloid attached posteriorly to a semirigid bony column. Within the single parabaloid are two smaller parabaloids containing the lungs and an asymmetrical area containing the contents of the mediastinum. Each of the smaller parabaloids has as its base a concave diaphragm. Attached to the top half of the large parabaloid on each posterior lateral surface are the shoulder girdles. The bony thorax is covered with muscle and the integument and is comprised of semicircular ribs arranged in parallel fashion attached to the sternum anteriorly and the axial column posteriorly. Ribs 1 to 10 eventually complete a circle, whereas 11 and 12 are not attached to the costal chondral junction anteriorly. There is a superior aperture to the parabaloid that is kidney shaped and is approximately 2 by 4 in (Fig. 12–1). The inferior aperture at the base is much larger and is irregularly shaped and occupied by the diaphragm. The first seven ribs are called true ribs

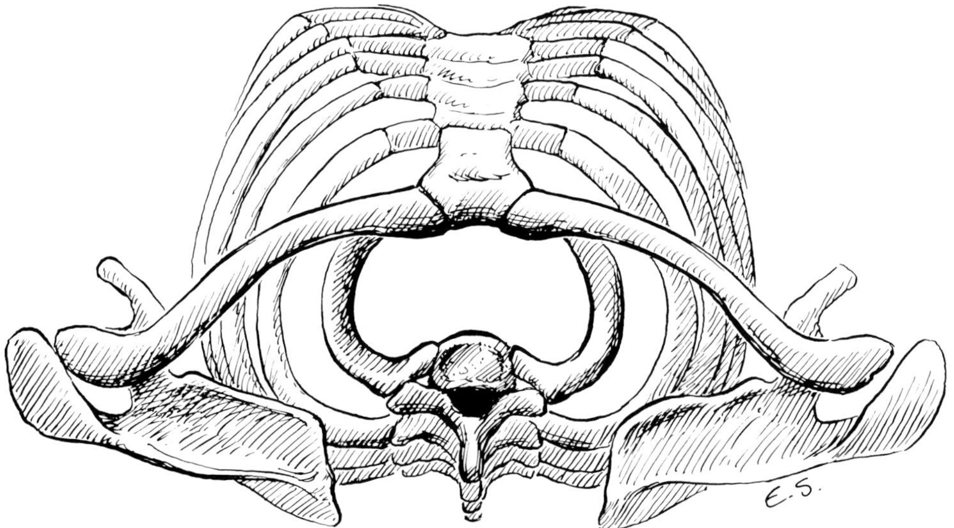

Figure 12–1. The thoracic outlet is approximately 2 × 4 in, yet contains all the major vessels destined for the head and upper extremities.

because their cartilages articulate with the sternum. The bottom five ribs are known as false ribs; however, ribs eight, nine, and ten do turn upward to join the costal cartilage, but the 11th and 12th ribs are free at their extremities and are referred to as floating ribs. The typical rib has a head with two facets that articulate with two vertebrae: the vertebra to which it corresponds numerically and the vertebra above it. The remainder of the rib is composed of a neck, a tubercle, and a shaft. Each rib receives its own nutrient vessel that enters just beyond the tubercle. Additional blood supply is obtained from the periosteal vessels.

The sternum is reminiscent of a Roman sword comprised of a short handle called the manubrium, a longer blade called the body, and a tip known as the xyphoid process. This shield-like bone joins the true ribs anteriorly and serves as a bony protective cover for the heart and great vessels. The sternum also serves as a very important attachment for the anterior muscles of the shoulder girdle and the strap muscles to the neck. Fractures of the sternum occur most frequently at the junction of the body and the manubrium where the bone is the thinnest.

The spaces between the semicircular parallel ribs are occupied by the intercostal muscles, which are important in ventilation. There are 11 intercostal spaces: the upper 9 are closed and the lower 2 remain open anteriorly. In addition to the muscles, there are an intercostal artery, vein, and nerve that are subject to injury from fractures or penetrating wounds. There is an important subcostal groove in each typical rib that is situated on the inner and inferior surface of the rib. Here is contained the intercostal vein, artery, and nerve. Posteriorly, the nerve is situated midway between the ribs, but from the angles of the rib forward, it lies in the subcostal groove. This is important to know when intercostal blocks are used. Additional blood supply to the chest wall is provided by the internal mammary arteries that arise from the subclavian artery and pass rostrally just inside the chest wall near the costochondral junctions. The mammary arteries and veins join the superior epigastric arteries coming from below.

The inner chest wall is lined by the parietal pleura, a glistening capsule that lubricates the movement of the visceral pleura during ventilation. The outer bony thorax is comprised primarily of muscular elements of the chest wall and the shoulder girdle.

During normal ventilation, the diaphragm's concave projection usually rises to approximately the fifth intercostal space during expiration. During maximum expiration, this may reach the fourth intercostal space. This introduces an important concept: the abdomen and thorax cannot be thought of as separate units. They represent a single unit, the torso. The lower rib cage is protection not only for the intrapleural contents but also the upper abdominal contents, primarily the liver and spleen. Injury to the lower chest either by penetrating or blunt trauma must be assumed to involve the abdominal viscera.

Other important anatomic structures include the 12 thoracic vertebrae. These vertebrae consist of a short, cylinder-shaped body, a bony arch, and a vertical spinous process. Extending laterally off the bony arch are the transverse processes that give partial attachment to the ribs. In addition, there are four small articular processes that interlock with the vertebrae above and below. The vertebral canal is formed by the posterior body of the vertebrae and the bony arch. This thoracic vertebral column is important because it protects the posterior mediastinum. The overlying paraspinous and rectospinous muscles on each side of the vertebral bodies provide additional protection, making posterior rib fractures much less common than those anterior to the angle of the rib.

The shoulder girdle serves as an ingenious attachment of the upper extremity to the bony thorax. There are two bones, the clavicle and the scapula, that serve as the rigid bony elements. The clavicle is attached directly to the sternal clavicular joint. The pectoralis major covers the anterior bony thorax on each side and arises medially along the sternal border and extends laterally and cephalad. Another portion of the muscle arises along the inferior surface of the clavicle, and both insert on the crest of the greater tubercle of the humerus. The scapula is a large triangular-shaped bone that has a spine projecting from its outer superior surface. Laterally there is a glenoid cavity that articulates with the humerus. The scapula's outer inferior surface serves as attachments for the teres minor, teres major, latissimus dorsi, and the large infraspinatus muscle. The medial edge serves as attachment to the levator scapula and both rhomboid muscles. The rhomboids, levator scapula, and the large subscapularis, which is on the costal surface of the scapula, serve to attach the scapula to the bony thorax medially along the vertebral column and chest wall. The importance of this shoulder girdle in thoracic injuries is that it protects the upper thorax so that ribs one to four are not easily fractured. Because of this extra protection, fractures found in this area imply a significant kinetic energy has been applied to the chest wall and intrathoracic injuries should be suspected.

Injuries to the upper thorax also may involve the great vessels as they exit from the thoracic outlet. On the right side is the innominate artery and its two branches, the common carotid and subclavian, which are draped over the first rib as they exit laterally with the brachial plexus. Similarly, on the left side the left common carotid and left subclavian artery are closely approximated to the first rib and clavicle. Thus, either penetrating or blunt injuries that involve the apex of the bony thorax may cause injury to the great vessels or brachial plexus.[4]

Other significant muscles that attach to the bony thorax include the abdominal muscles inferiorly that attach primarily to the costal margin and the ribs on the anterior lateral part of the lower chest wall. These include the rectus abdominis muscle medially, the external oblique, internal oblique, and transversus abdominis laterally. The posterior chest wall is covered by the semispinalis and longissimus intercostalis, which form the deep muscles of the back. The intermediate muscles are the rhomboids, the serratus posterior superior, the serratus posterior inferior, and the lumbar fascia. The superficial muscles include the trapezius and latissimus dorsi. The three layers posteriorly provide additional protection to the bony thorax. This area just inferior to the axilla is the thinnest part of the chest wall just inferior to the axilla, thus making it an ideal place to insert chest tubes.

MECHANISM OF INJURY

Chest wall injury falls into three main categories: penetrating, blunt, and blast. Penetrating injuries are further divided into stab wounds, gunshot wounds, and shotgun blasts. Stab wounds are relatively benign injuries unless an intercostal or internal mammary artery has been lacerated or unless a particularly vital structure within the thoracic cavity has been injured (Fig. 12–2) and rarely do they result in much morbidity. Gunshot wounds, on the other hand, can cause devastating injuries to the chest wall, particularly if they are from high-velocity weapons or close-range shotgun blasts. Table 12–2 lists common handguns and weapons with their respective muzzle velocities.

Terminal ballistics, the amount of energy imparted to tissues by the missile, largely determines the severity of the injury. The most widely accepted terminal ballistic theory is

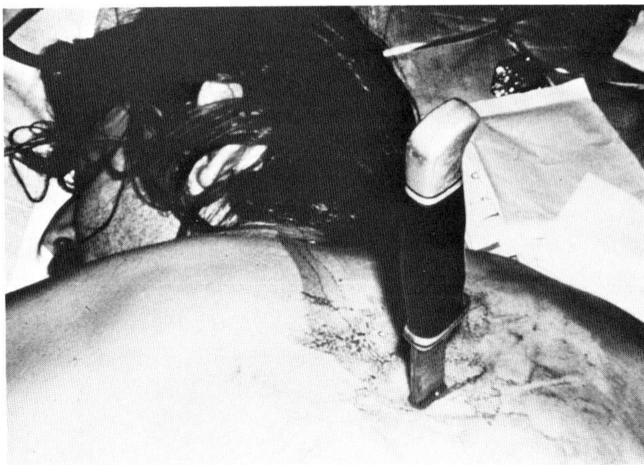

Figure 12–2. Some chest wall injuries can be quite dramatic, but even these can be managed with tube thoracostomy in most instances. In the prehospital setting it is generally best not to remove foreign bodies.

the kinetic energy theory that states that kinetic energy released through tissue equals mass times velocity squared, divided by twice the gravitational constant. This is expressed as:

$$KE = \frac{M(V_1 - V_2)^2}{2G}$$

where M is mass, V_1 is striking velocity, V_2 is exit velocity (residual), and G is gravity. This ballistic formula is thought to provide the best estimate of wounding capacity, and it thus follows that modest increases in velocity will result in tremendous increases in the kinetic energy of the missile and resultant killing and wounding power. A simple calculation using this formula demonstrates that a medium-velocity .22 magnum is capable of eight times the energy release of a relative low-velocity .38 revolver. Generally, weapons capable of generating a missile velocity in excess of 2000 ft/sec are said to be high-velocity weapons (see Table 12–2).

Table 12–2.   Average Muzzle Velocity of Common Weapons

WEAPON	FT/SEC
Handguns	
.22 short	1045
.22 magnum	2000
.38 caliber	1065
.357 magnum	1500
.45 colt	850
Rifles	
.22 long	1100
.30–30	2200
7.62 mm (M-14)	2400–2800
5.56 mm (M-16)	3250

Bullet design also is important, and to inflict the greatest possible tissue damage, a bullet should dissipate all of its energy to the tissue and have no residual exit energy. Missiles that disintegrate on impact, such as soft-point and hollow-nose bullets, cause extensive tissue damage. Some missiles, for example, can create a temporary cavity 30 times the size of the entering bullet, the size of this cavity being dependent on ballistics, type of bullet, yaw, and the tissue that is transgressed. The damage is worsened by secondary missiles or fragments of disintegrating bone and other tissue. This is further compounded in some instances by fragmentation of the bullet. Missile yaw and fragmentation within the tissue is very destructive, particularly when the velocity is greater than 2800 ft/sec.[6] These studies also show that it is not necessary to do radical debridement with wounds from high-velocity missiles as was once believed. Debridement of obviously dead tissue and delayed primary closure of the skin are the hallmarks of wound management.

Close-range shotgun blasts undoubtedly cause the most devastating injuries of any weapon to which civilians are normally exposed.[7,8] Sherman and Parrish[9] have classified shotgun wounds into three categories based on distance: Type 1, long range, or greater than 7 yards; type 2, close range, or 3 to 7 yards; and type 3, very close range, less than 3 yards. Type 1 injuries usually present as scatter types and may not even penetrate visceral cavities from distances greater than 40 yards. At 20 yards, penetration is increased, and yet expectant management sometimes may be warranted. Type 2 injuries usually involve damage to deep structures and require more aggressive management. In the chest wall, this may necessitate debridement of skin, muscle, and bony elements, leaving defects requiring temporary prosthetic closure or more permanent tissue closure. Type 3 wounds involve massive tissue injury and have an 85% to 90% mortality rate.

Blunt injury can be caused by direct impact, shear force, deceleration, and rotary force, the first two causing most of the problems to the chest wall. Direct impact may cause significant injury and severity can be estimated by knowing the force and duration of impact as well as the mass of the patient contact area. For this reason, fractures of four or more ribs represent a serious and often life-threatening injury even in the absence of other overt problems. Table 12–3 demonstrates the most common sites of injury from motor vehicle accidents; ejection, steering assembly impact, windshield impact, instrument panel impact, and rear collision account for most of these. The so-called crush injury also falls into this category. Crush injury is devastating to the chest wall, and in one study[4] crush injury caused flail chest or multiple rib fractures in 59% of the patients and an additional 12% had fractures of the sternum. Shock was present in 40% of the cases and nearly 10 U of blood were required in each case.

Shear force tends to produce degloving types of injuries, such as occur when the patient is run over by a large vehicle or a vehicle with lugs on the wheels. As the vehicle

Table 12–3. Distribution of Injuries After Motor Vehicle Accidents

INJURY	%
Encephalon	43
Chest	12
Abdomen, pelvis	9
Upper extremities	13
Lower extremities	23

From ref. 4.

passes over the body, the skin and subcutaneous tissues are pushed ahead, tearing nutrient blood supply from its muscular sources below. Subsequent extensive soft tissue loss is common after such injury. Associated fractures of the ribs may be compounded, creating further problems.

Deceleration injuries are associated most often with high-speed motor vehicle accidents and falls from heights. As the body decelerates, the organs continue to move forward at terminal velocity, tearing vessels and tissues from points of attachment. Although there may be extensive chest wall injury with impact, deceleration per se usually does not cause significant chest wall defects. Rotary forces also tend to cause tearing injuries from a tumbling type of action.

There have been studies using human cadavers in evaluating chest wall trauma.[10,11] The cadavers were subjected to deceleration impacted on a 6-in pad on the anterior chest surface. At a sled velocity of 16.8 mph, four rib fractures were caused at impact. At 18.5 mph, chest deflection was increased, resulting in extensive fractures. Other studies have confirmed that the older the patient, the more extensive the damage to the chest wall. Newman and Jones[12] studied impact, restraint use, and severity of injury after frontal, side, and roll-over impact. Unrestrained drivers had an incidence of four or more rib fractures of 47.4% for frontal, 59% for side, and 75% for roll-over impact. In comparison, restrained drivers had four or more rib fractures of 8.7%, 77.7%, and 50.0%, respectively. There was a correspondingly high association of intrathoracic injuries in these various categories. Not surprisingly, the same study showed a very close relationship between chest injuries (Abbreviated Injury Scale greater than 2) sustained in frontal impacts and speed of the automobile. In restrained occupants, rib fractures and sternal fractures were not seen until the car was traveling more quickly than 15 mph, whereas rib fractures were common in unrestrained occupants when the speed of the automobile was less than 10 mph. Significant rib fractures did not occur in the restrained persons until speeds of 30 mph were reached. In contrast, multiple rib fractures and significant intrathoracic injuries in unrestrained persons were quite common with speeds of 10 to 20 mph. In this series, there was only one death in restrained occupants, whereas unrestrained occupants accounted for seven deaths. Most of the deaths were secondary to associated lung contusions or rupture of the aorta or heart. These data are consistent with other investigative work.[13–15] Thus, injury to the chest wall as a sequela of blunt trauma is directly correlated to type of impact, speed of impact, age of the patient, and whether or not the occupant is restrained.

RELATIVE INCIDENCE

The exact incidence of chest wall trauma is unknown. We do know from a northeastern Ohio study[16] that the annual trauma incidence was 197 per 1000 population. We further know from Besson and Saegesser's[4] book that in a city of 200,000, four surgical casualties were admitted each day, primarily from motor vehicle accidents. Minor damage to the chest wall occurred in 24% of the cases seen in the emergency room. Major chest wall damage accounted for 34% of the admissions and flail chest accounted for 13%. This implies that injuries to the chest wall, whether minor, major, or severe, constitute the great majority of thoracic admissions to a hospital and that approximately one of every eight trauma admissions constitutes chest trauma. These numbers are probably most in keeping with a nonviolent urban or suburban area. In a large series of 585 thoracic trauma deaths,

Kemmerer and co-workers[17] showed that 39% of trauma admissions had significant rib fractures and another 5% had fractures to the sternum. Wilson and co-workers[18] showed an almost linear correlation between the number of ribs fractured and associated intrathoracic and intraabdominal injuries; there also seemed to be a close correlation of death in the number of ribs fractured. In their series, if there were more than seven ribs fractured, 68% had associated intrathoracic injury and 16% had intraabdominal injury. Their study also pointed out a valuable clinical lesson: if the patient with fractured ribs after blunt trauma is in shock and does not have a large hemothorax or pneumothorax to account for the reduced blood pressure, the bleeding must be in the abdomen.

Table 12–4 shows representative series and demonstrates the incidence of chest wall injury after blunt trauma. Most chest injuries involve the chest wall; with severe trauma, the mortality may be as high as 40%.[19] Undoubtedly, severe chest wall trauma is associated with significant intrathoracic trauma, which contributes to the mortality because there seems to be a correlation with ventilator time and mortality.[20]

PATHOPHYSIOLOGY

Open Pneumothorax

The pathophysiology of open pneumothorax has not drastically improved since the classic descriptions of Hewson and Larrey. Open pneumothoraxes often are called "sucking wounds of the chest," which is descriptive of their pathophysiology. There is a large hole in the chest wall that cannot be covered by the overlying subcutaneous tissue, muscle, or skin. As a consequence, with inspiration there is a movement of air into the pleural space. There is associated collapse of the lung and paradoxical motion of the mediastinum. There often is associated hemothorax and, if the defect in the chest wall is larger than the glottic opening, there will be more exchange of air through the injury site than through the glottis, resulting in progressive respiratory insufficiency and death.

Table 12–4.   Incidence of Chest Injuries After Blunt Trauma

INJURY	KEMMERER ET AL.[17] %	BESSON AND SAEGESSER[4] %
Rib fracture	39	47
Hemothorax	28	24
Lung laceration	10	21
Ruptured great vessel	10	4
Lung contusion	6	12
Lacerated diaphragm	5	7
Myocardial injury	6	7
Sternal fractures	5	22*
Lacerated trachea	1	5

*Steering wheel injuries.

Other Penetrating Wounds

Most stab wounds and gunshot wounds cause little or no damage to the chest wall. There may be associated rib fractures, but usually they are of little consequence to ventilation. The most likely associated injury leading to thoracotomy will be an injury to one of the intercostal vessels, which then bleeds into the pleural space. Similarly, penetrating wounds can cause injuries to the internal mammary arteries or the subclavian vessels as they exit over the chest apex. Exceptions to these general rules are shotgun blasts that, when fired at close range, can cause devastating chest wall defects leading to open pneumothorax and severe associated injuries to underlying structures. The open pneumothorax caused by shotgun blasts undoubtedly contributes to the high mortality from these wounds.

There is one warning regarding the pathophysiology of chest wall wounds. It usually takes an expert forensic pathologist to determine entrance and exit characteristics. Although sometimes the path may appear to be obvious, it is better for the physician to describe the wounds in great detail and leave the final determination to an expert. This has import in medicolegal testimony.

Other Wounds

Most other wounds of the chest wall, particularly those involving the integument, subcutaneous tissue, and muscle, do not cause major physiological derangements, the single exception being burns. A circumferential full thickness burn of the chest wall can cause major respiratory insufficiency secondary to a decrease in chest wall compliance. This should be easily recognizable and treated promptly with escharotomy.

Fractures to the Clavicle, Sternum, and Scapula

Fractures to the clavicle are common and rarely cause major pathophysiologic changes. Although painful, they usually do not embarrass ventilation and only rarely are associated with major vessel lacerations.

Fractures to the sternum are being reported with increasing frequency and constitute 5% to 10% of all thoracic injuries. Part of this increased incidence may be due to better recognition and to physicians being aware of the close association of fractured sternum to steering column trauma. Isolated sternal fractures usually do not cause major problems except pain; but, because of the painful sequelae, they may require operative management. Isolated sternal fractures are not common and usually are associated with other significant chest wall trauma, including flail chest. The most common associated injury is myocardial contusion, which can lead to significant arrhythmias and hemodynamic instability, which is discussed in Chapter 15.

The scapula is not commonly fractured. It is protected by a relatively thick coat of muscle and lies in a protected position. Therefore, when seen, fractures of the scapula are associated with a significant amount of kinetic energy imparted to that portion of the body and should make the clinician suspicious of significant associated injuries. Fractures involving the glenoid fossa and acromium, however, may have significant pathophysiologic consequences from an orthopedic standpoint.

Injuries to the Ribs, Including Flail Chest

As a consequence of the pioneering work by Stapp and his associates, we know that there is a high correlation between impact velocity and severity of chest wall trauma. There appears to be a linear relationship between ribs fractured and the pathophysiologic consequences. Other factors include age of the patient, location of the rib fractures, the presence of a flail segment, and associated injuries.

The one thing in common with almost all injuries involving the bony thorax is pain. Pain, in and by itself, can lead to decreased ventilation, decreased vital capacity, inability to clear secretions, and retention of carbon dioxide. As more ribs are fractured, there is a progression of pathophysiologic findings, including ventilation perfusion abnormalities, increase of respiratory work, hypoxemia, and a decrease in the functional residual capacity. These are especially common when multiple rib fractures result in flail chest (Fig. 12–3). It is at this time that the bellows actions of the chest wall muscles become reduced, leading to further abnormalities in ventilation. If the flail segment is large enough, there may be collapse of this segment during inspiration and shifting of the mediastinum toward the contralateral side on inspiration with a concomitant obstruction to venous return to the heart. Negative intrathoracic pressure is reduced, contributing to decreased ventilation.

Recently, there have been several articles pointing out the significance of associated injuries.[4,21–23] Clearly, when present, they do contribute to the pathophysiology. The most common associated injury is pulmonary contusion, which is associated with ventilation perfusion abnormalities; however, its occurrence may be less than previously thought.[24] There is an associated atelectasis and shunting of blood in larger contusions, a decrease in compliance and an increase in airway resistance, an associated decrease in pulmonary diffusion, and an increase in respiratory work that is additive to that contributed by the chest wall defect.

Ultimately, the combination of the pain, the decrease in ventilation, and the sequela of the associated injuries lead to retention of carbon dioxide, hypoxemia, and respiratory insufficiency. Although isolated rib fractures in the young, healthy patient may be of little consequence, isolated rib fractures in the elderly or those with preexisting pulmonary disease can lead to fatality due to progressive atelectasis and ventilatory insufficiency.

To sort out the variables that contribute to the pathophysiology of chest wall injury, we examined the records of 144 consecutive patients with chest wall injury during a 5-yr period at San Francisco General Hospital.[24] Most of the injuries (75%) were caused by motor vehicle accidents. The overall mortality rate was 25% (36 patients). The Injury Severity Score (IFS) averaged 32 ± 14^{SD} in the survivors, compared with 60 ± 14^{SD} in those patients who died, which also points out how severely injured these patients were. Interestingly, isolated pulmonary contusion or flail chest had a mortality rate of 16% each; however, the rate of combined pulmonary contusion and flail chest was 42%.

Signs and Symptoms

The patient's history can be extremely important in diagnosing chest wall injury, even for the unconscious patient. The paramedics should be questioned on how the patient was injured and the character of the patient's breathing during transport. If the paramedics give a history that the patient was extricated from behind the steering wheel, a strong suspicion of

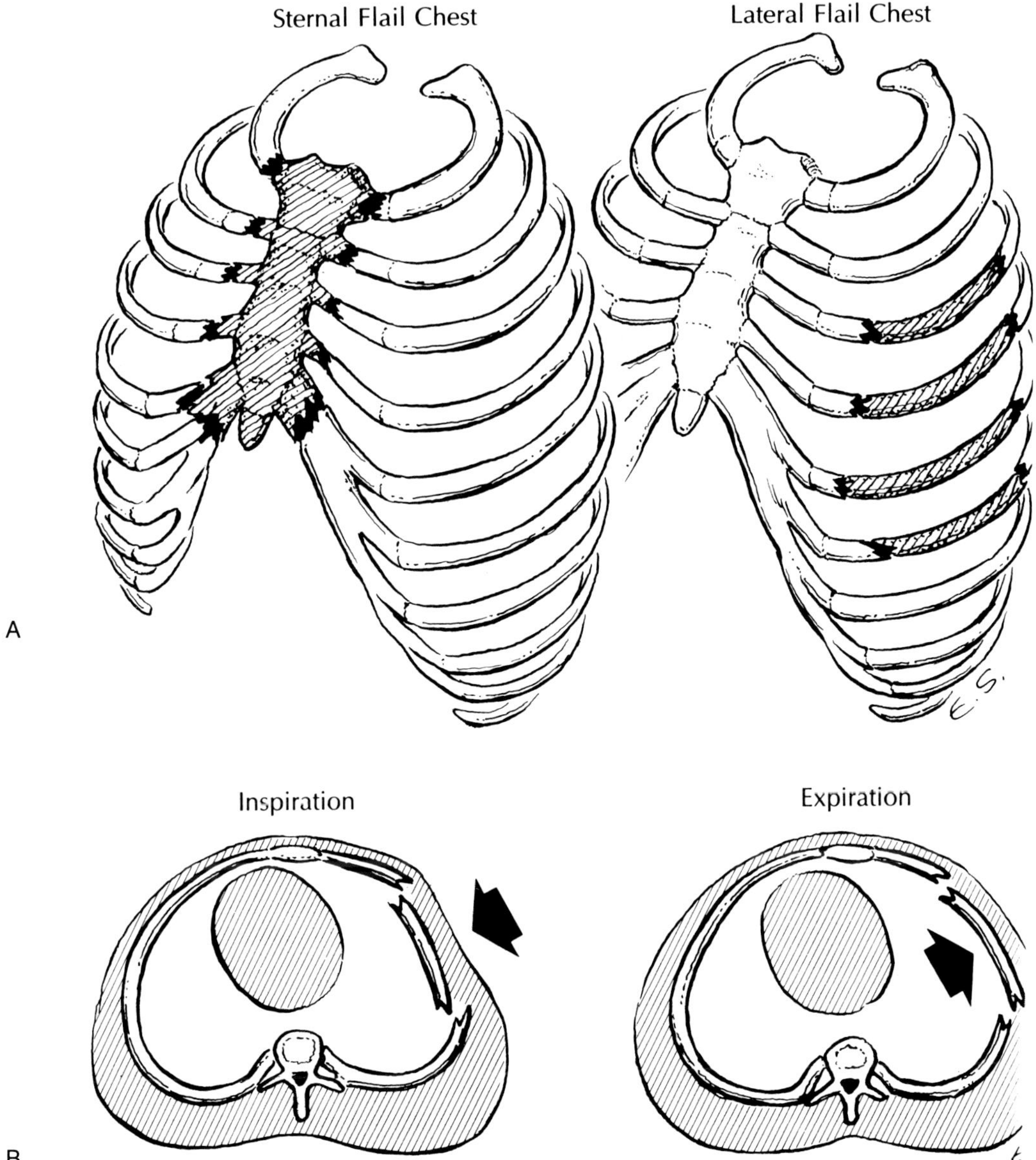

Figure 12–3. **A:** Flail chest can be either anterior involving the sternum or lateral involving the ribs. **B:** The inward movement of the flail segment with inspiration.

chest wall injury should be entertained. The paramedic's observations and treatment should be carefully noted, for they often direct the resuscitating surgeon to life-threatening airway and chest wall injuries. Observation of respiratory rate is extremely important as, except for the terminal patient, any ventilatory compromise will result in an increased respiratory rate. A slow, even rate of 20 or less is reassuring, 25 or more indicates pathology of some type, 30 or more indicates serious derangement, and 35 or more is an indication for immediate intubation and ventilatory support.

In the conscious patient, the hallmark of chest wall injury is pain, which is aggravated by coughing, deep breathing, and change of body position. The vital and consistent screening maneuver is to ask the patient to take a deep breath. If he/she can do so without discomfort, the probability of rib fracture or significant chest wall injury is negligible. With relatively minor chest wall injuries, the signs include localized palpable tenderness and compression pain; in addition, there may be crepitation upon palpation or auscultation.

In moderate and severe chest wall injuries, in addition to the pain, ventilatory insufficiency is common. Specific signs of ventilatory insufficiency include air hunger, cyanosis, use of the accessory muscles of ventilation, and a ventilatory rate faster than 25/ min. Less specific manifestations include those of generalized sympathetic discharge: anxiety, fear, agitation, tachycardia, and cold clammy skin. If the injury is severe, there may be a flail chest either laterally or anteriorly. Observation usually will confirm the presence of paradoxical motion of the chest wall with inspiration and expiration. A significant number of patients with flail chest may not manifest the problem initially, underscoring the need for repeated examinations in those with chest wall pain.

Chest radiographs have limited value and use in diagnosing chest wall injury (Fig. 12–4). In our experience, up to 50% of rib fractures may not be evident on plain roentgeno-grams. However, its routine use is advocated primarily to diagnose associated injuries, particularly intrathoracic complications. If fractures are demonstrated in the first three ribs, this signifies significant kinetic energy release and should raise the suspicion of associated injuries such as rupture of the thoracic aorta. Similarly, fractures demonstrated in ribs 8 through 12 should make one suspect intraabdominal injuries, primarily to the liver, spleen, and kidney. If a sternal fracture is suspected, a lateral film with attention to bony detail should be obtained.

Other laboratory tests may be of value, particularly if there are signs of ventilatory insufficiency as manifest by an increased respiratory rate. Under these circumstances blood gas determination should be routine. A carbon dioxide tension greater than 40 mm Hg in an acutely injured patient who does not have documented chronic hypercapnia must be taken as absolute evidence of ventilatory insufficiency. Hypoxemia usually indicates underlying associated lung injury. Vital capacity and inspiratory force also are useful measurements for the patient with chest wall injury, but these measurements usually are not performed in the emergency room. Parenchymal lung function can be assessed by computed tomography scan, oxygen tension to fractional inspired oxygen ratio, shunt fraction, and compliance; however, most of these require invasive monitoring and are performed in the intensive care unit.

The diagnosis of open chest wounds should be obvious. In addition to the local wound pain, there may be signs of ventilatory insufficiency if the patient has an associated pneumothorax. The larger the pneumothorax, the more significant the ventilatory insuffi-ciency. If the open pneumothorax is large, there often is associated hissing noise with

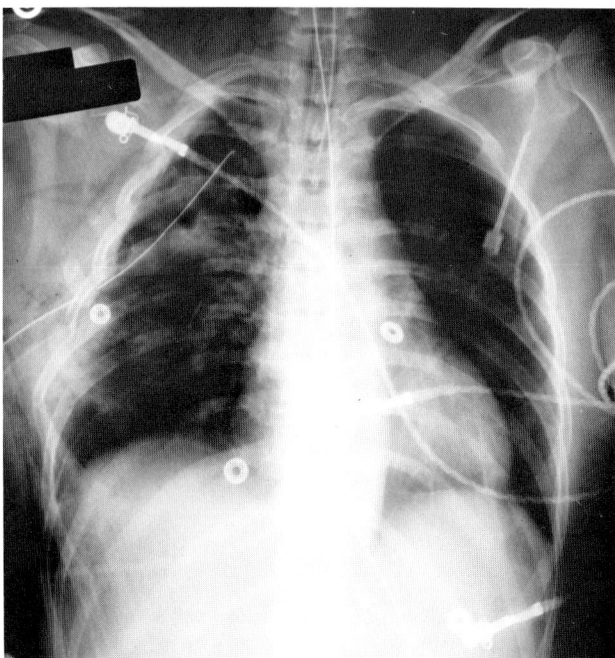

Figure 12–4.   Chest radiograph shows multiple rib fractures on the right with subcutaneous air dissecting over the entire hemithorax.

inspiratory and expiratory movement. A bloody froth is characteristic of air escaping from the open wound during expiration.

MANAGEMENT OF SPECIFIC INJURIES

The treatment of chest wall injuries is dependent on a stepwise prioritization of the patient. The first prioritization takes place immediately on seeing the patient. Within a few seconds, it can be determined whether the patient is hemodynamically stable or unstable, conscious or unconscious, and whether or not the patient has ventilatory insufficiency. In general, the unconscious patient or the patient who is hemodynamically unstable requires almost immediate airway intubation and establishment of ventilation. The timing will depend on the severity and the cause of the injuries.

Once the airway is established and ventilation ensured, other emergency treatment should be carried out. Open pneumothoraces should be closed with occlusive dressings. Flail segments of the chest wall should be stabilized by endotracheal intubation or mechanical ventilation, by temporarily placing sandbags next to the flail, or by turning the patient so that the flail segment is against the mattress. Chest tubes should be inserted to evacuate pneumothoraces and hemothoraces. If the patient remains unstable, further treatment is best carried out in the operating room. If, on the other hand, the patient is stabilized promptly, further diagnostic studies can be undertaken and treatment planned accordingly.

In the conscious hemodynamically stable patient, prioritization of treatment will be based on the presence of ventilatory insufficiency, associated injuries, and control of pain. In general, most patients with multiple rib fractures will require hospitalization for control of the pain and a period of observation to rule out associated injuries and complications of the pain.

There is no simple approach to treatment of patients with chest wall injuries. In general, we direct our attention to the treatment of pain, the presence or absence of ventilatory insufficiency, and the chest wall defect. The patient may have one or all of these problems, and therefore the treatment must be individually tailored.

Treatment of Pain

In general, strapping of the chest is not done because it may promote atelectasis and reduce vital capacity. At times, however, strapping may reduce pain and aid the coughing patient sufficiently so that the benefit outweighs the theoretical disadvantages. Occasionally, patients with single rib fractures may be managed effectively with oral analgesics, but, again, caution should be exercised, because most narcotics may adversely affect ventilation and clearing of secretions. A new, nonsteroidal, antiinflammatory drug, ketorlac (Toradol), may be a promising alternative to narcotics. The dosage is 30 to 60 mg intramuscularly as a loading dose and 15 to 30 mg every 6 hr. An oral form has been released and has a recommended dose of 10 mg every 6 hr.

Patients who are admitted to the hospital with chest wall injuries as part of their injury complex and have pain as a primary problem are optimally treated with epidural analgesia.[26,27] There are obvious contraindications to this management such as open wounds in the midline back, bleeding, or coagulation disorders. However, most surgeons and anesthesiologists prefer epidural analgesia for its excellent pain control. Wisner[27] showed a significant decrease in mortality and morbidity. In a randomized trial, he compared epidural fentanyl with intravenous infusions of fentanyl.[26] The epidural mode of treatment improved maximum inspiratory pressure and vital capacity. There were no significant changes in arterial blood gases with epidural fentanyl, but there was a decrease in Pao_2 and an increase in $Paco_2$ with intravenous fentanyl. As a result, many patients previously requiring ventilators for pain and ventilatory insufficiency can be managed now without them. Also, treatment of pain by epidural narcotic does not necessarily require intensive care, as most experienced ward nurses are qualified to administer this treatment. Suggested epidural narcotic orders by our pain service are shown in Table 12–5.

Alternatives to epidural narcotic analgesia include intercostal blocks and patient administrated analgesia (PCA). Intercostal blocks are administered by injection of 0.5% to 1.0% lidocaine with 1:100,000 epinephrine around the intercostal nerve to the involved segment, as shown in Figure 12–5. Usually the intercostal nerve above and below the injury should be injected as well. An alternative to lidocaine is bupivacaine hydrochloride, which provides longer relief.

Occasionally, *operative treatment* is indicated for minor to moderate chest wall injuries. Examples include separation of the costal chondral junction and sternal fractures. Costal chondral separation may not heal secondary to poor blood supply. If that is the case, excision of the cartilage may give dramatic relief of the pain. Sternal fractures also are

Table 12–5.   Acute Pain Service: Epidural Narcotic Standard Orders

1. Operating room dose: Drug ________________ Mg __________ Time __________
2. Drug for continuing epidural analgesia:
    A. PF morphine (1 mg/ml) ______________ mg every 6–12 hr.
    B. Fentanyl (10μg/ml normal saline) infuse __________ μg (__________ ml)/per hr.
    C. Other: Drug ________________ Concentration __________ Dose __________
        Interval __________
3. Fentanyl 50 μg (1.0 ml) into epidural catheter every 3 hr as needed for inadequate analgesia with prescribed dose above.
4. Maintain iv access (drip or heparin lock) for 24 hr after last dose of epidural narcotic.
5. Naloxone 0.4 mg at bedside.
6. **No narcotics or other CNS depressants** to be given except as ordered by the Acute Pain Service.
7. Monitoring: Respiratory rate and sedation scale every 1 hr for 1st 24 hr, and then every 4 hr.
8. Treatment of side effects:
    A. Call Acute Pain Service if sedation scale = 3.
    B. Call Acute Pain Service if respiratory rate is <8 breaths per min.
    C. Naloxone 0.4 mg iv stat for sedation scale = 3 plus respiratory rate <8 breaths per min. Call Acute Pain Service.
    D. Metoclopramide 10 mg iv q 6 h prn for nausea/vomiting. In addition, if age <60 yr, transdermal scopolamine patch to either mastoid area. Change every 72 hr as needed.
    E. Diphenhydramine 25 mg iv every 6 hr as needed for severe itching.
    F. For urinary retention, "in-and-out" bladder catheter as needed.
9. For inadequate analgesia or other problems related to epidural, call Acute Pain Service.
10. Triazolam 0.125 mg every 1 hr as needed. May repeat × 1.

Date ________________   ________________________________M.D.
Dr. ________________ on the APS was notified about this patient at __________ hr.

Appendix
Example of Bedside Sedation Scale

Sedation	Description
0 (none)	Alert
1 (mild)	Occasionally drowsy; easy to arouse
2 (moderate)	Frequently drowsy; easy to arouse
3 (severe)	Somnolent; difficult to arouse
4 (sleeping)	Normal sleep; easy to arouse

associated with a significant amount of pain and may be unstable. In both instances, an operative approach and wiring of the fracture will reduce morbidity (Fig. 12–6).

Treatment of Ventilatory Insufficiency

Ventilatory insufficiency can be categorized as minor, moderate, or severe.[28] Most importantly from a treatment standpoint, treatment can be divided into ventilatory and nonventilatory support. The indications for ventilatory management are shown in Table 12–6.[29–31] If at all possible, it is best to avoid ventilatory therapy, because chronic intubation and the

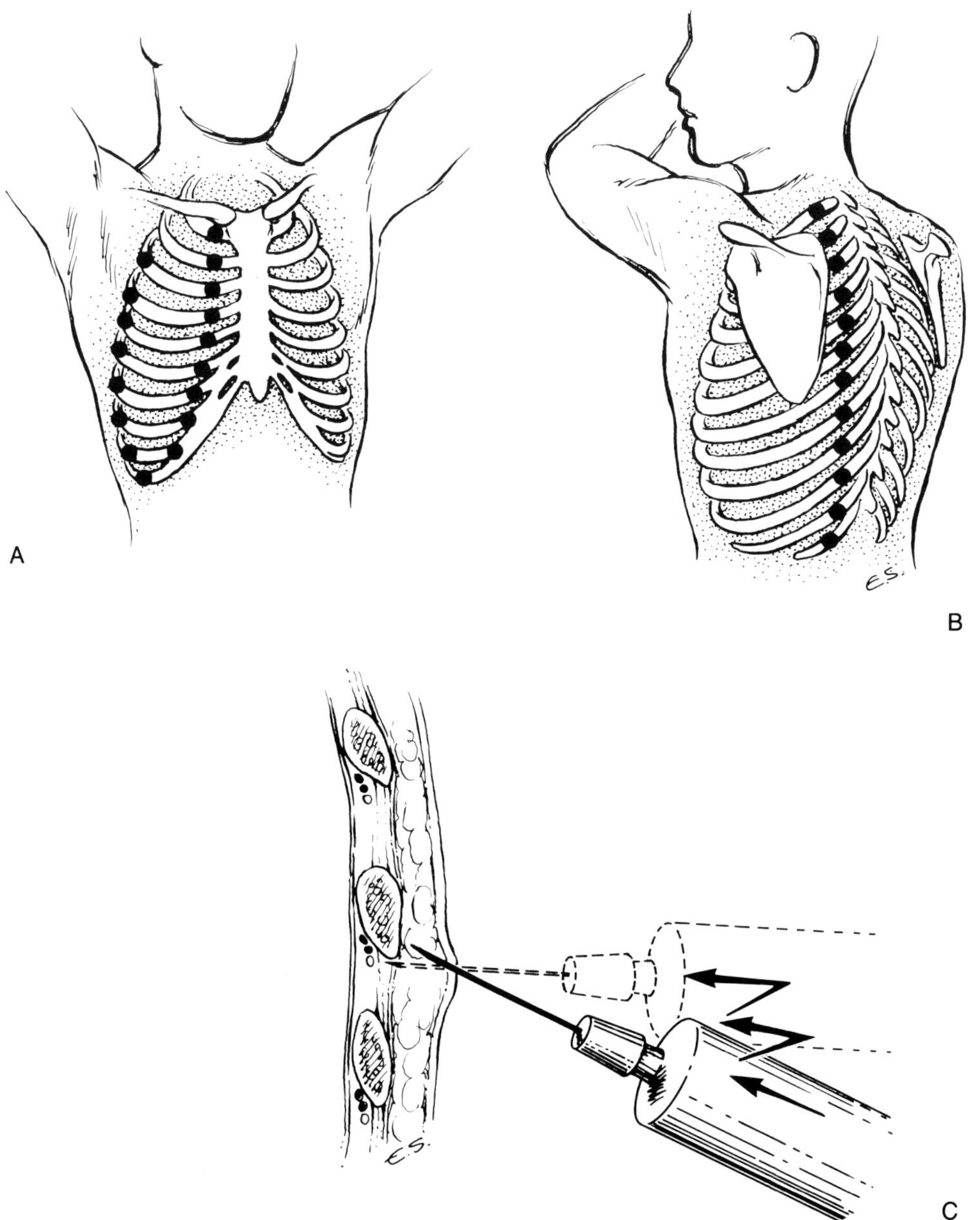

Figure 12–5. Intercostal blocks are placed strategically beneath the inferior border of the ribs as far posterior as possible for lateral fractures or anterior for separation of costochondral junctions and sternal fractures (**A**, **B**). The needle is advanced to the rib and "walked" off the inferior surface (**C**) and advanced 2 to 3 mm. One to 2 ml of local anesthetic is then injected.

use of ventilators set the stage for major complications, primarily pulmonary sepsis. If the patient meets the criteria outlined in Table 12–6, however, there often is no other recourse. Aggressive conservative management, on the other hand, may prevent the patient with moderate ventilatory insufficiency from falling into the severe category. This treatment includes adequate relief of pain, nasotracheal suction, incentive respirometers, chest physiotherapy, and supplemental oxygen to maintain the oxygen tension above 60 mm Hg.

There are some controversial adjunctive measures in treating ventilatory insufficiency that include restriction of intravenous fluids, steroids, diuretics, and salt-poor albumin.[32] It is not necessary to use any of these adjunctive measures. The resuscitation of the trauma patient should be based on maintaining flow to the critical organs. This is best determined by keeping atrial filling pressures as near normal as possible, maintaining adequate urinary output (>0.5 ml/kg/hr), and reversing the clinical signs of shock.[33,34] Once the patient has

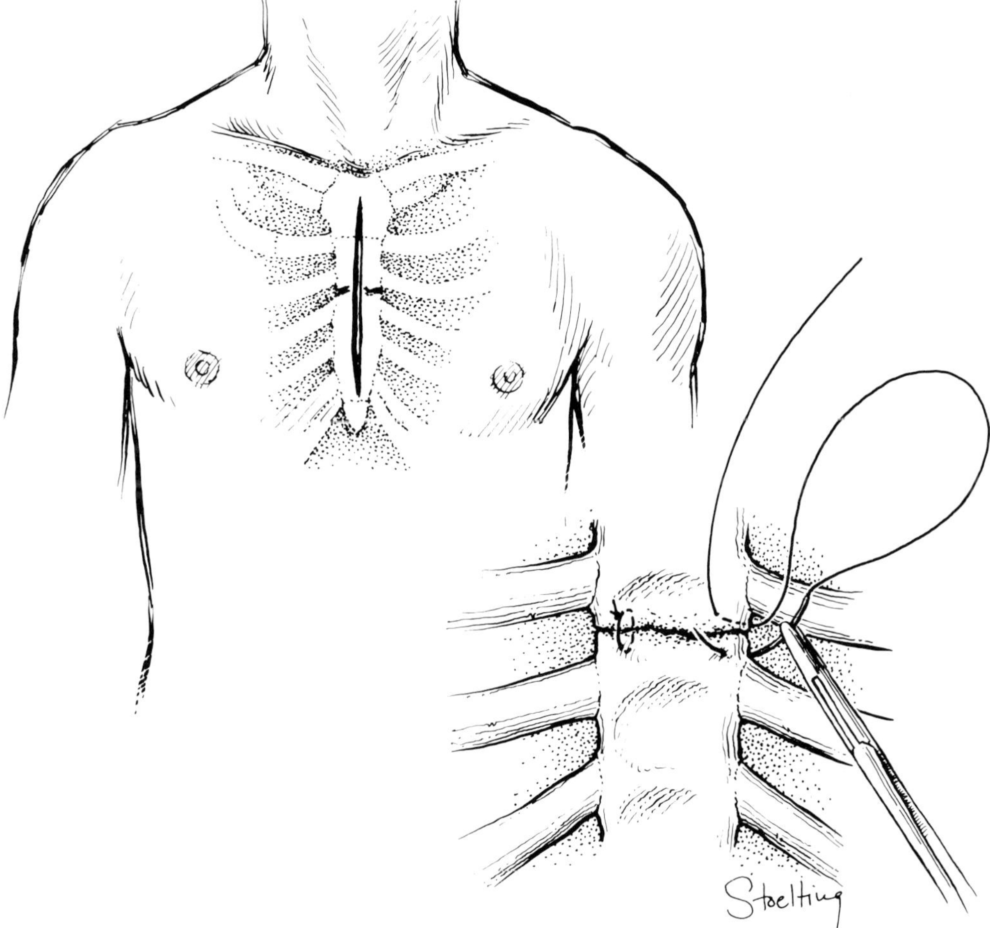

Figure 12–6.   Fracture of the sternum is located most commonly at the junction of the body and the manubrium. Repair, when indicated, is best accomplished with wire sutures.

Table 12–6. Indications for Mechanical Ventilation

VENTILATORY	NORMAL	VENTILATORY INDICATED
Respirations	12–20	>35
Carbon dioxide tension	35–40 mm Hg	>45 mm Hg
Vital capacity	65–70 ml/kg	<10–15 ml/kg
Maximum inspiratory force	−75–100 cm H_2O	<−25 cm H_2O
Parenchymal		
Alveolar to arterial oxygen tension difference	50–75 mm Hg	>350 mm Hg
Shunt	<5%	>15%
Wasted ventilation (V_d/V_t)	0.4–0.4	>0.6
Compliance	40–50 ml/cm H_2O	<30 ml/cm H_2O

been resuscitated, fluid management should be based on replacing sensible and insensible losses. Keeping the patient "dry" will not selectively reduce edema in the chest wall or in parenchymal lung injuries; the efficacy of diuretics in treating chest wall injuries and underlying pulmonary contusions is unproved. It is unrealistic to think that contusions of the chest wall or the lung can be selectively "dehydrated." The injudicious use of diuretics may volume deplete the patient and embarrass renal function. The administration of salt-poor albumin is equally controversial, and in one randomized study[34] was shown to affect adversely mortality and morbidity.

Steroids are extremely controversial; however, there is not a single randomized study demonstrating their efficacy. Most studies show that there are detrimental side effects to the steroids, including increased infection rates and impaired wound healing.

If the patient fails conservative treatment as documented by the values in Table 12–6, intubation and mechanical ventilation are indicated. This ventilatory support is discussed in more detail in Chapter 2.

Operative Treatment of Chest Wall Injuries

Operative management of chest wall injuries falls into two categories: treatment for open pneumothorax and treatment for rib and sternal fractures. The treatment of open chest wounds depends on the extent of the wound and the wounding agent. In general, stab wounds and low-velocity gunshot wounds require simple skin debridement, irrigation, and allowing the wound to heal secondarily, or delayed primary closure on the fifth postinjury day. More extensive wounds, particularly those caused by shotgun blasts, require major debridement and removal of foreign bodies, bone fragments, and wadding from the shell. If the wound is extensive enough that closure is impossible, a myocutaneous flap can be of great value. Pectoralis muscle, latissimi dorsi, and rectus abdominis flaps all lend themselves to covering chest wall defects. Synthetic materials such as Marlex are not used as commonly as they once were because of the advent of the much more satisfactory myocutaneous flaps. However, they may be of great value in acute management.

Operative stabilization of sternal fractures is indicated when there is severe pain or instability of the sternal fracture.[35] In general, this is best approached by an incision directly over the injury (limited midline sternotomy) and stabilization of the fracture segment with wire sutures. If there is a segmental fracture involving the sternum, it may be necessary to place a plate (Jerguson or Arbeitsgemeinshaft Osteosynthesefragen) over the fracture segment and secure it above and below the fracture lines.

Operative stabilization of rib fractures is not a new technique but has recently been reinstituted because of high morbidity or mortality in severe flail chest injuries.[14,36,37] It is used most advantageously when thoracotomy is required to treat associated injuries. There are many techniques for stabilizing rib fractures, including using Kirschner wires and wire sutures,[9] staples,[4] and steel plates[9] (Fig. 12–7). Our own experience has been confined primarily to plates that we wire across the flail segments. We have no experience with the Russian UKL staple or the Judet staples. Our technique is to use plates wired on every other rib and to secure the adjacent rib to the strutted rib with a chromic suture (Fig. 12–8). We also have used a single, horizontal plate augmented with a vertical plate (Fig. 12–9). Soft tissue, consisting of muscle and subcutaneous tissue, is then closed over the plate using monofilament sutures. The wounds are irrigated with antibiotic solutions (kanamycin and bacitracin).

The rationale of the operation is to minimize ventilator time if the chest wall injury is the primary indicator for ventilator treatment. It will not be of major benefit if the primary indication for ventilation treatment is the parenchymal lung injury or severe brain injury. In a personal experience with 12 patients, 2 of whom died from associated neurological injuries, it was found that patients spent an average of 8 days less on the ventilator than patients who did not have operative stabilization.

COMPLICATIONS

Complications of chest wall injury include dehiscence, rib pseudoarthrosis, intercostal neuralgia, chronic infection, respiratory failure, and pneumonia. Pseudoarthrosis is invariably secondary to nonunion of a rib fracture; surgical treatment will depend on whether or not it is clinically significant. Intercostal neuralgia usually is secondary to an intercostal nerve entrapped within a callous. If the patient does not respond to repeated nerve injection with lidocaine, alcohol infiltration of the nerve may give more long-lasting relief. An alternative is surgical transection of the nerve.

Chronic infection of the chest wall may follow midline sternotomy or thoracoabdominal or intercostal incisions. Reoperation, debridement, and good sternal fixation is required to treat the former. Intercostal incisions that are infected usually respond to opening the wound. The most difficult infection to treat is that involving the costal cartilages. These produce smoldering infections that are not responsive to antibiotics or conservative management. They usually require complete excision of the infected cartilage. Should the costal cartilage or infection of ribs six to ten be involved, extensive morbidity may be associated and major surgery involved. Myocutaneous flaps to fill the defect may be indicated.

In our experience, approximately 2% of patients who have had acute ventilatory insufficiency due to chest wall injuries will require readmission to the intensive care unit. These failures most often represent patients who did not get the intensive chest physical

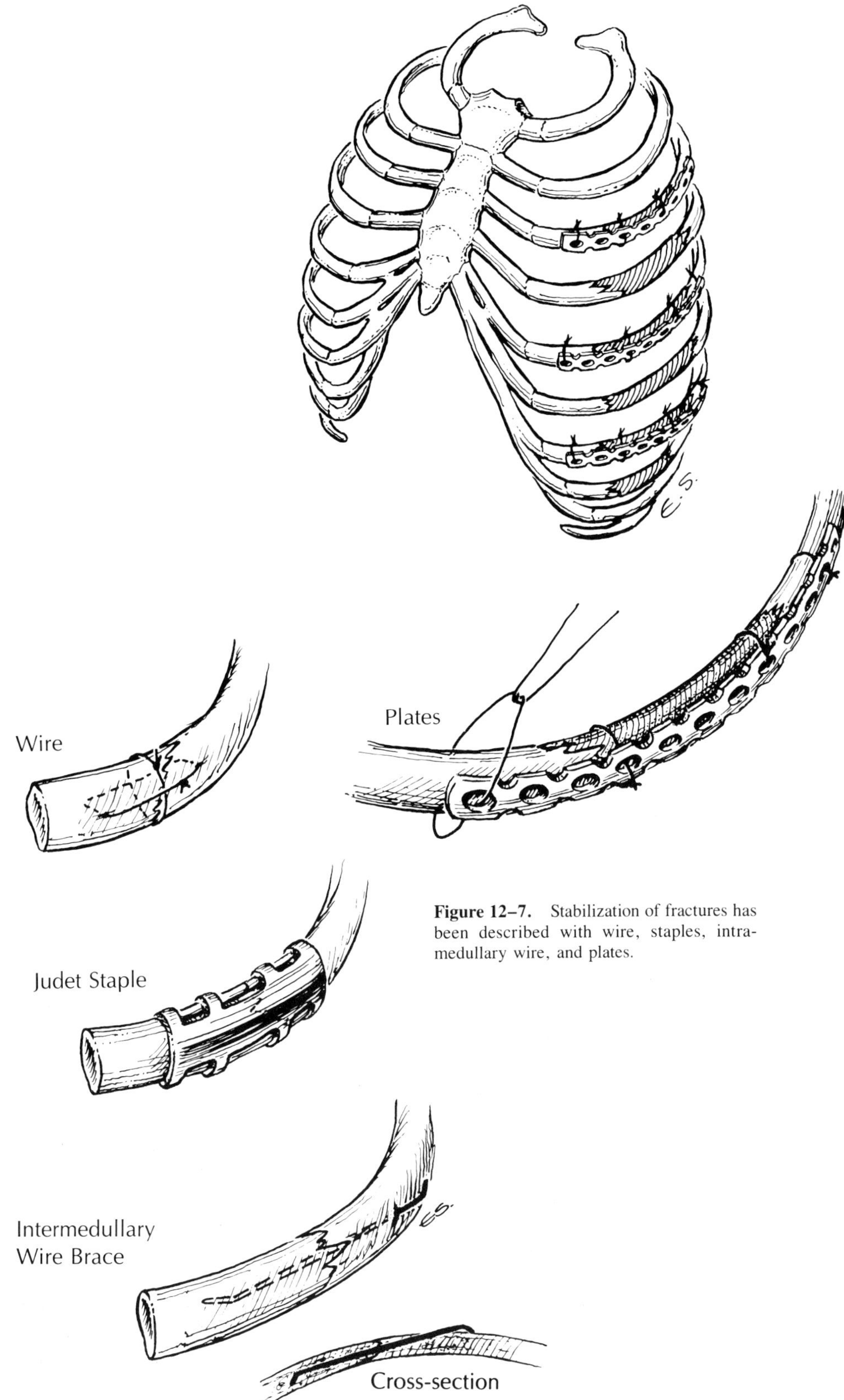

Figure 12–7. Stabilization of fractures has been described with wire, staples, intramedullary wire, and plates.

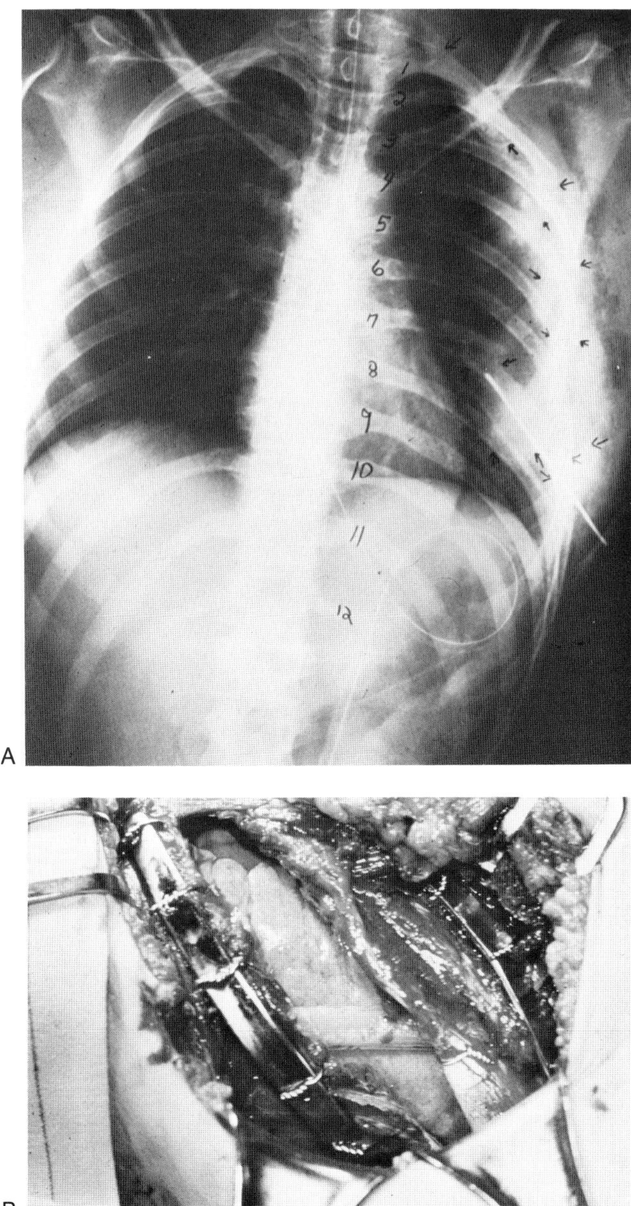

Figure 12–8. This 23-year-old flight attendant sustained a steering wheel injury to the anterior chest, primarily the left side. **A:** Extensive fractures are shown. **B:** Because of an associated extensive open pneumothorax, a thoracotomy was done and struts placed across the flail segment. She was weaned from the ventilator on postoperative day 3 and did well. (Figure continued on next page.)

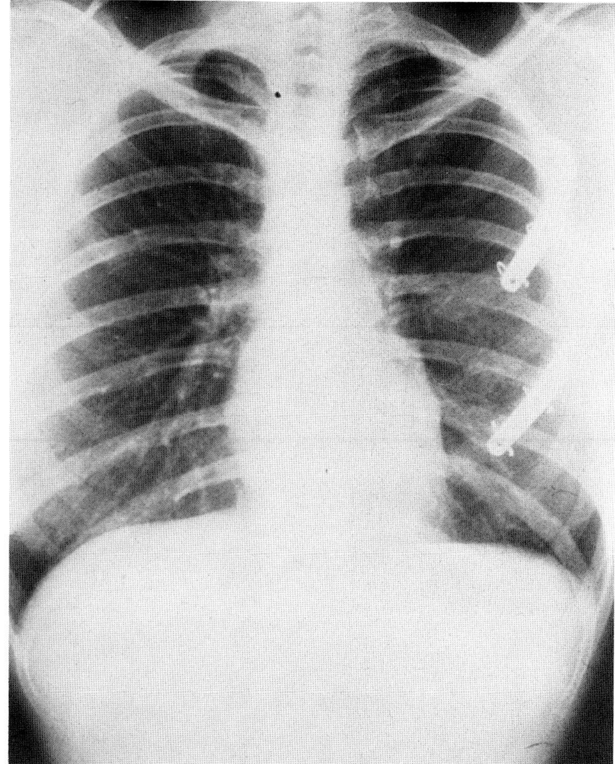

Figure 12–8, cont. **C:** A chest radiograph 2 yr after the injury.

therapy and suctioning on the wards that they previously had in the intensive care unit. Pneumonia also is a major contributing factor for the failure of these patients. Optimally, after extubation patients should be sent first to an intermediate care unit until it is clear that they can tolerate the less intensive ward nursing.

RESULTS

After minor chest wall injury, the outcome is generally quite favorable, except in the elderly in whom there may be significant morbidity and even mortality. Two recent studies show a clear relationship between age and outcome after chest wall injury.[20,38] One of these studies also shows the relationship between certain risk factors and flail chest injury.[38] An adverse outcome was associated with an increase in Injury Severity Score, associated injuries, blood transfusions, bilateral flail chest, and age greater than 50 years. In a study from the same institution,[18] long-term disability was found in more than 50% of patients with significant flail chest who had required ventilatory management. The patients had symptoms of chest tightness, chest wall pain, and dyspnea. Spirometry was abnormal in more than 50% of them. Most importantly, less than 40% of the patients had returned to work. Operative stabilization of the chest wall may minimize these long-term sequelae.

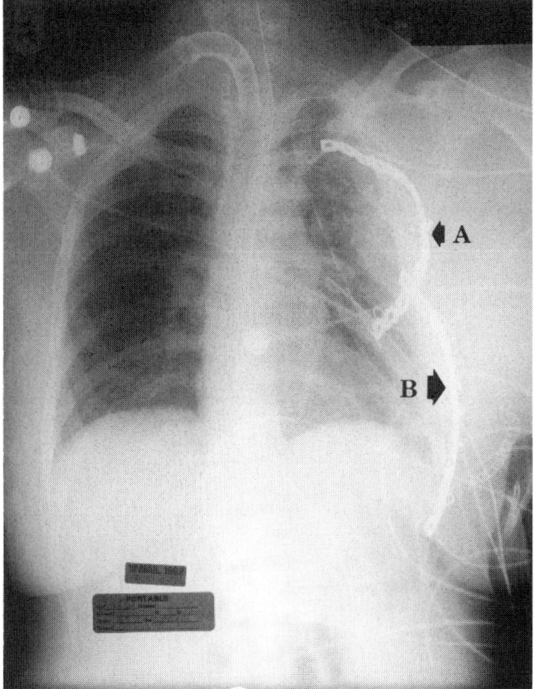

Figure 12–9. This 28-year-old woman sustained a severe flail chest in a motor vehicle accident. Six days postinjury the left chest was stabilized during thoracotomy. Bar A was wired on both sides of the segmental fracture involving the third rib. Bar B was wired to the anterior midportion of Bar A in a perpendicular manner and to rib nine, which was not involved in the flail segment. Each fractured segment under Bar B was then wired to the bar, thus giving stability to the entire flail segment. She was weaned from the ventilator 3 days later.

REFERENCES

1. Meade RH. *A History of Thoracic Surgery.* Springfield, IL: Charles C Thomas; 1961.
2. Dible HJ. *Napoleon's Surgeon.* London: William Heinemann Medical Books; 1970.
3. Beaumont W. *Experiments and Observations on the Gastric Juice and the Physiology of Digestion.* New York: Dover Publications; 1959.
4. Besson A, Saegesser F. *Color Atlas of Chest Trauma and Associated Injuries.* vol. I. Oradell, NJ: Medical Economics; 1983.
5. Harris GJ, Soper RT. Pediatric first rib fracture. *J Trauma.* 1990;30:343.
6. Fackler ML, Surinchak JS, Malinowski JA, Bowen RE. Wounding potential of the Russian AK-74 assault rifle. *J Trauma.* 1984;24:263.
7. Bender JS, Lucas CE. Management of close range shotgun injuries to the chest by diaphragmatic transposition: case report. *J Trauma.* 1990;30:1581.
8. Sherman RT, Parrish RA. Management of shotgun injuries; a review of 152 cases. *J Trauma.* 1963;3:76.
9. Thomas AN, Blaisdell FW, Lewis FR, Schlobohm RM. Operative stabilization for flail chest after blunt trauma. *J Thorac Cardiovasc Surg.* 1978;75:793.
10. Patrick LM, Anderson A. Three-point harness. Accident and Laboratory Data Companion, Proceedings of the 18th Stapp Car Crash Conference, Ann Arbor, MI, 1974.
11. Patrick LM, Mertz HJ Jr, Kroel CK. Cadaver knee, chest, and head impact wounds. Proceedings of the 11th Stapp Car Crash Conference, Society of Automotive Engineers, New York, 1967.
12. Newman RJ, Jones IS. A prospective study of 413 consecutive car occupants with chest injury. *J Trauma.* 1984;24:129.
13. Huelke DF. Steering assembly performance and driver injury severity in frontal crashes. S.A.E. 820474, Proceedings of the International Congress and Exposition, Detroit, 1982:1–30.
14. Paris F, Tarazona V, Blasco E, et al. Surgical stabilization of traumatic flail chest. *Thorax.* 1975;30:521.
15. Hobbs CA. Car occupant injury patterns and mechanisms. Supplementary Report 648. Crowthorne: Transport and Road Research Laboratory; 1981.
16. Barancik JI, Chatterjee BF, Greene YC, et al. Northeastern Ohio Trauma Study: 1. Magnitude of the problem. *Am J Public Health.* 1983;73:746.

17. Kemmerer WT, Eckert WG, Gathright JB, et al. Patterns of thoracic injuries in fatal traffic accidents. *J Trauma*. 1961;1:595.
18. Wilson RF, Murray C, Antonenko DR. Nonpenetrating thoracic injuries. *Surg Clin North Am*. 1977;57:17.
19. Schall MA, Fischer RP, Perry JF. The unchanged mortality of flail chest injuries. *J Trauma*. 1979;19:492.
20. Lee RB, Bass SM, Morris JA Jr, McKenzie E. Three or more rib fractures as an indicator for transfer to a Level I trauma center: a population base study. *J Trauma*. 1990;30:689.
21. Freedland M, Wilson RF, Bender JS, Levison MA. The management of flail chest injury: factors affecting outcome. *J Trauma*. 1990;30:1460.
22. Gaillard M, Herve C, Mandin L, Raynaud P. Mortality, prognostic factors in chest injury. *J Trauma*. 1990;30:93.
23. Garcia VF, Gotschall CF, Eichelberger MR, Bowman LM. Rib fractures in children: a marker of severe trauma. *J Trauma*. 1990;30:695.
24. Craven KD, Oppenheimer L, Wood LDH. Effects of contusion and flail chest on pulmonary perfusion and oxygen exchange. *J Appl Physiol*. 1979;47:729.
25. Clark GC, Schecter WP, Trunkey DD. Variables affecting outcome in blunt chest trauma: flail chest versus pulmonary contusion. *J Trauma*. 1988;28:298.
26. Mackersie RC, Karagianes TG, Hoyt DB, Davis JW. Prospective evaluation of epidural and intravenous administration of Fentanyl for pain control and restoration of ventilatory function following multiple rib fractures. *J Trauma*. 1991;31:443.
27. Wisner DH. A stepwise logistic regression analysis of factors affecting morbidity and mortality after thoracic trauma: effect of epidural analgesia. *J Trauma*. 1990;30:799.
28. Shackford SR. Blunt chest trauma; the intensivists perspective. *J Intens Care Med*. 1986;1:125.
29. Lewis F, Thomas AN, Schlobohm RM. Control of respiratory therapy in flail chest. *Ann Thorac Surg*. 1975;23:170.
30. Shackford SR, Virgilio RW, Peters RM. Selective use of ventilatory therapy in flail chest injury. *J Thorac Cardiovasc Surg*. 1981;81:194.
31. Shackford SR, Smith DE, Zarins CK, et al. The management of flail chest: a comparison of ventilatory and non-ventilatory treatment. *Am J Surg*. 1976;132:759.
32. Trinkle JK, Richardson DJ, Franz JL, et al. Management of flail chest without mechanical ventilation. *Ann Thorac Surg*. 1975;19:355.
33. Bongard FS, Lewis FR Jr. Crystalloid resuscitation of patients with pulmonary contusion. *Am J Surg*. 1984;148:145.
34. Lucas CE, Ledgerwood AM, Higgins RF, Weaver DW. Impaired pulmonary function after albumin resuscitation from shock. *J Trauma*. 1980;20:446.
35. Richardson DJ, Grover FL, Trinklke KJ. Early operative management of isolated sternal fractures. *J Trauma*. 1975;15:156.
36. Landercasper J, Cogbill TH, Lindesmith LA. Long-term disability after flail chest injury. *J Trauma*. 1984;24:410.
37. Schmit-Neuerbirg KP, Weiss H, Labitzke R. Indication for thoracotomy in chest wall stabilization. *Injury*. 1982;14:26.
38. Shorr RN, Rodriguez A, Indeck MC, et al. Blunt chest trauma in the elderly. *J Trauma*. 1989;29:234.

13

Pneumothorax and Hemothorax

F. WILLIAM BLAISDELL, M.D.

HISTORY: It was Galen, apparently, who first maintained that air is inhaled because of active expansion of the chest wall, passively followed by the lungs.[1] Dybkowsky showed that pleural liquid with suspended particles is pumped through stomata into the lymphatics by the respiratory movements and suggested that exchange of water and small solutes could occur also with the blood capillaries of the pleural membranes.[1] Starling showed that the pleural membranes are size-selective barriers through which the passage of liquids is determined by mechanical and osmotic forces, and that isotonic or even hypertonic saline solutions were absorbed.[2] Mayow is credited as providing the first clear description of pneumothorax.[1] Astley Cooper showed that air introduced into the pleural space is absorbed.[3]

In 1820, Carson described the first measurements of the refractive forces of the lung.[1] In a series of animal experiments, he showed that pressure inside the lung rose above atmospheric when the chest wall was opened and that under physiological conditions it pulls in the chest wall.[1]

Injuries to the chest are the major reason for mortality in all conflicts from ancient times to the present. Theodoric in 1267, speaking of chest wounds, said, "The stitches should be placed in accordance with the size of the wound so that the natural heat cannot escape in any way nor the air outside be able to enter."[4] With the advent of firearms during the Battle of Crecy in 1346, a new type of penetrating chest wound was introduced. In 1382, small guns were used against the Venetians, and the significance of gunshot wounds was recognized in the chronicles of these battles.[5] Methods of management of chest wounds improved with each succeeding war.[6–8] The most important treatable component of a gunshot wound to the chest was the open pneumothorax associated with it. The question of whether or not to close the wound remained difficult to answer. John deVigo in Rome in 1514 was the first surgeon to present his views on gunshot wounds to the chest, which he considered uniformly fatal and, in most part, untreatable.[5]

With regard to hemothorax, Paré (1545) believed in closing chest wounds when there was no blood or only a small amount of blood in the chest.[5] He also felt that those who kept the wound open when the amount of blood in the chest was considerable were right. The practice Paré followed, judging from his case records, was to keep the wound open for 2 or 3 days to allow the blood to escape and, if bleeding ceased, he closed the wound.

In contrast, Baron Larrey, Napoleon's surgeon, closed an 8-cm wound between the fifth and sixth ribs. This huge wound was hissing and exuding frothy blood. The patient was cold; the pulse was barely perceptible. Larrey closed the chest wound with adhesive plaster to hide it from the patient and his comrades. No sooner had the wound been closed than the soldier breathed more freely. In a few hours he became calm and in a few days he was cured. Larrey then referred to two other cases that he had managed similarly and concluded that his cases showed the value of immediate closure of an open wound as opposed to the recommendations of Paré.[5]

During the Civil War, Billings considered that traumatic pneumothorax could be treated by dilation of the chest wound or by thoracentesis. Billing's account of the Civil War gave credit to A. H. Smith for devising a valve made from a piece of intestine that, when applied to the wound, permitted blood and other fluid to escape but prevented the inflow of air.[5] By the final years of World War I, the controversy over whether or not to close chest wounds had resolved in favor of immediate closure. Closed tube drainage was added as a routine measure in World War II.

During the Civil War, no thoracenteses were done; by World War I, it was universally recognized that the aspiration of blood from the pleural cavity was important. During World War I, there was an occasional case of clotted hemothorax treated by surgery; this became standard practice by World War II. Mortality for chest wounds in the Civil War was 62.5%; in World War I, 24.6%; and in World War II, 12%.[5]

ANATOMY AND PHYSIOLOGY OF THE PLEURAL SPACE

The pleural cavities are lined by two serous membranes forming independent closed sacs into which each lung is mesially invaginated (Fig. 13–1). The sac is composed of connective tissue and lined with mesothelium, which secretes a small amount of serous fluid and lubricates its surfaces. In addition to collagen, there are elastic fibers and smooth muscle in the pleura. The parietal pleura lines the walls of the thorax where it is loosely attached and easily separated, whereas the visceral portion is intimately applied over the surface of the invaginated lung. The parietal pleura is extremely well innervated with somatic nerves, whereas the visceral pleura is not. The pleura is designed to facilitate excursion of the lungs against the walls of the thorax with a minimum of friction. The visceral pleura relates to the topography of the lung (Chapter 14).

The parietal pleura lies in contact with the ribs and the intercostal spaces. As the pleura extends from the parasternal area to the mediastinum, it forms a vertical sinus or cul de sac along the costal mediastinal line of the pleural reflection. The costal pleura cul de sac dips inferiorly in the groove formed between the costal wall and the diaphragm to form the costal diaphragmatic cul de sac or the inferior or costodiaphragmatic sinus. The costomediastinal and costodiaphragmatic spaces are invaded by the lung margins only in deep inspiration. During expiration, the pleural surfaces of the recesses are approximated.

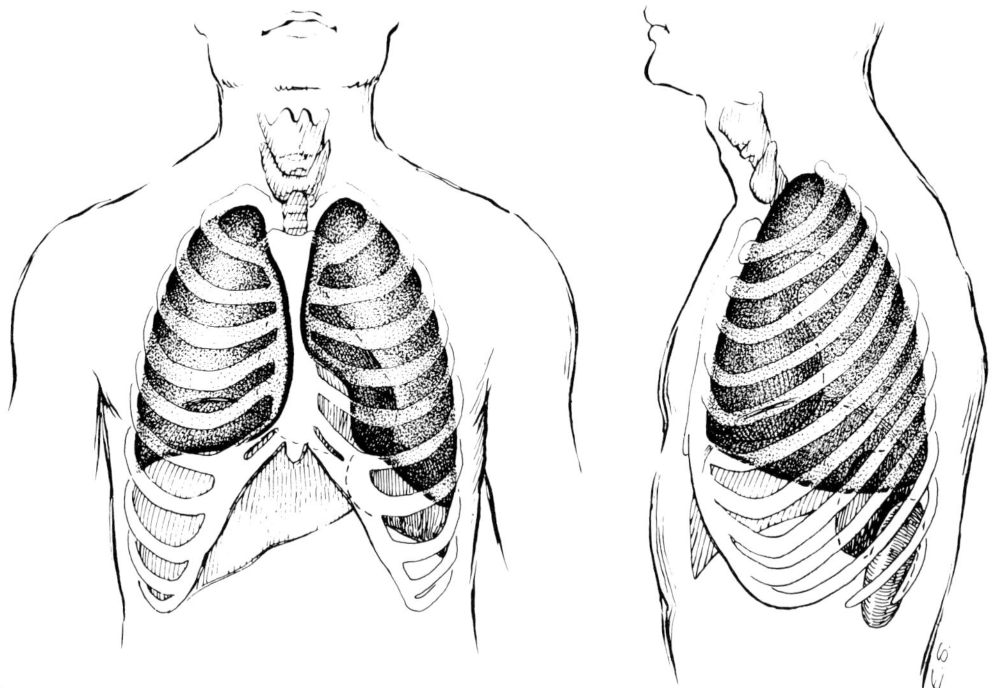

A

B

Figure 13–1.   The anatomy of the pleural space is depicted in the anteroposterior (**A**) and lateral (**B**) views (see text).

The pleural dome or cervical pleura projects upward and forward into the neck and is indicated on the surface by a curved line with an upward convexity drawn from the center of the sternoclavicular joint to the junction of the sternal and middle thirds of the clavicle. The apices of the lung during both inspiration and expiration fill the domes completely. The anterior and middle scalene muscles lie on the lateral surface of the cervical pleura before they attach to the upper surface of the first rib.

The subclavian artery lies in the groove on the medial and ventral aspects of the pleural dome. The internal mammary vessels, the first portion of the vertebral and the intercostal arteries, the inferior ganglion of the cervical chain, and the lower trunk of the brachial plexus rest on it also. The pleura encompasses the hilum in an oval fashion. The inferior extremity of the hilar pleura is continued to the diaphragm as a fold known as the pulmonary ligament. The hilum lies nearer the posterior than the anterior part of the mediastinum and is somewhat nearer the apex than the base.

The elastic recoil of the lungs produces a tendency for them to collapse when the pleural space is open and results in more or less constant negative pressure in the thoracic cavity. The pressure corresponds to the phase of ventilation. While the pleural cavities are closed, the lung is unable to recede form the chest wall unless there is an alteration in intrapleural pressure produced by fluid, blood, or air. When the parietal pleural cavity is open and air enters, the lung, diminished in volume, falls away from the chest wall, and the unopposed elasticity in the lung results in complete collapse. Collapse of one lung would not be of great significance, except that the mediastinum in the human is flexible and is capable of shifting rapidly with each breath. This can be incompatible with life because there is a tendency for the mediastinum to shift in the direction of the good lung. This compromises simultaneously the function of the good lung and produces pressure alterations in the great vessels and the heart. An inability to compensate for these alarming shifts retarded the development of thoracic surgery for many years. The pressure under normal, slow ventilation vary from -10 cm of water in inspiration to -2 cm with expiration. With more vigorous respiration, pressures of -15 during inspiration and 0 during expiration can be found.

The pleura is capable of absorbing particulate matter, and this is augmented by respiratory motion. Tagged red cells injected in the pleural space have been found to enter the vascular system, and, if blood remains liquid in the pleural space, it is capable of being completely absorbed. Oxygen is absorbed rapidly, but many days are required for the complete absorption of nitrogen from a large pneumothorax.

Although it was thought for many years that allowing the lung to collapse would slow bleeding from that organ, it is now evident that expanded lung tissue is a more effective tamponade for pulmonary vascular bleeding. With regard to through-and-through penetrating wounds, such as gunshot wounds of the chest, continued bleeding is much more likely from the systemic arteries of the chest wall than from the lung substance itself. Catastrophic hemorrhage from the lung is likely only from extensive wide-open, deep pulmonary lacerations. Whether or not air leak from lung laceration is tamponaded by the expanded ventilated lung is controversial, but the generally accepted view is that expansion of the lung against the chest wall results in more prompt sealing of the leak because of irritation and adhesion of the lung to the parietal pleura. However, under certain circumstances, the reverse may be true; persistent air leaks can sometimes be best controlled by allowing the lung to collapse before attempting reexpansion. Generally, however, both bleeding and air leaks are best managed by obtaining full expansion of the lung.

ASSESSMENT AND DIAGNOSIS

The relative incidence of hemothorax and pneumothorax after penetrating (Table 13–1) and blunt (Table 13–2) trauma was presented by Gray and associates[9] and by Harrison and co-workers.[10] In Shorr et al.'s series (Table 13–3), there were 287 cases of pneumothorax, hemothorax, or both.[11] Of 95 cases of pneumothorax, 54 were bilateral and 8 were tension pneumothoraces. Of 193 cases of hemothorax, 54 were unilateral, 17 bilateral, and 11 were delayed.

Rib fractures after major thoracic trauma in children may be absent despite catastrophic intrathoracic (or intraabdominal) injury.[12] This is because of the pliability of their chest wall and its inherent ability to recoil even from the most severe crush injury. Nakayama et al. noted that pulmonary contusion occurred with nearly equal frequency as did rib fractures—49.5% to 53%, respectively, after major thoracic trauma in children.[13] In their study, pneumothorax occurred in 37% of the children and hemothorax in 13%; all but 3 of the 105 cases were blunt trauma.

Most pneumothoraces or hemothoraces associated with blunt trauma in adults will be manifested by overt chest wall tenderness and pleuritic pain on deep inspiration. If there is penetrating trauma in the vicinity of the chest, pneumothorax and hemothorax are likely

Table 13–1.   Penetrating Injury—2917 Cases[9]

	#	PERCENT
Hemothorax	818	28
Pneumothorax	520	18
Hemopneumothorax	1244	42

Table 13–2.   Blunt Trauma Injury Type—203 Cases[10]

	#	PERCENT
Hemothorax	43	21
Pneumothorax	48	24
Hemopneumothorax	112	55

Table 13–3.   Chest Injuries in the Absence of Bony Thoracic Injury[11]

	NO. OF PATIENTS
Hemopneumothorax	44
Pulmonary contusion	35
Cardiac contusion	20
Ruptured diaphragm	10
Ruptured aorta	9
Cardiac rupture	4
Tracheobronchial injury	2
Pulmonary laceration	2
Greater vessel injury	1

complications and should be sought for. Remote injuries, particularly gunshot wounds, may pass in an unexpected direction and result in intrathoracic injury. Observation of the patient's breathing and the presence of chest discomfort with ventilation are the most valuable clues leading to the recognition of thoracic injury.

Pneumothorax

The recognition of pneumothorax is not difficult. Careful auscultation of the chest inevitably will reveal absent or decreased breath sounds on the side of the pneumothorax. In the noisy emergency room and where there is assisted ventilation, it may be difficult to be sure of these changes. There usually will be hyperresonance to percussion with pneumothorax. Unfortunately, this sign is often equivocal. Dullness to percussion usually is present with significant hemothorax. Although dullness occurs on dependent portions of the lung, in the supine patient these portions of the lungs are adjacent to the examining table as often the patient with significant hemothorax cannot sit up for definitive examination.

For these reasons chest radiograph should be used immediately in the assessment of all trauma patients. Pneumothorax occasionally may be missed, particularly if the emergency radiograph is of poor quality or if subcutaneous air obscures lung detail. Recent experience with computed tomography (CT) in evaluating pulmonary contusion confirms that plain chest radiography misses pneumothorax more than previously suspected. The radiograph should be inspected for lung markings extending to the periphery, because failure to recognize even a small pneumothorax may have significant consequences later on. If the patient is in extremis, particularly if a chest radiograph is not immediately available, a small incision made into the pleural space will confirm the diagnosis as a gush of air escapes. If the surgeon is operating within the abdomen, inspection of the diaphragm will provide clues to the presence of a pneumothorax and the diaphragm can be opened to confirm or rule out the diagnosis.

Pneumothorax can result from open chest wall injury, lung laceration, bronchial or tracheal tear, and esophageal rupture. Subcutaneous emphysema and mediastinal air also are manifestations of bronchial tear and lung rupture in addition to pneumothorax. Air leak from the lung can result in tension pneumothorax, ordinary pneumothorax, and subcutaneous and mediastinal emphysema.

Tension pneumothorax is a catastrophic, immediately urgent problem. The high pressures in the ipsilateral chest result not only in complete collapse of the corresponding lung but in a shift of the mediastinum and compromise of the function of the opposite lung, the severity of the compromise depending on the pressure within the pleural space. If the patient is receiving anesthesia and the pneumothorax is not suspected, the change in compliance will result in the anesthesiologist using higher and higher pressures in an attempt to obtain adequate ventilation. This results in progressively more severe shifts of lung and compromise of not only pulmonary function but also venous return. The clinical condition should always be suspected in any patient with chest trauma who deteriorates suddenly. The trachea will shift to the side away from the tension, the neck veins will be distended, blood pressure ultimately will decrease, and oxygenation will be compromised (Table 13–4). The patient will be profoundly agitated if spontaneously breathing, and the anesthesiologist will note marked decreasing compliance if the patient is on mechanical ventilation.

A *simple pneumothorax* develops in most instances when an intrapleural air leak occurs. That is, the air leak results in progressive collapse of the lung until ventilation of the ipsilateral lung decreases sufficiently to seal the leak. Depending on the size and location of the air leak, this may occur almost immediately, with just a small rim of air surrounding the lung being evident. Alternatively, the lung may collapse almost completely to a fist-sized mass centering on the hilum. In most instances, the lung collapse is somewhere in between these extremes. A rim of air of approximately 1 cm around the lung is referred to as a 10% pneumothorax, and when the volume of the lung on the anteroposterior chest radiograph

Table 13–4.   Diagnosis of Tension Pneumothorax

Percussion tympany—ipsilateral
Breath sounds—ipsilateral
Tracheal shift—contralateral
Radiograph
Needle or tube

appears to occupy only half of the pleural space, it is referred to as a 50% pneumothorax. Because of the contour of the chest, a 10% pneumothorax actually may be closer to a 50% loss of lung volume and a 50% pneumothorax to an 80% to 90% loss of lung volume (Fig. 13–2).

If the patient's pulmonary status was normal before injury, a 10% pneumothorax may be well tolerated. There may be minimal dyspnea, although usually the patient will have a vague feeling of chest discomfort. As more of the lung collapses, the patient will become apprehensive and progressively more dyspneic. The patient will be noticeably so with a pneumothorax of 50%, the point of maximal collapse when the patient is spontaneously breathing and a tension pneumothorax is not present.

Subcutaneous emphysema and *mediastinal emphysema* are far more common with blunt trauma than with penetrating trauma. Subcutaneous emphysema often occurs in conjunction with pneumothorax when there has been major injury to the chest wall and air escapes from the pleural space through the intercostal muscles and at the site of rib fractures. Subcutaneous emphysema can be recognized on radiographs. Physical examination also can detect subcutaneous emphysema for it produces a sensation similar to that of palpating crinkling tissue paper. The subcutaneous air may obscure the pleural lung markings on the radiograph and make the diagnosis of associated pneumothorax difficult. There may be no associated pneumothorax, on occasion, if the damaged portion of the lung is trapped outside the chest wall (Fig. 13–3). Blunt traumatic rupture of the lungs occurs most often on the pleural surface, but the rupture may involve that portion of the lung facing the major bronchi and hilar vessels. In the latter instance, air extends back along the bronchi into the mediastinum and subsequently into the deep cervical region, from there up into the face and down over the chest. This type of emphysema also is a manifestation of bronchial or tracheal rupture. Characteristically, the emphysema of major tracheal or bronchial rupture markedly worsens when positive pressure ventilation is used. When a patient is spontaneously breathing, the most likely source of mediastinal and cervical air is from a rupture of the lung substance. This is of significance because a rupture of the lung substance does not require surgical treatment.

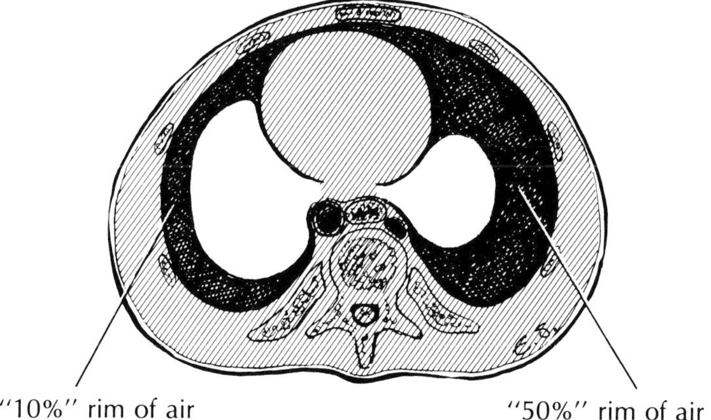

Figure 13–2.   Cross-section of the chest depicts why the "10%" pneumothorax actually compromises 50% of lung volume and a "50%" pneumothorax compromises 90% of lung volume.

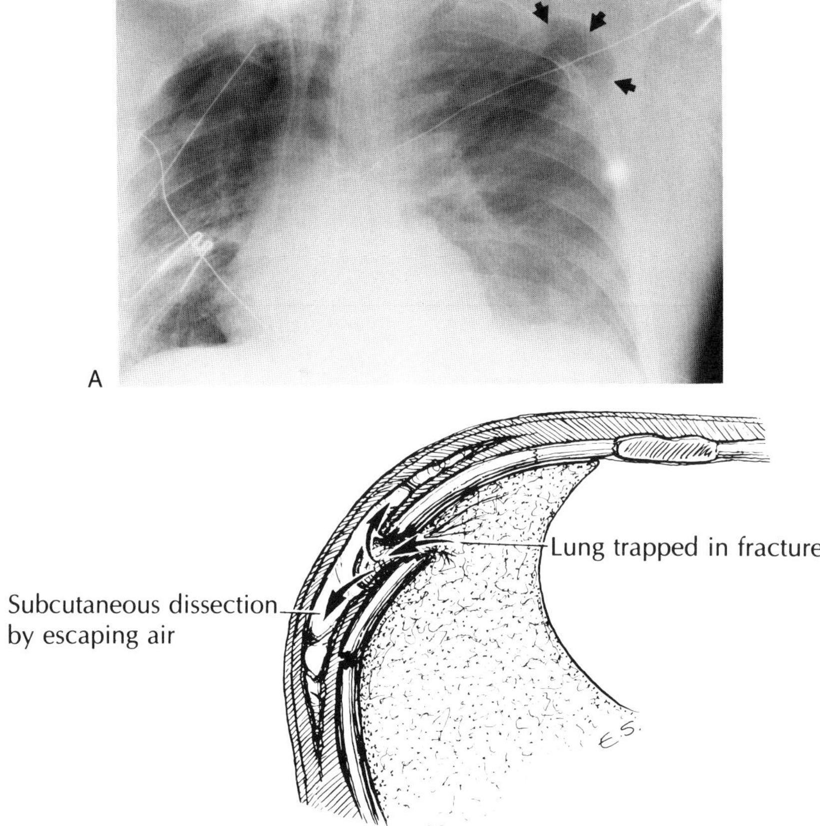

Figure 13–3. Depicts the appearance of the chest radiograph when a piece of lung is trapped in the fracture site (**A**). In this circumstance, the trapped lung may act as a one-way valve (**B**) so that with dramatic subcutaneous emphysema air is pumped into the subcutaneous tissue on inspiration.

An *open, sucking chest wound* or, rarely, a diaphragm rupture associated with a viscus injury such as stomach rupture may be responsible for lung collapse. In an open, sucking chest wound, closure of the wound with petroleum jelly–covered gauze and an occlusive dressing combined with chest tube and suction is the initial treatment. Laparotomy and viscus repair combined with diaphragm repair is definitive treatment for a ruptured diaphragm. In both cases, contamination of the pleural cavity is likely, and irrigation and cleansing of the pleural cavity is appropriate, enlarging the incision as necessary.

Hemothorax

Hemothorax can occur secondary to bleeding from the chest wall, bleeding from the lung or major hilar vessels, or from mediastinal structures including the heart and great vessels. Most importantly, bleeding can have its source in the abdomen.

In the upright patient, blood tends to accumulate on the diaphragmatic surface, and

300 to 400 ml of blood in the pleural space usually is enough in the upright position to cause blunting of the costophrenic angle on an x-ray. If the patient is supine when the x-rays are made, the blood is readily recognized by a graying of the involved pleural space, the relative degree depending on the amount of blood (Fig. 13–4). If there is a question of preexisting disease, the nature or presence of fluid may be in question. If the fluid shifts on x-ray when the patient is changed to an upright or decubitus position, this will document that the liquid is fluid. Needle thoracentesis will provide information on the nature of the fluid, if it is in doubt. Also, bleeding in the chest wall, which inevitably is associated with rib fractures, may dissect under the pleura and simulate hemothorax, but this blood usually is clotted and cannot be removed by needle or tube.

The source of blood in the chest is most commonly from systemic vessels of the chest wall, the intercostal and the internal mammary arteries, and their corresponding veins. Another source of bleeding is from the abdomen through a laceration of the diaphragm. This is particularly true of stab and gunshot wounds that involve the lower half of the thorax. Of course, large systemic vessel injury and cardiac injury may, on occasion, be the source of hemorrhage, but these are rare clinical problems because most injuries to major systemic vessels such as the aorta are immediately fatal. The exceptions are small penetrating wounds from low-caliber handguns, stab wounds less than 1 cm in size, and blunt traumatic ruptures with incomplete separation of all vessel layers.

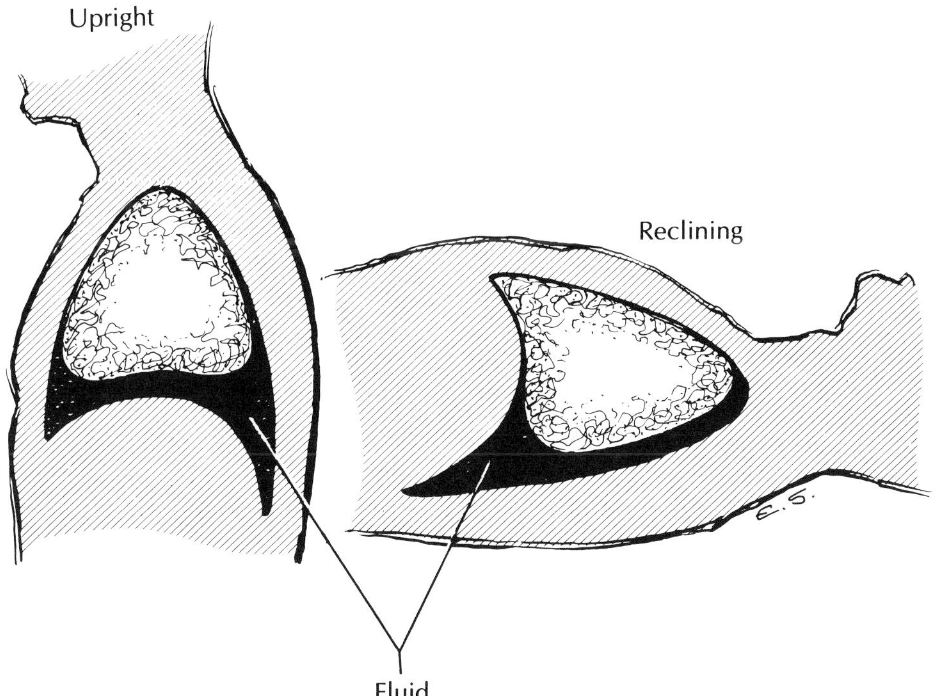

Figure 13–4. Depicts the distribution of intrapleural fluid in the upright (**A**) as opposed to the supine position (**B**).

In our experience, 80% to 90% of the major blood loss associated with hemothorax comes from systemic vessels and only 10% to 20% comes from vessels in the lung substance. The reasons for this is that the lung is capable of tamponading the low-pressure bleeding and the mean pressure in the pulmonary artery is at best only 15 mm Hg and in the pulmonary veins about 5 mm Hg. Correspondingly, lower pressures follow overt hemorrhage. Hilar vascular injuries with massive hemothorax usually are immediately fatal and therefore are not common clinical problems. Such concepts greatly influence the management of hemothorax, because intercostal arteries and internal mammary arteries, the most common sources of ongoing bleeding, are relatively small vessels, usually bleed at a modest rate, and are much more capable of spontaneous tamponade than larger systemic vessels.

MANAGEMENT OF PNEUMOTHORAX AND HEMOTHORAX

Pneumothorax

The treatment of tension pneumothorax is immediate decompression (Fig. 13–5). The insertion of several large-bore needles or even just a small decompressive incision without the insertion of a chest tube will relieve the problem. The needle should be inserted or an

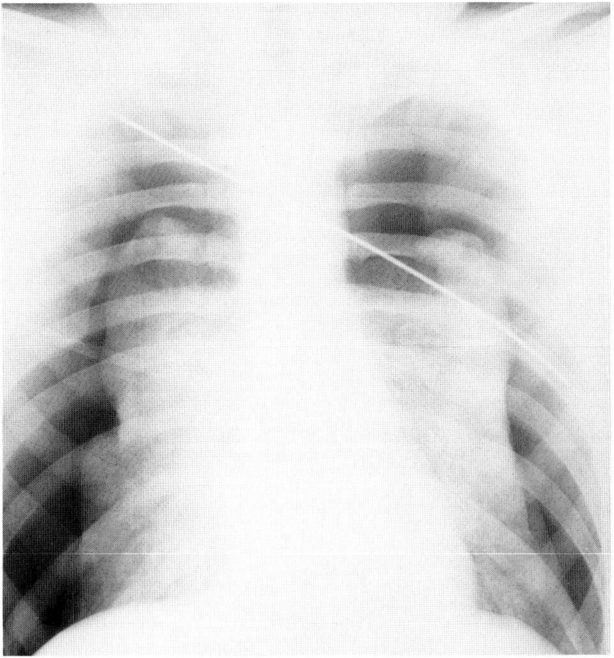

Figure 13–5.   The appearance of bilateral tension pneumothorax. The patient was admitted in extremis with distended neck veins. An immediate chest radiograph showed massive collapse of both lungs. The patient responded promptly when bilateral chest tubes were placed.

incision should be made in an intercostal space immediately superior to the rib. Appropriate sites would be in the area from the sternal angle (second rib) to the pectoral groove (sixth interspace), from 2 cm lateral to the sternum to the posterior axillary line (Fig. 13–6).

An immediate gush of air from the needle, the incision, or chest tube confirms the diagnosis, and this should be followed by the insertion of a large-bore chest tube and the establishment of suction drainage. If the patient does not respond immediately, it is usually appropriate to place another chest tube in the same or even the opposite pleural space.

Ordinary pneumothorax is treated similarly to tension pneumothorax, but treatment is not so urgent. If the diagnosis is suspected but the patient is not in extreme distress, it may be appropriate to wait for confirmation by chest radiography. This avoids the problem of placing chest tubes in patients with preexisting pulmonary disease or directly into or over an area of adhesions. Although the optimal location for chest tubes is generally considered to be anterior for treatment of pneumothorax, chest tubes can be placed anywhere within the area described previously. Because hemothorax often is present, the midaxillary line is considered optimal because there are no major muscles in the way and because blood is more difficult to drain than air and hemothorax accumulates posteriorly in the supine patient. In the patient with mild to moderate collapse, a 24F to 28F chest tube may be sufficient, although a larger tube is always appropriate and is more effective in draining blood.

The technique for insertion of chest tubes is described in Chapter 21. It basically involves making an incision over the appropriate intercostal space and advancing a pointed clamp into the pleural space and spreading it until a hole is made of sufficient size to admit the index finger or, at least, the little finger. If the hole is not large enough, as the tube is advanced it may skid off the plane in front of the ribs and pass circumferentially around the chest wall. On the anteroposterior chest radiography, the tube may appear to lie in the pleural space when in fact it is extrapleural.

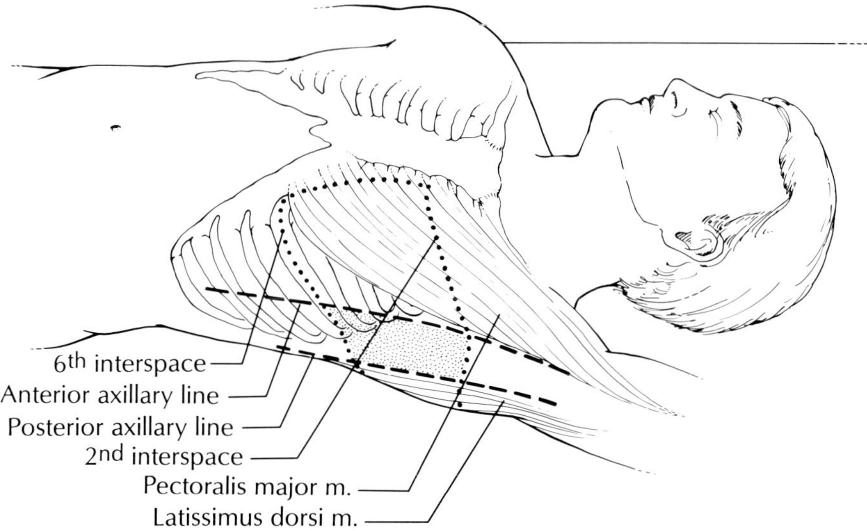

Figure 13–6.   Diagram illustrates the optimal area for chest tube insertion (dotted line). The doubly shaded area is preferred in most instances because overlying chest wall musculature is minimal and both air and blood are drained well.

The chest tube should be connected to suction drainage, and 10 to 15 cm of negative pressure applied. In almost all cases, this will result in the immediate expansion of the lung, although, on occasion, major air leaks may compromise expansion. In these circumstances, the choice is to increase the negative pressure to 20 to 25 cm of water or insert a second chest tube connected to a separate drainage system and suction. Almost all leaks can be controlled in this way. However, if prompt reexpansion does not occur, open thoracotomy may be necessary on the basis that a major lung laceration or segmental bronchial injury may be responsible for the leak. Moreover, whenever a major leak is present, bronchoscopy should be performed to assess the integrity of the tracheobronchi tree. Whenever doubt exists about tracheobronchial injury or when there is such a large air leak that full lung expansion cannot be obtained, the patient should be taken to the operating room for bronchoscopy and thoracotomy.

In persistent or recurrent lung leaks in which there is incomplete lung expansion, thoracotomy usually is indicated. Alternatively, a day or two of collapsed lung may be tried in refractory cases to see if the lung will seal under these circumstances. However, after penetrating trauma when contamination of pleural space can be assumed, the best protection against infection of the pleural space (empyema) is to ensure immediate complete expansion of the lung. Thoracotomy with plication of the lung leak should be used if complete expansion is not accomplished by nonoperative means.

Mild *subcutaneous emphysema* can be ignored, but occasionally subcutaneous emphysema reaches dramatic proportions and the patient can assume a gross appearance that is offensive and perhaps even dangerous. The most virulent forms of subcutaneous emphysema occur when a portion of lung is trapped in the chest wall. The chest wall then acts as a one-way valve that decompresses into the subcutaneous tissue with inspiration as the chest wall opens slightly and closes when the chest wall laceration collapses during expiration. If the area of lung leak can be located, an incision made over the area will decompress the emphysema. The incision is covered with gauze containing petrolatum, and the intrapleural portion of the injury treated with a large chest tube.

Subcutaneous emphysema whose origin is the mediastinum can be decompressed by a tracheostomy-type incision consisting of a small transverse incision placed just above the suprasternal notch and carried down through the deep cervical fascia. This usually produces immediate, dramatic relief by stopping the dissection of air.

Although smaller bronchopleural fistulas will almost always close with supportive treatment, larger fistulas can present a major challenge. The most difficult problems with pleural fistulas occur in association with pulmonary resection. In this instance, the persistent space is vulnerable to contamination and infection (empyema).

Major persistent bronchopleural fistulas are best treated with surgery. The leak should be closed by primary suture assisted by coverage with viable adjacent tissue such as a flap of pleura or intercostal muscle. Associated infection should be treated with systemic antibiotics. Infection control may be facilitated by irrigation of the pleural space with antibiotic solution. Resection of nonfunctional lung combined with bronchial resection also may be successful, particularly if infection can be controlled preoperatively and prevented postoperatively.

On occasion, a major bronchopleural fistula may develop in which surgical treatment may be contraindicated. It may be the result of delayed recognition of the bronchial leak in which associated contamination may compromise successful closure. These leaks are best managed with high-suction pressures or simultaneous use of several chest tubes in an attempt to keep the lung expanded.

Despite a surgeon's best efforts, a rare case treated either by conservative means or by surgery will have a persistent bronchopleural leak. After several weeks of closed chest tube drainage, the bronchopleural fistula tract becomes encased in a fibrous tract. At this point, open drainage can be utilized without fear of lung collapse by cutting off the tube just outside the chest wall and leaving the remainder in place. Later the tube may be withdrawn slowly, leaving a straight bronchopleural cutaneous fistula that, in the absence of a large empyema, will tend to close with time. When lung tissue has been removed and the space that the fistula decompresses is large, permanent open drainage of the chest is appropriate in poor-risk cases. A thoracoplasty with collapse of the chest wall can be used alternatively in good-risk cases.

Permanent open drainage is facilitated by using an Eloesser flap. This involves making a small dependent thoracotomy incision and removing segments of one or two ribs over the dependent portion of the cavity and inserting a skin flap into the tract to maintain its patency (Fig. 13–7).

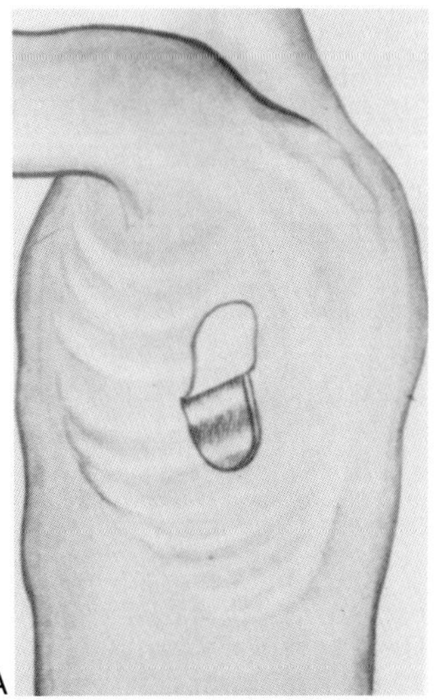
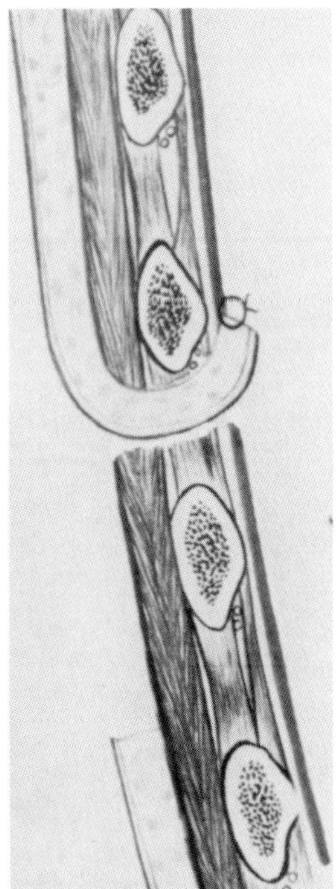

Figure 13–7.   A, B: Eloesser flap technique. A section of rib is removed from an area overlying the most dependent portion of the empyema cavity and the skin flap is turned in and sutured to the pleura to maintain patency of the sinus. (Reprinted with permission from Eloesser.[23])

Hemothorax

A hemothorax that consists of 500 ml or more of blood in the pleural space is best treated by tube drainage. This is particularly true if the hemothorax is recognized soon after injury. At this point bleeding must be assumed to be ongoing and the insertion of a chest tube permits both the monitoring of the rate of bleeding and the immediate decompression of the blood to prevent a clotted hemothorax.

With the patient upright for a chest radiograph, 500 ml of blood can be recognized because the sulcus is obliterated. On the supine film, blood produces a slight but distinct graying on the radiograph. On the lateral decubitus film, a significant rim of fluid can be seen between the chest wall and the lung amounting to 1 cm or more.

When draining a hemothorax, a large-bore chest tube of 32F to 36F is appropriate for the average adult. The chest tube is best placed between the anterior and posterior axillary line in approximately the sixth to seventh interspace (which corresponds to the nipple line anteriorly). The tube should be advanced posteriorly. This is facilitated by allowing a pneumothorax to develop during the placement of the tube so that the collapse of the lung will facilitate directing the tube.

Generally, one tube is sufficient, because failure of blood to empty completely signifies the presence of either a clotted hemothorax or subpleural clotted blood and additional chest tubes are usually of no value. If the tube is placed during surgery to drain major ongoing bleeding and particularly if the patient has developed coagulopathy, it may be prudent to insert two tubes rather than one to decrease the likelihood that additional tube drainage or reoperation will be required.

Bleeding from the chest usually occurs at a modest rate. As opposed to intraabdominal hemorrhage, most thoracic bleeding can be treated by closed methods without resorting to thoracotomy. Ninety to 95% of hemothoraces will respond to this regimen.

Because transfusion itself carries a risk, certain arbitrary guidelines have been developed by most trauma surgeons regarding the management of thoracic bleeding (Table 13–5). If the patient presents in shock with a major hemothorax and 1000 ml of blood drains immediately after insertion of the chest tube, the patient should be taken promptly to the operating room. The exception might be patients with other injuries requiring evaluation who respond to shock resuscitation and in whom the bleeding, after the initial gush, decreases to a modest and tolerable rate. If the circulatory status can be stabilized with intravenous fluid, time may be made available for a diagnostic procedure such as CT, aortography, or laparotomy. With the completion of these procedures, if bleeding has stopped and the chest radiograph is reasonably clear, conservative management can be continued.

Any bleeding that reaches 1500 ml and is still continuing should be treated by open

Table 13–5. Bleeding Indications for Thoracotomy

Shock plus hemothorax opacification
Blood loss exceeding 1500 cc
Clotted hemothorax
Blood loss 200 ml/hr for 3–4 hr

thoracotomy. In most instances, this will ensure the most rapid recovery with the least morbidity. The requirement for thoracotomy to control bleeding, however, varies greatly in reported series, from 5% to 25%, depending on the institution.[14–16]

In addition, a clotted hemothorax that results in opacification of a hemothorax on x-ray or that appears to occupy space equivalent to 500 to 1000 cc is best treated by early thoracotomy, preferably in the first day or two after injury. This will result in improved pulmonary function and greatly decrease the risk of a complicating empyema.[17]

Additional arbitrary guidelines are helpful, particularly if the patient is seen immediately after the accident and the initial drainage is modest. If subsequent to the insertion of the chest tube the bleeding rate is 200 ml an hour for more than 3 to 4 hr, thoracotomy is indicated. Bleeding at this rate usually will require a transfusion and its attendant risk. Bleeding less than 100 ml an hour rarely requires treatment by operation unless associated lesions are present that require surgical treatment. Continued bleeding at 100 ml an hour usually is the result of coagulopathy, not major vessel hemorrhage. The failure of bleeding to stop is an indication for hematologic evaluation and medical treatment of any coagulopathy that is detected. This may consist of platelet infusion, with or without coagulation factors.

In all instances, the drainage should be monitored with chest radiographs every 6 to 12 hr for the first 24 hr. The slowing of drainage from the chest tube can be associated with the development of the clotted hemothorax. If the chest radiograph remains clear, then the rate of bleeding is adequately assessed by the chest tube. But if the chest radiograph shows progressive opacification, then immediate surgical treatment is appropriate to ensure control of the hemorrhage and the evacuation of the blood clot. This is particularly important in penetrating trauma, because these injuries are contaminated from the start. For this reason, prophylactic antibiotics should be initiated in the emergency room and continued for 24 to 48 hr postinjury. The presence of residual clot may lead to empyema or to chronic inflammation and the development of a fibrous peel that traps the lung and impairs function.

OPERATIVE TECHNIQUE

The incision generally used for most thoracic trauma is either anterior thoracotomy or anterolateral thoracotomy. This is because in the blunt trauma patient, simultaneous laparotomy frequently is necessary. Even when penetrating trauma involves the upper chest, the source of bleeding may well be abdominal, as the diaphragm can move with exhalation as high as the fifth interspace. Liver injuries, in particular, can bleed into the right chest and not into the abdomen, especially when the bare area of the liver is involved. Peritoneal lavage or even exploratory laparotomy in these circumstances could be negative and yet proper control of the liver hemorrhage will require the abdominal approach. Moreover, the unstable patient tolerates full lateral thoracotomy poorly. Should the anesthesiologist require additional lines for monitoring unexpected complications or should a double lumen endotracheal tube be required, these are best accomplished in the supine position.

Thoracotomy technique is described in Chapter 21. At thoracotomy, all blood and clots should be evacuated from the pleural space and packs placed to isolate any bleeding. Although it is appropriate to inspect the lung and the mediastinum initially, the chest wall at the site of a knife or missile penetration or beneath fractured ribs usually is the source of ongoing bleeding.

The treatment of pulmonary lacerations is described in Chapter 14 and bronchial and tracheal lacerations in Chapter 11. Bleeding whose source is the abdomen should be treated by laparotomy. Chest wall hemorrhage is best secured by suture of the appropriate intercostal bundle or internal mammary vessels, both proximal and distal to the area of bleeding. When the location of the penetrating wound is posterior and low in the chest, such as the eighth to tenth interspace, the bleeding point may not be accessible from the anterior thoracotomy approach. After assessing for the presence or absence of other lesions, it may be appropriate to close the anterior thoracotomy, roll the patient on his/her side, and explore the area of injury directly with a small intercostal incision.

Generally, any chest tube placed before surgery can be left intact. If the tube is large bore, that is, 32F or larger in the adult, it may be all the drainage that is necessary in the patient with penetrating trauma. But if the patient has had blunt trauma or multiple injuries or has developed a coagulopathy as manifested by continued oozing from all wound sites, the placement of two chest tubes is indicated. One should be placed transversely across the diaphragm and the other up along the spine.

Full expansion of the lung should be allowed before closure of the chest to check for any missed air leaks. Pouring saline into the pleural cavity may facilitate locating the source of the air.

Pneumothorax can be treated by oversewing the site of lung injury (Chapter 14). The depths of any major laceration should be investigated for small bronchial leaks that can be directly sutured. In these instances, fine monofilament, nonabsorbable sutures such as 4-0 or 5-0 proline may be appropriate to repair the bronchus or plicate it. Small lacerations from penetrating objects can be left open or they can be closed with fine pleural sutures. Larger lacerations involving the margin of the lung are best treated by plication, with running, locking mattress sutures of synthetic collagen and a fine needle or by collapsing the lung and closing the laceration with a stapling device. If blebs should be present and are the source of the air leak, they should be plicated with running mattress sutures or by stapling.

If there is a major pleural leak remaining at the completion of repair, more than one chest tube may be appropriate to ensure lung expansion. In this instance, one of the tubes should be anterior and one lateral or posterior. Each tube should be connected to an independent drainage system to ensure that both tubes function.

POSTOPERATIVE CARE

Chest tubes are connected to water-seal suction drainage. Usually 10 to 15 cm suction is appropriate for the management of pneumothorax or hemothorax whether or not an operation has been performed. The suction should be continued until the air leak has stopped. Drainage of blood may or may not be facilitated by suction, but suction should be continued for the first 24 hr. When fluid drainage has decreased below 100 cc for 24 hr and the air leak has stopped, the chest tube should be placed on water-seal drainage. No recurrence of the pneumothorax at 24 hr is an indication for removal of the chest tube, unless associated drainage exceeds 100 ml, as described previously.

Patients with penetrating trauma rarely require mechanical ventilatory support for more than a few hours postoperatively, whereas patients with blunt chest trauma and multiple rib fractures may require positive pressure ventilation for several days or until the chest wall stabilizes and ventilatory mechanics are adequate to ensure spontaneous ventilation (Chapter 12). The patient is then weaned from the ventilator, as described in Chapter 2.

To facilitate adequate ventilation, the use of epidural analgesia is appropriate. After chest wall injury or thoracotomy, most patients will have severe pain when taking a deep breath or attempting to cough. The use of epidural catheter analgesia provided by morphine or fetanyl has constituted a major advance in the management of chest injuries in the past decade and has resulted in significant decrease in respiratory complications.

Twenty-four hours of prophylactic antibiotics are generally indicated, starting preoperatively. One gram of a cephalosporin preoperatively and then 1 g every 6 hr for 24 to 48 hr is indicated.

The hematocrit should be monitored every 6 hr for the first 24 hr in patients with major injuries. Major bleeding or hemothorax should be treated by reoperation. The indications for surgery are similar to those for initial bleeding. The partial thromboplastin time, prothrombin time, and platelets should be assessed for the presence of a platelet defect or coagulopathy (see Complications section). Profuse oozing that develops on the operating table is most often due to a platelet defect; 0.1 unit of platelets per kg is appropriate to treat this defect. If platelet packs can be obtained, they are optimally administered at the completion of the definitive portion of the operation and before incision closure. If not available, they can be administered immediately postoperatively. In the absence of disseminated intravascular coagulation (DIC), coagulopathies are unusual, and most bleeding problems will be the result of defective platelet function or hypothermia.

COMPLICATIONS

The complications of hemothorax and pneumothorax are persistent bleeding, recurrent hemothorax, major air leaks with or without pulmonary collapse, empyema, bronchopleural fistula, and reexpansion pulmonary edema.

Coagulopathies are treated by administration of platelet packs. Occasionally fresh frozen plasma may be necessary. Most coagulopathies are initiated by DIC and are best modified or prevented by maintaining circulatory volume and a dynamic circulation. The vicious cycle that results in the perpetuation of DIC consists of bleeding, hypotension, and hypovolemia leading to a clotting tendency, further depletion of clotting factors, further bleeding, and hypovolemia. Replacement of coagulation factors and platelets without correcting hypovolemia results in "feeding the fire" of DIC. The administration of 10,000 U of heparin intravenously may modify the rate of clotting factor consumption and permit the restoration of levels of clotting factors sufficient for adequate hemostasis.

Recurrent hemothorax is best treated by the insertion of additional chest tubes, preferably in the area of blood accumulation. Arbitrarily, bleeding associated with reopacification on the chest radiograph or exceeding 500 ml in the first postoperative hours should be treated by reoperation.

Persistent air leaks, if associated with lung collapse and persistent pneumothorax, should be treated by the insertion of additional chest tubes and increasing the amount of suction. Large leaks should be operated on as previously described and major lung lacerations and bronchial tears identified and treated.

Maintaining full lung expansion is the best means of avoiding empyema. Caplan et al. noted that 16% of all patients who had chest tubes placed for drainage of fluid in the pleural cavity developed subsequent empyema.[18] They found that if the empyema complicated prior hemothorax, the infection, usually occurring about 10 days after chest tube insertion, was due to *Staphylococcus aureus.* When empyema complicated pneumothorax, the infection was usually due to a gram-negative organism colonizing the upper respiratory tract and occurred an average of 4 days after chest tube insertion. In his study, 17 of 31 patients whose empyema followed trauma had resolution of the infection after antibiotics and chest tube drainage, 11 patients died secondary to infection or intercurrent disease, and 12 patients required open surgical drainage or decortication. If the patient becomes febrile, drainage from the chest tube should be cultured, as should any peritube skin drainage, and appropriate antibiotics initiated. Additional chest tubes should be inserted as necessary to remove any fluid collections.[19] If chest opacification is still evident on the x-ray, decortication of any fibrin peel on the lung should be done to facilitate lung reexpansion. This is best done early, within the first postoperative week, but may be done relatively easily any time up to 6 weeks postoperatively. After this time, the infected fibrin peel assumes a fibrous consistency, making decortication difficult, although not impossible.

Reexpansion pulmonary edema is a complication that follows sudden reexpansion of a collapsed lung. It is most apt to occur when reexpansion of the lung has been delayed. Its frequency increases with the extent and duration of the collapse and is more apt to occur in younger patients and is less frequent in patients over age 40 years. The manifestations are cough, pulmonary edema with foaming sputum, agitation, tachycardia and tachypnea, and a white-out of the corresponding lung on chest x-ray. Mahfood and associates[20] reported a 21% mortality in 53 cases of reexpansion edema. Matsura et al.[21] analyzed 146 cases of spontaneous pneumothorax reexpanded by chest tube and found an incidence of 14% of reexpansion pulmonary edema. The etiology is speculative, but Matsura et al.[21] believe it is related to increased capillary permeability in lungs damaged by hypoxia.

RESULTS

The mortality associated with either simple hemothorax or pneumothorax should be low and relate primarily to the chest wall and associated visceral injuries. In blunt trauma with hemothorax, bleeding is not commonly from the chest wall. After blunt trauma, hemorrhage can be appreciable, but most of the mortality relates to impaired ventilation and inability to clear secretions caused by the chest wall injury. Harrison and associates[10] found that the mortality among 96 patients having only one or two ribs fractured was 16% compared with that of 27.5% among 120 patients with three or more rib fractures. Mortality in their series related to mechanism of injury: 50% for those hit by automobiles, 24% for those involved in automobile accidents, and 9% for the victims of falls. The mortality rate for bilateral hemothorax was 57%. Harrison's group[10] found a mortality rate of 20% for simple pneumothorax and a 33% rate for tension pneumothorax.

For penetrating trauma, the mortality and morbidity rates are negligible for chest wall injuries and relate to the cause of the trauma, usually knife or bullet, and to the associated injuries. Gray and associates,[9] for example, found that the mortality after gunshot wounds to the chest was nearly five times that of stab wounds (7.6% vs. 1.7%).

Graham and co-workers[14] had mortality rates of 29 deaths in 373 cases of hemothorax (7.7%).[14] Drummond and Craig[22] reported 7 deaths in 114 patients with hemothorax (6%); Griffith and associates,[15] 2 deaths in 107 cases (1.8%); and Weil and Margolis,[16] 6 deaths in 395 cases (1.5%). Most of the deaths in all series were in patients who presented in shock.

In patients with pneumothorax alone, Gray and colleagues[9] reported a mortality rate of 1.4%; in hemopneumothorax, the rate was 4.3%.

After major thoracic injury in children, Nakayama et al. found an overall mortality rate of 6.7% in 105 cases,[13] 1 out of 3 following penetrating trauma, and 5 out of 102 with blunt trauma. In three of these deaths, he found pneumothorax contributed to the problems, but only one, a tension pneumothorax, was the direct cause of death.

In summary, mortality rates in all series have improved progressively in recent years, presumably due to better prehospital organization and prompt emergency room and operative treatment.

REFERENCES

1. Agostini E. Mechanics of the pleural space. *Physiol Rev.* 1972;52:67.
2. Starling EH, Tubby AH. On absorption from and secretion into the serous cavities. *J Physiol (Lond).* 1894;16:140.
3. Davy J. Observations on air found in the pleura in a case of pneumothorax—with experiments on the absorption of different kinds of air introduced into the pleura. *Phila Trans Royal Soc Lond, Ser B.* 1823;1113:498.
4. Campbell E, Coltan J. *The Story of Theodoric.* vol I. New York: Appleton-Century-Crofts; 1955.
5. Meade RH. *A History of Thoracic Surgery.* Springfield, IL: Charles C Thomas; 1961.
6. Carter BN, DeBakey ME. Current observations on war wounds of the chest. *J Thorac Surg.* 1944;13:271.
7. McNamara JJ, Messersmith JK, Dunn RA, et al. Thoracic injuries in combat casualties in Viet Nam. *Ann Thorac Surg.* 1970;10:389.
8. Valle AR. An analysis of 2,811 chest casualties of the Korean Conflict. *Dis Chest.* 1954;26:623.
9. Gray AR, Harrison WH, Couves CM, et al. Penetrating injuries to the chest. *Am J Surg.* 1960;100:709.
10. Harrison WH Jr, Gray AR, Couves CM, et al. Severe non-penetrating injuries to the chest. *Am J Surg.* 1960;100:715.
11. Shorr RM, Crittenden M, Indeck M, et al. Blunt thoracic trauma: analysis of 515 patients. *Ann Surg.* 1987;206:200.
12. Bender TM, Oh KS, Medina JL, Girdnay BR. Pediatric chest trauma. *J Thorac Imag.* 1987;2:60.
13. Nakayama DK, Ramenofsky ML, Rowe MI. Chest injuries in childhood. *Ann Surg.* 1989;210:770.
14. Graham JM, Mattox KL, Beal AC Jr. Penetrating trauma of the lung. *J Trauma.* 1979;19:665.
15. Griffith GL, Todd ER, McMillin RD, et al. Acute traumatic hemothorax. *Ann Thorac Surg.* 1978;26:204.
16. Weil PH, Margolis IB. Systematic approach to traumatic hemothorax. *Am J Surg.* 1981;142:692.
17. Coselli JS. Reevaluation of early evacuation of clotted hemothorax. *Am J Surg.* 1984;148:786.
18. Caplan ES, Hoyt NJ, Rodriguez A. Empyema occurring in the multiply traumatized patient. *J Trauma.* 1984;24:785.
19. Stavas J, van Sonnenberg E, Casula G, Wittich GR. Percutaneous drainage of infected and noninfected thoracic fluid collections. *J Thorac Imag.* 1987;2:80.
20. Mahfood S, Hix WR, Aaron BL. Reexpansion pulmonary edema. *Ann Thorac Surg.* 1988;45:340.
21. Matsura Y, Nomimura T, Murakami H. Clinical analysis of reexpansion pulmonary edema. *Chest.* 1991;100:1562.
22. Drummond DS, Craig RH. Traumatic hemothorax. *Am Surg.* 1967;33:403.
23. Eloesser L. An operation for tuberculous empyema. *Surg Gynecol Obstet.* 1935;60:1096.

14

Pulmonary Injury: Laceration, Contusion, Hematoma, Pneumatocele, and Traumatic Asphyxia Blast Injury

F. WILLIAM BLAISDELL, M.D.

HISTORY: The management of thoracic injuries has only been definitive since the advent of World War II. Before that time, survival from a chest injury related more to luck on the part of the patient than to any aspect of surgical care.[1] As far as can be determined, the first description of lung injury was found in a treatise of Theodoric in 1266 who said: "While I was living in Bologna, a certain Domicellus, a Bolognan of normal birth was cured by the hand of Master Hugo, part of his lung being torn away and Master Roand was there to witness it."[2]

The experience in 1822 of William Beaumont in treating his former patient, Alexis St. Martin, is better known for Beaumont's gastric fistula observations than for his management of the life-threatening chest injury. The wound was caused by a discharge of a gun within a yard or so of St. Martin's chest, "fracturing and carrying away the anterior half of the 6th rib, lacerating the lower portion of the left lobe of the lung, diaphragm, and penetrating the stomach." Beaumont saw St. Martin 20 or 30 minutes after the accident and found a portion of the lung herniating out of the chest wall, "lacerated and burnt and below this a portion of the stomach." He reduced the lung, quickly closed the wound, and so saved the patient's life.[3]

In the 18th century, Hewson[4] called attention to the mechanism of pulmonary rupture following contusion of the chest. In 1886, Ashurst wrote about the rupture of thoracic viscera without rib fracture. He said he had reported 30 such cases, 19 of whom died.[5]

In 1889, Holmes, consulting surgeon to St. George's Hospital in London, said: "All penetrating wounds of the chest, if small, should be closed at once and dressed antiseptically. If the wound is large and the lung evidently extensively injured, it is a better plan not to close the external wound completely, but to insert a large drainage tube to carry off the blood into an antiseptic dressing and so prevent its accumulation in the pleural cavity."[5] In 1916, Mentz reported removal of foreign matter from the lung and pointed out the relative safety of thoracotomy.[5]

During the London bombings in World War II, blast injuries became common. Benzinger wrote, "In these cases, the blast wave produced hemorrhagic lesions of the lungs. The symptoms were out of all proportion to the evidence of injury. There was respiratory difficulty, cyanosis, restlessness, and a cough productive of frothy blood and sputum. Physical signs were restricted respiratory movements, muffled and distant breath sounds, and the Roentgen ray signs were of disseminated pneumonia. The lung bases were more involved than the apices. At autopsy there were hemorrhagic areas in the lungs, with capillary bleeding in the alveolar spaces and sometimes massive hemorrhages in the hilar regions."[6]

At the end of World War II, Burford and Burbank called attention to the appearance of "wet lungs" following thoracic injuries.[7] They also noticed that wet lungs not only followed thoracic injuries but also abdominal and head injuries. This phenomenon was subsequently identified as the acute respiratory distress syndrome during the Vietnam War.[8]

The lung is a surprisingly resilient structure. Because of its low mass, missiles pass readily through its substance, little kinetic energy is released, and minimal injury results. Moreover, the lung is like a giant sponge and readily envelopes and tamponades injured vessels within its substance. As a result, injuries to the lung, whether from blunt or penetrating trauma, are not commonly the source of mortality. The primary exceptions are major contusions, blast injuries, and air embolism, which are relatively rare in civilian trauma. It is the associated injuries to heart, systemic vessels, abdominal contents, and chest wall that account for most of the morbidity and mortality associated with thoracic trauma.

ANATOMY

The *right lung,* which constitutes about 55% of the lung mass, is composed of three lobes: the upper, middle, and lower (Fig. 14–1). Two fissures usually are present on the right: the oblique fissure, which separates the lower lobe from the upper and middle lobes, and the horizontal fissure, separating the upper lobe from the middle lobe. The oblique fissure begins posteriorly on the right at the level of the fifth rib, runs obliquely downward and forward approximately parallel to the course of the ribs, and ends anteriorly at the diaphragm in the vicinity of the sixth costochondral junction. The horizontal fissure begins

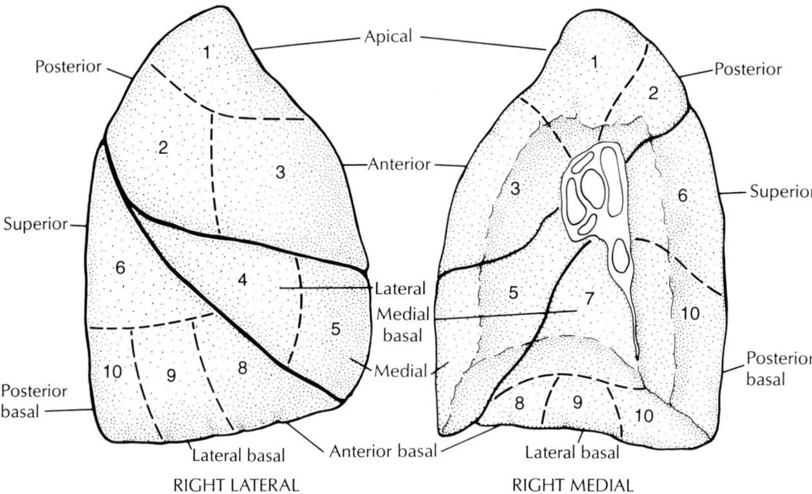

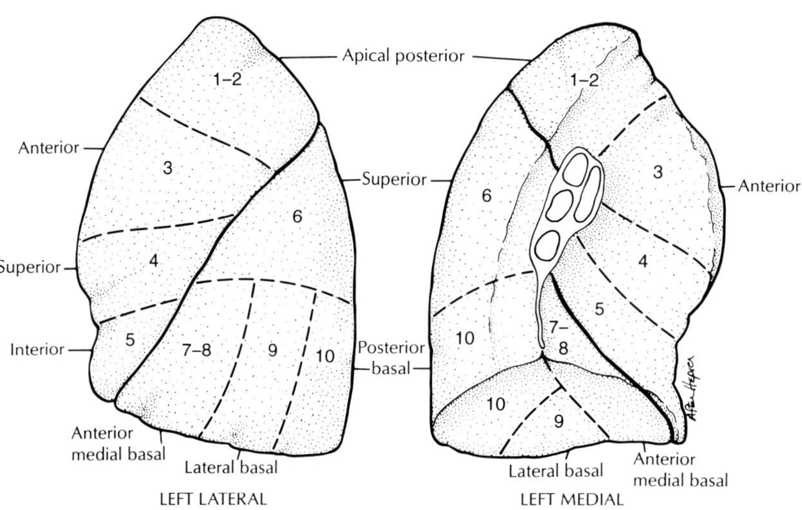

Figure 14–1. The segmental anatomy of the lung. **A:** There are 10 segments on the right lung as opposed to eight segments on the left lung.

in the oblique fissure in the region of the midaxillary line at the level of the sixth rib and extends anteriorly to the costochondral junction of the fourth rib. Each lobe of the right lung is divided into several anatomic units or segments: the upper lobe into three, the middle lobe into two, and the lower lobe into five (each segment is supplied by the segmental bronchus as described in the previous chapter).

The *left lung* is composed of two lobes. The oblique fissure divides the two lobes.

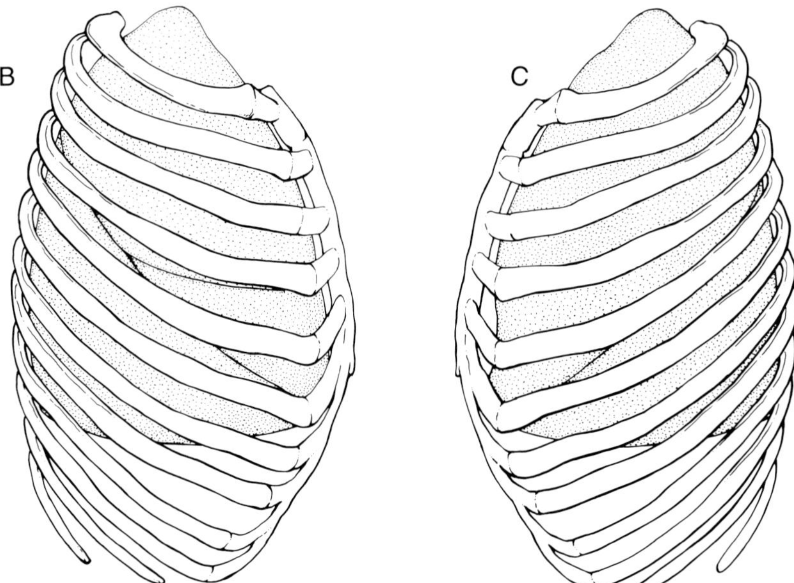

Figure 14–1, cont.   **B:** The relationship of the fissures to the chest wall on the right. **C:** The relationships to the left chest wall.

Anatomically it is approximately a mirror image of the right lung (Fig. 14–1). The lingula of the left upper lobe corresponds to the middle lobe on the right but is fused with the upper lobe in most instances. The segments of the left lobe correspond to the bronchi: four in the upper lobe and four in the lower lobe, two fewer than on the right lung.

Variations in the fissures occur: there may be complete fusion or the fissure may be partially fused. Fusion, when it occurs, is more apt to occur posteriorly, so there may be difficulty demarcating the superior segment of the lower lobe from the posterior segment of the upper lobe on the right lung and the apical posterior from the superior lobe on the left lung.

In the absence of inflammation, each lung lies free in its pleural cavity and is covered by a smooth, glistening *pleura.* The major vascular structures and the bronchi attach the lung to the mediastinum, with the pleural reflection of the lung being continuous with that of the mediastinum. The *pulmonary ligament,* sometimes referred to as the inferior pulmonary ligament, extends from the diaphragm to the inferior pulmonary vein and anchors the lower half of the lung below the hilum to the mediastinum.

The major vascular structures are the *right* and *left pulmonary* arteries that pass superiorly in the hilum and the right and left superior pulmonary veins. The *superior pulmonary vein* lies in the anterior hilum, slightly overlapping anteriorly the pulmonary artery; it supplies the upper and middle lobe on the right and the upper lobe on the left (Fig. 14–2); the *inferior pulmonary vein* lies posterior to the superior pulmonary vein and drains the lower lobe on both sides. Detailed anatomy of the arteries and veins is described under Pulmonary Resection in this chapter.

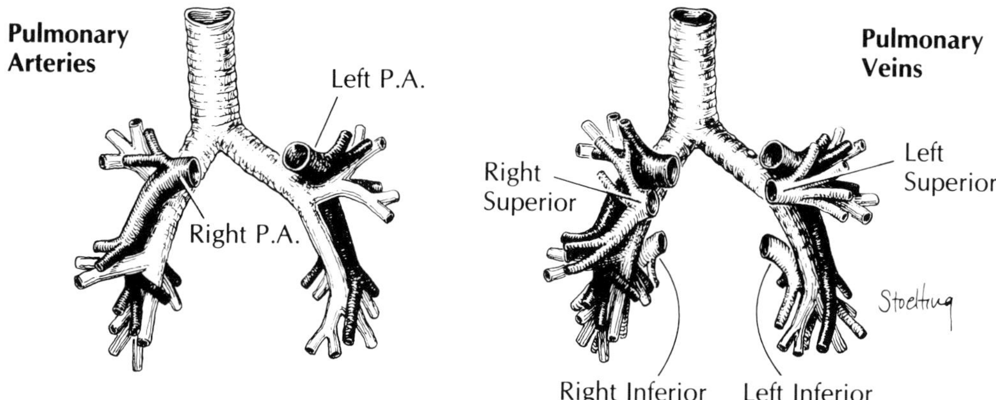

Figure 14–2.   The relationship of the pulmonary artery to the bronchi.

ETIOLOGY AND INCIDENCE

The causes of pulmonary injury are multiple. They include blunt trauma to the chest wall, with or without rib fractures; penetrating trauma from knives, guns, or sharp objects, such as glass; blast injuries, such as those occurring with explosions; and compression of the chest against a closed glottis.

The incidence of lung injuries and their frequency relative to other injuries of the chest varies. In Vietnam, two-thirds of the casualties with penetrating chest trauma had a significant lung injury.[9] In Graham and associates'[10] experience with thoracic injuries, 373 of 666 patients had penetrating wounds of the lung; of these 666 patients, 244 had chest wall injury only; the remainder had multiple intrathoracic injuries. Stab wounds accounted for 221 of the injuries; gunshot wounds, 133; and other penetrating injuries, 17. Associated injuries to other organs occurred in one-third of these patients; 91 patients required thoracotomy.

With regard to blunt trauma, Mogissi[11] reported 182 patients with chest injury: 16 cases had lung contusion (8.8%); eight cases had lung laceration (4.4%). In a series of blunt chest trauma cases reported by Carr,[12] pulmonary contusion was the most common parenchymal finding. Kemmerer and co-workers[13] found pulmonary lacerations in more than 10% of traffic deaths (60 of 585), more than 50% of whom died before reaching the hospital. Jenkins and associates[14] found that 13 of 210 patients with blunt trauma had pulmonary lacerations.

In 127 patients without thoracic bony injuries, Shorr et al.[15] found 35 instances of pulmonary contusions, 44 instances with hemopneumothorax, and 2 isolated instances of pulmonary laceration.

Nakayama et al.[16] found that rib fractures were much fewer in children, whose injuries primarily relate to blunt trauma, due to the high compliance of their chest wall. In 105 cases, they found a 49.5% incidence of rib fractures versus a 53.3% incidence of pulmonary contusion. Pneumothorax occurred in 37.1%; hemothorax in 13.3%; and associated head, abdominal, and orthopedic injuries were present in 68.5% of these children.

SPECIFIC LESIONS

The lesions of the lung that follow chest injury can be classified as lacerations, contusions, hematomas, pneumatoceles, blast injury, traumatic asphyxia, and torsion of a lung or lung lobe.[17–21]

Lacerations of the lung can be defined as tears in the pulmonary parenchyma that present on the external surface of the lung. *Contusions* of the lung represent bruises of the lung, which essentially are hemorrhages into the pulmonary parenchyma. These can be the result of penetrating injuries (such as gunshot or knife wounds), blunt chest wall compression, or rib penetration. *Hematomas* consist of gross disruption of the subpleural parenchyma of the lung or laceration of the deep substance of the lung. *Pneumatoceles* are air cysts that result, as do hematomas, from gross disruption of lung; usually there has been disruption of a small bronchus with intraparenchymal accumulation of air. *Blast injury* is produced by an explosive external force that is transmitted through the tracheobronchial tree to the lung parenchyma and results in diffuse hemorrhages throughout major portions of the lung. *Traumatic asphyxia* is a similar but more dramatic lesion that is produced by forceful compression of the chest wall against a closed glottis. Such a compression results in diffuse parenchymal injury of a type similar to that produced by blast injury but with a marked explosive increase in upper body venous pressure. As a result, traumatic asphyxia results in widespread hemorrhagic manifestations of the face, neck, and upper extremities.[21] Finally, disruption of the lung's hilar attachments can result in rotation or torsion of a lung or a lung lobe with resultant vascular compromise or bronchial obstruction.

Pulmonary Laceration

Blunt trauma sufficient to produce lung laceration requires great force. Such lacerations either result from penetration by a rib or represent bursting-type tears from severe chest crush.[22] All penetrating trauma, by definition, produces at least a small laceration of the lung once the chest cavity is entered to any appreciable degree. Such a small laceration is rarely of clinical consequence and usually is not identifiable on chest radiographs unless pneumothorax has resulted.

Gunshot wounds may be surrounded by an area of lung contusion that results in a radiologic density on chest radiographs. These and smaller lacerations produced by rib fractures from blunt trauma may, on rare occasion, be associated with hemoptysis, but the usual manifestation is pneumothorax or hemothorax. In hemothorax, the most significant portion of the bleeding usually is from chest wall and not from lung tissue itself because the lung is an effective hemostatic organ and lung tissue is capable of tamponading the relatively low-pressure pulmonary vascular bleeding quite effectively.

With more severe lung lacerations, hemoptysis is common.[22] In Mogissi's[11] series, a lung laceration was identified in 4.4% of 182 patients with chest trauma, and hemoptysis was present in every case identified as having a significant lung laceration. Hemopneumothorax is the typical manifestation, although often the hemopneumothorax is modest to minimal. All cases of blunt trauma in Mogissi's series that were associated with major lung lacerations had rib fractures. In addition to indirect signs of hemopneumothorax, on radiographs there usually was a well defined opacity in the lung substance that often had an upward convexity.[11]

Treatment

Treatment involves the immediate placement of one or more chest tubes to drain any hemothorax that is present and reexpand the collapsed lung. With penetrating trauma, further specific treatment is required in only about 5% of the cases. Operative intervention may be required for persistent bleeding or for a clotted hemothorax.[23–25] In most instances of penetrating trauma, the source of bleeding, if continuous, is the chest wall and not the lung.

Failure of the lung to expand, major air leak,[24] clotted hemothorax, massive, ongoing bleeding, or severe hemoptysis suggest deep lung lacerations[26] and represent indications for operation. In a number of instances, air embolism[27] with hypotension, arrhythmias, or cardiac arrest constitute indications for operative treatment for patients with massive injury.

When thoracotomy is necessary, approximately half of large pulmonary lacerations can be treated by suturing major bleeding points and air leaks in the lung. Suture control of major air leaks may require plication of lung tissue with or without resection of small amounts of devitalized lung. In approximately 50% of these operative cases, pulmonary resection may be required to control hemoptysis or control bleeding from major vascular or bronchial tears.

If air embolism is suspected, the hilum should be occluded with a vascular clamp or a tourniquet until the source of air leak can be identified and repair or resection performed.[27] The anesthesiologist should raise the systemic pressure by the temporary use of pressor agents to facilitate the flushing of any air identified in the coronary arteries. Systemic anticoagulation may be of benefit, if used temporarily, because clotting has been shown to aggravate the vascular obstructive problems associated with coronary air embolism. A formal lobectomy or even pneumonectomy occasionally may be required if the lung is badly damaged or hemorrhagic. This would be the case after high-velocity missile injuries with extensive hemorrhage to the lung.

Pulmonary Contusion

Pulmonary contusion can be defined as direct damage to the lung from external trauma (Fig. 14–3).[26] This can be due to penetrating wounds or blunt chest wall trauma.[15,18,26] Most pulmonary contusions are small and relatively benign (Fig. 14–4); that is, the hemorrhage is local and juxtaposed to the site of rib fractures. A visible manifestation on x-ray is that of an infiltrate in the involved segment or lobe of lung that results from diffuse hemorrhage into lung tissue. This bleeding that results from direct trauma occurs immediately after the injury. If an infiltrate is not manifested on the initial chest radiograph, subsequent appearance of one usually is not due to pulmonary contusion. Aspiration, pneumonia, or atelectasis should be suspected and are more likely causes.

Hemorrhage in the lung substances can continue for hours; the radiologic manifestations will be that of a progressive infiltrate. Hemoptysis often (but not always) is present when there has been a major lung contusion.

Pulmonary contusion must be differentiated from aspiration of gastric contents, bronchial secretions, and blood from the mouth or throat. Aspiration usually does not produce immediate changes in the chest radiograph because the onset of infiltrates usually

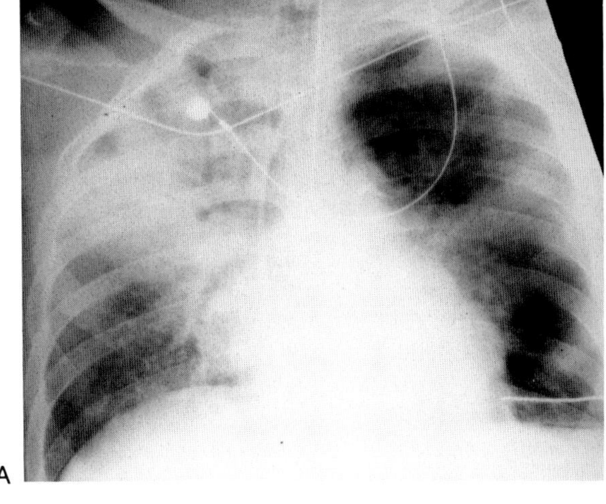

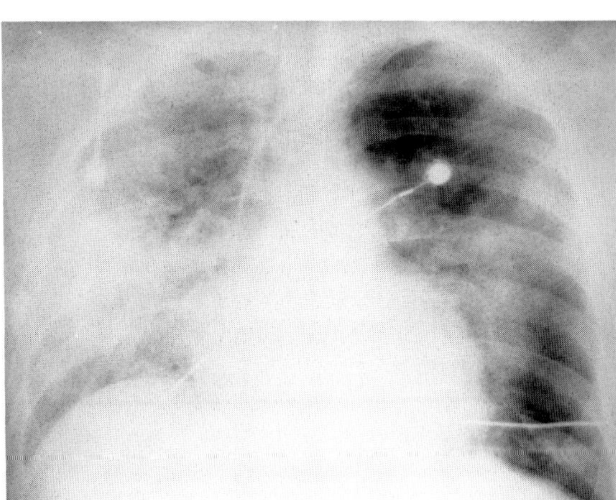

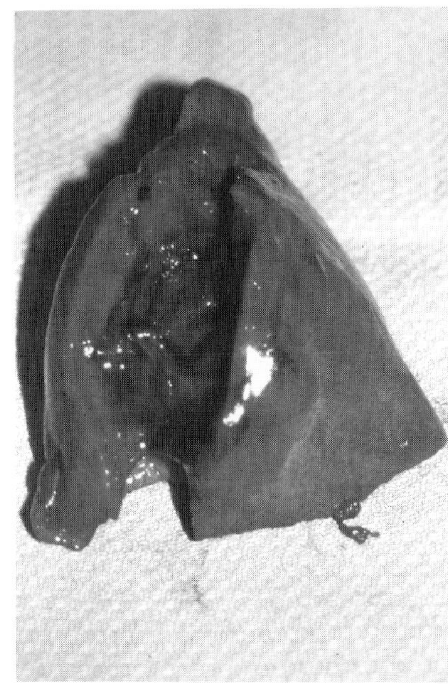

Figure 14–3. Pulmonary contusion. **A:** The infiltrate as noted on the chest radiograph at the time of the patient's presentation to the emergency room. **B:** The infiltrate has progressed 24 hr later. **C:** Gross appearance of a resected hemorrhagic lung lobe.

requires a number of hours. Aspiration is manifested by abundant tracheobronchial secretions, by the presence of particulate matter, or blood in the tracheobronchial tree.

Contusion is the most common overt pulmonary parenchymal injury. In Shorr et al.'s[15] series of 127 patients without bony thoracic injury, 35 patients had pulmonary contusion. Nakayama et al.[16] found in children, in whom nearly all lesions are blunt, that 53% had contusion and a lesser percentage had rib fractures.

The diagnosis of pulmonary contusion is easily made. If penetrating trauma is the source, then the pulmonary infiltrate will surround the site of lung penetration and will spread circumferentially from this area. Ordinary handgun wounds cause minimal lung damage because little energy is transmitted to tissues and the area of hemorrhage or contusion is limited to the small area surrounding the penetrating injury. If a major vascular

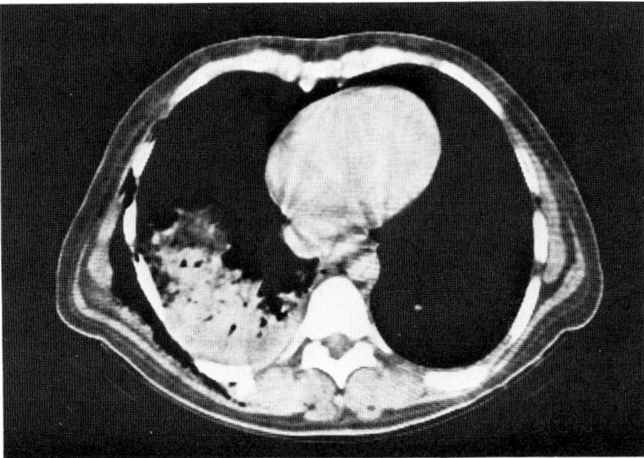

Figure 14–4. CT scan shows the appearance of the lung in a patient with what appeared to be a minimal contusion on chest radiography.

structure is injured near the hilum of the lung, there may be massive hemorrhage into the lung tissue and the tracheobronchial tree. Under this circumstance, hemoptysis will occur. Surprisingly, injury to vascular structures within the substance of the lung, except for specific locations near the hilum, is rarely associated with massive hemorrhage because the pulmonary arterial and venous pressures are low and lung tissue is capable of tamponading bleeding—blood flow tends to proceed through the normal low-resistance main channels instead of leaking into the substance of the lung.

When there is extensive damage to the chest wall or a high-velocity missile is involved, the underlying contusion can be virulent. When the contusion involves the major portion of a lung lobe, the immediate and late morbidity and mortality may be considerable due to intrabronchial bleeding and/or pulmonary arteriovenous shunting of blood.

In most instances, blunt thoracic wall trauma that produces contusion is associated with significant lacerations of the lung and the parallel manifestations of hemothorax, pneumothorax, or hemopneumothorax.

Treatment

Treatment usually is simple because the lung substance tends to limit hemorrhage and the pulmonary reserve in the average trauma patient with a small lesion usually is excellent. Pulmonary contusion, in the absence of other significant injuries, may produce variable alterations in pulmonary function and in some instances may be life threatening. In the absence of a need for operative intervention, resolution of the infiltrate usually occurs within a week or two on simple supportive care. When there are severe associated chest wall injuries, these may require endotracheal intubation and mechanical ventilation or even open thoracotomy to control massive intrapleural hemorrhage. The presence of other major injuries, shock, and secondary changes in the lung such as the respiratory distress syndrome may be superimposed on the pulmonary contusion. In this instance, management is dictated by the status of pulmonary function. Assessment and reassessment of pulmonary function should be done following such injury, and mechanical ventilatory support with endotracheal intubation started based on standard clinical criteria.

In certain specific injuries, particularly high-velocity missile injuries or massive chest wall injury, the substance of a lobe or an entire lung may be badly damaged and the ability to oxygenate blood is compromised by large amounts of nonventilated lung.

In the Vietnam conflict, Fischer and associates[28] found that pulmonary resection was necessary in the management of many with severe contusion; it lessened morbidity and improved survival. In our experience with civilian injuries, pulmonary resection is not required commonly and unless there are severe lacerations of lung in which bleeding into the pleural space is a concomitant problem.

Bleeding into the airway constitutes an indication for rapid operative intervention. Bleeding from the hilum should be controlled initially by the application of a hilar vascular clamp or snare. After assessment of the injury, vascular repair, segmentectomy, lobectomy or, rarely, pneumonectomy may be necessary. The final indication for excision relates to difficulty oxygenating the patient because of a large shunt in a major contusion limited to one lobe or one lung. A trial of pulmonary artery occlusion at the time of thoracotomy may be required to determine the patient's tolerance of the procedure.

Hematomas

Pulmonary hematomas may be difficult to differentiate from pulmonary contusions because surrounding most hematomas there is also blood extravasation into the substance of lung. Hematoma is a space-occupying lesion occurring in a rent in the substance of the lung. This rent can be the result of a penetrating injury, with hemorrhage from a major vessel in the interior of the lung, or can be the result of a crush injury, with disruption of a portion of a substance of the lung.[29] The lesion usually is asymptomatic but may be associated with hemoptysis. A radiographic picture of a hematoma may be difficult to distinguish from a picture of a contusion; characteristically, the associated contusion resolves first, leaving a sharply defined, round density, the hematoma, on the x-ray (Fig. 14–5). This then resolves slowly in several weeks. Computed tomography (CT) scan also can be helpful in differentiating between contusion and hematoma.

Treatment

The treatment of the lesion is conservative; no specific treatment is indicated in the absence of other pulmonary complications such as severe hemoptysis, hemothorax, or pneumothorax. Occasionally, secondary infection or failure of an apparent hematoma to resolve weeks after injury may require surgery to rule out a preexisting lung lesion.

Pneumatocele

A pneumatocele, an uncommon lesion resulting from penetrating trauma or from blunt trauma, is a cyst-like cavity that fills with air rather than blood; usually it is the result of a small bronchial injury associated with disruption of lung substance and is aggravated by positive pressure ventilation. An appreciation of the incidence of the lesion is now possible because of CT scans.[30] The patient may develop hemoptysis. If the lesion becomes

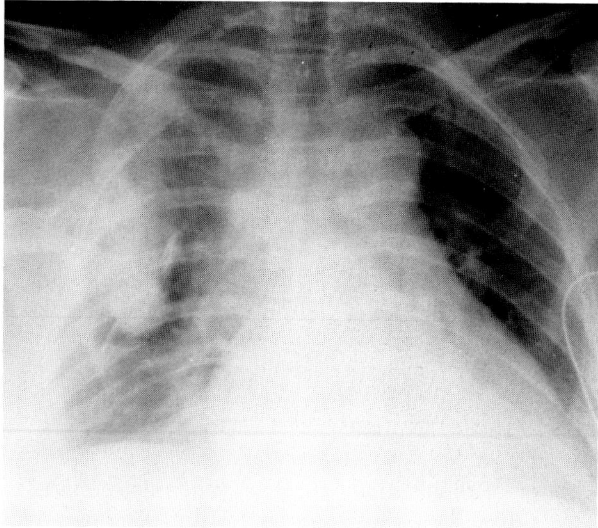

Figure 14–5. A pulmonary hematoma appears as a discrete density on chest radiography, as opposed to the diffuse infiltrate seen with contusion.

secondarily infected, pulmonary abscess may result, as manifested by systemic signs or large amounts of purulent sputum. Operative treatment usually is not required unless the patient fails to respond to antibiotic therapy or develops empyema. Pulmonary resection may be indicated (on rare occasions) for persistent hemoptysis or for failure of parenchymal infection to resolve with conservative management.

Blast Injury

Blast injury of the lungs is caused by the transmission of pressure waves through the tracheobronchial tree from a nearby explosion.[31] Benzinger[6] noted that when the chest wall was protected from the blast and the airway exposed via a tracheotomy, experimental animals survived. His studies emphasized the importance of simultaneous compression of the chest wall and diaphragm at the time the pressure wave moved through the airway.

The symptoms of blast injury are those of progressive respiratory failure: the development of moist, bubbling rales. Cough is typically ineffective. Bronchial fluid spreads rapidly throughout the nondamaged areas of the lung and progressive atelectasis develops. A chest radiograph demonstrates diffuse infiltrates through both lungs (Fig. 14–6). Pneumomediastinum or pneumothorax, or both, may be present.

The severity of the injury depends on the magnitude of the explosion and the proximity of the patient to the incident. The pulmonary damage consists of rupture of the alveoli and capillaries and interstitial and intraalveolar hemorrhage. It is a diffuse, contusive type of lesion in which there also may be bronchovenous fistulas that may result in air emboli and sudden death.[32]

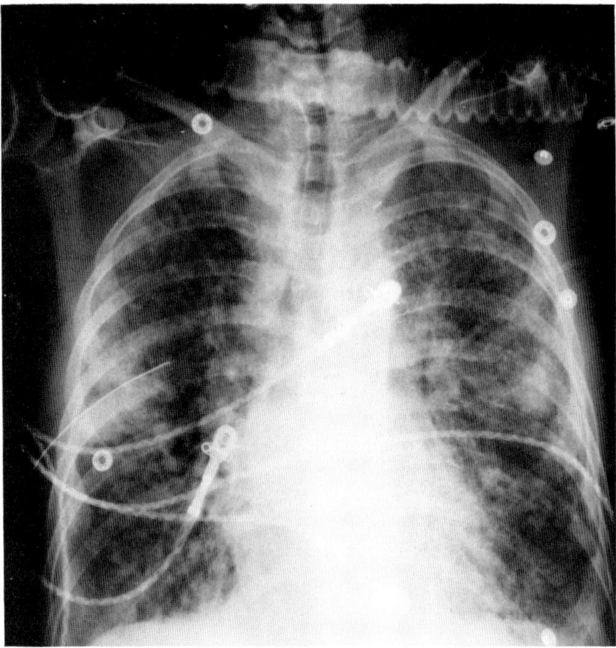

Figure 14–6.   Blast injury of the lung closely resembles contusion, but the infiltrate usually is diffuse throughout both lungs.

Treatment

Treatment involves endotracheal intubation, mechanical ventilation, positive end-expiratory pressure, and increased oxygen concentration as necessary to maintain arterial oxygenation. Chest tubes should be used to drain hemothorax and pneumothorax to expand the lungs and optimize function. In desperate cases, extracorporeal membrane oxygenation, as advocated by Steiner et al.[33] may be of benefit.

Traumatic Asphyxia

Traumatic asphyxia results from severe, sudden compression of the chest against a closed glottis or tracheobronchial tree.[19,34] A compressive force sufficient to cause a sudden rise in pressure in all the great veins in the upper half of the body results in the transmission of the high pressure into small venules and capillaries of the head and neck. These temporarily become massively engorged, leading to diffuse extravasation of blood into adjacent tissues. At the same time, the force often results in diffuse interstitial hemorrhage within the substance of the lung that may seriously compromise oxygenation. This combination results in a startling appearance of the patient. There is a triad of signs: a cyanotic hemorrhagic appearance of the skin of the head and neck, subconjunctival and scleral hemorrhages, and petechiae seen scattered over the craniocervical area. Associated cerebral hemorrhage results in alterations in cerebral function or unconsciousness, and mortality is high in the first few hours from progressive cerebral and pulmonary edema.

Mechanical ventilatory support provides a means of preventing progressive deterioration of pulmonary function in most patients. If death does not occur in the first few hours, most patients survive, and prognosis at this point is related to associated injuries.

Permanent cerebral sequelae are unusual, perhaps because, as speculated by Kirsh and Sloan,[35] the brain is protected by the rigid structure of the cranium, which resists the sudden increase in venous pressure; in addition, the large venous sinuses at the base of the brain dampen the transmission of pressure.

Lung Torsion

Torsion of the lung is extremely rare.[4,36] The three cases cited in the literature involved a whole lung or lung lobes. Torsion of pulmonary tissue was in either direction and occurred as a complication of lung trauma in each instance. It is most apt to occur in children because of the compressibility and resiliency of the thoracic cage. Daughtery[36] postulated that sudden compression of the lower chest wall displaces the lower lobe upward, tearing the inferior pulmonary ligament and, when the pressure is increased, the aerated upper lobe rotates to occupy the high-vacuum space created in the lower thorax.

The diagnosis can be made by a history of blunt chest trauma combined with evidence of increasing hemothorax or opacification of a hemothorax on an x-ray despite tube thoracostomy. Stratmeier and Barry[37] reported that the initial chest radiograph shows peculiar striations in the midlung field extending from the hilus laterally and sweeping upward toward the apex in a curving fashion. However, the common finding is atelectasis secondary to bronchial obstruction and pulmonary contusion. Venous engorgement occurs rapidly.

The key to successful treatment is early diagnosis. This involves operation before irreversible damage occurs so that detorsion, rather than resection, can be done. If there is any significant delay, infarction of lung is the result and treatment requires resection. The bronchial tree may be flooded with bloody secretions when the torsion is corrected; this requires the attention of the anesthesiologist and preferably the use of a double lumen tube to protect the good lung.

PULMONARY RESECTION

The indications for pulmonary resection have been previously described.[10,22,28,37,38] In many instances, severe contusion, air embolism, massive bleeding, and intrabronchial bleeding require immediate thoracotomy and the application of a vascular clamp across the pulmonary hilum to temporarily control the problem. Powell et al. advocate a hilar snare as giving more secure hemostasis.[39] If repair of the injury so controlled is not possible, then lobar or total lung resection is indicated. In other instances (Table 14–1) in which there is a badly mangled lung or lobe but no active bleeding, the operative procedure can be performed with more deliberation.

Although a posterolateral incision is the general approach of choice for elective pulmonary resection, the anterolateral incision is optimal in most trauma instances because

Table 14–1.   Indications for Lung Resection

Severe intrabronchial hemorrhage
Severe lobar contusion
Major lobar artery or venous injury
Major intraparenchymal bronchial injury
Air embolism
Torsion of lung with infarction

the trauma patient often is unstable and tolerates a supine position better than a lateral position. Moreover, should unsuspected pathologic changes be found or sudden deterioration occur, the abdomen is readily entered. The supine position also has an advantage in that it provides access to either chest and, in certain types of penetrating trauma, unexpected pathology may require entering the opposite pleural cavity.

If time permits, the patient is positioned supine with a pad under the shoulder and buttock of the side to be entered (Chapter 21). In general, the optimal anterolateral incision is made in the pectoral or inframammary groove, curving upward medially to follow the contour of the rib and obliquely upward laterally to the posterior axillary line, still parallel to the direction of the ribs.

The pectoral muscle inserts on the sixth rib, and the fifth interspace is the optimal location for general thoracic exploration in the trauma patient. Therefore, after the skin incision is made, the pectoral muscle is detached from the sixth rib and an incision is made through the intercostal muscles and pleura to enter the chest cavity. Although the incision usually is carried out from the parasternal area to the posterior axillary line, the intercostal muscles and pleura can be undercut to the paravertebral area. This is done using partially opened scissors, chisel fashion, along the top of the sixth rib at least as far posteriorly as the angle of the rib. Should exploration suggest pathologic changes in the opposite chest, the sternum can be transected and the incision carried into the opposite pleural cavity by using a mirror incision on the opposite side.

Once pulmonary resection is found to be necessary, additional exposure usually is required. This is obtained by cutting costal cartilages of the rib above and below the fifth interspace incision. In addition, the skin incision can be curved upward along the parasternal line and additional cartilages cut as high as the second rib if necessary to provide exposure of the pleural cavity to the apex of the lung.

The pulmonary hilum lies in the anterior half of the chest, and the ability to carry out pulmonary resection is not at all compromised by the anterior approach, which provides immediate exposure of the heart and the intrapericardial vasculature of the lung and access to all of the anterior hilar structures of the lung.

If a hilar clamp has been required to control lung bleeding, it may be appropriate to open the pericardium and dissect the lung vessels from within the pericardial cavity. This permits vascular control with the hilar clamp or tourniquet still in place.

Technique of Pneumonectomy

The basic principles for emergent left or right pneumonectomy are essentially the same. The control of bleeding from the lung involves control of the hilum. This is readily done by the immediate application of a vascular clamp of the DeBakey-Crafoord type. If a clamp can be placed a few centimeters away from the mediastinal pleura, extrapleural dissection of the pulmonary artery can be carried out. Pulmonary arteries to both right and left lung lie in the anterosuperior portion of the hilum. The pulmonary artery on both sides is partially overlapped anteriorly by the superior pulmonary vein. If a hilar clamp is in place, congestion of the lung is not a problem and the superior pulmonary vein can be divided first. This greatly improves access to the main pulmonary artery. If proximal placement of the hilar clamp is required, the pericardium should be opened and dissection of the superior pulmonary vein carried out within the pericardium. The vein usually can be encircled rapidly and controlled adjacent to the atria with a small vascular clamp and the pulmonary vein divided. The vein is best controlled with a running over-and-over baseball stitch of 3-0 or 4-0 Prolene. Control of the pulmonary artery is readily accomplished within the pericardium; with a vascular clamp applied proximally, the artery is divided to preserve a cuff of tissue distal to the proximal clamp. This cuff can be oversewn with a double row of running 3-0 or 4-0 Prolene sutures.

The only major remaining pulmonary vascular structure is the inferior pulmonary vein. This is found by mobilizing the inferior surface of the hilum by dividing the pulmonary ligament and carrying the dissection upward until the vein is encountered. The inferior pulmonary vein lies relatively posterior in the hilum just anterior to the esophagus. It can be encircled from within the pericardium or dissection carried out extrapericardially depending on the ease of access. The cardiac side of the vein is oversewn with 3-0 or 4-0 Prolene sutures, as previously described. At this point, unless there is a major bronchial tear, the hilar clamp can be removed if it has been applied and the right or left bronchus divided. Ready access to the right main bronchus may require division of the azygus vein to expose the right main bronchus above the takeoff of the upper lobe bronchus. Several bronchial arteries may be encountered entering the hilus of the lung from the posterior mediastinum. These can be clamped and ligated independently. The bronchus is divided proximally just distal to the carina using 4.8-ml staples and the lung specimen removed.

The exposure of the left main bronchus near the carina is more difficult because of the surrounding aortic arch. In addition, the ligamentum arteriosum extends from the aorta opposite the subclavian artery to the left pulmonary artery at the point where it emerges from the mediastinum. The aorta can be retracted and the dissection carried proximally until the carina is identified. The left main stem bronchus should be divided with the stapler 5 to 10 mm distal to the carina; care should be taken to ensure that no compromise of the right main bronchus occurs.

Lobar Resection

In emergency circumstances, any one of the five major lobes of the lung can be resected. Segmental or wedge resections may be appropriate under certain circumstances. The gross anatomy of the lobes requires much more attention with lobectomy than with pneumonectomy. The right main pulmonary artery occupies the anterior and superior portion of the hilum and curves downward and medial to the right upper lobe bronchus. It gives off a large anterior segmental branch within the mediastinum. The superior segmental branch of the right lower lobe and the branches to the middle lobe come off nearly opposite one another at the juncture of and deep within the major and minor fissures.

The left pulmonary artery is attached to the undersurface of the aorta opposite the subclavian artery by the ligamentum arteriosum (the residual ductus), which joins the left pulmonary artery just as it emerges from the mediastinum. The pulmonary artery gives off a large branch into the anterior segment of the upper lobe just as it emerges from the mediastinum. As opposed to the right side, the left pulmonary artery curves downward and posterior to the left main stem bronchus. The left main bronchus is approximately 3 cm long before the takeoff of the upper lobe bronchus and then continues downward, giving off first the superior segment bronchus and terminating in the remaining segmental bronchus. The fissure between the upper and lower lobe usually is complete on both sides. The most common location for fusion lies posteriorly. The minor fissure between the upper and middle lobe on the right often is fused and may even be nonexistent. These anatomical planes can be developed by sharp dissection, by utilization of a coagulation current, or by ultrasonic techniques.

The arteries run deep in the interior of the lobes and segments they supply. The superior pulmonary vein drains the upper and middle lobes of the lung in the case of the right lung and, on the left, it drains the entire upper lobe, including lingula. The anterior segment is drained by a large vein that crosses over and anterior to the pulmonary artery. The inferior pulmonary vein lies relatively posterior in the hilum and drains the lower lobe. As opposed to the arteries, the veins tend to run in the periphery of the lobes, segments, and lobules of the lung.

The origin of the right upper lobe bronchus is just at or distal to the carina and lies laterally and posterior to the pulmonary artery. The bronchus to the middle and lower lobes lies in the posterior hilum.

Right upper lobectomy may be relatively easily carried out (Fig. 14–7). The primary problem involves dissecting the pulmonary artery in such a fashion as not to compromise the blood supply of the middle or lower lobe. If vigorous bleeding should occur during dissection of the right pulmonary artery, intrapericardial control permits exposure, dissection, and repair of any inadvertent lacerations in a dry field. The phrenic nerve should be identified anteriorly, the vagus nerve posteriorly, and the dissection of the hilum carried out in the interval between these two nerves. The vein draining the anterior segment crosses over the pulmonary artery and is often best divided early to permit exposure of the pulmonary artery. The anterior segmental artery is the first branch of the pulmonary artery. It is a large vessel, often emerging from the pulmonary artery as it passes through the mediastinal pleura. It can be encircled, ligated proximally in continuity, divided distally, and ligated.

At this point, it is appropriate to dissect the major and minor fissure, remembering that the confluence of major vascular structures occurs deep within the fissure at the juncture of the major and minor fissures. In most instances, the pulmonary veins lie posterior in the fissure and under the pulmonary artery. The artery is recognized by the large branch to the middle lobe and should be preserved to avoid the need for middle lobectomy. If the vein is anterior, as may be the case, branches entering the upper lobe can be divided. If any doubt exists as to the nature of the vessel, blood can be aspirated, utilizing a small syringe. Dark blood indicates a pulmonary artery; bright red, the pulmonary vein. This distinction requires emphasis, because mistaking the pulmonary artery for branches of the pulmonary vein may result in inadvertently dividing the arterial supply to the lower lobe. Should bleeding develop during this portion of the dissection, rather than clamping and ligating vessels whose identity is unknown, it is preferable to control the artery and vein within the

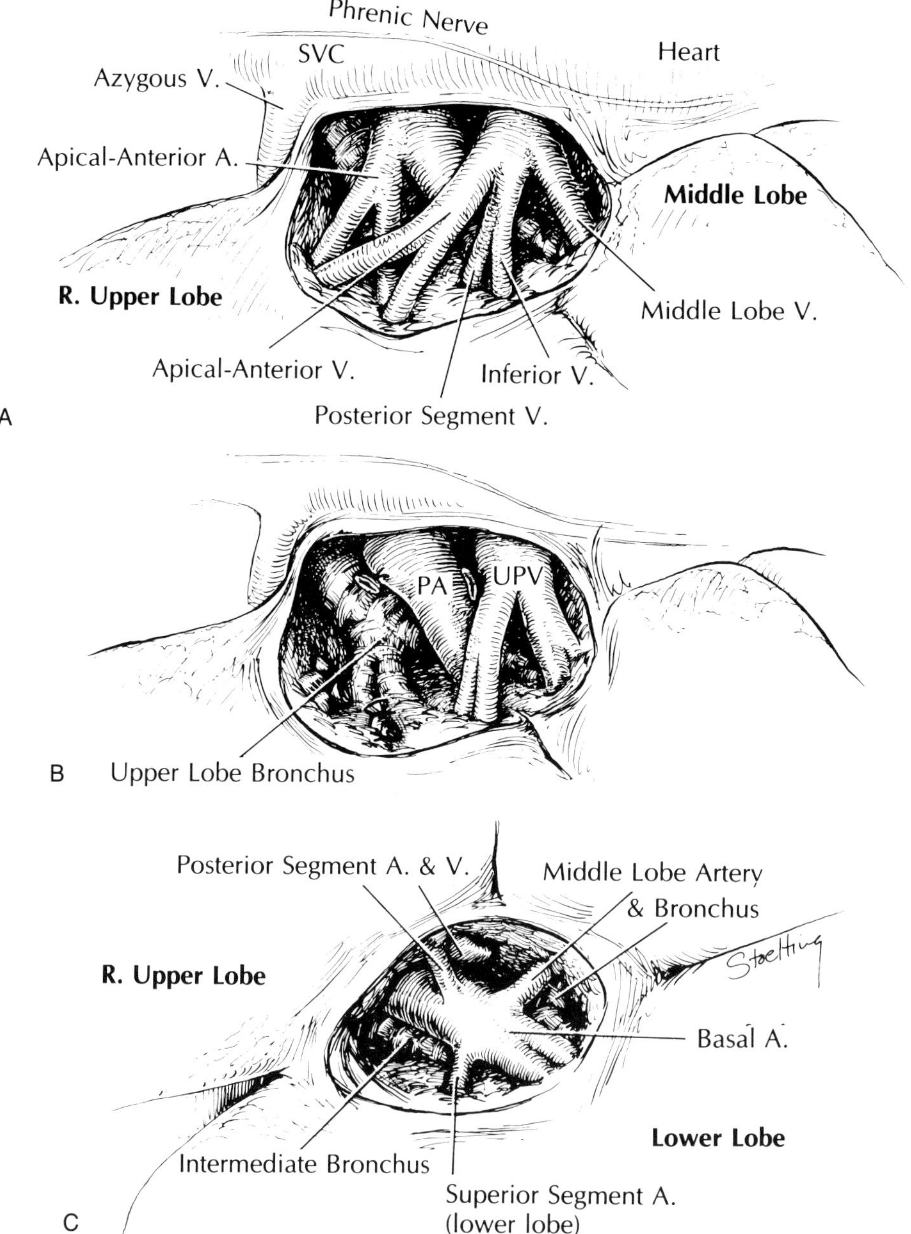

Figure 14–7.   Anatomy encountered during right upper lobectomy. **A:** The right hilum as exposed anteriorly. **B:** The hilum as seen anteriorly and above. **C:** The anatomy seen during dissection of the minor fissure.

pericardium and then, in a dry field, carry out the dissection to identify the precise structures. Also, any injuries to the major vessels that resulted from the trauma may be repairable by using this technique. The upper lobe is gradually peeled away from the main pulmonary artery as the venous branches are divided anteriorly and from within the fissure. This should leave the upper lobe attached only to the upper lobe bronchus. Dissection of the upper lobe bronchus should be carried out sufficiently to identify the middle and lower lobe bronchi. The upper lobe bronchus should be cleared for approximately 1 cm and transected with a stapler utilizing 3.5- or 4.8-mm staples 2 to 3 mm from its origin.

Middle lobectomy is approached by dividing the pleura anterior to the hilum and then dissecting the major and minor fissure around both sides of the lobe (Fig. 14–8). Branches of the pulmonary artery entering the lobe superiorly and those from the pulmonary vein are divided, leaving the middle lobe attached to the relatively long middle lobe bronchus. This is dissected to identify the lower lobe bronchus above and below the takeoff of the middle lobe bronchus. A stapler is applied adjacent to the lower lobe bronchus, and the middle lobe is removed.

Right lower lobectomy involves dissection of the major fissure until the pulmonary artery is identified deep within the fissure at the junction of the major and minor fissures (Fig. 14–9). If there has been injury to the lower lobe artery and bleeding obscures the field, the right pulmonary artery can be dissected at the superior aspect of the hilum or within the pericardium and temporarily controlled by a vascular clamp. The pulmonary artery branch to the middle lobe comes off opposite and anterior to the superior segmental branch to the lower lobe. Therefore, the superior segment artery should be ligated independently, followed by the rest of the artery distal to the middle lobar vessels.

The inferior pulmonary vein drains the lower lobe and is identified by dissecting the pulmonary ligament from below until the pulmonary vein can be identified, encircled, divided, and both ends oversewn. At this point, the dissection is carried far enough into the hilum to separate the lower lobe from the middle lobe. The junction of the middle and lower lobe bronchi is then identified, cross-clamped, and divided distal to the middle lobe takeoff with the stapler. The superior segmental bronchus to the lower lobe may require separate ligation because its posterior takeoff is very close to the anterior takeoff at the middle lobe bronchus.

Left upper lobectomy is similar to that of right upper lobectomy (Fig. 14–10). The anterior segmental artery comes off a bit more distally on the pulmonary artery than the one on the right. It can be identified by opening the pleura investing the anterior and superior portion of the hilum. The vessel is then divided and ligated. The anterior portion of the hilum can then be opened and the pulmonary vein encircled. If either the pulmonary artery or vein has been injured, dissection can be carried out intrapericardially with a clamp across the hilum of the lung. Once intrapericardial control of the pulmonary artery and the superior pulmonary vein has been obtained, the hilar clamp can be removed and the individual vessels exposed directly. The major fissure should be dissected down to the pulmonary artery and the bronchus. As opposed to the right lung, the pulmonary artery lies lateral to the upper lobe bronchus. A segmental branch to the superior segment of the lower lobe lies opposite the lingular branches and in the fissure. The lingular branches come off anteriorly and can be encircled and divided. The resection is then carried back along the pulmonary artery to interrupt additional branches to the posterior and apical segments of the upper lobe. The superior pulmonary vein is then divided, and the proximal end oversewn with running 3-0 or 4-0 Prolene sutures, leaving the upper lobe attached only to

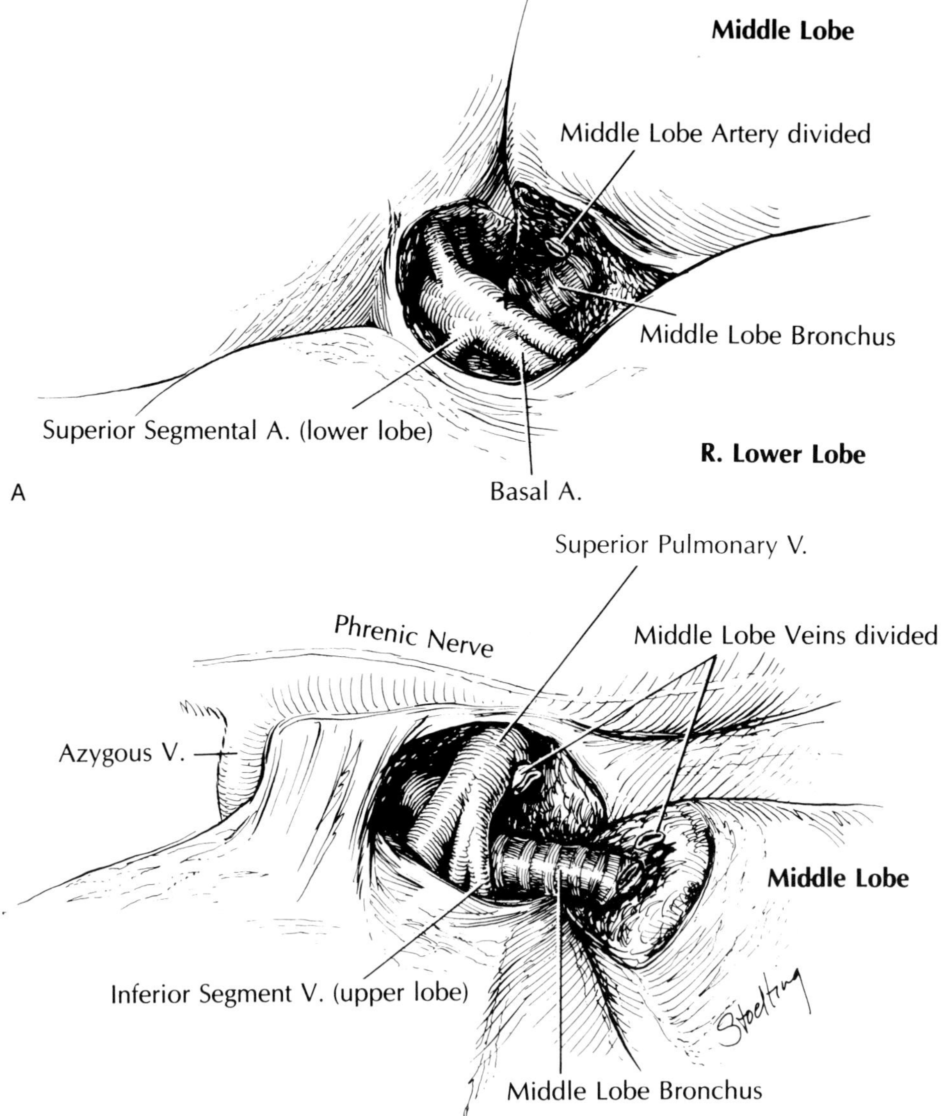

Figure 14–8. Middle lobectomy. **A:** The anatomy as seen through the minor fissure. **B:** The anatomy seen from behind and below.

the upper lobe bronchus. Dissection is carried down to identify the left main bronchus above and the lower lobe bronchus below. A stapler is then applied across the bronchus just at its takeoff from the main bronchus, the bronchus is transected, and the resection is completed.

Left lower lobectomy is similar to, but a mirror image of, that of the right lower lobe (Fig. 14–11). Precautions and anatomy are essentially the same. The lingular branches of the pulmonary artery must be identified and preserved.

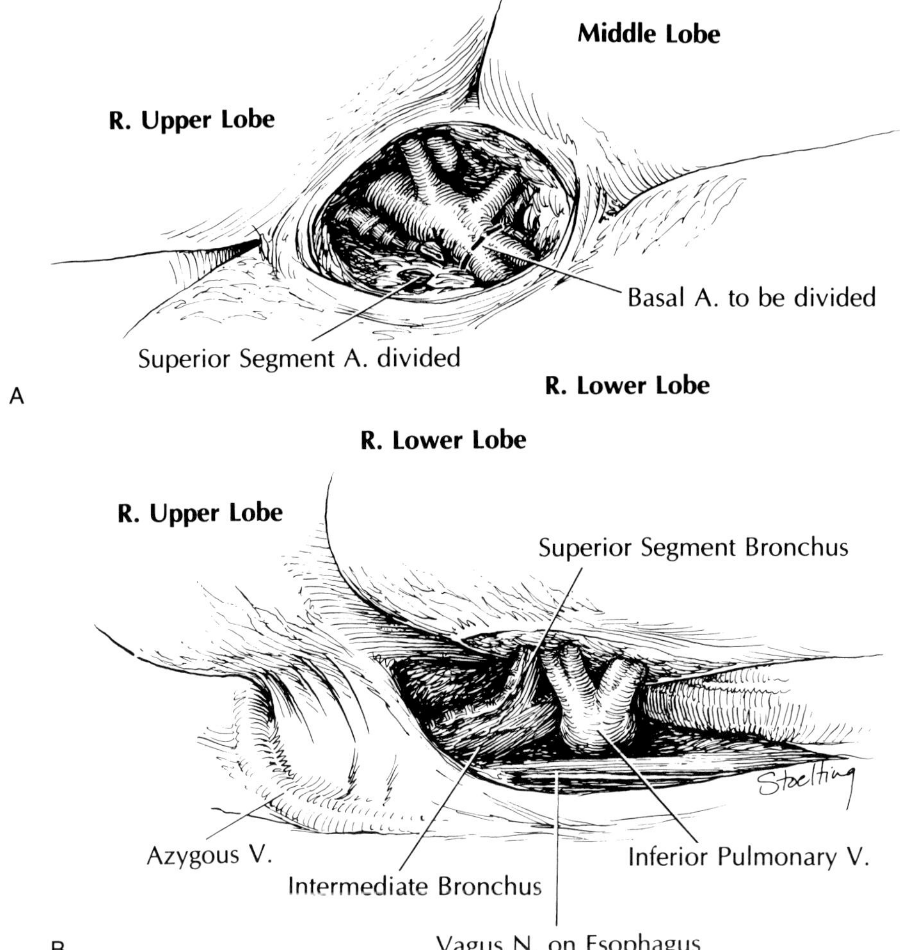

Figure 14–9.   Right lower lobectomy. **A:** The anatomy as seen through the major fissure. **B:** The anatomy as seen from behind and below.

Segmental and *wedge resection* very often can be used to treat damaged lung. Although classic anatomic dissection can be done in most instances, the resection is appropriately carried out by trimming away obviously devitalized and injured tissue. If possible, the resection should not be carried into the root of the lung where major segmental bronchi and vascular structures may be encountered, because this might risk compromise of nondamaged portions of the lung.

The principle is this: When major vascular structures are involved in the area near the hilum, lobectomy or pneumonectomy usually is the best choice to control hemorrhage and remove devitalized lung. When major air leaks are present that involve major segmental bronchi, lobectomy usually is the treatment of choice. When bleeding involves areas of the lung away from the hilum, nonanatomic segmentectomy or wedge resection may be indicated.

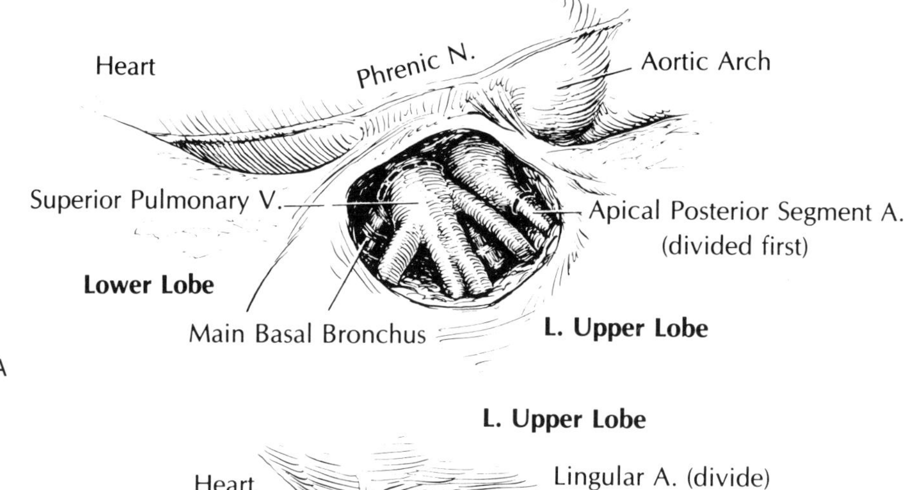

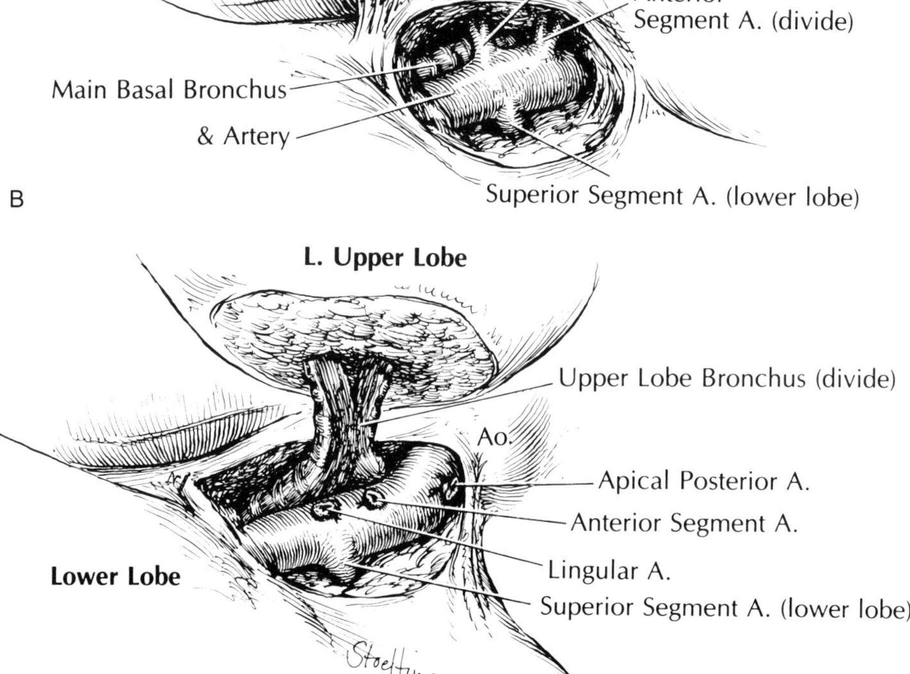

Figure 14–10.   Left upper lobectomy. **A:** The hilar anatomy as seen anteriorly. **B:** The anatomy as seen from above and behind. **C:** The final stages of resection before division of the upper lobe bronchus.

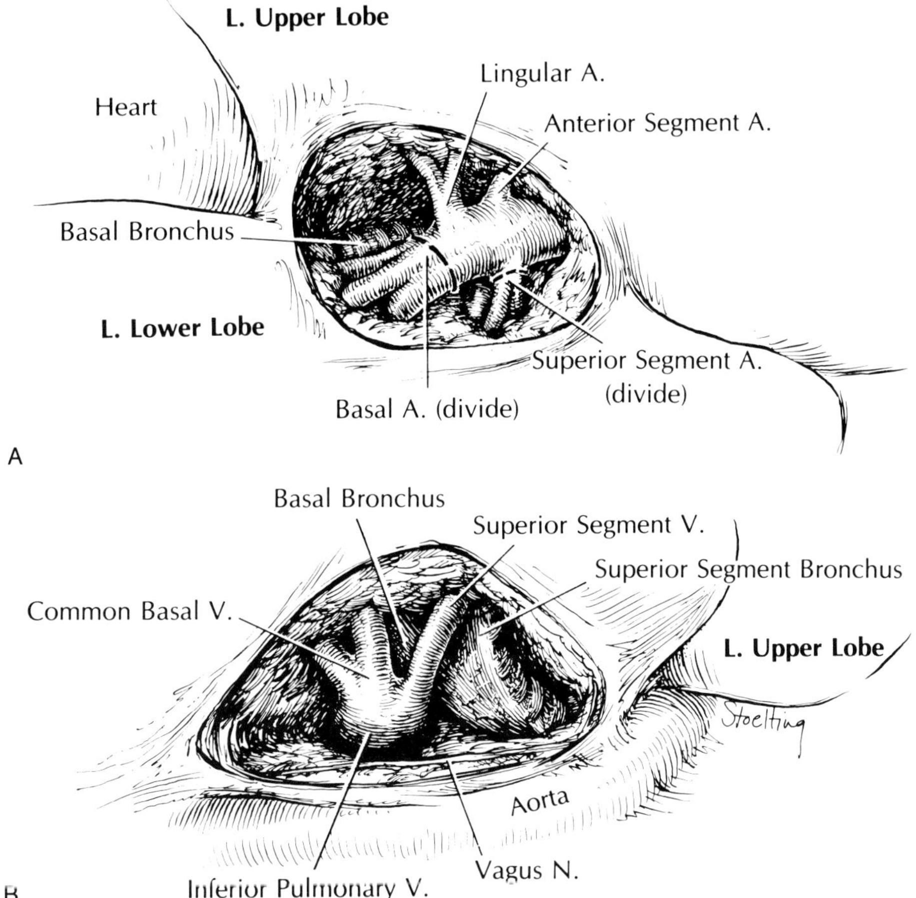

Figure 14–11.   Left lower lobectomy. **A:** The anatomy as seen through the major fissure. **B:** The anatomy as seen from behind the lower lobe.

A vascular clamp can be placed across the portion of the lung to be incised, and a running mattress suture of synthetic collagen is used to plicate the raw surface of the lung behind the clamp. Any large vessels or bronchi that are encountered should be ligated individually. Alternatively, staples can be applied in a V fashion and resection performed within the V.

After completion of a pneumonectomy or lobectomy, hemostasis is carefully assessed. Bronchial arteries that may not have been previously identified may be the source of continued oozing and should be identified and clamped and ligated. Pleura or pericardium may be mobilized and used to cover the bronchial stump after pneumonectomy. After upper lobectomy, the inferior pulmonary ligament should be divided to permit upward displacement of the lung. After pneumonectomy for trauma, it is appropriate to place one modest-sized chest tube in the pleural space to monitor bleeding and to permit control of the mediastinum. If bleeding is not a major problem postoperatively, the tube should be removed in 12 to 24 hr to avoid contaminating the empty pleural space.

One or two chest tubes should be placed after lobectomy, depending on the status of the pleural space. If bleeding or air leak is considerable, two large-bore chest tubes are indicated. One can be placed anteriorly in the second or third interspace in the midclavicular line, the other posteriorly in the posterior axillary line. Another option is to place both laterally, one directed superiorly into the apex, the other, a right angle tube, is directed posteriorly.

The ribs are then approximated with #1 pericostal absorbable synthetic collagen sutures. The intercostal muscles are approximated with running collagen suture. The muscle layers are approximated with similar running sutures. The subcutaneous tissue is closed with a fine suture and the skin closed with clips or sutures.

POSTOPERATIVE CARE

The one or two large-bore chest tubes that should have been placed before chest closure should be connected to suction drainage with a negative pressure of approximately 10 cm of water. Postoperative chest radiographs should be obtained to verify expansion of the lung and to ascertain that intrathoracic blood is being drained appropriately.

Opacification of the chest as seen on radiography usually means a clotted hemothorax. This is best treated by reoperation, removal of the clot, and control of bleeding.

Failure of the lung to expand is associated with a major air leak and requires the insertion of a second chest tube, if there is not one already in place, or increasing the suction to 20 cm of water. Failure of the lung to expand fully at this point can be accepted temporarily but, if the lung has not expanded after 24 hr either an additional chest tube should be inserted or a reoperation should be done to control the air leak. Each chest tube should be attached to a separate drainage system; otherwise, it is likely that only one chest drainage tube will function.

After major chest injuries, mechanical ventilation using an indwelling endotracheal tube is indicated until the patient demonstrates good mechanical and parenchymal function. Chest wall instability, if present, may require a week or more of mechanical support before sufficient stability is obtained. Ventilator weaning can be attempted by intermittent mandatory ventilation and noting the patient's ability to maintain reasonably normal blood gases on the progressive increase in spontaneous ventilation that is required.

Blood loss and circulatory status should be monitored carefully. If the injury is limited to the chest, the rate of blood loss is monitored by measuring and replacing chest drainage volume for volume to the nearest 500 ml. Chest radiographs should be taken regularly of unstable patients to ensure that chest drainage is effective and blood is not accumulating in the chest. The hematocrit level should be maintained at or above 30%.

Urine output assessment is crucial to document adequate renal perfusion. This is verified as adequate if urine output is between 0.5 and 1 ml/kg/hr. Less than this amount implies inadequate cardiac output and inadequate renal perfusion; higher than this amount suggests that intravenous fluid administration is more rapid than necessary. A minimal or marginal urine output usually implies persistent hypovolemia. A response to a 500-ml fluid bolus verifies this. However, if doubt exists regarding adequacy of volume therapy, a Swan-

Ganz catheter should be passed to permit assessment of pulmonary wedge pressure. This is particularly appropriate in the treatment of multiple or complex injuries. When there is major lung damage or the respiratory distress syndrome has developed, there may be progressive dissociation of left- and right-sided cardiac pressures so the central venous pressure becomes unreliable as a guide to fluid therapy.

In the older patient with underlying heart disease or the young patient with myocardial contusion, the cardiac filling pressures may be high yet cardiac output inadequate to maintain renal and peripheral perfusion. In these instances, cardiotonic agents such as low-dose dopamine or dobutamine may be administered to stimulate cardiac function.

Tracheobronchial secretions should be removed by suctioning as appropriate. This may require almost constant attention if the patient has aspirated or is bleeding into the tracheobronchial tree. Secretions should be assessed periodically by Gram's stain and culture when they become abundant or purulent so that developing infections can be recognized and treated promptly with specific antibiotics.

Chest radiographs should be obtained daily, as long as the patient requires critical care, to ensure that expansion of the lung is complete and to monitor the appearance or disappearance of infiltrates.

As chest tubes cease to function, as manifested by disappearance of air leaks and a drop in daily drainage below 100 ml, suction can be discontinued and the tubes left to water seal. After 24 hr, if no air leak is present, drainage is minimal, and pulmonary expansion is maintained, chest tubes can be removed.

Because chest tubes placed under emergency circumstances may have been contaminated during insertion, the drainage sites should be left open rather than closed by suture. This is because any contamination of the chest tube tract in which the skin has been closed can only drain back into the pleural cavity, setting the stage for empyema. For this reason the patient is asked to take a deep breath and strain against a closed glottis while the tube is quickly removed. A pad of gauze containing petrolatum should be applied immediately to the drain site and this held in place by a 4 × 4 gauze square taped only at its margins. This permits the gauze to act as a flap valve so that secretions from within the chest cavity or tube tract can drain to the outside for an additional period after tube removal.

COMPLICATIONS

The complications of pulmonary injury in the conditions discussed include bleeding, with or without hemothorax; persistent air leak, with or without pneumothorax; progressive cardiorespiratory failure; persistent hypovolemia; pneumonia; lung abscess, empyema; and air embolism.

Bleeding is a frequent complication of pulmonary parenchymal injury. Major intratracheal bleeding with persistent gross hemoptysis lasting more than 1 or 2 hr is an indication for reoperation to treat parenchymal or bronchial lesions. In these instances, pulmonary resection may be necessary. Intraparenchymal bleeding in the absence of severe intrabronchial or intrapleural hemorrhage usually can be managed expectantly. Progressively falling blood gases in the immediate postinjury period may require an operative intervention and pulmonary resection if progressive consolidation of lung lobe is seen on radiography. Intrapleural hemorrhage should be decompressed by one or more chest tubes.

Progressive opacification of the chest on an x-ray or hemorrhage from a chest tube in excess of 500 ml an hour for more than 1 or 2 hr after chest surgery demands reexploration, as does bleeding in excess of 200 ml/hr for more than 6 hr.

Massive air leak in the postinjury or postoperative period also is an indication for operative intervention. Large lung lacerations, bronchial tears, or unligated smaller bronchi usually are found that can be dealt with by suture or ligature. Moderate air leaks can be treated expectantly with one or more large-bore (32F or greater) chest tubes. If pulmonary expansion can be maintained, leaks usually will seal in several days. If lung expansion cannot be obtained or maintained on this regimen, prompt surgical intervention is indicated. Air leaks can be troublesome, particularly in patients with stiff lungs or those having underlying obstructive airway disease. Reoperation carries the greatest risk for this group; expectant treatment for 7 to 10 days or even longer usually is appropriate.

Progressive respiratory failure management involves careful monitoring of blood gases, chest radiographs, and the clinical condition of the patient. In the nonintubated patient, tachypnea is the warning sign. A respiratory rate >30/min demands arterial blood gas monitoring and supplemental oxygen. If progressive deterioration occurs, as manifested by a persistent respiratory rate >35/min, or an oxygen tension of 70 cannot be maintained with supplemental oxygen, endotracheal intubation with mechanical ventilation should be initiated. Oxygen concentrations should be increased as necessary to maintain a normal oxygen tension, with the tidal volume adjusted to normalize the carbon dioxide. Positive end-expiratory pressure of 3 to 5 cm of water should be used. Once oxygen concentration reaches 40% to 50%, increasing levels of positive end-expiratory pressure should be used to control the progressive atelectasis.

Hypovolemia is a relatively common complication. Although overhydration should be avoided, underhydration or hypovolemia is far more dangerous because it increases the tendency for vascular permeability alterations and hence ultimately results in aggravation of the interstitial edema. If any doubt exists about the adequacy of cardiovascular function or volume status, a Swan-Ganz catheter should be passed and pulmonary artery wedge pressures and cardiac outputs assessed. Cardiotonic agents should be titrated to normalize cardiac output and peripheral perfusion as judged by the warmth of the extremities and the urine output.

Pneumonia, or some type of pulmonary infection, is a frequent complication in patients with massive injury. Depression of immune function is likely in this group, which has a tendency to develop diffuse interstitial pulmonary infections. With lesser injuries, particularly those confined to the chest, bronchopneumonia is the usual infectious complication. Neither are prevented by prophylactic antibiotics, which are best reserved to treat specific infections when they develop. It is impossible to sterilize the tracheobronchial tree, and the use of broad-spectrum antibiotics prophylactically ensures that a resistant, often virulent infection will supplant infections with the body's own organisms.

Chest radiograph and sputum cultures should be assessed every day or two. Gram's stains should be obtained when the sputum appears purulent. Smears should be obtained routinely every day as long as the patient's condition is critical. The onset of signs of sepsis, with the development of purulent sputum and with or without abnormalities on the chest radiograph, dictate treatment with the most appropriate antibiotic for the organism identified on smear or culture.

Lung abscess may complicate intraparenchymal hematomas or severe anaerobic lung infections. The abscess may drain spontaneously into the tracheobronchial tree and produce confluent pneumonia or it may rupture into the pleural space, resulting in empyema. Prophylactic antibiotics probably do not have a role to play in preventing secondary infection in hematomas. However, early operative treatment of badly damaged lung with excision of destroyed pulmonary tissues may favorably alter the course of a patient. The indication for antibiotic treatment is the development of septic complications or a change on the chest film that suggests the onset of infection. Closed drainage may be appropriate as an initial management if the abscess is well delineated and not responding to treatment.[40] Open drainage is rarely required unless there is associated empyema.

Empyema prevention involves complete reexpansion of the lung. One or more chest tubes should be inserted as necessary to obtain full pulmonary reexpansion. Residual clotted hemothorax may be an indication for operation to prevent secondary infections and the development of empyema. Prompt treatment of empyema by appropriate placement of one or more large-bore chest tubes directly into the collection provides definitive treatment in most instances. Failure to reexpand the lung fully may result in the development of a fibrous peel that may require decortication weeks or months later to control infection, free up the trapped lung, and optimize pulmonary function.

Air embolism is a well documented complication of injury to cervical veins and to injuries of the intrathoracic superior and inferior vena cavae. In these veins, pressure is negative during the inspiratory phase of ventilation. Thomas and Roe[27] were the first to recognize the significance of pulmonary air embolism after lung lacerations. They documented that this is a frequent cause of morbidity and mortality after thoracic injury, and they speculated that the laceration of pulmonary parenchyma and small bronchi may be associated with simultaneous laceration of small pulmonary veins that run in the periphery of lobes and segments. Air leaking out of the damaged lung can be sucked into adjacent pulmonary veins. Even more importantly, introduction of positive pressure ventilation pushes air out of the lacerated lung under increased atmospheric pressure and provides the possibility of pushing it into an adjacent open pulmonary vessel.

A sudden deterioration of a patient with chest wall injury, particularly in the absence of overt bleeding, suggests the possibility of air embolism and demands immediate thoracotomy (Table 14–2). Aspiration of air from the heart or careful inspection of the coronary arteries under these circumstances often will reveal the characteristic air bubbles that are diagnostic of air embolism. These bubbles produce an air trap, obstruct coronary blood flow, and result in ventricular fibrillation and cardiac arrest. Systemic air emboli may lodge in cerebral vessels and cause secondary cerebral complications, although this has not been as well documented as coronary air embolism.

It is apparent that the hypovolemic patient with a large pulmonary laceration is most susceptible to air embolism. Because these patients usually are resuscitated with mechani-

Table 14–2. Diagnosis of Air Embolism

Chest injury, no obvious head injury, but focal neurologic signs
Fundoscopic examination
Sudden cardiovascular collapse after endotracheal intubation
Froth, blood gas deteriorization

cal ventilation at a time when pulmonary vascular volume is extremely low, it is relatively easy to force air into lacerated pulmonary veins.

It is not appropriate to treat air embolism secondary to pulmonary lacerations as one would treat air embolism from systemic veins. The latter involves rolling the patients left side down to trap air in the right ventricle. Air entering through pulmonary veins goes directly into the left heart. Therefore, the head-down position (Trendelenburg's position) is presumably optimal. Air entering the left ventricle should be trapped in the apex of the ventricle where it can be slowly absorbed or aspirated by cardiocentesis or allowed to move slowly by small increments into the circulation.

Although closed needle aspiration of the ventricle can be tried, the most direct treatment is immediate thoracotomy, opening the pleural space on the side of the presumed injury and clamping the pulmonary hilum. This provides simultaneous control of the lung laceration, decompresses the pleural space, permits exposure of the injured vessels, and allows suture control of the air leak. Air within the heart can be aspirated under direct vision with a needle. The anesthesiologist should administer pressor agents to obtain a high systolic pressure. This tends to drive the air bubbles through the coronary arteries. Systemic anticoagulation with heparin may be of value by decreasing the tendency for the air to activate intravascular clotting. If the patient has not arrested, the prognosis is good and relates to the associated injuries.

RESULTS

The results that follow lung injury relate more to associated injuries than to the lung injury itself. Pulmonary contusion morbidity relates directly to the magnitude of the contusion. Lobar contusion can result in severe hypoxemia if vascular reflex vasoconstriction is absent, allowing continued perfusion of alveolar consolidated lung lobe.[18] Moreover, major pulmonary contusion can cause serious long-term respiratory dysfunction. Kishikawa et al.[17] found that functional residual capacity remained significantly reduced for up to 6 months after injury and changes could still be detected in patients in the supine position injured 1 to 5 years previously.

With traumatic asphyxia, Rosato et al.[19] found that associated injuries were the factor accounting for morbidity and mortality; there was a direct relationship to the injury severity score. In the same series, there were three cardiac injuries in eight cases of traumatic asphyxia and one death from cardiac rupture.

Overall mortality from major thoracic injuries will vary with the nature of the series. Mortality after penetrating trauma to the lung is minimal except for hilar injuries, which usually are immediately fatal. Blunt parenchymal injuries are inevitably associated with chest wall injuries and parenchyma. Injury severity parallels the magnitude of chest wall injury. Shorr et al.[15] found in their analysis of 515 blunt chest trauma cases that there was a 36% morbidity rate and a 15.5% mortality rate. For severe contusion associated with blunt chest injuries, they found a 28.6% rate of mortality.

In patients who recover from major thoracic injury, severe long-term disability is minimal in our experience and that of others. Livingston and Richardson[41] studied 28 patients surviving severe chest injury. Although pulmonary function was markedly abnormal 2 weeks after hospital discharge, rapid improvement was noted in all parameters by 4 months and, at later follow-up 1 to 11 yr later, disability was present in less than 5%.

REFERENCES

1. Duval P. *War Wounds of the Lungs.* Bristol, England: John Wright; 1918.
2. Campbell E, Colton J. *The Surgery of Theodoric.* vol. I. Translated from the Latin by Campbell and Colton.
3. Beaumont W. *Experiments and Observations on the Gastric Juice and the Physiology of Digestion.* Pittsburg, NY: FP Allen; 1833.
4. Hewson W. *The Works of William Hewson, FRS.* Gulliver G, ed. London: Sydenham Society; 1846.
5. Meade RH. *A History of Thoracic Surgery.* Springfield, IL: Charles C Thomas; 1961.
6. Benzinger T. Physiologic effects of blast in air and water. In *U.S. Air Force Aviation Medicine WW II.* vol II. Washington, DC: Department of the Air Force; 1950.
7. Burford TH, Burbank B. Traumatic wet lung: observations on certain physiologic fundamentals in thoracic trauma. *J Thorac Cardiovasc Surg.* 1945;14:415.
8. Eiseman B, Ashbaugh DG. Pulmonary effects of nonthoracic trauma. *J Trauma.* 1968.
9. McNamara JJ, Messersmith JK, Dunn RA, et al. Thoracic injuries in combat casualties in Vietnam. *Ann Thorac Surg.* 1970;10:389.
10. Graham JM, Mattox KL, Beall AC Jr. Penetrating trauma of the lung. *J Trauma.* 1979;19:665.
11. Mogissi K. Lacerations of the lung following blunt trauma. *Thorax.* 1971;26:223.
12. Carr RE. Injuries to the pulmonary parenchyma and vasculature. In: Daughtry DC, ed. *Thoracic Trauma.* Boston: Little, Brown; 1980.
13. Kemmerer WT, Eckert WG, Gathright JB, et al. Patterns of thoracic injury in fatal traffic accidents. *J Trauma.* 1961;1:595.
14. Jenkins MT, Jones RF, Wilson B, Moyer CA. Congestive atelectasis. *Ann Surg.* 1950;132:372.
15. Shorr RM, Crittenden M, Indeck M. Blunt thoracic trauma: analysis of 515 patients. *Ann Surg.* 1987;206:200.
16. Nakayama DK, Ramenofsuy ML, Rowe MI. Chest injuries in childhood. *Ann Surg.* 1989;210:770.
17. Kishikawa M, Yoshiona T, Shimazu T, et al. Pulmonary contusion causes long-term respiratory dysfunction with decreased functional residual capacity. *J Trauma.* 1991;31:1203.
18. Wagner RB. Effect of lung contusion on pulmonary hemodynamics. *Ann Thorac Surg.* 1991;52:51.
19. Rosato RM, Shapiro MJ, Keegan MJ. Cardiac injury complicating traumatic asphyxia. *J Trauma.* 1991;31:1387.
20. Johnson RS. Pulmonary laceration complicating closed chest injury. *Br J Dis Chest.* 1967;61:205.
21. Hankins TR, McAslan TC, Shin B, et al. Extensive pulmonary laceration caused by blunt trauma. *J Thorac Cardiovasc Surg.* 1977;74:519.
22. Richardson JD. Indications for thoracotomy in thoracic trauma. *Curr Surg.* 1985;42:361.
23. Bender TM, Oh KS, Medina JL, Girdany BR. Pediatric chest trauma. *J Thorac Imag.* 1987;2:60.
24. Pierson DJ. Persistent bronchopleural air leak during mechanical ventilation. *Respir Care.* 1982;17:408.
25. Conn JH. Thoracic trauma. *J Trauma.* 1963;3:22.
26. Fulton RL, Peter ET, Wilson JN. The pathophysiology of pulmonary contusions. *J Trauma.* 1970,10.719.
27. Thomas AH, Roe BB. Air embolism following penetrating lung injuries. *J Thorac Cardiovasc Surg.* 1973;66:533.
28. Fischer RP, Geiger JP, Guernsey JM. Pulmonary resection for severe pulmonary contusions secondary to high velocity missile wounds. *J Trauma.* 1974;14:293.
29. Errion AR. Pulmonary hematoma due to blunt non-penetrating thoracic trauma. *Am Rev Respir Dis.* 1963;88:384.
30. Tacino I, Miller MH. Computed tomography in blunt chest trauma. *J Thorac Imag.* 1987;2:45.
31. McCaughey W, Coppel DL, Dundee JM. Blast injuries of the lungs. *Anaesthesia.* 1973;28:2.
32. Zuckerman S. Experimental studies of blast injury to the lungs. *Lancet.* 1940;2:219.
33. Steiner RB, Adolph VR, Heaton JF. Pediatric extracorporeal membrane oxygenation in posttraumatic respiratory failure. *J Pediatr Surg.* 1991;26:1011.
34. Jongewaard WR, Cogbill TH, Landercasper J. Neurologic consequences of traumatic asphyxia. *J Trauma.* 1992;32:28.
35. Kirsh MM, Sloan H. *Blunt Chest Trauma: General Principles and Management.* Boston: Little, Brown; 1971.
36. Daughtery DC. Traumatic torsion of the lung. *N Engl J Med.* 1961;256:318.
37. Stratmeier EH, Barry JW. Torsion of the lung following thoracic trauma. *Radiology.* 1954;62:726.
38. Scannel JG. Pulmonary resection—anatomy and techniques. In Glenn WWL, ed. *Thoracic and Cardiovascular Surgery.* 4th ed. Norwalk, CT: Appleton-Century-Crofts; 1983.
39. Powell RJ, Redan JA, Swan KG. The hilar snare, an improved technique for securing rapid vascular control of the pulmonary hilum. *J Trauma.* 1990;30:208.
40. Yellin A, Yellin EO, Lieberman Y. Percutaneous tube drainage: the treatment of choice for refractory lung abscess. *Ann Thorac Surg.* 1985;39:266.
41. Livingston DH, Richardson JD. Pulmonary disability after severe blunt chest trauma. *J Trauma.* 1990;30:562.

15

Cardiac Injury: Contusion, Tamponade, Laceration, Rupture, Internal Derangement, and Foreign Bodies

DAVID M. FOLLETTE, M.D.

HISTORY: Since the earliest time, the unique vulnerability of the heart to trauma has been noted. Homeric stories often referred to the fatal aspects of heart wounds. In Pupel's translation of the Iliad (Grube) "Patroklos wounded Sarpedon with a javelin—the insulting victor with disdain bestrode the prostrate prince, and on his bosom trod: The weapon from his panting heart, the reeking fibers clinging to the dart. From the wide wound gushed a stream of blood, and the soul issued in the purple flood."[1]

Although Holerius in the 16th century questioned the belief that all heart wounds are fatal, it was Tourby in 1642 who found a scar in the heart of a man who had been wounded by a sword 4 years earlier (Table 15–1).[1]

In 1855, Purple published an article describing 42 recorded cases of heart wounds. He found that all wounds examined were not immediately fatal and that, although the right ventricle was most frequently injured, the duration of life was greater if the left ventricle was the one involved.[2]

In 1878, Fischer published a series of 452 heart injuries. A number of these recovered spontaneously.[1] In 1871, Collender successfully removed a needle from the heart.[1]

In September 1895, Cappelen[3] in Christiania operated on a patient with a heart wound and sutured it. Although the patient died 2½ days later, the case attracted much attention because of the temporary survival and the demonstrated feasibility of suturing the heart.

In 1897, Ludwig Rehn[4] of Frankfurt am Main reported the case of a young man who was stabbed in the heart, in the right ventricle, which was successfully repaired. By 1903, Ricketts of Cincinnati was able to report that 20 of 56 wounds of the heart had been successfully operated on.[1] In 1926, Claude Beck[5] worked out the technique for control of cardiac bleeding by stopping cardiac inflow through manual compression of the great vessels via an approach through the transverse sinus. He also emphasized digital control of the bleeding point during placement of cardiac sutures and described the optimal technique for suturing the heart.[5]

In 1935, Bigger[6] reported a series of cardiac wounds and advocated midline sternotomy as the best approach to the heart. He classified wounds into two types. In the first, the wound of the heart was not associated with a free wound into the pleural cavity. The symptoms were a result of the accumulation of blood in the pericardial cavity and the development of cardiac tamponade. The second type of cardiac wound consisted of free communication of the wound in the heart with the pleural cavity. These patients inevitably died of hemorrhage before treatment could be instituted.[6]

The most extensive study of blunt trauma of the heart was that of Bright and Beck in 1935.[7] All but a few patients died. According to them, the first survivor was a 23-year-old man reported by Moullin and Mansel in 1895. He had had a football injury that resulted in tamponade that was decompressed surgically.

In 1917, Escaude and Brueg[8] in France wrote that seven bullets had been removed from patients in which the bullet was embedded in the myocardium. Four patients were cured by the operation; in one, the bullet migrated to the hypogastric vein from which it was successfully removed.[8]

The greatest technical advance in thoracic trauma management during World War II was said by Meade to have been that of Harken, who removed 56 foreign bodies from the heart, 13 from the cardiac chambers themselves. Harken had no deaths, and all patients recovered completely; he credited his success to the ready availability of large quantities of banked blood.[9]

ANATOMY OF THE HEART

The heart lies in the anterior mediastinum, extending roughly from the level of the third costal cartilage to the sternoxiphoid junction. When evaluating the possibility of cardiac

Table 15–1.   Historical Cardiac Trauma

Tourby (1642)	Spontaneous survival
Collender (1871)	Needle removal
Purple (1855)	42 injuries
Cappelan (1855)	First suture
Rehn (1897)	First success
Escaude and Broeq (1917)	Removal of intracardiac bullets

injuries, projection of the anatomy of the heart on the anterior chest is appropriate (Fig. 15–1). The superior border of the heart is represented by a line drawn across the sternum at the level of the third costal cartilage from points 2.5 cm lateral to either sternal margin. This represents the clinical base of the heart or its line of demarcation from the great vessels. The normal extreme left margin of the heart lies at a point just inferior to the nipple in the left fifth intercostal space.

The location and shape of the heart varies with the changes in position of the diaphragm. When the diaphragm is high, the heart lies in a horizontal plane, and the long axis of the base and apex form a wide angle to the midsternal plane. In a long thorax with a low-placed diaphragm, the heart hangs in a more dependent position in the chest cavity, its base apex line forming a more acute angle with the midsternal line.

The anterior projection of the right atrium reaches from the third to the sixth costal cartilage about 1 to 2 cm lateral to the right sternal border. The right ventricular margin generally runs just lateral to the left margin of the sternum. Most of the anterior surface of the heart is represented by the right atrium and its auricular appendage superiorly and the right ventricle below. Only a small strip of left ventricle at the cardiac apex is seen from a

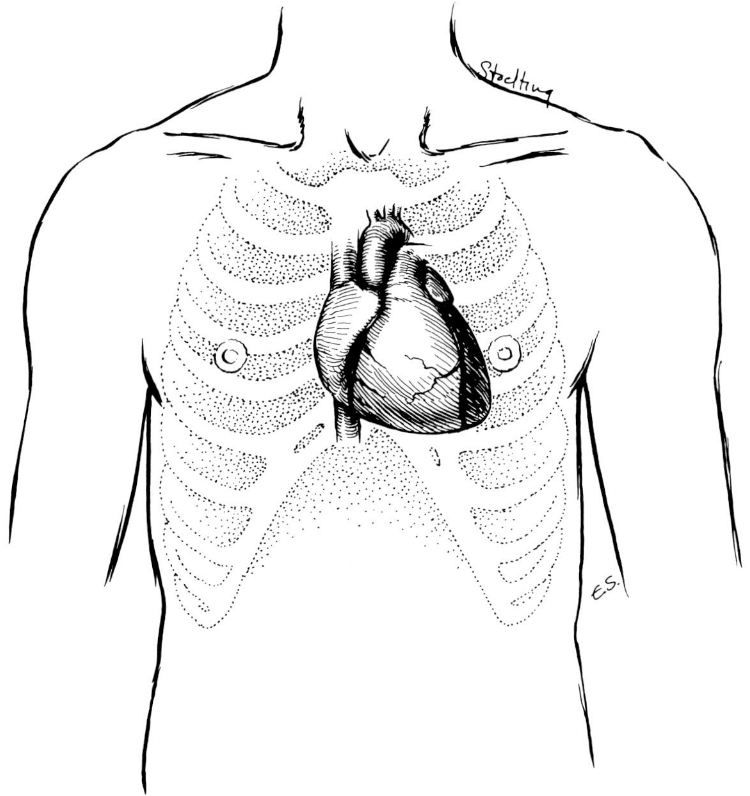

Figure 15–1.   Location of the heart relative to chest anatomy. The right atrium and ventricle comprise most of the anatomy anteriorly.

direct anterior view. The relative location of the intracardiac anatomy including the valves is shown in Figure 15–2.

The definitive anatomy of the heart and the intrapericardial great vessels is shown in Figure 15–3. The anterior surface of the heart is represented by the right ventricular outflow tract superiorly on the left and the right atrium on the right. The right ventricle constitutes two-thirds of the anterior surface of the heart when visualized on direct anteroposterior view, with only a small wedge of left atrium exposed near the apex of the heart at the level of the sixth interspace and seventh rib just inside the midclavicular line.

The right lateral view of the heart shows that it is composed in the upper half by the superior vena cava posteriorly (Fig. 15–3), the aorta above and anteriorly, and the right atrium anteriorly and below the aorta with its auricular appendix projecting forward toward the sternum. The lower half of the right lateral cardiac surface is composed of the right ventricle anteriorly and small portion of the inferior vena cava inferiorly and posteriorly.

As reviewed from the left lateral position (Fig. 15–3), the left atrial appendage projects anteriorly to the pulmonary hilum and lies anterior to the pulmonary artery. The left atrium constitutes a large portion of the superior portion of the pericardial contents. The left ventricle constitutes the inferior two-thirds of the lateral border and most of the posterior aspect of the heart. The left atrium constitutes the remainder. The pulmonary veins, both right and left, drain into the left atrium at the posterior aspect of the heart behind the vena cava on the right and in front of the descending aorta on the left.

The aorta takes origin from the left ventricle behind the pulmonary artery and crosses under the main pulmonary artery, then anterior and to the right of this vessel. The

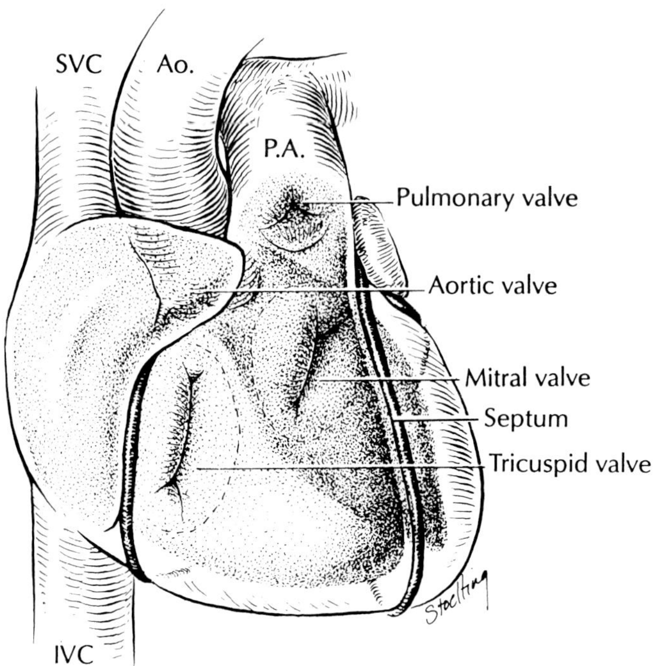

Figure 15–2.   The gross cardiac anatomy with the location of the cardiac valves.

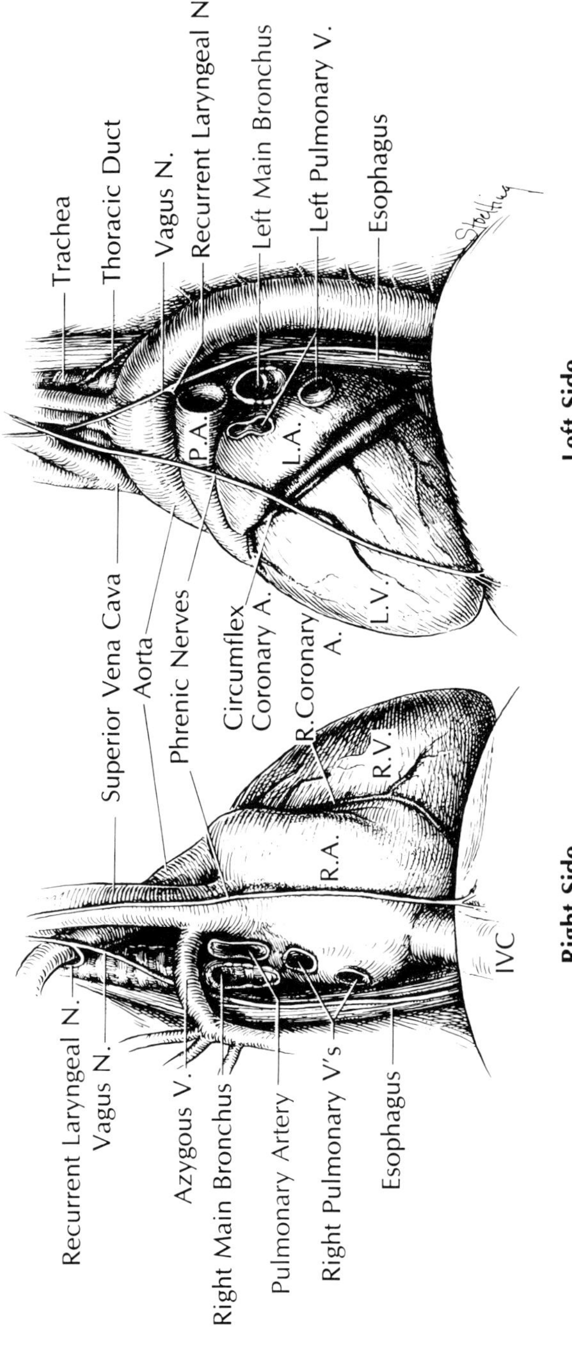

Figure 15–3. The external anatomy of the heart as viewed from the right, anterior, and left, corresponding to the exposure seen from right lateral thoracotomy, median sternotomy, and left lateral thoracotomy.

pulmonary artery extends upward to the left and branches under the aortic arch; the right pulmonary artery passes under the ascending aorta. The right lateral cusp of the aortic valve is the only cusp not providing a takeoff point for a coronary artery. The anterior lateral valve sinus provides the site of origin for the right coronary artery. The right coronary artery extends laterally and posteriorly in the atrioventricular groove, then descends laterally in the posterior interventricular groove to the apex of the heart.

The left main coronary artery takes origin in the sinus of the left posterior coronary cusp, passes in the arteriovenous groove behind the pulmonary artery for a short distance, and, at the anterior interventricular junction, bifurcates into the anterior descending and the circumflex coronary arteries. The anterior descending artery extends downward in the groove between the two ventricles along the anterior surface of the heart to its apex. The circumflex coronary artery extends laterally and posteriorly in the atrioventricular groove, giving rise to marginal branches to the left ventricle and extending nearly to the posterior descending coronary artery.

The pericardium encircles the heart, is attached to the diaphragm inferiorly, and extends onto the right and left pulmonary arteries. It encompasses the ascending aorta and extends upward to where it is reflected off the inferior surface of the aortic arch. It encircles both ventricles, the origins of the pulmonary veins, and the superior and inferior vena cavae. It is supplied by blood vessels from the internal mammary artery.

The phrenic nerve passes down the lateral pericardium on each side anterior to the hilum of the lung to extend onto the diaphragm. The vagus nerves, after giving off recurrent laryngeal branches to the larynx, pass downward posterior to the pulmonary hilum and give rise to pulmonary and cardiac branches before descending into the abdomen and the esophagus.

ETIOLOGY AND INCIDENCE

Traumatic injuries to the heart are of two distinct types: blunt and penetrating. Most of these cardiac injuries are due to penetrating trauma.[10]

Blunt injuries are secondary to compression, deceleration, blast, direct blows to the chest, or increased intravascular pressure associated with compression of abdominal contents. Any action that transports kinetic energy to the heart may cause injury. Automobile accidents are the most common cause of blunt cardiac trauma. The mechanism is most often the steering wheel; the thoracic contents are compressed between the sternum and vertebrae during sudden deceleration (Fig. 15–4). It has been estimated that nearly 900,000 cases of cardiac trauma occur each year in automobile accidents.[11] In individuals with severe chest trauma, usually with sternal and rib fractures, the incidence of blunt cardiac injury may average 30%.[12,13]

Most patients who survive blunt cardiac trauma are in the younger age group. The resiliency of the chest wall in younger patients can result in no associated bony trauma in one-third, even though they have cardiac injury. Thus, the absence of visible trauma may result in delay of the diagnosis of potentially severe cardiac injury. The cardiac damage from blunt trauma includes the types outlined in Table 15–2. The excellent autopsy review of Parmley and co-workers[14] of primary blunt cardiac injury details more fully the pathologic states found. If one looks at all blunt thoracic trauma, cardiac trauma is somewhat rare. In a recent review from the Maryland Institute of Emergency Medical

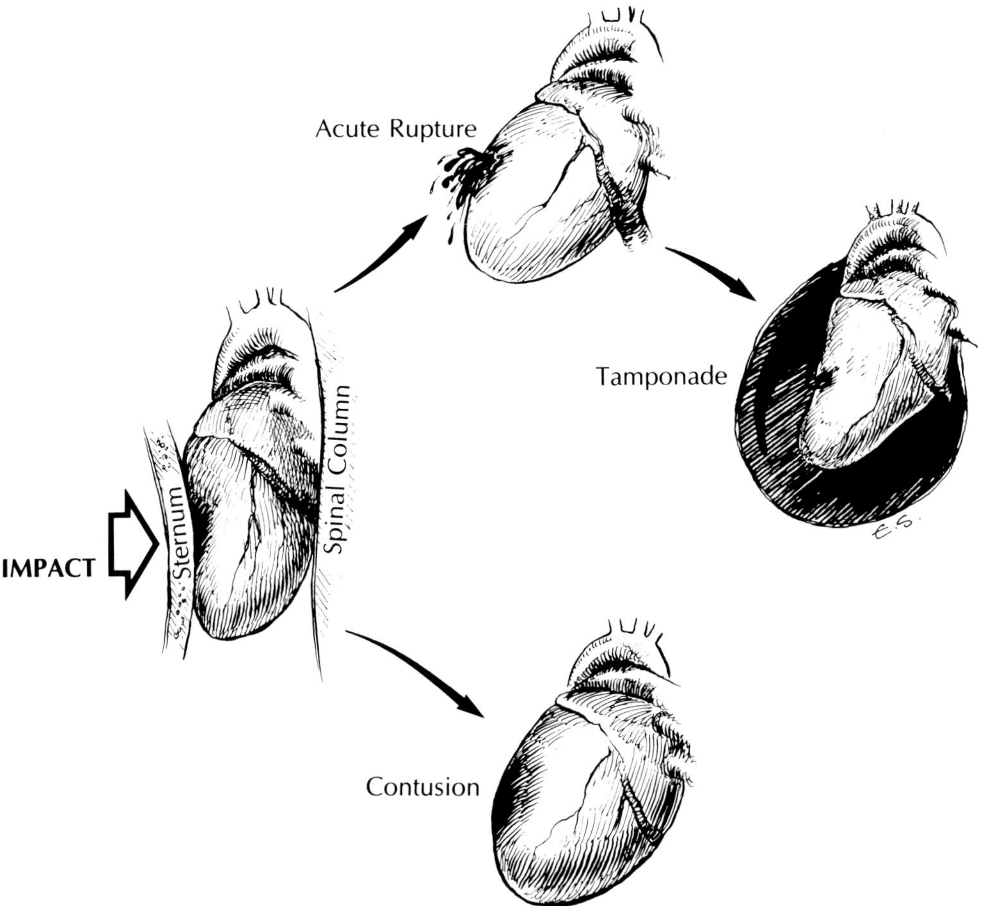

Figure 15–4. Mechanism and nature of blunt cardiac injury. The impact may result in acute rupture, tamponade, or contusion.

Services, blunt cardiac injuries represented less than 10% of total cases of blunt thoracic trauma.[15]

Penetrating injuries are caused by knives, missiles, or bullets. Knife wounds constitute the most common type of penetrating injury presenting to the emergency room, presumably because gunshot wounds are more immediately lethal.

Penetrating wounds of the heart produce a similar spectrum of myocardial, pericardial, and coronary artery injuries, including laceration of cardiac chambers, septa, valves, coronary arteries, and great vessels (Table 15–3), and may result in fistula formation. Aside from such wounding agents as penetrating missiles, fractured ribs, and sternal fragments, migratory foreign bodies also have been known to produce cardiac problems. Except for the massive destructive nature of shotgun wounds, most patients with penetrating wounds to the contents of the pericardial sac have a far better survival rate than those with blunt trauma, for less tissue damage is sustained.

Table 15–2. Types of Blunt Cardiac Injury

Myocardial
  Contusion
  Infarction
  Rupture
  Septal perforation
  Intracardiac shunts
  Arrhythmias
Coronary arterial
  Perivascular hematoma
  Intimal laceration
  Thrombosis
  Division
Valvular
  Rupture of valve cusps
  Rupture of papillary muscles or chordae tendinae
Pericardial
  Hemopericardium, cardiac tamponade
  Traumatic pericarditis, postpericardiotomy syndrome
  Constrictive pericarditis
  Pericardial rupture
  Cardiac herniation

PATHOPHYSIOLOGY

The extent of the injury to the pericardium often determines the survival of the patient in penetrating injuries to the heart. In general, patients with penetrating cardiac trauma who survive to reach the hospital have some degree of pericardial tamponade. If the myocardial injury produces insignificant bleeding, a small laceration in the pericardium may quickly become occluded with clot or adjacent tissue and prevent exsanguination while simultaneously reducing cardiac distention and, thus, the rate of myocardial bleeding. Patients who present to the emergency room with pericardial tamponade tend to have a better survival rate than patients with equivalent degrees of shock who do not.[16,17] However, a large tear in the pericardium may allow exsanguination through rapid emptying of the contents of the pericardium into the thorax. This type of injury is most commonly associated with a gunshot wound and can result in a high mortality.[18] Wounds of the thick muscular myocardium, when slit-like or linear, frequently seal with clot before large volumes of blood are lost. However, hemorrhage from atrial wounds seldom spontaneously stops, and slow but persistent bleeding is the rule in those who survive the immediate injury.

Frank myocardial infarction secondary to direct extensive myocardial damage or due to coronary artery injury may occur after blunt trauma. This can lead to ventricular aneurysm formation, ventricular rupture, scarring, or endocardiac thrombus formation with its potential of systemic embolization. Blunt trauma to the chest also can lead to combined injuries to both the heart and great vessels. Several cases of simultaneous rupture of the heart and the aorta have been reported.[19] Pseudoaneurysm of the thoracic aorta and rupture of the ventricular septum[20] and tricuspid valve[21] have been seen. Acute aortic valvular incompetence[22] and injuries to the pulmonary veins and left atrium[23] have been documented as well.

Table 15–3.   Penetrating Cardiac Trauma

Myocardium
  Laceration
  Perforation
  Septal perforation
  Intracardiac shunt
  Infarction
Coronary arteries
  Laceration
  Division
Valve
  Incompetence
Tamponade
Hemothorax

Recently a great deal of emphasis has been placed on the importance of wearing a seat belt. Although seat belts definitely save lives, they do not prevent cardiac injury, especially in high-speed motor vehicle accidents. It is interesting to note that patients who die from ventricular rupture with a seat belt in place generally have left ventricular rupture, whereas nonbelted drivers usually have right ventricular injury.[24] A person in a motor vehicle accident can suffer significant blunt cardiac injury even though wearing a seat belt.

In patients sustaining significant blunt trauma, traumatic asphyxia may occur. This syndrome has a triad of symptoms that occurs on the head and neck. Patients often present with striking petechiae, subconjunctival hemorrhage, and cranial/cervical cyanosis. It has been recognized recently that up to a third of these patients also may have a significant cardiac injury. Therefore, any patients who present with the classic signs of traumatic asphyxia should have a thorough evaluation to exclude a cardiac diagnosis as well.[25]

DIAGNOSIS

Because of the variety of physical forces that can result in cardiac trauma, the extent of damage may not be readily assessable or even recognizable in view of the often distracting and life-threatening injuries sustained. Thus, it is important in all patients with potential cardiac injuries that the diagnosis be considered and a thorough physical examination be carried out, with attention directed toward those signs that may establish the diagnosis of a cardiac injury. Both penetrating and blunt trauma can produce acute changes, but *penetrating trauma* is statistically a much more common cause of acute changes.

The accurate diagnosis of cardiac injury requires a careful review of the factors causing the injury. In cases of penetrating wounds, knowledge of the type of instrument used, including direction of the force applied and the angle of entry and exit, all facilitate diagnosis, exposure, and treatment of the injury. For this reason, entrance and exit sites of wounding agents should be indicated with radiopaque material that will show on the chest and abdominal x-ray films.

Rapid assessment of hemodynamic parameters including pulse, blood pressure, and neck vein status should be done. Venous pressure should be measured by central vein catheter placement. A chest radiograph, electrocardiogram, and blood gas analysis should be obtained. Simultaneously, blood should be drawn for typing and cross-match. A urinary catheter should be placed to monitor urinary output as a guide to vital organ perfusion. Objective signs of cardiac tamponade, such as Beck's triad,[5] which includes pulsus paradoxus, muffled heart sounds, and neck vein distention, often are missing.[26] The lack of changes noted on radiographs or electrocardiograms should not divert the examiner's attention away from the possibility of underlying cardiac injury. In selected cases, an echocardiogram may be beneficial in the assessment of precordial trauma.[27] Manifestations of cardiac injuries common to both blunt and penetrating trauma are given in Table 15–4.

Pericardiocentesis (Fig. 15–5) may facilitate the diagnosis of tamponade, but its use as definitive treatment is not condoned, except as a form of temporary therapy. Its use is of greatest value in the diagnosis and treatment of chronic or late-appearing pericardial effusions. Even if emergency pericardiocentesis is attempted, the examining physician must understand that false positive or negative results occur in at least one-third to one-half of patients.[26,28]

Pericardiocentesis is easily accomplished with an 18- or 20-gauge spinal needle or an equivalent-sized plastic sheathed needle. This is advanced directly upward from the left paraxiphoid position aiming 45° posteriorly. Blood coming from the hub of the needle or the small syringe during aspiration may be either from the pericardial space or a cardiac chamber. Twenty-five to 50 ml of blood should be aspirated, if possible. A prompt improvement in vital signs is diagnostic of an intrapericardial location. Although a failure of the aspirated blood to clot also is a manifestation of pericardial blood, this requires 5 to 10 min of observation, which is not practical under urgent, life-threatening circumstances.

An alternative to ascertain if blood aspirated came from a cardiac chamber is to connect the nub of the exploring needle to the chest lead of the electrocardiogram and constantly record the electrocardiogram as the needle is advanced. A giant electrocardiographic complex (current of injury) indicates contact of the needle tip with the myocardium, whereas aspiration of blood and no change in the electrocardiographic reading indicates that the needle tip is in the pericardial space. At this point a guidewire should be passed through the needle and the needle withdrawn. Over the wire, a plastic catheter can then be inserted safely and the pericardial fluid aspirated. If echocardiography is available, this can be a useful adjunct in determining how completely the pericardial space has been emptied. Placement of the indwelling plastic catheter is advantageous if thoracotomy is delayed because it permits repeated or continuous decompression of the pericardial space.

Clinically, *blunt cardiac injury* can be divided into two types: acute and subacute. The *acute type* is the catastrophic injury that causes death immediately or soon after if surgical

Table 15–4.   Manifestations of Cardiac Injuries

Tamponade
Hemorrhage
Shunts
Foreign body
Myocardial failure
Arrhythmias
Valve insufficiency
Myocardial ischemia

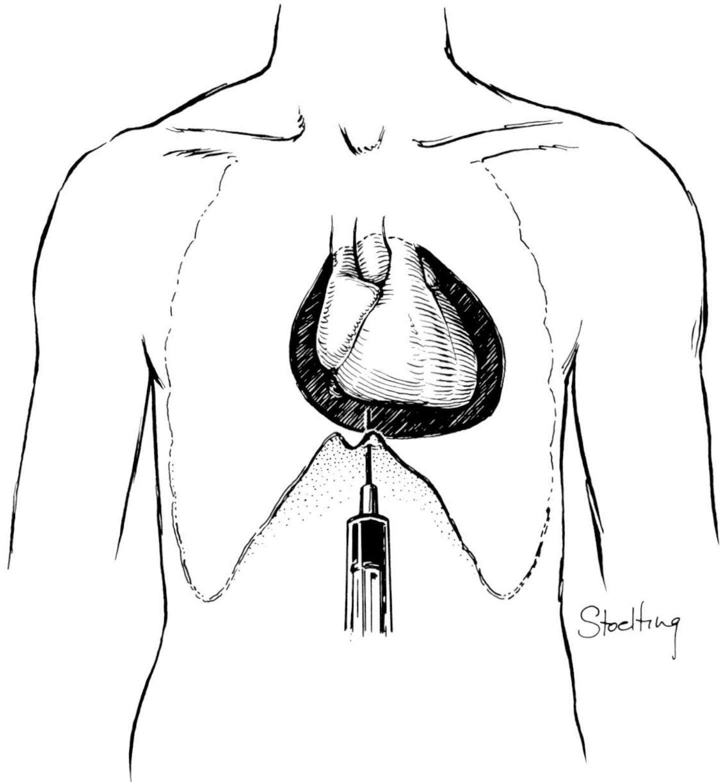

Figure 15–5. Technique of pericardiocentesis. The aspirating needle is advanced upward from the paraxiphoid area toward the sternal notch at an angle of 45° to the skin.

intervention is not undertaken (Table 15–5). These injuries are cardiac chamber rupture with acute pericardial tamponade, combined chamber and pericardial rupture with bleeding into the pleural cavity, and acute myocardial damage with cardiogenic shock. The diagnosis of acute injury usually is not difficult to make because the patient presents in severe shock refractory to rapid fluid resuscitation and remains in shock. A chest radiograph will identify the chest as the source of hemorrhage. Neck veins, if distended, help identify acute pericardial tamponade. However, if hypovolemic shock is associated, distended neck veins may never become apparent. Acute injuries, although lethal in themselves, usually have 6 to 10 associated solid organ and soft tissue injuries.

The *subacute type* of blunt cardiac injury may not cause immediate death but may diminish cardiac reserve and put the patient at risk for death from cardiac and hemodynamic complications (Table 15–5). The subacute injuries include myocardial contusion, subacute pericardial tamponade, myocardial infarction, valvular injury, intracardiac shunts, mural thrombi, and arrhythmias (Table 15–5).

The diagnosis of these injuries may be difficult because of other associated injuries, the lack of physical evidence of chest and cardiac trauma, and the nonspecificity or nonsensitivity of electrocardiography, creatine kinase (CK) isoenzymes, chest radiograph, and technetium pyrophosphate scans. In contrast to the patient with acute cardiac injury, the

Table 15–5.   Cardiac Injuries

Acute
Cardiac chamber rupture and tamponade
Pericardial and cardiac chamber rupture
    and exsanguination into the pleural space
Myocardial contusion with heart failure

Subacute
Cardiac contusion without heart failure
Myocardial infarction
Subacute pericardial tamponade
Valvular injury
Intracardiac septal defects
Mural thrombus
Cardiac arrhythmia

patient with a subacute injury has an average of 3.5 other associated soft tissue and solid organ injuries. Typically, this type of patient responds quickly to fluid resuscitation. This, however, may lead to a false sense of security and compromise the prompt recognition of the cardiac injury. On physical examination the chest wall may show little evidence of injury despite extensive underlying damage. Sternal tenderness is present in most patients with subacute cardiac injuries and is a key finding. The cardiac examination may be normal and distended neck veins present in only 30% of patients with pericardial tamponade. A new murmur or rub is the most frequent sign of cardiac damage in subacute injuries.

The *chest radiograph* will not be helpful in the acute stage of myocardial contusion, infarction, or valve injury. On *electrocardiographic* readings, diffuse ST-T changes frequently attributed to cardiac contusion instead may be due to acute anemia, hypovolemia, electrolyte disturbances during rapid fluid resuscitation, increased sympathetic or vagal tone, or tachycardia. New Q waves or heart block are reliable signs of significant cardiac injury (Fig. 15–6). Serial electrocardiographs are necessary to confirm injury in any patient

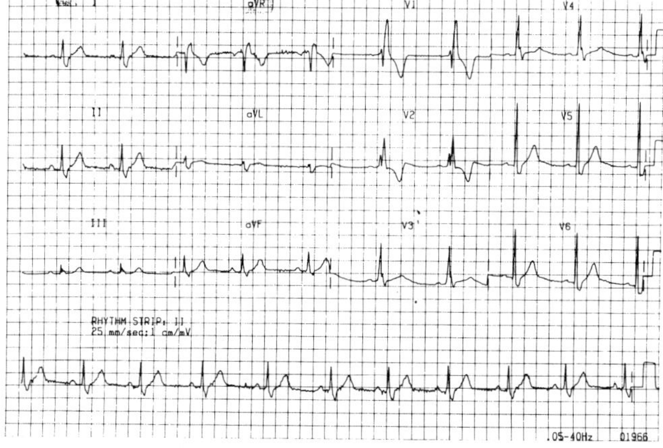

Figure 15–6.   Electrocardiogram in a patient with myocardial contusion. In this instance, left bundle branch block is seen.

and allow the physician to follow improvement or regression of electrical activity, but they do little to confirm immediately the presence of an acute injury.

The *CK isoenzymes* are not specific or sensitive for cardiac injury and impart a significant delay in making the diagnosis if they are used. The total CK value frequently is elevated into the thousands in patients with blunt trauma. The CK MB fraction frequently is elevated as well. The increase in total CK activity is principally due to skeletal muscle injury. Once believed to be specific for cardiac tissue, the MB fraction is found in significant amounts in skeletal muscle, urinary bladder, liver, stomach, pancreas, prostate, uterus, colon, small bowel, lung, and other tissue. It also is found in abnormally elevated amounts in the serum of athletes in training. It is therefore difficult to interpret the significance of the presence of the MB fraction in the serum of patients with blunt trauma. In addition, the CK MB fraction does not discriminate between injured chambers and will not detect valvular damage, coronary artery injury, pericardial effusion, or mural thrombus. It cannot be used to quantitate cardiac function.

A number of studies have illustrated the poor sensitivity of the *technetium pyrophosphate* scan for the detection of myocardial contusion.[29]

Another screening test currently available for blunt cardiac injury is the *two-dimensional echocardiogram*. It provides information on wall motion, septal motion, valvular and chordae integrity, pericardial effusion, mural thrombi, and ejection fraction (see Chapter 6). Although several reports have confirmed its efficacy in humans for detecting a spectrum of cardiac lesions,[30] it may not be that helpful in the diagnosis of myocardial contusion.[31] A new modality in the diagnosis of blunt as well as penetrating cardiac trauma is the use of transesophageal echocardiography. This test can give more accurate information on valvular lesions, septal defects, the degree in intracardiac shunt, and the possibility of concomitant injury to the great vessels[32] (see Chapter 6). If the echocardiogram demonstrates abnormal wall motion, then coronary angiography may be appropriate to assess the integrity of the major coronary arteries.

The aspect of cardiac injury that determines survival is the degree of remaining cardiac reserve at the time there is an increase in cardiac demand. When cardiac demand from the sequelae of multiple associated injuries becomes greater than cardiac output, circulatory collapse occurs. The best way to quantitate and monitor cardiac function is with the use of a *Swan-Ganz pulmonary artery catheter* (Chapter 2). Starling curves can be constructed and serial cardiac indices followed. Mixed venous samples can be drawn from the pulmonary artery port of the catheter to make the diagnosis of a traumatic left-to-right shunt. Any blunt trauma patient with unstable vital signs, an abnormal echocardiogram, or persistent hypoperfusion should have a pulmonary artery catheter inserted.

SPECIFIC INJURIES

Pericardial Injury

The most common acute cardiac emergency seen in the patient with penetrating or blunt trauma is acute *pericardial tamponade*. The pericardium is a closed fibrotic sac, relatively unyielding, that contains the heart, the distal portions of the vena cava, and the great vessels as they arise from the heart. The relatively rigid pericardium will not tolerate an acute accumulation of blood or fluid without significant hemodynamic consequences. The most common cause of acute tamponade in the trauma patient is chamber wall or coronary artery laceration, both having high immediate mortality.

The presence of Beck's triad,[5] defining cardiac tamponade, is useful when present and consists of paradoxical pulse, muffled heart sounds, and neck vein distention. Unfortunately, it is not routinely found even in the presence of severe acute pericardial effusion and tamponade.[26] In as many as one-third of patients seen with hemodynamically significant pericardial tamponade, blood pressure is unobtainable because of hypovolemic shock due to associated injuries. In the uncooperative or hypoxic thrashing patient, it is often impossible to assess the paradoxical pulse even if the blood pressure can be measured. The noisy environment of the emergency suite often does not allow the identification of subtly muffled heart sounds despite other evidence of pericardial tamponade, and neck vein distention is present initially in less than one-third of patients.

The classic sign on the chest radiograph is the "water bottle sign." On the upright film, the inferior margins of the heart may bulge outward, giving the appearance of a slumping canvas bottle of water (Fig. 15–7). In the acute injury situation, this sign often is minimal or absent. When tamponade is recognized, the treatment consists of immediate pericardial aspiration or surgical decompression.

Traumatic pericarditis results from accumulation of fibrin and extravasated red cells accompanied by sympathetic effusion after blunt chest trauma. Patients present with pericardial friction rub and have ST-T wave abnormalities on the electrocardiogram. Delayed cardiac tamponade after blunt chest trauma does occur, but it is unusual and

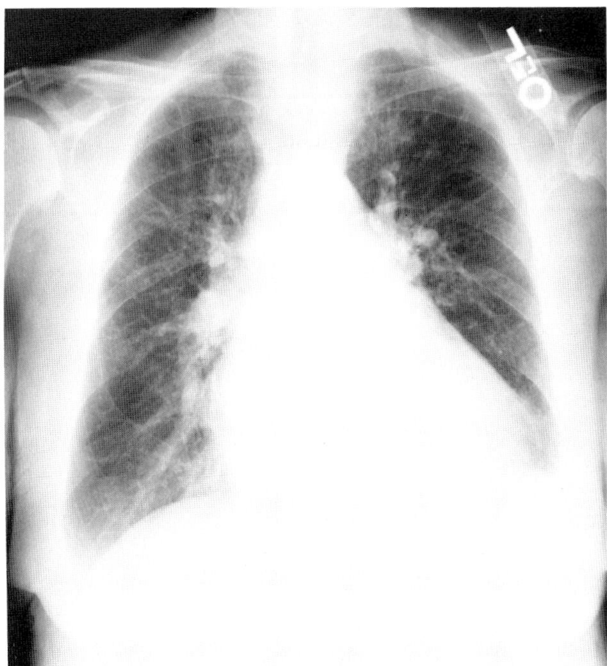

Figure 15–7.   Marked enlargement of the cardiac shadow. Aspiration of the pericardium confirmed pericardial tamponade.

usually can be handled by pericardiocentesis with the placement of a drainage catheter.[33] The onset of late tamponade often is insidious and the diagnosis confused with myocardial infarction, sepsis, or pulmonary embolization. Patients often will present with nausea, vomiting, marked fatigue, and shortness of breath. This particular symptom complex should alert the physician to the possibility of late cardiac tamponade syndrome.

The occurrence of this symptom complex or other signs of low cardiac output in an individual with blunt chest trauma alerts the physician to late pericardial effusion. Delayed tamponade also has been reported in patients after penetrating chest trauma and often presents in an insidious fashion such as seen in patients with blunt trauma.[34] Suggestion of pericardial tamponade requires a physical examination to check for clinical signs of tamponade. Electrocardiograms may demonstrate low voltage; however, the key to diagnosis is the demonstration on chest x-ray of marked cardiomegaly and the presence of pericardial effusion on an echocardiogram. In cases where constrictive pericarditis is suggested, a cardiac catheterization may be necessary to firmly establish the diagnosis.

Postpericardiotomy syndrome may occur after either penetrating or blunt trauma. It often presents with an insidious, low-grade fever, elevated erythrocyte sedimentation rate, nonspecific ST-T wave changes on an electrocardiogram, and unexplained chest pain. Again, echocardiography may be helpful to establish the diagnosis. Treatment consists of nonsteroidal agents such as Indocin or Motrin. Occasionally, treatment with corticosteroids may be necessary.

Pericardial Laceration

Pericardial laceration, single or multiple, can occur after blunt injury as an isolated event but more often is associated with extensive cardiac damage. The pericardium may rupture on the diaphragmatic or pleural surfaces. The latter is more common. It tends to occur on the left and parallel to the course of the phrenic nerve. Evisceration of the heart between the edges of the pericardial sac has been reported, with torsion of its great vessels acutely reducing cardiac output. Radiographic findings of an abnormal cardiac silhouette and air within the pericardium or below the heart that may be free or due to interposed lung should make the diagnosis. The lung in a normal expanded state prevents complete herniation of the heart. Thus, there is more likely to be hemodynamic compromise when there is simultaneous rupture of the pericardium and ipsilateral pneumothorax. Another complication of both penetrating and blunt trauma to the pericardium is the development of a tension pneumopericardium. This has been reported to occur after blunt and penetrating trauma.[35,36] Treatment of this condition usually consists of placement of a catheter in the pericardium.

Myocardial Contusion and Infarction

Myocardial contusion occurs in 20% of patients with severe chest trauma,[11] in 15% to 17%[12] of autopsied subjects of automobile accidents, and in as high as 76% of patients with severe multiple organ trauma.[13] It is a lesion that results primarily from blunt trauma.

The spectrum of pathologic lesions ranges from localized areas of ecchymoses a few millimeters in size on the epicardial surface of the heart to widespread myocardial fiber disruption. Extravasation of red blood cells and edema fluid results in reduced local microcoronary circulation. Diminished perfusion in areas of contusion may result from simultaneous coronary artery injury or damage to smaller vessels within the contusion and may lead to tissue necrosis and infarction. Because the injuries are acute, there is no opportunity for arterial collateral formation as occurs with slow, progressive atherosclerotic occlusions. Thus, the interruption of normal myocardial perfusion superimposed on direct tissue damage may result in a reduction in myocardial reserve, secondary not only to the injury but to the local tissue hypoxia.

Hypotension or hypovolemic shock in the multiple-organ injured patient further compromises coronary perfusion. Altered respiratory dynamics result in hypoxia and hypoxemia, a further challenge to myocardial function (Chapter 2). Myocardial insufficiency secondary to loss of myocardial reserve due to hypoxia, hypovolemia, and the stresses of trauma may tax the heart to a point where cardiac failure can occur after apparent trivial intrathoracic injury. Provided the work demanded of the heart does not exceed the reserve, the hemodynamic response of the heart, although marginal transiently, usually will respond to the body's needs. However, heightened hemodynamic demands after trauma in the presence of compromised myocardial blood flow results in clinical deterioration or significantly depressed cardiac output in more than half of patients with blunt cardiac trauma.[37]

In infants involved in automobile accidents, there is a significant potential for cardiac injury. Restraining car seats are equipped with horizontal bars that may impinge on the chest wall in deceleration accidents. These infants, because of their age, may not be able to express symptoms. As a result, the diagnosis is easily missed.[38]

The *diagnosis* of myocardial contusion can be difficult. The classic symptoms of significant myocardial contusion are limited to angina-like precordial pain found in one-fourth of patients. The accompanying chest pain may not be relieved by nitroglycerin.

The problem of identifying myocardial contusion in the multiple-organ injured patient relates to the lack of specific clinical signs pointing to significant cardiac injury. After blunt trauma to the heart, arrhythmias occur in as many as 20% of patients.[37] These may represent the only diagnostic clue that the heart has been injured. They consist of supraventricular tachycardia or atrial fibrillation, often with spontaneous reversion to normal sinus rhythm (Table 15–6). Repetitive ventricular ectopic beats leading to ventricular fibrillation are rare. Conduction defects are also uncommon but, if they do occur, may be a result of injury to the sinus nodal artery or the right coronary artery. These vessels usually supply blood flow to the bundle of His and its branches. The conduction defects may range from bundle branch block to complete heart block.

Often the diagnosis of myocardial contusion is entertained only after the electrocardio-

Table 15–6.   Myocardial Injury, Electrocardiograhic Changes

Ventricular premature complexes
Right bundle branch block
Paroxysmal atrial tachycardia
Inverted T waves
Nonspecific ST-T
Sinus tachycardia
Sinus bradycardia

gram and enzyme studies done on admission are checked serially to detect changes. Diagnosis, however, can be difficult. Other tests that have been used include pyrophosphate scanning, radionucleotide assessment of ventricular function, and echocardiography. A number of studies have documented that although these tests can document myocardial contusion, they do not significantly alter the management or the outcome once the diagnosis is established.[31,39–42] Electrocardiogram remains the best diagnostic test to predict the severity and the clinical impact of myocardial contusion.[43,44] Electrocardiographic changes usually consist of ST-T wave alterations returning to normal within 2 to 3 weeks. Often the initial electrocardiographic reading is normal and ST-T wave changes will develop within 4 hours. It is unusual for significant changes to occur after this period of time.[43] Transmural myocardial infarction can occur and new Q waves support this diagnosis. The actual incidence of electrocardiographic evidence of cardiac injury after blunt chest trauma has been estimated between 17% and 38%.

The *treatment* of myocardial contusion is supportive and expectant, with bed rest, supplemental oxygen, and careful monitoring of hemodynamics, including left ventricular filling pressures and cardiac output. These measures of cardiac function will dictate fluid and drug therapy. The most common cause of early death after myocardial contusion is arrhythmia, normally ventricular tachycardia or fibrillation. These can be managed with lidocaine intravenously. The key to success, however, is diagnosis. Thus, careful monitoring is essential in patients who demonstrate significant evidence of heart block, bundle-branch block, premature ventricular contractions (PVCs), and other conduction abnormalities. If no evidence of cardiac failure or further arrhythmias occurs during observation in the emergency department, these patients can be observed in unmonitored beds.[31]

Coronary Artery Lacerations

Wounds to coronary arteries present with pericardial tamponade and electrocardiographic abnormalities, including evidence of myocardial ischemia and often an associated hemothorax, and usually are the result of penetrating injuries, although on rare occasions they may be the result of blunt trauma.

Proximal right and left main coronary artery divisions after penetrating trauma are fatal, as often are lacerations to the left anterior descending or left circumflex arteries proximal to the first major branches.

The acute division of a major coronary artery may result in myocardial failure, shock, ventricular ectopic activity, and often either tamponade or exsanguination. Laceration of distal small coronary arteries may produce an area of infarction. Arrhythmias or chronic aneurysm formation may follow, depending on the location of the wound and presence of collaterals.

The left anterior descending coronary artery that lies beneath the sternum is the site of most blunt injuries. The right coronary artery also is vulnerable, usually within 2 cm of its origin. The right coronary artery can also be damaged directly by torsion of the heart, with displacement of the cardiac mass caudally and to the left. This produces a stretch injury to the proximal artery just distal to its origin.

Complete occlusion or severance of a main coronary artery at the time of blunt injury usually results in death. In survivors with coronary injury, intimal damage, intramural hemorrhage, or perivascular contusion can lead to late critical narrowing and thrombosis.

Hemodynamic deterioration or even sudden death may occur days to weeks after the injury, with extensive or progressive hypoperfusion of a large segment of myocardium.

The *diagnosis* of coronary artery injury is most commonly made if acute pericardial tamponade is present because surgical treatment of the tamponade leads to discovery of the lesion. Unexplained arrhythmias or evidence of myocardial ischemia may lead to diagnostic work-up, including angiography, or to emergency surgery.

The late development of an aneurysm of the ventricle more often follows distal coronary artery laceration or widespread myocardial contusion, as after shotgun blasts or tangential gunshot wounds. The signs and symptoms of an aneurysm may be due to reduced cardiac output, arrhythmias, or systemic embolization. There may be electrocardiographic evidence of transmural injury and an abnormal radiograph of the cardiac silhouette.

Survivors of coronary artery laceration may develop not only myocardial infarction and ventricular aneurysm but, more rarely, coronary artery and cardiac chamber fistulas. This latter entity appears late due to slow reabsorption of adjacent traumatized myocardium in continuity with a coronary artery injury. Elective repair is indicated in almost all such occurrences.

The *treatment* of myocardial infarction secondary to coronary artery trauma is expectant and conservative. Few cases of myocardial infarction after blunt chest trauma have been well documented by angiography; thus, the need for immediate coronary artery bypass is rarely recognized. The extensive nature of associated organ injuries contraindicates heparinization and the use of thrombolytic agents. In view of the extent of myocardial wall damage associated with blunt coronary artery injury, thromboendarterectomy or percutaneous transluminal dilation probably will not be successful. Delayed coronary arteriography, after recovery, may be totally unrevealing due to subsequent resolution of the intraluminal thrombosis.

Myocardial Laceration and Rupture

Lacerations of the myocardium most commonly result from penetrating trauma, that is, knives rather than guns. Myocardial rupture is a lesion of blunt trauma, and only a small percentage of patients with these injuries survive to reach the hospital.

The chambers most often involved with penetrating injuries are the anterior, more exposed, right ventricle, followed in lesser frequency by the left ventricle, right atrium, and left atrium. The mortality from injuries to the left ventricle is twice that of the right,[26] and the prehospital mortality from penetrating trauma is 60% to 80%.[1,45–47]

Myocardial rupture often is the immediate cause of death at the scene of an automobile accident and is an autopsy finding in approximately two-thirds of immediate fatalities.[14] Delayed cardiac rupture may occur 1 to 2 weeks after blunt trauma at the height of myocardial necrosis. It may follow faulty scar formation in the nutritionally deprived multiple-organ damaged patient.

The reduced incidence of isolated atrial rupture relates to the ability of blood to be translocated from the atrium into the compliant systemic or pulmonary venous bed.

In the review of Parmley and associates[14] of patients with blunt cardiac chamber rupture who reached the hospital and for whom survival times were available, 13 patients with damage to the atria lived for 30 min to 3 days and one patient with right ventricular rupture survived 6 hr.

The *diagnosis* of acute cardiac laceration or transmural rupture is suggested by shock disproportionate to suspected blood loss or other organ injuries. It is manifested most often by acute pericardial tamponade.

The *treatment* of myocardial laceration or rupture should be immediate surgery. Emergency thoracotomy for trauma to the heart should be performed in the operating room rather than the emergency room if at all possible. Blunt injuries to the heart requiring immediate thoracotomy in particular often are complex, consisting of multiple injuries. The patient with blunt cardiac injury usually has a large number of associated solid organ and soft tissue injuries. There are rarely insufficient personnel, equipment, instruments, lighting, suction, and exposure in the emergency room to perform simultaneous cardiac and abdominal surgery that may be required to save these patients (see section on Operative Therapy).

Shunt Formation

Because of the embryonic development of the heart (i.e., a tubular structure twisting upon itself in three directions and the central location of the valvular tissue each to the other and to each heart chamber), complex intracardiac fistulas can occur secondary to penetrating trauma.

Aortic/right ventricular shunts, coronary artery/intracavitary shunts, and aorto-pulmonary shunts often are found after penetrating wounds. Ventricular septal defects and aortic valve damage are also complications of wounding missiles. Although the diagnoses have been difficult to obtain in the past during the initial examination, with the advent of interoperative transesophageal echocardiography, it is now possible to make a precise diagnosis of these conditions. A minute fistula, if associated with little tissue damage, may seal, but those associated with widespread myocardial necrosis enlarge.[48]

After penetrating wounds about the heart, the presence of a precordial murmur, right ventricular lift with or without a thrill, and congestive failure suggest the presence of a shunt. If a shunt is identified at the time of initial operative procedure, primary repair usually is not attempted unless the patient has significant hemodynamic compromise. Any clinical deterioration should prompt use of diagnostic studies and emergency repair should be considered. Elective operative therapy is indicated after recovery of the major traumatic insult if the patient maintains a persistent shunt of greater than 1.5 to 1. A shunt of this magnitude may lead to the development of pulmonary hypertension, valvular incompetence, and may serve as a nidus for endocarditis.

Fistula communication between the aortic root and the right-sided cardiac chambers or left atrium are generally clinically significant and require elective surgical repair. Associated conduction defects may accompany these sequelae of penetrating wounds or their surgical management, and thus careful electrophysiologic studies are indicated pre-operatively.

Blunt cardiac injury may produce intracardiac shunts due to disruption of the ventricular septum, usually at the apex or, less commonly, the atrial septum. Because of the extensive force required to disrupt cardiac septa, immediate mortality associated with such injuries is high, often due to simultaneous free wall rupture. Septal rupture also has been associated with traumatic rupture of the aorta.[20] It also has been associated with traumatic rupture of the tricuspid valve causing acute tricuspid regurgitation.[23]

The etiology of an acute septal rupture is presumed due to the application of a compressive force during ventricular diastole leading to an acute rent in the septum. Late rupture may occur in the course of convalescence due to the reabsorption of a septal hematoma accompanied by significant necrosis. This latter disruption can occur several weeks after injury and may be the cause of delayed onset of murmurs and congestive heart failure or sudden death in the otherwise untoward convalescence from blunt trauma. The diagnosis requires a high index of suspicion. Such intracardiac lesions present with the sudden onset of a holosystolic thrill and right ventricular lift along the left sternal border accompanied by acute cardiac decompensation secondary to left-to-right shunt. The resulting volume overload in an already compromised myocardium is a potentially lethal situation. Echocardiography is of great value in diagnosis when this lesion is suspected.

In the case of small ventricular septal defects, spontaneous closure may occur. However, should hemodynamic decline occur, immediate cardiac catheterization to delineate the extent of the injury and anatomic location may be required before repair using cardiopulmonary bypass.

Valve Injuries

The aortic valve is most commonly injured by penetrating trauma, followed in frequency by the mitral and, least often, the pulmonic and tricuspid. The classic signs of valvular deficits may not be immediately recognized due to the presence of more obvious life-threatening external wounds. Low cardiac output and hypovolemia further obscure the extent of valvular damage until reasonable cardiac function is established. Thus, close observation, repeated examination, and appropriate monitoring of patients receiving penetrating wounds is mandatory (Chapter 2). The presence of new cardiac murmurs, thrills, or deterioration in clinical status should prompt diagnostic studies. The symptoms of valvular incompetence vary from none to progressive clinical decline. Injuries to cardiac valves, even if identified immediately, usually can be observed until stabilization of the patient and subsequent cardiac catheterization establishes the anatomic loss and extent of hemodynamic derangement.

With regard to blunt injury, the rapid displacement of blood secondary to crushing, burial, or other compressive injuries during ventricular diastole may lacerate cardiac valve leaflets, papillary muscles, or chordae tendinea and lead to insufficiency of the valve. Of the cardiac valves, those on the left side of the heart are most vulnerable to such injury. The valve cusp damaged most often usually is either the left coronary or the noncoronary aortic leaflet. The location of such injury suggests not only rapid displacement of blood volume at an inappropriate time in the cardiac cycle, but also a torsional effect on the aortic root due to rapid displacement of the cardiac mass. This often leads to a tear of one of the cardiac cusps and acute aortic regurgitation. No attempts of valve repair have been successful. In most cases, a valve replacement is necessary.[22]

Injuries to the mitral valve occur secondary to acute compression of the heart during the period of maximum diastolic filling, with resultant bursting of valve tissue. Similarly, any sudden increase in intraaortic pressure that leads to laceration or leaflet rupture also may result in stretching and hematoma formation within the papillary muscle. This may alter papillary muscle function to a point at which valvular insufficiency results. Should the papillary muscle be completely disrupted, acute onset of congestive failure occurs and is an ominous prognostic sign. The rare instance of tricuspid valve involvement is better tolerated than that of left-side valve damage.[23]

The *diagnosis* of a significant valvular injury is made when congestive heart failure continues with the acute development of a characteristic valvular insufficiency murmur. Confirmation of valvular injury can be made by two-dimensional echocardiography at the bedside. The most accurate determination, however, will be seen by the use of a biplane transesophageal echo probe that can accurately define the degree and severity of the valvular injury as well as the amount and quantity of regurgitation. Cardiac catheterization may be necessary, however, in younger patients who are not at risk for coronary artery disease. Transesophageal echo provides the necessary information to plan surgical treatment.

Treatment can be supportive in the absence of congestive heart failure, but usually surgery is indicated if any significant valvular insufficiency is recognized.

Foreign Bodies

Projectiles often are fixed in the cardiac tissue at the time of the wounding. Some may serve as a source of bacterial endocarditis. In others, the migration of the missile into a cardiac chamber, the pulmonary circulation, or the systemic circulation may occur.[49] The potential for migration of missile emboli with distal limb or organ gangrene or infarction requires the location and removal, if possible, of the foreign body at the initial operation. Moreover, the introduction of bits of clothing, tissue, or bone fragments carried by the wounding agent into the pericardial space may result in a purulent pericarditis. After shotgun injuries, missile embolization to the right ventricle often occurs.[50] These do not require removal because subsequent embolization to the lung is not harmful. Embolization of shot to the left ventricle is potentially serious and must be removed because embolization to cerebral arteries has been reported.[50]

OPERATIVE THERAPY

The treatment of all patients with penetrating or nonpenetrating wounds near the heart who present with tamponade or shock is immediate thoracotomy. This can consist of either anterolateral thoracotomy, which can be carried transsternally into the opposite chest, as necessary, or midline sternotomy. Once the possibility of cardiac injury is recognized, the patient should be transferred immediately to the operating room where simultaneous resuscitation and evaluation of the patient's status can be undertaken. If in the initial phases of evaluation and resuscitation in the emergency department the patient develops cardiac arrest, an emergency room thoracotomy is indicated (Chapter 3). If a patient has a recordable blood pressure and relatively stable hemodynamics, time is available for definitive evaluation and subsequent operation under optimal circumstances in the operating room.

The problems that relate to cardiac injury are primarily those of hemopericardium with tamponade; hemopericardium with free pleural cavity decompression with hypovolemic shock; cardiac failure due to myocardial contusion, arrhythmia, infarction, intracardiac shunts, or valvular insufficiency; and intracardiac foreign bodies. There is a small group of patients who sustain multiple penetrating injuries who present with hemodynamic changes who initially require exploratory laparotomy. Use of the subxiphoid or transdiaphragmatic pericardial window often can be helpful in establishing a definitive diagnosis of a cardiac injury.[51] (Chapter 21)

Cardiac Tamponade

When diagnosed, cardiac tamponade should be treated by emergency room thoracotomy if cardiac arrest is present or immediately impending (Fig. 15–8).[52,53] Otherwise, tamponade should be treated by a definitive thoracotomy if the patient's condition permits transport to the operating room. If a surgeon capable of treating tamponade is not present or the operating room is not immediately available, cardiac tamponade can be treated with pericardiocentesis (see previous section). Placement of an indwelling plastic catheter in the pericardial space permits intermittent aspiration of blood, depending on the patient's condition. Fibrin precipitated in the pericardial space may prevent adequate decompression,

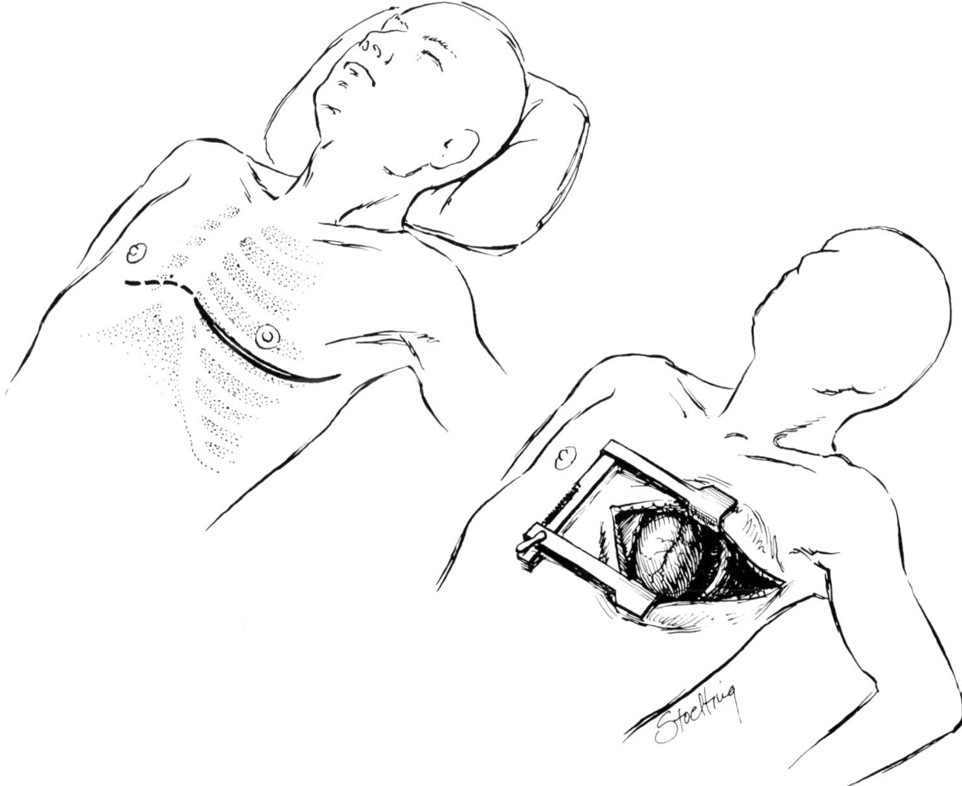

Figure 15–8. Emergency thoracotomy for acute pericardial tamponade is best accomplished using anterior thoracotomy carried out in the sixth interspace (pectoral or submammary groove). Costal cartilages can be cut as necessary to facilitate exposure or the incision can be carried across the sternum into the right anterior chest to facilitate exposure of cardiac lesions.

and the alternative, under these circumstances, is to pass an additional catheter or replace the existing one.[28]

If the patient has had blunt trauma in which the primary injury appears limited to the heart or if the patient has had penetrating cardiac trauma without associated injuries, the surgical approach can be either a midline sternotomy or anterior thoracotomy on the side of the presumed injury. If there is any question about an associated abdominal injury, the thoracic incision can be combined with a midline upper abdominal incision that permits simultaneous abdominal evaluation. The midline sternotomy incision is carried from the manubrium to the xiphoid. The anterior thoracotomy incision extends from the parasternal area to the posterior axillary line (Chapter 21). Sternal retractors are placed, gross bleeding controlled, and the pericardium entered. Whenever the surgeon suspects tamponade, the pericardium must be opened because the appearance of the pericardium may be deceiving. The only sure way to rule out tamponade is to inspect the interior of the pericardial space (Fig. 15–9). Treatment of the tamponade is, of course, resolved with opening the pericardium and evacuating the contained clot. Lacerations of the heart should be identified and bleeding controlled by finger pressure and the laceration sutured to control secondary hemorrhage.

Occasionally, the surgeon may be exploring the abdomen for trauma and the patient deteriorates for unexplained reasons. Tension pneumothorax must be ruled out and may require bilateral tube thoracostomies. If the patient is still unstable, the next procedure is to make a pericardial window through the diaphragm to rule out undiagnosed pericardial tamponade. If found, the midline incision should be extended up the sternum or a separate left anterior thoracotomy done. This also illustrates why it is so important always to prepare and drape the entire torso of trauma cases.

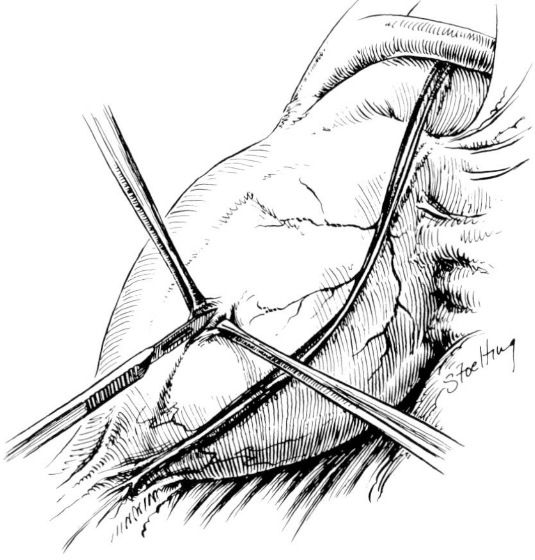

Figure 15–9. Technique for opening the pericardium. The pericardium is grasped with forceps or hemostats and opened longitudinally, taking care to identify the phrenic nerve that passes anterior to the pulmonary hilum.

Myocardial Laceration with Intrapleural Hemorrhage

The primary indication for operation in this instance is the ongoing blood loss. The heart usually is not recognized in advance as the source of bleeding, and, unless transport of the patient and treatment is rapid, mortality is the rule. Occasionally, the initial hemorrhage will have ceased with loss of intracardiac volume and a drop in diastolic pressure that allows the heart muscle and clot to tamponade the bleeding. However, with resuscitation raising intracardiac pressure, hemorrhage may recur. Indications for thoracotomy are the failure of a patient to respond to resuscitation, hemorrhage from the pleural space in excess of 1000 ml, or ongoing persistent bleeding from the chest tube. Usually, the side of the bleeding is the most appropriate thoracic cavity to open using anterior thoracotomy. If additional exposure of the heart is indicated, transverse sternotomy is done, carrying the incision into the opposite chest cavity until adequate exposure has been obtained. The pericardium should be explored by opening it longitudinally, avoiding the phrenic nerve, and the bleeding site controlled by digital pressure followed by appropriate sutures.

In many instances, the lesion that was the source of the hemorrhage will no longer be bleeding. The reason for this is that lacerations compatible with survival are inevitably modest in size and spontaneous cessation of hemorrhage often occurs as heart muscle swelling and clot combine to tamponade the injury.

If a bleeding point is ascertained, this should be controlled digitally until full evaluation of the heart can be accomplished. It must be remembered that penetrating lesions may be through and through and there may be a duplicate lesion in the posterior aspect of the heart. If there is evidence of bleeding posteriorly, the hand can be wrapped around the heart as the fingers search for the source of the hemorrhage or the heart can be temporarily lifted upward and the posterior portion of the ventricles inspected. Dislocation of the heart compromises the cardiac output and may result in cardiac arrest if the circulation has been marginal. Intermittent inspection of posterior lesions can be accomplished once intravascular volume is restored and the posterior laceration closed by temporary dislocation of the heart for a minute or two and accepting the adverse impact on the circulation. In rare instances, inflow occlusion may be necessary to give a dry field (Fig. 15–16). Attempts at rapid closure of cardiac lacerations are ill-advised because heart muscle is friable and a readily treatable lesion can be converted into an irreversible one if coronary arteries are compromised or sutures tear and increase the size of the laceration.

Techniques in closure vary with the chambers of the heart. The most commonly injured, the right ventricle, is composed of relatively thin, friable, cardiac muscle. Lacerations that are 5 mm or less can be controlled with simple atraumatic sutures carefully placed and tied gently. Blood loss should be accepted during placement of the sutures to facilitate exposure. Lacerations larger than 5 mm or in which sutures tear or are holding poorly should be closed with Teflon felt bolsters (Fig. 15–10). This prevents the sutures from cutting through the friable myocardium. Pericardium also can be used as bolsters and avoids the risk of leaving a foreign body in the pericardial space with its potential for infection.

When lacerations occur adjacent to coronary arteries, coronary vessels should be undersewn by mattress sutures (Fig. 15–11) with or without the use of bolsters.

Laceration of the left ventricle, which is thicker and has more intrinsic integrity, usually can be closed with simple sutures (Fig. 15–12). Bleeding sites can be controlled with finger pressure and sutures are placed more or less blindly under the finger, then tied

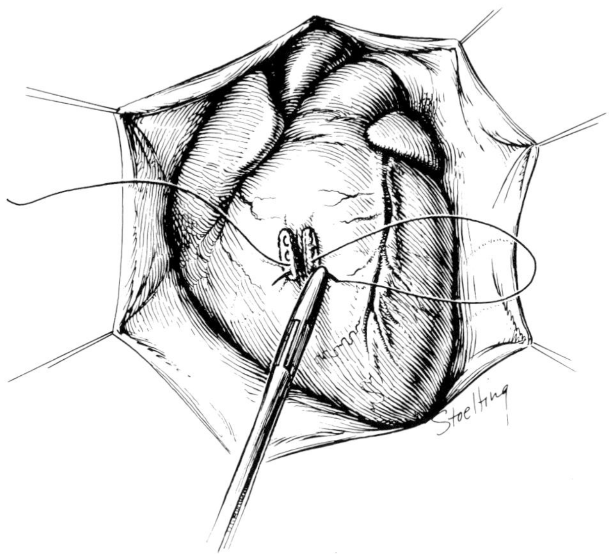

Figure 15–10. Technique for suturing the right ventricle using Dacron or Teflon felt bolsters.

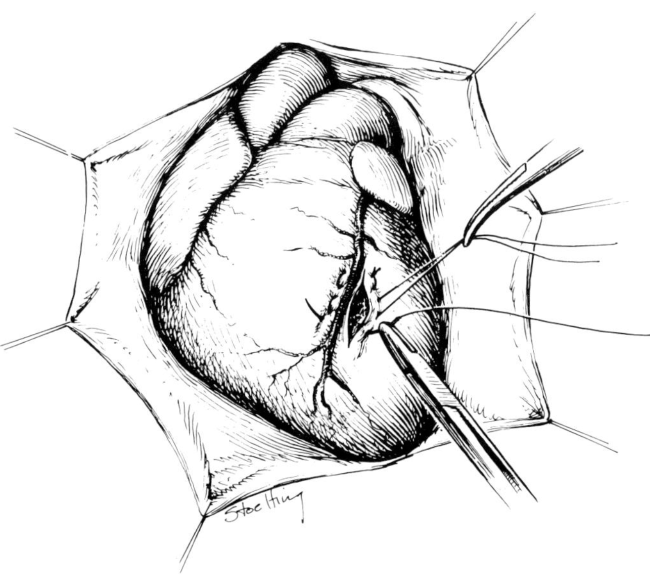

Figure 15–11. Technique used for suturing lacerations adjacent to coronary arteries. Mattress sutures are placed so as to undersew the artery.

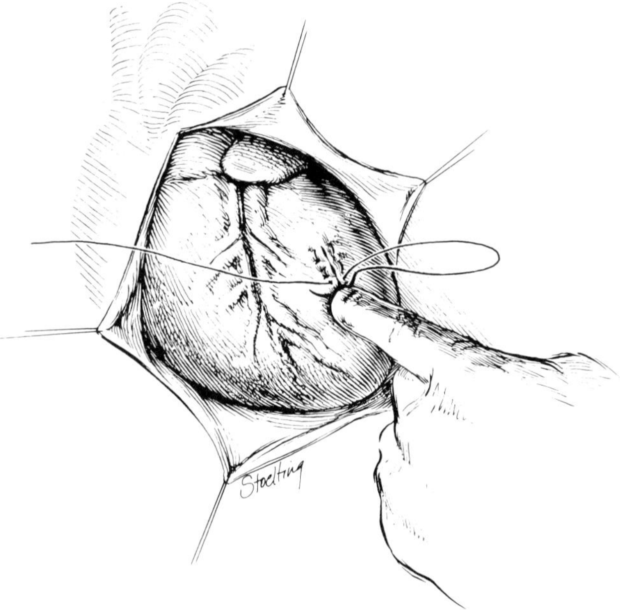

Figure 15–12.   Direct suture of the myocardium. This technique is most often possible when the laceration involves the thick-walled left ventricle.

one by one. If the myocardium begins to tear, Teflon felt bolsters as are used for right ventricular injuries may be required.

Atrial injuries, because these are low-pressure chambers, often can be closed temporarily by the judicious application of a vascular clamp (Fig. 15–13). Vascular forceps can be used to grab the edges of the laceration to facilitate the application of the clamp. When the clamp has been placed, fine 5-0 Prolene sutures can be used in running fashion to provide definitive closure. Alternatively, if the application of vascular clamps is not feasible, the laceration can be approximated under the occluding finger, as with ventricular injuries, or tamponaded by inserting a balloon catheter (Fig. 15–14).

Coronary Artery Lacerations

Lacerations of the main coronary arteries, that is, the right, left main, left circumflex, and anterior descending, usually are immediately fatal. If the rare case occurs of major coronary artery injury, repair is mandatory.[54] Vessel bleeding can be controlled temporarily by finger pressure or by atraumatic vascular forceps. The vessels are then isolated and controlled with traction tapes or with small bulldog clamps. If magnification is available, this greatly facilitates repair, which should be carried out with fine 7-0 Prolene sutures to provide intima-to-intima approximation. Alternatively, saphenous vein bypass can be carried out (Fig. 15–15). This, however, requires the use of cardiopulmonary bypass. If bypass is available, difficult or complicated lesions can be treated. Use of cardioplegia during aortic

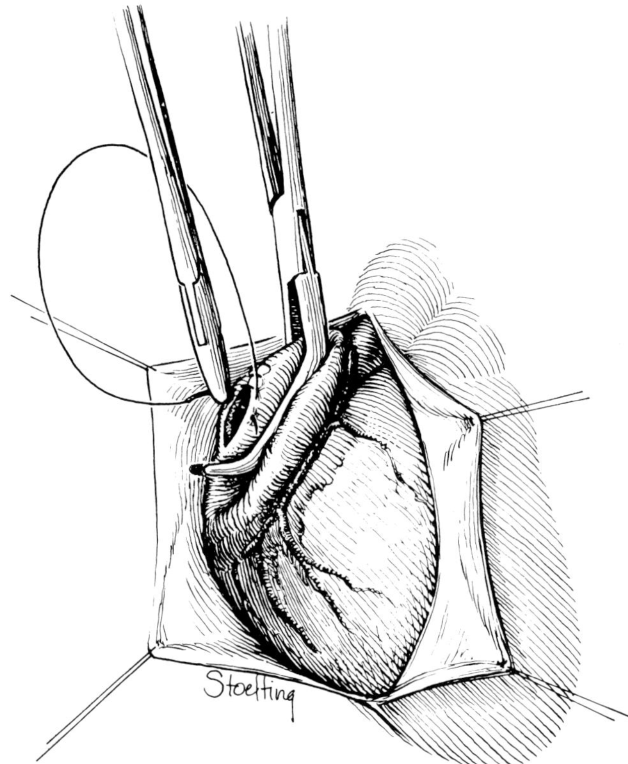

Figure 15–13.   Technique that can be used when the laceration involves the atrium. The laceration is grasped initially by forceps or a Babcock-type clamp and then a partially occluding type clamp applied while the laceration is sutured.

cross-clamping can greatly facilitate the repair. Cardioplegia allows precise repair in a bloodless field and improved postoperative myocardial function.[55] If after repair there is evidence of depressed myocardial function, continuing the patient on cardiopulmonary support may allow significant recovery of the myocardium, which may be only stunned and not irreparably injured.[56] An alternative that can be used when cardiopulmonary bypass is not available is to fibrillate the heart using low-voltage current from the defibrillator and massage intermittently to maintain circulation between the application of sutures. Lesions involving the distal third of the right coronary, the anterior descending, and the circumflex coronary or marginal vessels can be treated by ligation.

Intracardiac Shunts and Valve Injuries

Because most traumatic cardiac lesions result from penetrating trauma, the surgeon has an opportunity to inspect the heart during a course of repair of the lacerations associated with penetrating trauma. The use of a sterile stethoscope permits direct auscultation of the heart during surgery. This facilitates the identification of the murmurs related to traumatic atrial

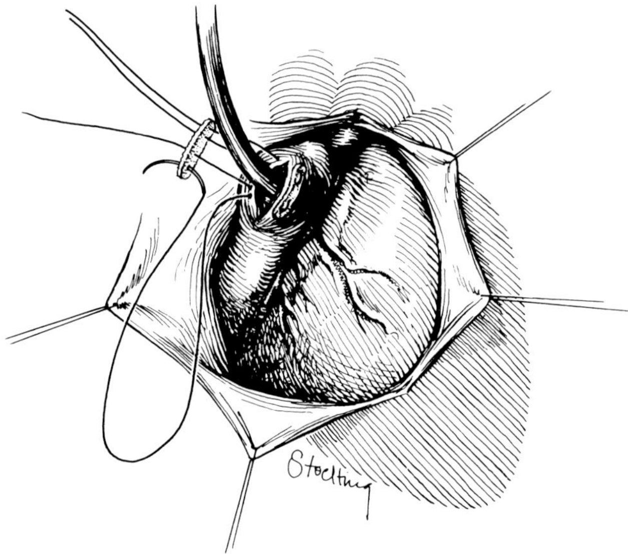

Figure 15–14.   A small atrial laceration also can be controlled temporarily with a balloon catheter while sutures are placed.

or ventricular septal defects and valve lacerations or insufficiency related to chordae or papillary injury. Cardiac failure, which persists after adequate resuscitation in the patient with penetrating trauma, also should lead to the suspicion that an intracardiac lesion is present. Interoperative transesophageal echocardiography should be considered under these circumstances.[16]

Injuries to cardiac valves and intracardiac shunts should be treated expectantly. Unless total disruption of a valve or overwhelming volume overload occurs, emergency intracardiac surgery is seldom warranted.

In a minority of circumstances, refractory congestive failure or even cardiac arrest may ensue. Proper treatment of the lesions may require cardiac catheterization for definitive diagnosis. In a large percentage of cases, however, an accurate diagnosis can be obtained when a transesophageal echocardiogram is done. Once an accurate diagnosis has been established, definitive repair using cardiopulmonary bypass may be necessary.

In desperate circumstances when no heart-lung machine is available and it is difficult to control bleeding from posterior lacerations or when intracardiac lesions result in the patient not responding to attempts at resuscitation, an alternative can be tried. This consists of inflow occlusion of the superior and inferior vena cavae using encircling tapes and tourniquets (Fig. 15–16). The tapes are pulled up, an atriotomy incision is made that can be contained by a vascular clamp, the heart fibrillated as previously described, the atrium entered, and the lesion identified. One or two sutures can be placed within 2 to 3 min of allotted time. The atrium is then filled with saline and the atrial clamp reapplied. The preceding can be repeated as often as necessary to repair the lesion. Intermittent cardiac compression can be given or the heart defibrillated for a 10-min period between inflow occlusion. Such patients inevitably have already developed mild hypothermia, because they have received rapid transfusion of cold blood and their body temperature is lower than

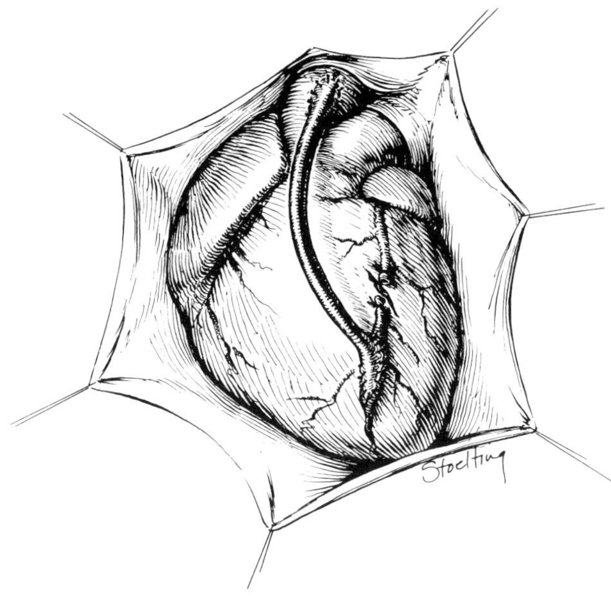

Figure 15–15. A laceration of a major coronary artery can be treated by repair or autogenous vein bypass, as depicted.

normal. The surgeon has 3 to 4 min of intracardiac inspection possible with the use of intermittent caval occlusion. However, if the patient can be resuscitated and transferred to a center where cardiopulmonary bypass can be carried out, this, of course, is the optimal choice.

Cardiopulmonary bypass is best done through a midline sternotomy, although a transverse sternotomy incision can be used if necessary to convert an anterior thoracotomy into an appropriate incision for cardiac exposure and cannulation. Standard cardiopulmonary bypass is instituted with either a femoral arterial or ascending aortic input line with both cavae isolated and cannulated for venous return. Because intracardiac repair in trauma cases usually is not complicated and support may be required initially while other lesions are being treated, the use of inferior caval cannulation through the femoral vein combined with femoral artery perfusion may be appropriate. This method also facilitates treatment of lesions such as aortic rupture in which complete cardiac isolation is not necessary. It is possible that in the future new systems of percutaneous cardiopulmonary support may find expanded use in a patient suffering significant cardiac trauma.[16]

Almost all septal defects can be repaired with simple suturing techniques. Small valve lacerations can be repaired with interrupted or running sutures. When gross papillary muscle disruption has compromised the mitral valve, mitral valve replacement may be the most appropriate treatment.

With any penetrating cardiac injury, the possibility of an air embolus exists. This also can occur with injuries to the vena cava or pulmonary veins. The surgeon may note small air bubbles in the coronary arteries (see Fig. 15–17). The best treatment is to raise the blood pressure with cardiotonic drugs to drive the air through the coronary vasculature.

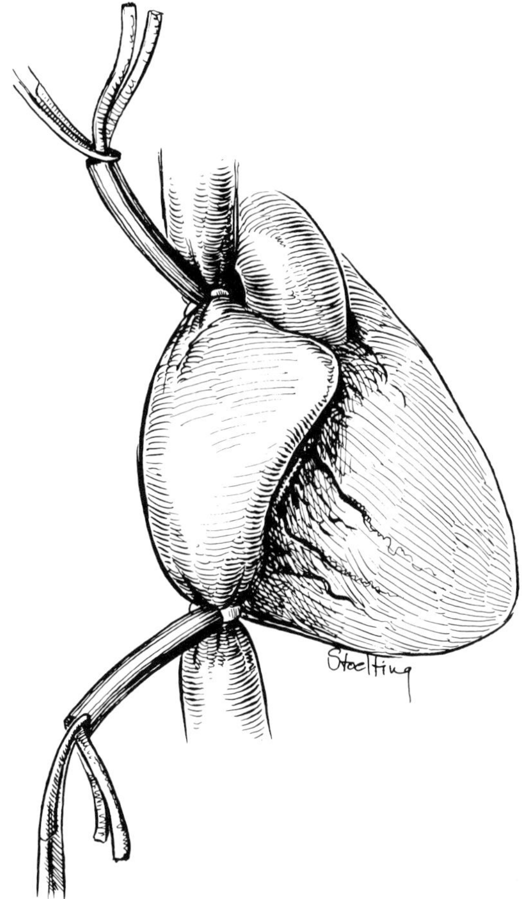

Figure 15–16. Inflow occlusion may, in rare instances, be of value by facilitating exposure of relatively inaccessible lesions. Occlusion times should not exceed 2 or 3 min.

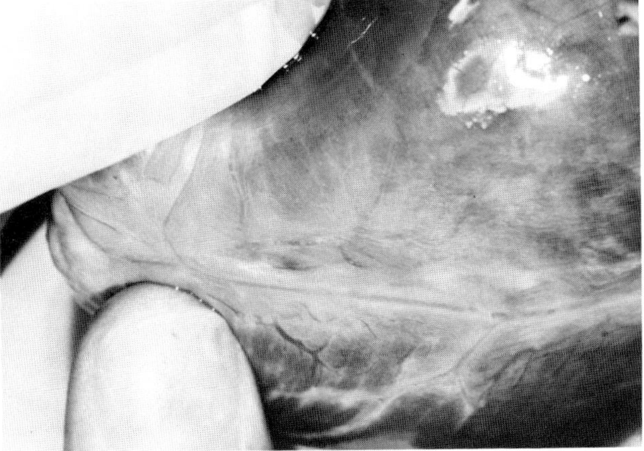

Figure 15–17. Coronary air embolism can be seen in this photograph. Raising aortic root pressure with pressor agents facilitated the passage of the air and relieved the obstruction.

Intracardiac Foreign Bodies

Intracardiac foreign bodies may be identified in the course of emergency exploration for cardiac laceration and tamponade (Fig. 15–18). Most often these are bullets from low-velocity handguns. Techniques for extraction of foreign bodies without coronary bypass were described by Harken[9] during World War II. In most instances, the location of foreign bodies are best identified radiologically, and definitive removal carried out under full cardiopulmonary bypass. It is possible by positioning the patient to move the foreign body into a location where it can be isolated and simply extracted from an atrial appendage. In rare instances in which the cardiac foreign body can be palpated through the wall of the ventricle, the small foreign body can be isolated by the placement of sutures through the myocardium. A small incision can then be made in the heart and the bullet or foreign body popped from the ventricular cavity as the isolating sutures are pulled up. Those foreign bodies located within the substance of the myocardium, most common in the left ventricle, can be isolated at the site of injury by deep-placed sutures. An incision is made over the foreign body, avoiding major coronary arteries, and the material extracted, after which the sutures are tied.

POSTOPERATIVE CARE

Postoperative management of patients after thoracotomy for cardiac wounds is often surprisingly simple. Once the defect has been repaired, prompt recovery is the rule. Patients should be monitored in a critical care setting with therapy aimed at restoration of hemodynamic stability by using necessary volume, pharmacologic, and respiratory support.

If the patient is hemodynamically unstable, a Swan-Ganz catheter should be passed into the pulmonary artery to monitor central pressures and to ascertain the need for volume therapy or cardiotonic agents. Close attention needs to be paid not only to pulmonary pressures but also to cardiac output, systemic vascular resistance, and pulmonary vascular resistance. Appropriate treatment should be determined only after an accurate assessment of all hemodynamic parameters. In most instances, the patient will require increased volume to maintain adequate preload. However, if significant cardiac instability is present, as manifested by elevated filling pressures, cardiac support with inotropic drugs and afterload reduction may be necessary. To evaluate whether the patient's cardiac output is adequate or inadequate, the urine output, arteriovenous oxygen difference, and assessment of systemic acidosis are all useful guides.[57] If adequate cardiac perfusion cannot be obtained, consideration for placement of an intraaortic balloon should be given. The device can now be placed percutaneously and can be used despite cardiac irritability and hemodynamic instability.[58]

Patients may develop a variety of cardiac rhythms. These need to be diagnosed accurately and treated appropriately. If ventricular dysrhythmias are present, the usual treatment is with lidocaine. However, certain patients may continue to have severe ventricular irritability and, if they do, treatments with other antiarrhythmic drugs such as bretylium may be indicated.

Blood gases should be monitored closely and pulmonary support used. In general, patients should be left intubated in the early postoperative phase until their cardiac and

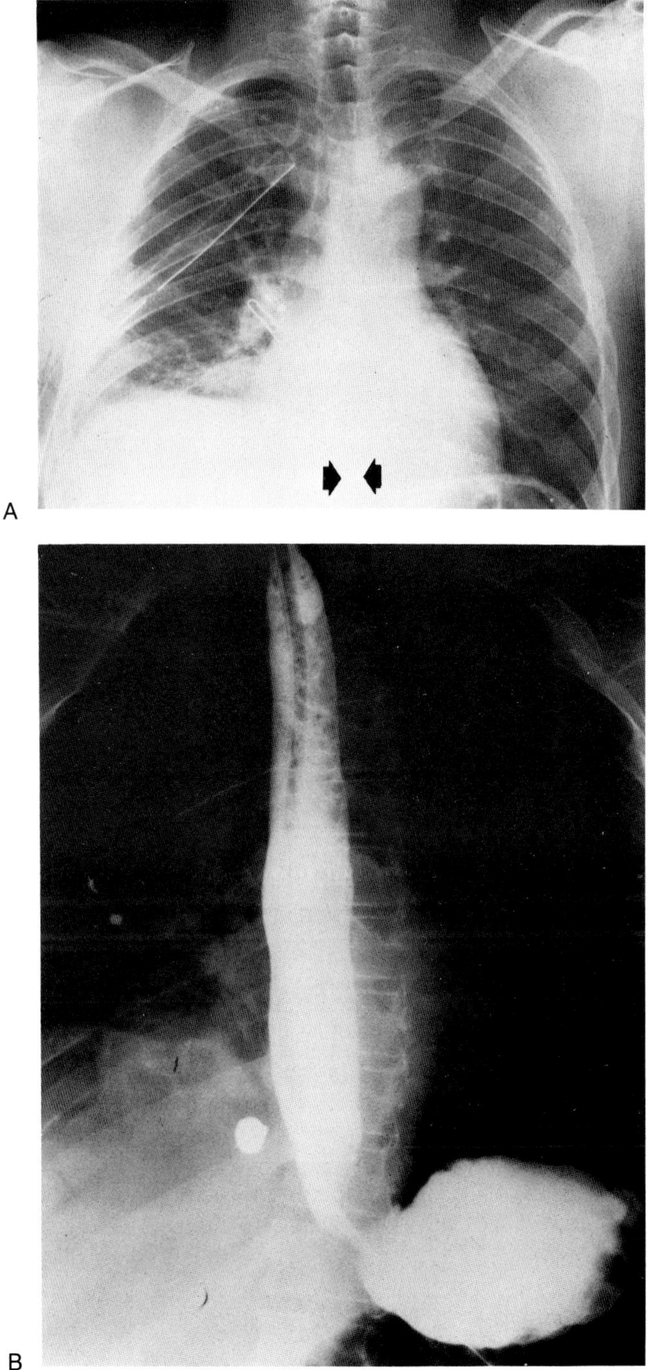

Figure 15–18.   An intracardiac foreign body is seen on the anteroposterior chest radiograph between the two arrows (**A**). The location is seen more easily on an overpenetrated view carried out with an esophogram (**B**).

pulmonary functions can be adequately assessed. Respiratory settings should be adjusted to provide optimal blood gases, with the oxygen tension kept between 70 and 90 by appropriate adjustment of oxygen concentration in the inspired gas. If oxygen concentrations greater than 50% are required, positive end-expiratory pressure should be adjusted upward. Carbon dioxide tension should be controlled by adjusting the respiratory rate or the tidal volume of the ventilator. It may be necessary under certain circumstances to use not only positive end-expiratory pressure but also pressure support and inverse ratio ventilation. It may be necessary to perform postoperative bronchoscopy if the patient is exhibiting evidence of lobar or segmental collapse. The endotracheal tube should be left in place postoperatively until it is ascertained that pulmonary function is adequate and the cardiac status is stable.

COMPLICATIONS

The complications after cardiac injuries are relatively few. These consist of myocardial failure secondary to compromised coronary circulation or direct cardiac contusion. These are treated by appropriate support similar to that used for myocardial infarction, including careful monitoring of fluid therapy using Swan-Ganz catheters and cardiotonic agents such as dobutamine and low-dose dopamine. (see Chapter 2)

Intrapericardial bleeding postoperatively may be manifested by excessively high filling pressures to maintain cardiac output. Echocardiographic evaluations should be used and pericardiocentesis carried out as indicated. If a good response does not follow, reoperation to evacuate blood and clots is indicated.

If the patient manifests persistent cardiac failure and does not respond to conservative management, more sophisticated diagnostic studies such as cardiac catheterization or transesophageal echocardiography should be carried out to accurately define the cardiac pathology. Chronic infections of the pericardial space can occur and may require aggressive treatment with a median sternotomy, removal of any devitalized bone and tissues, and placement of either pectoralis or rectus muscle flaps to ensure adequate closure. Fortunately these infections are extremely rare. Postoperative pericarditis usually is sterile and responds to treatment with nonsteroidal agents or, in rare circumstances, corticosteroids. If inadequately treated, chronic constrictive pericarditis and cardiac failure may occur.

RESULTS

The survival rates of patients with successfully repaired cardiac wounds who leave the operating room alive are very good. Late mortality is uncommon, even in those patients who have undergone emergency room thoracotomy. Simple cardiac injuries have a high survival rate despite cardiac arrest. Many patients who are seen with penetrating stab wounds of the heart will have blood pressures above 70 mm Hg. Survival after emergency thoracotomy of those patients who are alert and conscious is 70% to 80% with stab wounds and 33% with gunshot wounds.[26] The causes of death are shown in Table 15–7.

Even in patients with penetrating injuries who present with no signs of life or who are agonal, emergency thoracotomy accompanied by appropriate resuscitative maneuvers will achieve a survival rate of 15% to 30%.[18,26,51,52] In patients who present with blunt trauma

Table 15–7. Cardiac Injury, Causes of Death[59]

CAUSES OF DEATH	NO. OF DEATHS
Hemorrhage	12
Ventricular fibrillation and low cardiac output	8
Tamponade	1
Brain injury	1
Respiratory distress syndrome	1
Sepsis	3

and no signs of life, however, the chance of revival after emergency thoracotomy is extremely low.[59,60] Cardiac injuries associated with ventricular fibrillation before or upon opening the chest have extremely high mortality, as is true of patients requiring thoracotomy after blunt trauma to the heart.

REFERENCES

1. Meade RH. *A History of Thoracic Surgery.* Springfield, IL: Charles C Thomas; 1961.
2. Purple SS. Statistical observations on wounds of the heart. *NY J Med Collat Sci.* 1855;14:411.
3. Cappelan A. Vulnus cordis. *Nord Mag Laegevidensk.* 1856;6:285.
4. Rehn L. Uebr. Petrierend Herzwunden and Herznaht. *Arch Klin Chir.* 1897;55:315.
5. Beck CS. Wounds of the heart: the technique of suture. *Arch Surg.* 1926;1:205.
6. Bigger IA. Wounds of the heart. *Int Clin.* 1934;1:133.
7. Bright EF, Beck CS. Contusions of the heart. *JAMA.* 1935;104:109.
8. Escaude F, Brueq P. Deux case de projectile inclas dans les parois du coeur et bien tuleres. *Rev Chir (Paris).* 1917;53:268.
9. Harken DE. Foreign bodies in and in relation to the thoracic blood vessels and heart. *Surg Gynecol Obstet.* 1946;83:117.
10. Mattox KL, Feliciano DV, Burch J, Beall Jr AC, Jordan Jr GL, DeBakey ME. Five thousand seven hundred sixty cardiovascular injuries in 4459 patients. *Ann Surg.* 1989;209(6):698.
11. Jones JW, Hewitt RL, Drapanas T. Cardiac contusion: a capricious syndrome. *Ann Surg.* 1975;181:567.
12. Kissane RW. Traumatic heart disease. *Circulation.* 1952;6:421.
13. Sigler LH. Trauma of the heart due to nonpenetrating chest injuries. *JAMA.* 1942;119:855.
14. Parmley LF, Manion WC, Mattingly TW. Nonpenetrating traumatic injury to the heart. *Circulation.* 1958;18:371.
15. Shorr RM, Crittenden M, Indeck M, Hartunian SL, Rodriguez A. Blunt thoracic trauma: analysis of 515 patients. *Ann Surg.* 1987;206(2):200.
16. Follette DM. Penetrating cardiac injuries—a look to the future. *Ann Thorac Surg.* 1991;51:701.
17. Moreno C, Moore EE, Majure JA, Hopeman AR. Pericardial tamponade: a critical determinant for survival following penetrating cardiac wounds. *J Trauma.* 1986;26(9):821.
18. Attar S, Suter CM, Hankins JR, Sequeira A, McLaughlin JS. Penetrating cardiac injuries. *Ann Thorac Surg.* 1991;51:711.
19. Howanitz EP, Buckley D, Galbraith TA, Murray KD, Myerowitz PD. Combined blunt traumatic rupture of the heart and aorta: two case reports and review of the literature. *J Trauma.* 1990;30(4):506.
20. Brown PS Jr, Nath R, Votapka T, et al. Traumatic ventricular septal defect and disruption of the descending thoracic aorta. *Ann Thorac Surg.* 1991;52:143.
21. Moront M, Lefrak EA, Akl BF. Traumatic rupture of the interventricular septum and tricuspid valve: case report. *J Trauma.* 1991;31(1):134.
22. German DS, Shapiro MJ, Willman VL. Acute aortic valvular incompetence following blunt thoracic deceleration injury: case report. *J Trauma.* 1990;30(11):1411.
23. McKeown PP, Rosemurgy A, Conant P. Blunt traumatic rupture of pulmonary vein, left atrium, and bronchus. *Ann Thorac Surg.* 1991;52:787.
24. Santavirta S, Arajärvi E. Ruptures of the heart in seatbelt wearers. *J Trauma.* 1992;32(3):275.

25. Rosato RM, Shapiro MJ, Keegan MJ, Connors RH, Minor CB. Cardiac injury complicating traumatic asphyxia. *J Trauma.*1991;31(10):1387.
26. DeGennaro VA, Bonifils-Roberts EA, Ching N, Nealon TF. Aggressive management of potential penetrating cardiac injuries. *J Thorac Cardiovasc Surg*. 1980;79:833.
27. Freshman SP, Wisner DH, Weber CJ. 2-D echocardiography: emergent use in the evaluation of penetrating precordial trauma. *J Trauma*. 1991;31(7):902.
28. Symbas PM, Harlattis N, Waldo WJ. Penetrating cardiac wounds: a comparison of different therapeutic methods. *Ann Surg*. 1976;183:377.
29. Potkin RT, Werner JA, Trobaugh GB, et al. Evaluation of non-invasive tests of cardiac damage in suspected cardiac contusion. *Circulation*. 1982;66:627.
30. Tenzer ML. The spectrum of myocardial contusion: a review. *J Trauma*. 1985;25(7):620.
31. Wisner DH, Reed WH, Riddick RS. Suspected myocardial contusion: triage and indications for monitoring. *Ann Surg*. 1990;212(1):82.
32. Shapiro MJ, Yanofsky SD, Trapp J, et al. Cardiovascular evaluation in blunt thoracic trauma using transesophageal echocardiography (TEE). *J Trauma*. 1991;31(6):835.
33. Solomon D. Delayed cardiac tamponade after blunt chest trauma: case report. *J Trauma*. 1991;31(9):1322.
34. Aaland MO, Sherman RT. Delayed pericardial tamponade in penetrating chest trauma: case report. *J Trauma*. 1991;31(11):1563.
35. Hudgens S, McGraw J, Craun M. Two cases of tension pneumopericardium following blunt chest injury. *J Trauma*. 1991;31(10):1408.
36. Demetriades D, Levy R, Hatzitheofilou C, Chun R. Tension pneumopericardium following penetrating trauma: case report. *J Trauma*. 1990;30(2):238.
37. Doty DB, Anderson AE, Rose EF, et al. Cardiac trauma: clinical and experimental correlations of myocardial contusion. *Ann Surg*. 1974;180:452.
38. Golladay ES, Donahoo JS, Haller JA. Special problems of cardiac injuries in infants and children. *J Trauma*. 1979;19:526.
39. McLean RF, Devitt JH, Dubbin J, McLellan BA. Incidence of abnormal RNA studies and dysrhythmias in patients with blunt chest trauma. *J Trauma*. 1991;31(7):968.
40. Dubrow TJ, Mihalka J, Eisenhauer DM, et al. Myocardial contusion in the stable patient: what level of care is appropriate? *Surgery*. 1989;106(2):267.
41. Fabian TC, Cicala RS, Croce MA, et al. A prospective evaluation of myocardial contusion: correlation of significant arrhythmias and cardiac output with CPK-MB measurements. *J Trauma*. 1991;31(5):653.
42. Healey MA, Brown R, Fleiszer D. Blunt cardiac injury: is this diagnosis necessary? *J Trauma*. 1990;30(2):137.
43. Foil MB, Mackersie RC, Furst SR, et al. The asymptomatic patient with suspected myocardial contusion. *Am J Surg*. 1990;160:638.
44. Norton MJ, Stanford GG, Weigelt JA. Early detection of myocardial contusion and its complications in patients with blunt trauma. *Am J Surg*. 1990;160:577.
45. Abbott JA, Cousineau M, Cheitlin M, Thomas AN, Lim RC. Late sequelae of penetrating cardiac wounds. *J Thorac Cardiovasc Surg*. 1978;75:510.
46. Beall AC, Patrick TA, Ikies JE, Bricker EL, DeBakey ME. Penetrating wounds of the heart: changing patterns of surgical management. *J Trauma*. 1972;12:468.
47. Suggs WL, Rea WJ, Ecker RR, Webb WR, Rose EF, Shaw RR. Penetrating wounds of the heart: an analysis of 459 cases. *J Thorac Cardiovasc Surg*. 1968;56:531.
48. Thandroyen FT, Matisonn RE. Penetrating thoracic trauma producing cardiac shunts. *J Thorac Cardiovasc Surg*. 1981;81:569.
49. van Arsdell GS, Razzouk AJ, Fandrich BL, Skahudo M, Schmidt CA. Bullet fragment venous embolus to the heart: case report. *J Trauma*. 1991;31(1):137.
50. Skipper R, Debski R. Intramyocardial shotgun pellets diagnosed on initial emergency room chest x-ray: case report. *J Trauma*. 1990;30(12):1609.
51. Mayor-Davies JA, Britz RS. Subxiphoid pericardial windows—helpful in selected cases. *J Trauma*. 1990;30(11):1399.
52. Baker CC, Thomas AN, Trunkey DD. The role of emergency room thoracotomy in trauma. *J Trauma*. 1980;20:848.
53. Ivatury RR, Shah PM, Ito K, Ramirez-Schon G, Suarez F, Rohman M. Emergency room thoracotomy for the resuscitation of patients with "fatal" penetrating injuries of the heart. *Ann Thorac Surg*. 1981;32:377.
54. Espada R, Whisennand HH, Mattox KL, Beall AC. Surgical management of penetrating injuries to the coronary arteries. *Surgery*. 1975;78:755.
55. Follette DM, Mulder DG, Maloney JV Jr, Buckberg GD. Advantages of blood cardioplegia over continuous coronary perfusion or intermittent ischemia—experimental and clinical study. *J Thorac Cardiovasc Surg*. 1978;76:604.

56. Follette DM. The role of coronary artery bypass grafting after acute myocardial infarction. *Cardio Newsmagazine of Contemporary Cardiology.* 1992;(April):84.
57. Buckberg GD, Robertson JM, McConnell DH, Brazier JR. Determinants of myocardial performance and the adequacy of subendocardial blood flow. In: Utley JR, ed. *Perioperative Cardiac Dysfunction.* Baltimore: Williams & Wilkins; 1985:139–158.
58. Ammons MA, Moore EE, Moore FA, Hopeman AR. Intra-aortic balloon pump for combined myocardial contusion and thoracic aortic rupture. *J Trauma.* 1990;30(12):1606.
59. Mattox KL, Koch LV, Beall AC Jr, et al. Logistic and technical consideration in the treatment of the wounded heart. *Circulation.* 1975;51&52(Suppl 1):210.
60. Fulda G, Brathwaite CEM, Rodriguez A, Turney SZ, Dunham CM, Cowley RA. Blunt traumatic rupture of the heart and pericardium: a ten-year experience (1979–1989). *J Trauma.* 1991;31(2):167.

16

Aortic Injury

HERBERT A. BERKOFF, M.D.
EDWARD J. HURLEY, M.D.

HISTORY: Vesalius, in 1557, first described blunt traumatic rupture of the aorta.[1] The first successful treatment of an aortic injury was apparently performed in 1922 by a Russian surgeon, Dshanelidze, who repaired an 8-mm puncture wound of the intrapericardial ascending aorta in a 20-year-old man.[2] In 1947, Strassman collected 72 cases of aortic injury from the literature.[3] The first successful treatment of blunt traumatic rupture of the thoracic aorta was apparently that of Bahnson, who operated on a chronic posttraumatic aneurysm in 1952, carrying out an aneurysmorrhaphy (Fig. 16–1).[4] In 1956, Gerbode and co-workers[5] operated on four patients with posttraumatic descending aneurysm using pump oxygenator support and had success with three using homograft interposition. The initial successful repair of an acute transection was attributed to Forsee and Blatte[6] in 1958, who recognized and repaired the ruptured aorta of a 21-year-old airman 3 days after the injury by using left heart bypass. The first classic series of the natural history of thoracic aortic injury was that of Parmley and co-workers,[7] who in 1958 reported 275 patients with rupture of the aorta from nonpenetrating causes. Since that time, many series have reported increasing success with the management of traumatic aortic rupture, with salvage rates now being commonly 90%.[1,8–10]

ANATOMY

The thoracic aorta is conveniently divided into the ascending, transverse arch, and descending thoracic aorta (Fig. 16–2). The ascending aorta is, for a good portion of its extent, intrapericardial. The pericardium envelops the aorta medially to the innominate artery and extends two-thirds of the way up the anterior and lateral portion of the ascending aorta.

At its origin from the heart just above the aortic valve, the aorta lies posteriorly and to the right of the pulmonary artery and ascends to the right over the right pulmonary artery, coming to lie just posteriorly to the right second and third intercostal spaces and the parasternal line. In its caudal portion, the superior vena cava lies to the right and posterior to

298

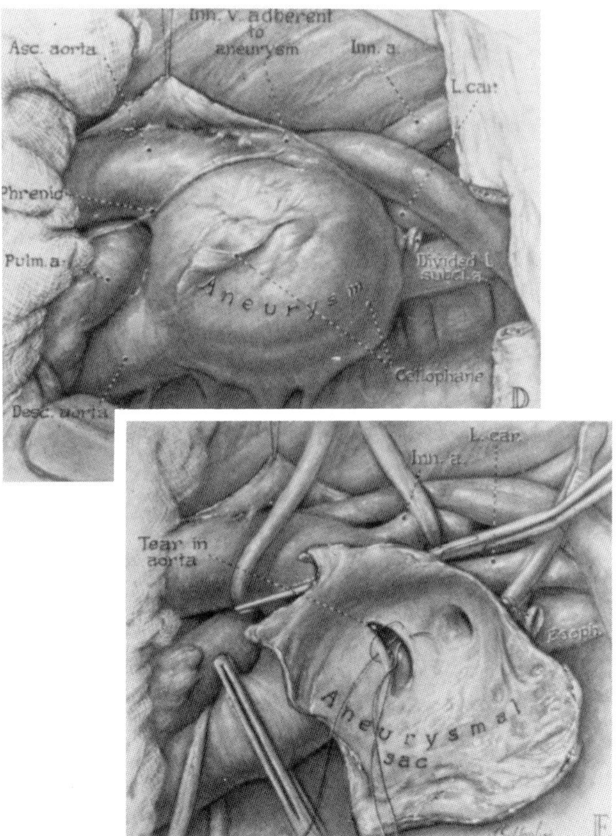

Figure 16–1. First repair of a traumatic rupture of the aorta. (Reprinted with permission from Bahnsen.[4])

the aorta, with the vena cava becoming progressively more anterior as the angle of the sternum at the level of the second rib is reached. The left innominate vein passes superior to the cranial surface of the transverse arch. The only two branches of the ascending aorta are the right and left coronary arteries.

The transverse arch of the aorta begins at the level of the innominate artery, which is relatively anterior in its origin, and passes transversely and dorsally posterior to the left innominate vein and obliquely toward the vertebral column. The left carotid artery normally arises from the aorta 1 cm distal to the innominate artery, taking its origin from the aortic arch as the latter passes anterior to the trachea. One of the most common anatomic variations is the sharing of left carotid artery and the innominate artery of a common origin from the aorta. The transverse arch ends with the subclavian artery on the left and above and the ligamentum arteriosum medially and below. The left subclavian artery normally arises posteriorly 1 to 2 cm distal to the left common carotid. The subclavian artery then passes obliquely to the left in the left chest, lying in a fold of mediastinal pleura.

The origin of the descending aorta arises anterior and to the left of the vertebral column at the level of the fourth thoracic vertebra and then descends toward the diaphragm, affixed to the left vertebral sulcus by investing mediastinal pleura. The esophagus lies to the right

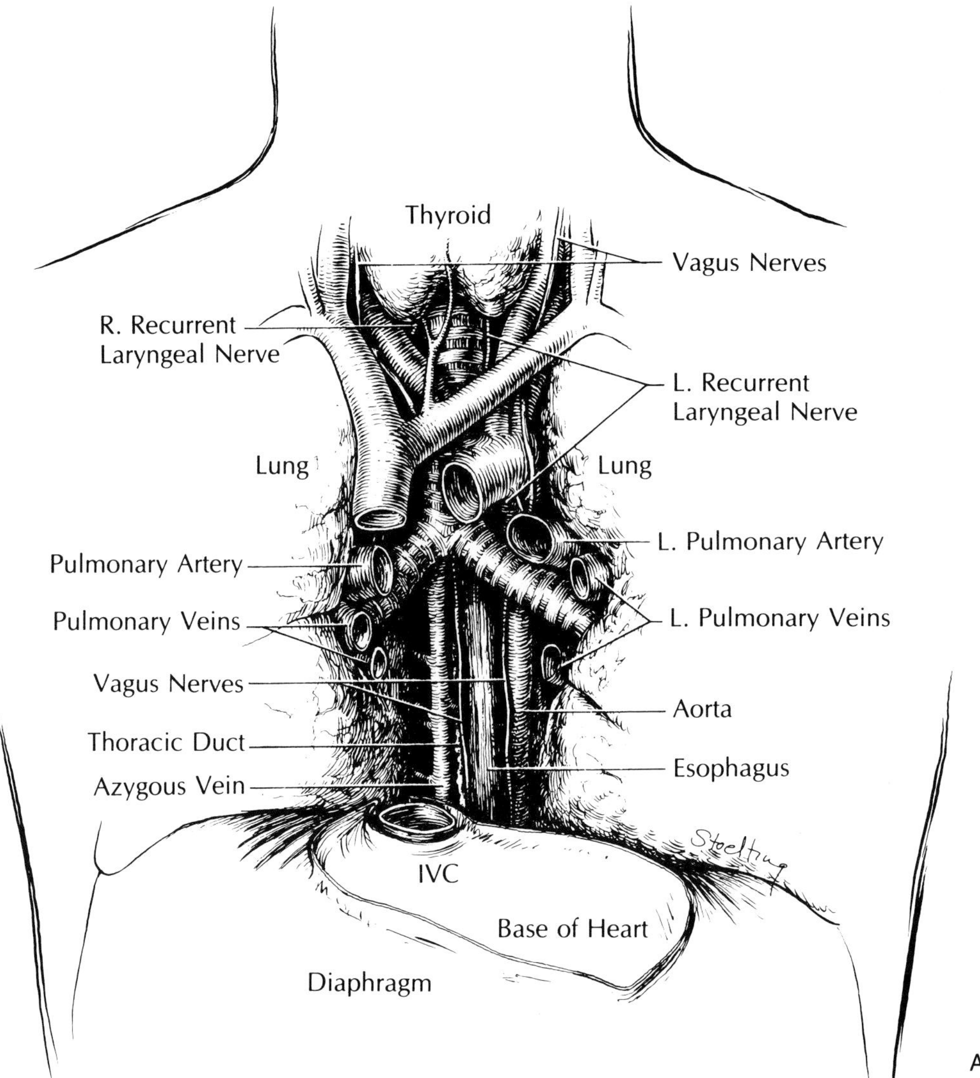

Figure 16–2.   The relative location of the ascending, transverse arch, and descending thoracic aorta is shown in this diagram. **A:** anterior view.

of the descending aorta, and the thoracic duct lies posteriorly between the aorta and the esophagus. The vagus nerve in either chest passes downward behind the hilum of the lung. On the left, the main vagus trunk gives rise to the recurrent laryngeal nerve as it crosses the aorta at the level of the ligamentum arteriosus. The latter passes caudal to the ligamentum and ascends posteriorly to the aorta and into the neck lateral and anterior to the esophagus. On the right, the recurrent nerve encircles the right subclavian artery at its origin from the innominate artery and ascends into the neck lateral to the vertebral bodies. The descending aorta averages approximately 20 cm in length and extends from the fourth thoracic vertebra

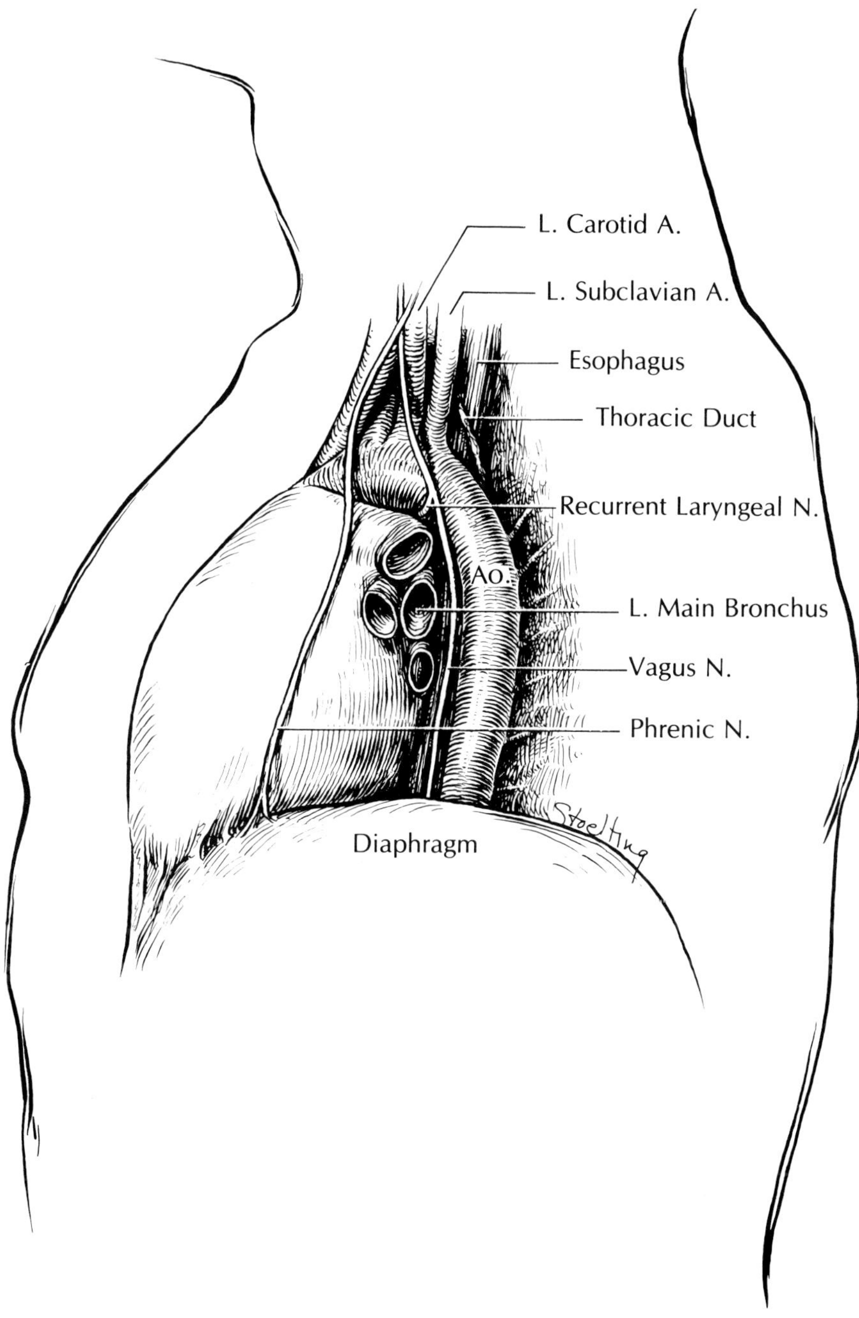

B

Figure 16–2, cont. **B:** left lateral view (see text).

to the aortic hiatus at the level of the 12th thoracic vertebra. The heart, within the pericardium, lies anteriorly and to the right of the descending thoracic aorta. The esophagus passes obliquely forward in the lower mediastinum and enters the abdomen through the esophageal hiatus, just anterior to the aorta. The azygous and hemizygous veins and the thoracic duct pass through the aortic hiatus of the diaphragm, with the hemizygous on the left, the azygous on the right, and the thoracic duct posterior to the aorta.

Nine pairs of intercostal arteries normally arise from the posterior and medial portion of the aorta and branch into either hemothorax in the intercostal groove beneath the lower border of each rib. In addition, several pairs of bronchial arteries variably originate from the arch or descending aorta and proceed directly to the hilum of the lung. Four or five segmental esophageal arteries pass from the descending aorta to the esophagus at intervals along its length.

The intercostal arteries provide critical blood supply to the spinal cord in 20% or more instances. This apparently is because the anterior spinal artery that supplies the spinal cord longitudinally is discontinuous in many instances, the anterior portion of the cord being supplied segmentally from the intercostal arteries. The most critical of these appears to lie at the T8–T12 area, where a large intercostal or intercostals supply a critical collateral, the artery of Adamkiewicz.

MECHANISM OF INJURY

The ascending aorta is the largest portion of the thoracic aorta in diameter and also the most vulnerable to penetrating injury.[1,12,13] In patients who survive to reach the emergency room, the mechanism of injury usually is a stab wound with ice pick or a narrow knife because penetrating wounds larger than 1 cm usually are immediately fatal. Every series of penetrating trauma describes survival from a bullet wound from small caliber handguns, whereas injuries from larger caliber gunshot wounds are rarely compatible with patient survival long enough to reach the hospital.

Blunt traumatic rupture most commonly occurs due to deceleration injury from automobile accidents, falls from heights, and motorcycle and airplane accidents.[3,7,9,14–16] Blunt injury to the aorta and great vessels, in general, results from accidents involving sudden horizontal or vertical deceleration. Horizontal deceleration produces traumatic rupture of the aorta distal to the origin of the left subclavian artery at the level of the ligamentum arteriosum (the aortic isthmus) in 95% of patients who survive long enough to have the diagnosis made. In 2% to 3%, the rupture occurs in the ascending aorta above the aortic valve. In the remainder, the tears occur at the level of the diaphragm or at multiple levels (Fig. 16–3).[7] Vertical deceleration produces injuries not only of the ascending aorta but to the aortic arch vessels, more commonly the innominate, less often the left subclavian, secondary to acute lengthening of the great vessels at their origin.

In addition to deceleration, whether horizontal or vertical, other mechanisms of blunt injury may be incriminated in aortic or great vessel injury. Compression of the chest with rapid displacement of the heart downward and to the left may produce ascending aortic rupture. Upward displacement of the heart and mediastinal structures from a cranially directed impact to the lower chest may rupture the descending aorta, an injury noted in patients sliding forward and under a dashboard overhang.

In certain injuries to the great vessels, hyperextension of the head with extreme

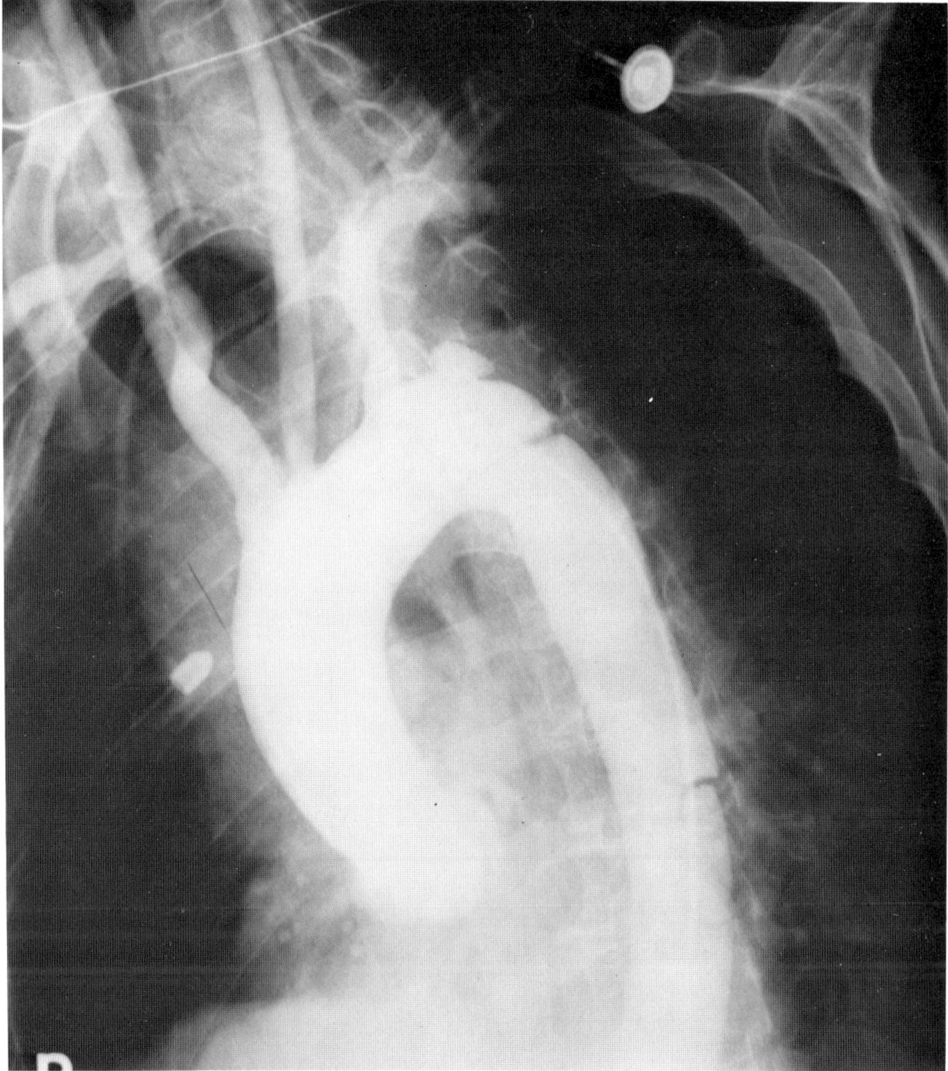

Figure 16–3.   Aortogram shows three tears in the thoracic aorta. The upper two were repaired utilizing a graft replacement and the lower lesion by direct suture.

rotation of the cervical spine produces partial or complete avulsion of the great vessels as they arise from the arch of the aorta.

Coroners' statistics show that the vast majority of traumatic aortic ruptures are immediately fatal.[3,9,17] Although those involving the ascending aorta are nearly 100% fatal, between 10% and 20% of the patients with injuries involving the proximal descending aorta survive long enough to reach the hospital, permitting diagnosis and treatment. Parmley and co-workers[7] in a review of 125 patients with aortic transection found 20% lived for more than 1 hr. Of those surviving 1 hr, 30% died in 6 hr, 40% by 24 hr, 72% by 8 days, and 90% by 10 weeks (Table 16–1). The formation of a pseudoaneurysm in surgically untreated

Table 16–1. Aortic Injury[7]

Dead on arrival	237
Died 1st day	12
Died 2–7 days	11
Died 2nd week	5
Died 3rd week	2
Survivors*	8

*All developed aneurysms.

survivors also has inherent hazards; 50% will be symptomatic within 3 yr, and late rupture has been known to occur as early as 6 months or as late as 3 decades after injury.

Between 10% and 25% of all deaths from automobile accidents are caused by aortic disruption, 20% of whom will have multiple transections.[7,18–20] In fact, Voigt[17] found that aortic rupture was present in one-third of a large series of fatal automobile accidents in Sweden.

In our experience in a large university hospital that sees all regional major trauma and in which there was only a relatively modest referral practice of acute injuries, the incidence of a penetrating or blunt aortic rupture constituted at most 1% to 2% of all major thoracic injuries.

DIAGNOSIS

The primary initial clinical manifestation of penetrating trauma to the aorta is intrathoracic hemorrhage with shock. If the intrapericardial portion of the ascending aorta is involved, cardiac tamponade often is the presenting sign. The presence of distended neck veins and an elevated central venous pressure indicates that the patient's shock is not due to hypovolemia, which is often the initial presumption, but secondary to diminished cardiac output from the pericardial tamponade. Massive bleeding into the mediastinum and into the right pleural space occurs with extrapericardial ascending thoracic aortic injuries and into either pleural space or mediastinum with penetrating injuries of the transverse arch. Left hemothorax most often follows descending aortic injuries. Spontaneous closure of small penetrating aortic injuries must occur for survival. With the decrease in blood pressure after the initial hemorrhage, adventitial fragments tend to swell and fold into the area of injury. With resuscitation and restoration of intravascular volume and subsequent increase in arterial pressure, bleeding may recur. This will be manifested by a brief clinical response to administration of fluids, with a temporary increase in blood pressure followed by a precipitous return of hypotension due to bleeding into one or both pleural cavities or the mediastinum. In some instances, such as those associated with penetrating injuries from narrow instruments or small-caliber gunshot wounds, adventitial tamponade of the bleeding site may be effective enough to preclude hemorrhage, even when the blood pressure is increased with fluid infusions. Delayed hemorrhage may occur hours or days after initial injury, or a false aneurysm may form, which may gradually enlarge with time.

The key to diagnosis of *penetrating wounds* of the aorta or great vessels is a high index of suspicion when a wound passes near any major intrathoracic vessel. As a general rule, whenever there has been such an injury, especially accompanied by major hemorrhage, aortography must be performed on an emergency basis, for when a wound of an artery occurs in proximity to a major body cavity such as the pleural space, sudden exsanguination can occur before the injury is recognized and before definitive vascular control can be obtained. On rare occasions, simultaneous injury to the aorta and contiguous vessels, such as to an adjacent cardiac chamber, pulmonary artery, or vena cava, may result in the development of an arteriovenous fistula as the artery decompresses into a low-pressure chamber (Fig. 16–4). In these instances, a continuous murmur often accompanied by a thrill may be heard or palpated over the site of injury. For this reason, auscultation and palpation of vessels at the base of the neck should be done in every patient with major penetrating thoracic or cervical trauma.

The successful diagnosis of *blunt traumatic aortic rupture* requires a high index of suspicion after any major deceleration injury. As many as one-third of patients who survive to be seen in trauma units with traumatic vascular rupture present with no external evidence of thoracic trauma, thereby giving a false sense of security to the examining physician. Many of the patients are unconscious at the time of admission because of associated head injuries and as many as 50% arrive in shock. Thus, in an unconscious patient with vascular collapse but with no external evidence of thoracic trauma or underlying vascular injury, there may be a delay in the diagnosis of aortic or great vessel damage.

The recognition of blunt trauma to the aorta or great vessels depends on suspecting the diagnosis in an individual who presents with a history of torsional, shearing, compressive, or deceleration forces despite the presence or absence of other obvious injuries (Table 16–2). If complete transection of the aorta has occurred, the patient usually does not survive to reach the emergency department but, in the 10% to 20% who do, the integrity of the adventitia may contain the hemorrhage (Fig. 16–5). The administration of fluids with restoration of cardiac output and blood pressure may lead to a secondary hemorrhage, often fatal, before diagnostic procedures can be completed. This usually will be manifested by the development of a left hemothorax, because by far the most common traumatic aortic injury is that just distal to the subclavian artery. Strong pulses in the upper extremities combined with weak pulses in the lower extremities occasionally may occur because the divided intima and media may act to partially obstruct the flow of blood to the lower half of the body distal to the site of the tear. In most instances, the large, contained mediastinal hematoma may result in proximal hypertension and distal hypotension due to a combination of intrusion of the hematoma on the aortic lumen, stimulation of arch baroreceptors by the hematoma, and activation of the renin mechanism. As many as 50% of patients with acute, contained traumatic transection of the aorta will have upper extremity systolic blood pressure greater than 150 mm Hg and diastolic pressures as high as 100 mm Hg. The hypertension may continue to exist postoperatively from 2 to 12 days, with an average of 4 days from the onset of the injury, despite adequate surgical repair. Paraplegia or partial to complete anterior or spinal artery hypoperfusion secondary to avulsion or occlusion of intercostal arteries also may be an initial manifestation of aortic injury. The complete list of symptoms and signs of aortic rupture are given in Table 16–2.[7,10,19,21]

The classic radiographic manifestation of traumatic aortic rupture is mediastinal widening, as seen on the chest film. This is the single most valuable aid in diagnosing possible aortic injury because the injury is almost always associated with hemorrhage into the mediastinum (Fig. 16–6). Although various forms of thoracic trauma, such as sternal fracture, may rupture small vessels in the mediastinum and produce a mediastinal

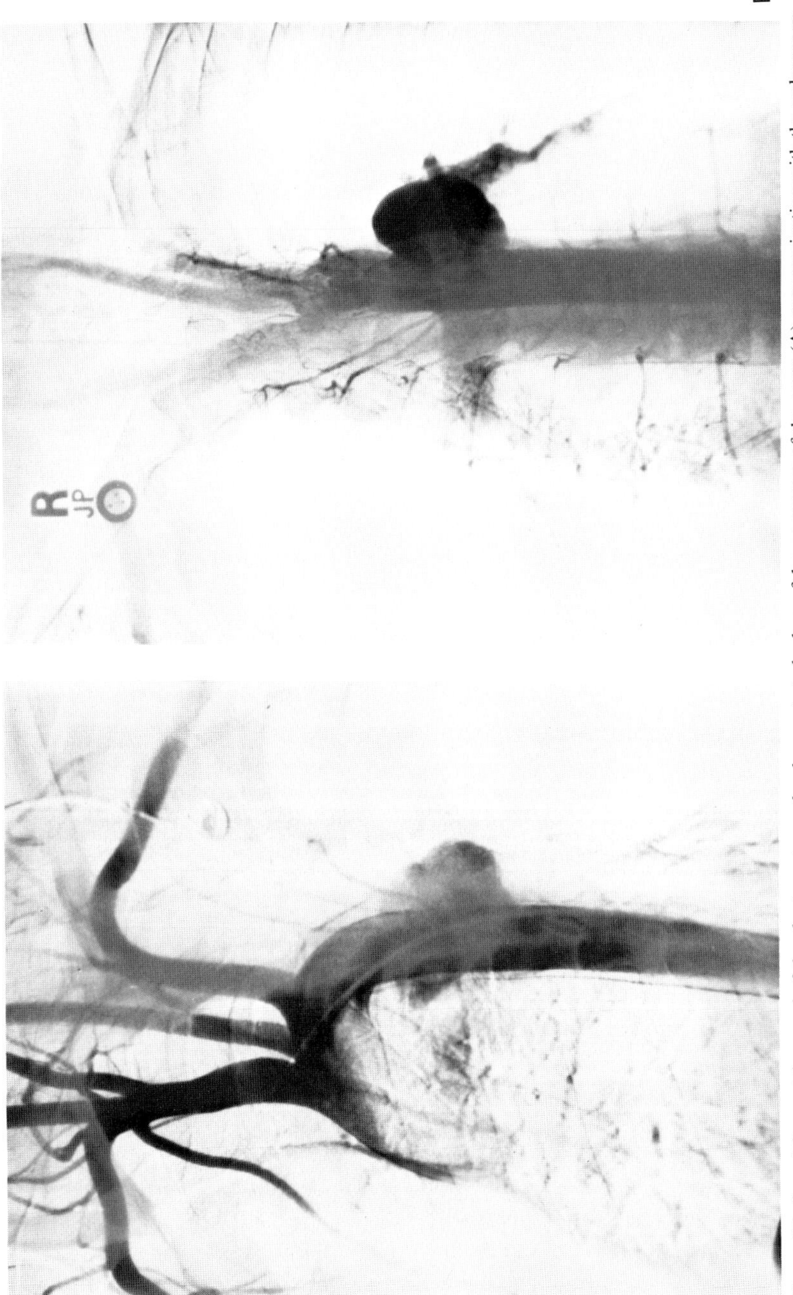

Figure 16–4.   After a stab wound of the chest, aortography demonstrated a large false aneurysm of the aorta (**A**) communicating with the pulmonary artery (**B**).

Table 16–2. List of Symptoms and Signs of Aortic Rupture

Symptoms
Retrosternal pain
Interscapular pain
Hoarseness
Dyspnea
Dysphagia
Paraplegia
Distal ischemia
Signs
Sternal fracture
Fracture of upper ribs
Fracture or dislocation of thoracic spine
Fullness or hematoma at base of neck
Tracheal deviation
Hypertension in arms
Hypotension in legs
Bruits in chest and neck
Hemothorax
Stridor

hematoma, any widening of the mediastinum should and must be considered presumptive evidence of aortic damage until proved otherwise. Because the mediastinum is magnified on the anteroposterior radiograph used most frequently with injured patients, there may be a false impression of mediastinal widening. As a result, only 25% to 35% of patients with radiographic mediastinal widening will prove to have actual transection of the thoracic aorta or disruption of the great vessels.

Aneurysms and periaortic hematomas involving the ascending aorta tend to project in silhouette into the right pleural space. In addition to radiographic evidence of mediastinal widening, the radiographic signs (Table 16–3) or aortic rupture are mediastinal hemorrhage noted as a widened mediastinal stripe in 90% of patients; apical hematoma, most often observed as early obliteration of the medial aspect of the left upper lobe; shift of the trachea to the right; compression and downward displacement of the left main stem bronchus to greater than the normal 40%; blunting of the contour of the aortic knob; variable amount of blood in the left chest; and obliteration of the aortic window on lateral film. There may be deviation to the right of a nasogastric tube in the esophagus by the periaortic hematoma. A left pleural effusion unassociated with rib fractures or pulmonary contusion may be found in 10% to 15% of patients with an aortic injury.

The confirmation of the diagnosis of aortic rupture in a stable patient is best made with selective thoracic aortography and is mandated in all cases of suspected aortic tears, considering the lethal outcome of untreated transections. The angiographic catheter should be passed from a femoral artery up into the proximal ascending aorta so that the entire thoracic aorta from the aortic valve to the diaphragm and its major branches can be visualized. Although the performance of retrograde aortography via the femoral artery conjures up the possibility of lethal complications, this has not resulted in rupture of the false aneurysm at the time of dye injection. As previously indicated, a small percentage of cases may involve the ascending aorta or the arch, or multiple injuries may be present. Therefore, sufficient concentration of dye injected with the pressure injector with the patient

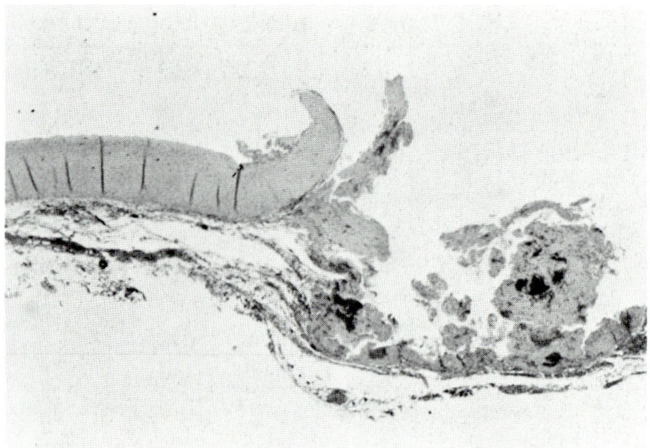

Figure 16–5.   Microscopic section of an aortic injury shows that the integrity of the aorta has been maintained by the adventitia.

in the right posterior oblique position is needed to visualize adequately the aortic arch, isthmus area, and the descending aorta to the level of the diaphragm (Fig. 16–7). In most cases of transection of the aorta at the isthmus, the aortogram will demonstrate a pseudoaneurysm formation, without extravascular dye, near the ligamentum arteriosum. Often the intimal flap can be seen or internal tears visualized as filling defects within the lumen. Medial dissection also may accompany the transected aorta and can be noted by aortogram.

The appearance of the ductus diverticulum, particularly in children, must be considered in the differential diagnosis of isthmal widening and not be misinterpreted as an aneurysm on the aortogram. The ductus diverticulum is smooth-walled and limited to the inferiomedial aspect of the aorta without evidence of intimal irregularity.

Computed tomography (CT) or magnetic resonance (MR) scanning using contrast media may be the examinations of choice in the future as they may be more readily available than angiography.[22] But, utilizing present CT technology, a small intimal tear may be obscured by dense aortic contrast when the tear is partial and the injury is not seen in profile. Moreover, there must be a sufficient number of scanning cuts so the area of injury is not missed. For these reasons, the gold standard for diagnosis at the present time is conventional aortography.

Most patients with traumatic thoracic rupture will have associated injuries. The most serious of these are head injuries and cervical or thoracic spine fractures or dislocations. Thoracic rupture should be suspected in patients with major deceleration injuries who present with altered consciousness or in the conscious patient who complains of cervical pain. CT scans of the head are indicated in the former and cervical and thoracic spine films demonstrating all cervical and thoracic vertebrae are mandatory in the latter. Multiple rib fractures, with or without flail chest, are common findings associated with traumatic aortic injuries, as are pneumothorax, hemothorax, and pulmonary contusion. Fractures of the first two ribs, which are strong, short, and relatively well protected and require considerable violence to fracture, are associated with aortic injury in 5% to 15% of these injuries.

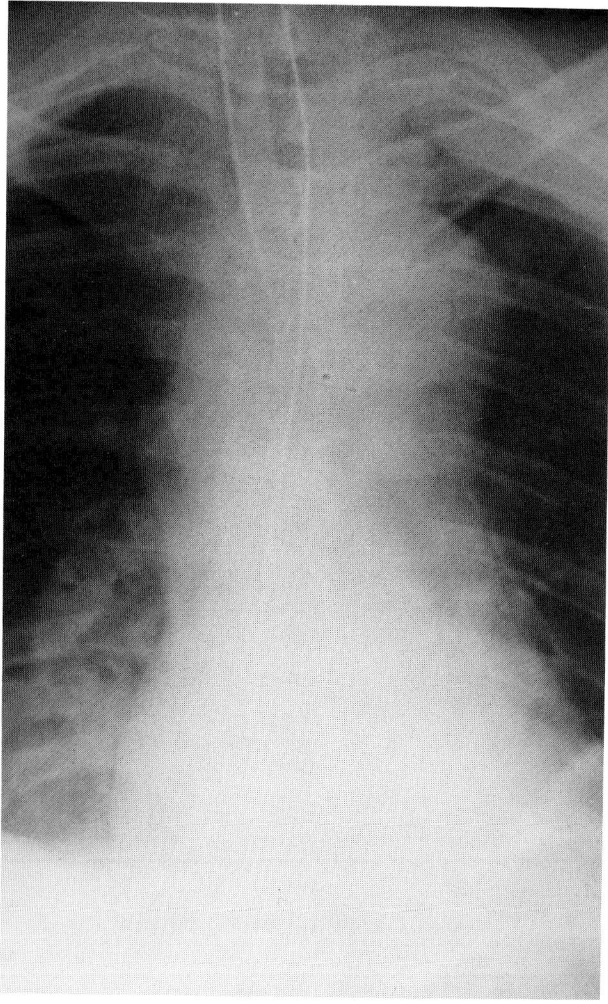

Figure 16–6.   This chest radiograph shows mediastinal widening as well as deviation of the trachea to the right. In addition, there is left apical capping. Aortography verified the presence of aortic rupture.

Intraabdominal injuries, specifically of spleen, liver, and kidney, may be present, as may pelvic and lower extremity fractures. Fleming and Green[9] found that 50% of their patients with acute thoracic aortic rupture had major intraabdominal injuries. The Parkland Hospital Group in Dallas had a similar experience, with 48% of their patients with aortic transection having associated intraabdominal injuries.[8] In patients with multiple organ system injury, assessment of the surgical priorities to be undertaken is mandatory. If the patient is exsanguinating, immediate left thoracotomy is indicated. However, if the patient shows evidence of a stable intrathoracic process but has associated intraabdominal organ damage with or without a positive peritoneal lavage, laparotomy should take precedence over management of potential thoracic injuries. This is because abdominal injuries usually can be managed more quickly and, if untreated, markedly complicate the management of

Table 16–3. Radiographic Changes

Mediastinal widening
Prominent aortic knob
Aortic outline obliteration
Aortic window obliteration
Tracheal deviation
Depression of left bronchus
Widening of paravertebral stripe
Deviation of esophagus
Hemothorax

the aortic injury.[8] In most instances, ongoing signs of blood loss in the absence of overt hemothorax are more likely to be related to the abdominal injury than the thoracic injury. As a matter of principle, a patient should not be lost from an easily treatable injury while attempting to manage a more complex injury such as aortic rupture.

Of those 10% to 20% of patients with aortic injuries who survive long enough to reach the emergency department, approximately half will develop massive secondary hemorrhage within the first 24 hr after admission and resuscitation. Most of the remainder will develop free rupture in the following several days. The 5% to 10% of patients with aortic transection who survive without specific treatment leave the hospital only to manifest a chronic pseudoaneurysm at a later date. Therefore, whenever traumatic rupture of the aorta is suspected by history or reconstruction of the events of the accident or physical signs on radiography, evaluation by aortography should proceed quickly. Should the patient develop manifestations of massive hemorrhage before or during definitive studies, the diagnostic testing (including aortography) should be aborted and the patient taken directly to the operating room for exploration.

PRINCIPLES OF MANAGEMENT

Surgical treatment results in a 90% survival rate of patients who are stable at initiation of the operation; thus, surgical management is indicated in all but a few instances. Exceptions may consist of patients with presumed fatal associated injuries, such as massive head injury or older patients with severe preexisting medical problems. In these instances, hypotensive therapy using the technique advocated by Wheat[22] and others[23] may be appropriate. As indicated previously, 5% to 10% will survive and leave the hospital if the injury is either not recognized or conservative management is elected.

As soon as aortic injury is suspected, the patient should be typed and cross-matched and 6 to 10 U of blood obtained. Blood pressure control, as just indicated, should be initiated while assessment is continued and diagnostic studies are performed. Many of these patients are hypertensive, and every effort should be made to control systolic thrust. If the patient can tolerate it, systolic pressure should be controlled at 100 to 120 mm Hg. Inadequate urine output or development of arrhythmias or myocardial ischemic changes may dictate a higher pressure (see Chapter 7 for drug therapy).

One of three principles of operative management should be selected: a) repair of the thoracic aorta without any type of bypass, b) the use of a local plastic shunt with

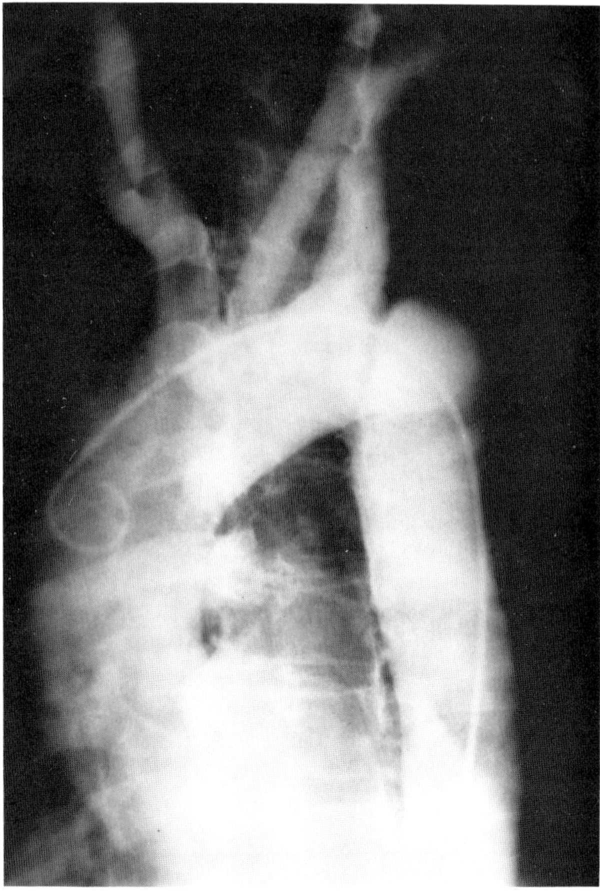

Figure 16–7.   The aortogram demonstrates the most common location for aortic rupture: the level of the isthmus just distal to the subclavian artery.

incorporated heparin bonding, or c) some type of pump support.[4,5,24–30] The last can consist of either cardiopulmonary bypass using standard cannulation of the superior and inferior vena cavae, left femoral vein to femoral artery bypass with oxygenation, or left atrial-to-femoral artery bypass, with or without an oxygenator.

Crawford and associates[24,25] have demonstrated the feasibility and safety of simple cross-clamping of the thoracic aorta in repair of thoracic injuries with control of blood pressure proximally with antihypertensive agents such as nitroprusside. However, even though they demonstrated that there is no difference in morbidity or mortality regardless of technique, if prolonged aortic occlusion times are necessary, some form of bypass should be used to reduce the risk of ischemic complications. Simple cross-clamp without shunt or pump is best reserved for those instances in which the patient is exsanguinating pre-operatively or who during the course of thoracotomy develop free hemorrhage into the pleural space before institution of bypass. Systemic anticoagulation may or may not be appropriate in certain patients, depending on the associated injuries, particularly potential head injury; however, newer pump setups require very little heparin and can be used safely in nearly all resuscitations.

The heparin-bonded shunt can be used optimally in those instances in which any anticoagulation might compromise the patient (Fig. 16–8).[29] The proximal end of the shunt can be placed in the apex of the left ventricle, in the ascending or transverse arch, or in a branch such as the left subclavian artery. The distal end is then inserted into the descending thoracic aorta or an exposed femoral artery. The disadvantages of the shunt are that the proximal placement in the aorta requires opening the mediastinum and exposing the proximal aorta, which may decompress the periaortic hematoma and resultant hemorrhage before proximal and distal control has been obtained. The proximal aortic insertion also results in a second vascular injury in the aorta that must be repaired. Plus, it is hard to ascertain if the shunt is functioning and how much flow it is providing to the distal aorta. Although the use of the heparin-bonded shunt is a relatively simple technique, it is best applied in those situations in which cardiopulmonary bypass is not available.[31,32]

The third technique involves the use of a pump, with or without an oxygenator. The advantages are that the pump-oxygenator can be used to support the myocardium in the case of associated myocardial injuries, blood and other volume expanders can be rapidly infused

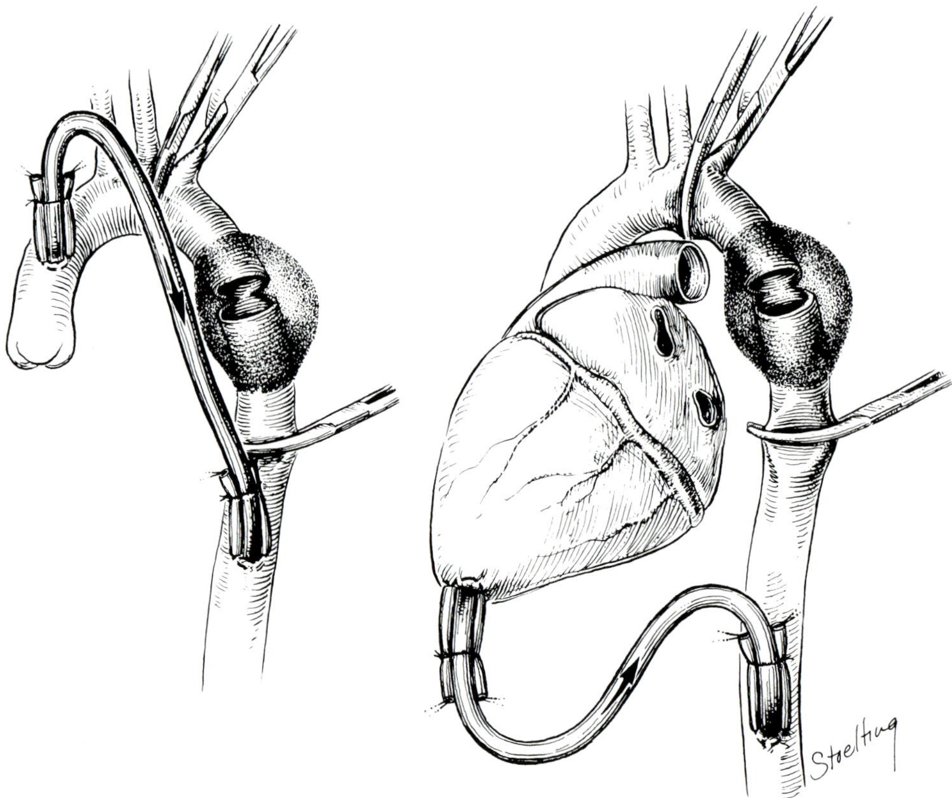

Figure 16–8.   Depicts the use of a heparin-bonded shunt to bypass the area of injury during aortic occlusion for repair.

through the cannula from the pump, and suction can be used to retrieve and immediately return blood lost during the procedure. Moreover, more precise control of proximal and distal perfusion and pressures is possible with pump support.

Lesions of the aortic arch or ascending aorta require full cardiopulmonary bypass using conventional anterior sternotomy and caval or right atrial cannulation and descending aorta or femoral artery return to permit complete diversion of blood from the heart and the operative field.

In cases of descending aortic injuries, in its simplest form with the use of a pump alone, the pericardium is opened and the left atrium is cannulated through the atrial appendage. Oxygenated blood is pumped from the left atrium to the femoral artery or into the descending thoracic aorta (Fig. 16–9).

Another alternative to divert blood around the site of aortic cross-clamp is to use femoral vein-to-artery cannulation, providing arterialization of the blood with the use of an oxygenator in the line (Fig. 16–10). This permits the patient to be placed on bypass before entering the chest. Modifications of the system are now available so that femoral-femoral bypass can be accomplished simply and quickly with high flow rates and *minimal* heparinization. Both oxygenators and heat exchangers with low clotting properties can be added easily to the circuit to provide maximum protection to organs distal to the aortic clamp. This circuit can be ready and in place as the chest is being opened.[33]

With any of these techniques, it is important to control the proximal aortic pressure because, with the application of a clamp to the thoracic aorta, there is simultaneous elevation in afterload, obstruction of distal flow, and activation of the renin mechanism due to distal hypotension superimposed on the already altered baroreceptor mechanism. This tends to produce a severe increase in proximal aortic pressure, with attendant complications of this altered afterload on the probably already compromised left ventricle and on cerebral vessels. Any increase in left ventricular diastolic pressure increases myocardial oxygen demand. Such an increase in individuals whose myocardium has already been depressed by periods of hypotension and metabolic acidosis may result in an insidious increase of left ventricular end-diastolic pressure, elevation of pulmonary venous pressure and pulmonary edema, and fatal myocardial depression.[13] One approach to this problem is the use of a right radial artery catheter and a distal aortic or femoral artery catheter to monitor proximal and distal pressure. In addition, the use of a left atrial pressure line or Swan-Ganz catheter is useful to constantly monitor left atrial pressures. This permits the judicious use of pharmacologic agents, nitroglycerin, or nitroprusside to control afterload.

SURGICAL TREATMENT

Injuries of the ascending aorta and proximal portion of the aortic arch are best approached in the conventional manner for open heart surgery using an anterior midline sternotomy incision. In instances in which the site of injury has not been ascertained preoperatively, the thoracic cavity in which there is ongoing hemorrhage should be entered using an anterolateral thoracotomy. An anterolateral thoracotomy can be converted into a transverse sternotomy by transecting the sternum at the fourth or fifth interspace and extending the incision into the appropriate intercostal space in the opposite chest. This provides good access to the entire anterior mediastinum, the ascending aorta, and the proximal arch.

As most *penetrating trauma* consists of simple injuries, cardiopulmonary bypass

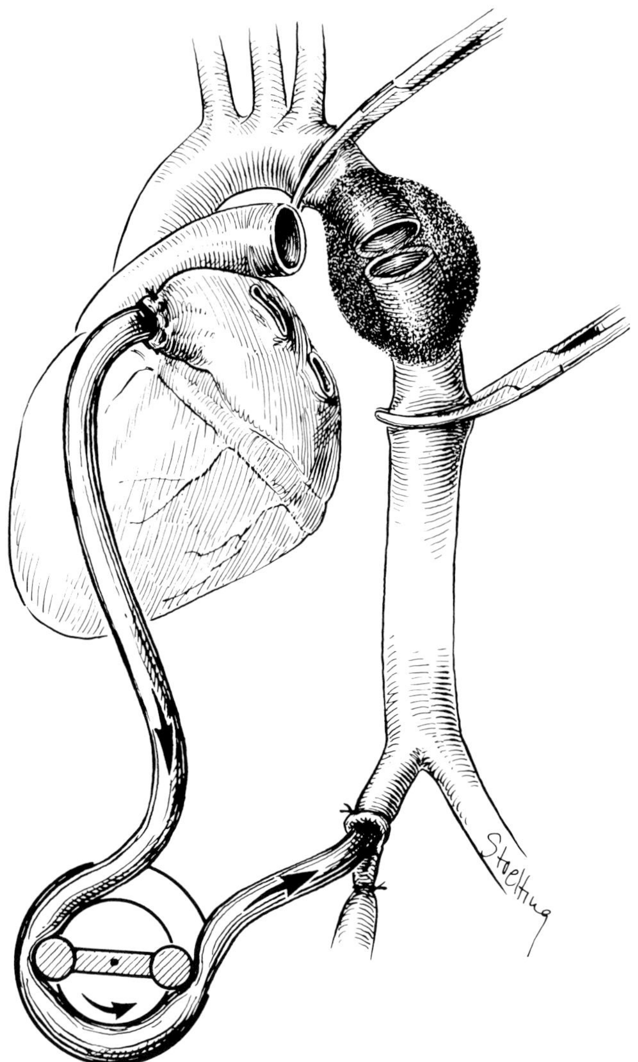

Figure 16–9. An alternative technique for aortic bypass. This requires a pump and anticoagulation but permits bypass to be carried out before approaching the aorta.

usually is not necessary. Small lacerations can be controlled with digital pressure and sutured directly, or a partial occluding clamp can be applied and the injury repaired in a dry field. If the aorta is friable, some type of bolster such as Dacron or Teflon felt can be incorporated into a mattress suture or used as a circumferential wrap about the site of injury after suture closure of the wound.

Generally, our favored incision for almost all penetrating intrathoracic injuries is an anterolateral thoracotomy. If this incision is used, the left shoulder and left hip are elevated slightly with pads to bring the patient to a slightly oblique position (Fig. 16–11). The left arm is suspended on the anesthetist's stand or left at the side. The skin incision is placed in

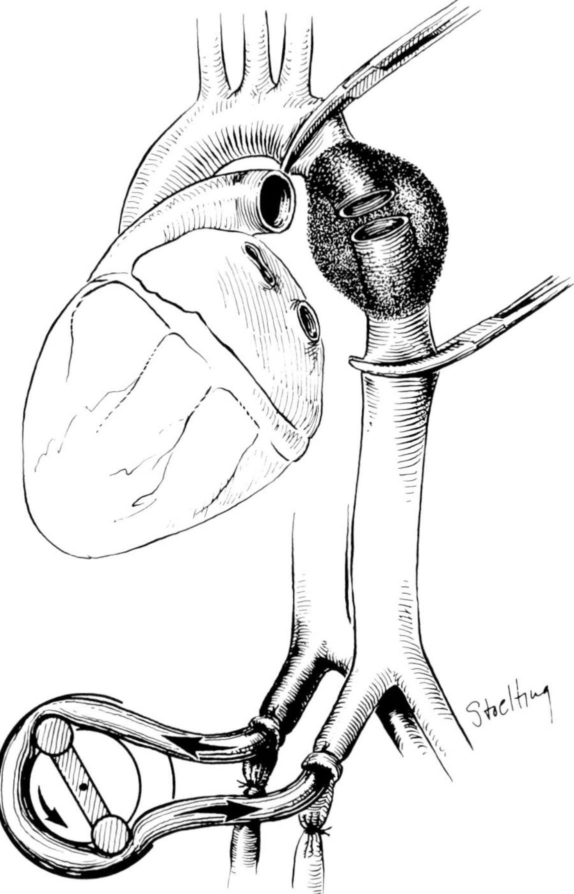

Figure 16–10. Femoral vein to femoral artery bypass requires the use of an oxygenator that may be appropriate when dealing with ascending or arch lesions.

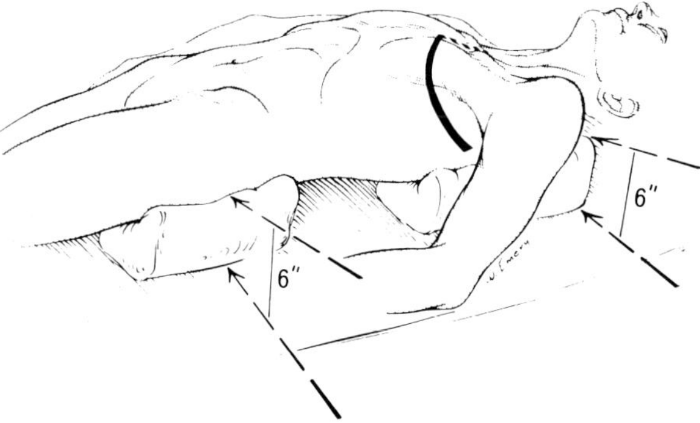

Figure 16–11. This is the position of choice when dealing with the multiply injured patient. It permits simultaneous laparotomy as well as adequate exposure of the proximal descending aorta.

the pectoral or inframammary groove, then extended upward, laterally paralleling the direction of the ribs. Medially, the incision is curved upward in the parasternal line as high as necessary. The pectoralis major is taken down from its attachments to the sixth rib and the fourth or fifth interspace is entered. The skin incision usually extends to the posterior axillary line, but the muscles of the chest wall can be undercut with the chest cavity partially open. The intercostal muscles can be divided with the scissors nearly to the vertebrae and the costal cartilages of the third, fourth, and fifth ribs cut anteriorly, if necessary, for exposure. This opens up a flap of chest wall, permitting generous exposure of the entire pleural cavity. The advantage of this incision is that the unstable patient does better in the supine position and immediate access to the heart and control of all the great vessels is available.

Blunt traumatic ruptures usually require the repair of the entire circumference of the aorta. This is best done with some type of shunt or bypass in place, as described previously. We have, in certain desperate situations, used venous inflow occlusion and immobilized and temporarily occluded the superior and inferior vena cavae. This gives a reasonably dry field for periods of 3 to 4 min at a time. Rarely blunt injury will lend itself to isolation by a partial occluding clamp.

The most common sites of blunt nonpenetrating injuries are in the distal arch beyond the left carotid artery and in the descending aorta. Surgical exposure of the distal arch and the descending aorta is best accomplished through the left chest. This can be done by using a standard posterolateral thoracotomy through the fourth interspace with the pelvis rotated backward 45° and the left hip fully extended to allow access to the femoral vessels, if necessary. The operative management in the stable patient with descending aortic injury should include the use of a double lumen endotracheal tube to allow selective collapse of the left lung and provide for adequate ventilation in the lateral thoracotomy position. Its use reduces the amount of intraoperative pulmonary manipulation required for exposure that may worsen the accompanying pulmonary contusion (see Chapter 7).

In dealing with blunt rupture at the descending thoracic aorta, the initial maneuver is to assess the location of the hematoma in the mediastinum. If this involves the apex of the chest, as is true of most ruptures of the proximal descending aorta, proximal control is best initiated by opening the pericardium and isolating the ascending aorta. Dissection is then carried distally, encircling the aortic arch, either between the innominate and left carotid artery or between the left common carotid and the left subclavian artery, avoiding entering the mediastinal hematoma at the site of injury and thus releasing its tamponade effect on the disrupted aorta. The mediastinal pleura is opened over the descending thoracic aorta distal to the hematoma to permit the descending thoracic aorta to be encircled with a tape at some convenient spot away from the site of injury to ensure distal control. The mediastinal pleura is then opened between the vagus and phrenic nerves after these are identified. The phrenic nerve is mobilized to permit retraction away from the field. The location of the vagus nerve is sought to allow preservation of it and the recurrent laryngeal nerve as the dissection approaches the ligamentum arteriosum. With the aorta previously encircled, the dissection is carried progressively distally to identify the subclavian artery. If not done previously, the arch is encircled just proximal to the subclavian artery. The mediastinal hematoma usually is entered at this point by opening the pleura over the area of presumed injury.

Should a pump or shunt be indicated, all preparations for its implementation, including heparinization, should be completed at this point in case unexpected hemorrhage occurs. If a noninjured segment of the aorta distal to the subclavian artery is clearly identified, this is encircled, as is the aorta immediately distal to the area of the injury. Pump support is then instituted. Vascular clamps are then applied proximally and distally, the periaortic hematoma entered, and the injury assessed. The proximal clamp often must be placed proximal to the left subclavian artery, which also is clamped to obtain an adequate proximal cuff for suturing.

Infrequently, there may be only a partial tear of the intima and media of the aorta, in which instance the occluding clamps should be applied approximately 1 cm on each side of the laceration, the laceration trimmed, and then approximated as an assistant maintains constant apposition of the vascular clamps to permit tension-free closure using 4-0 braided polyester or monofilament Prolene sutures (Fig. 16–12).

When the artery is completely transected, the divided ends tend to retract. In such cases, the edges of the tear of the aorta are trimmed and any loose fragments of adventitia

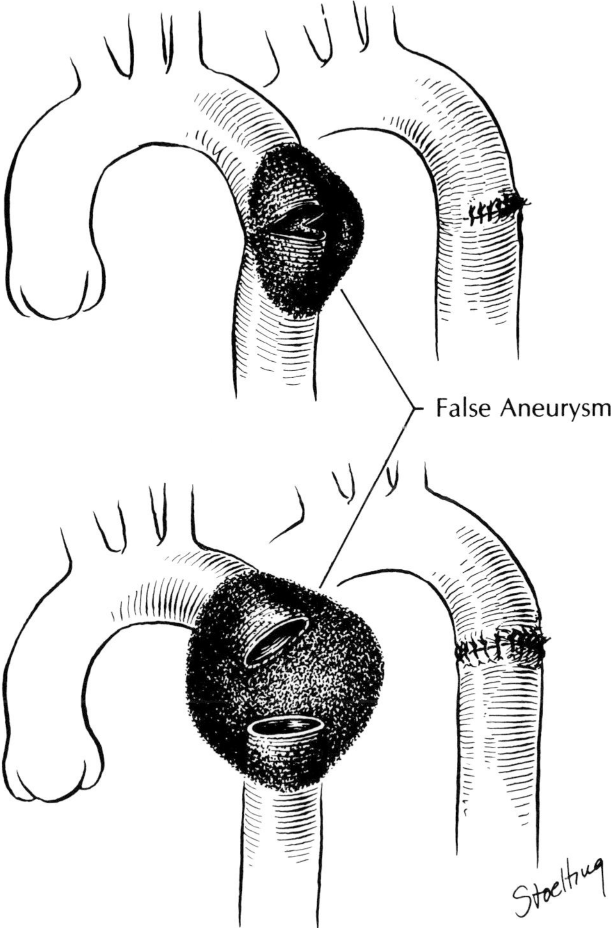

Figure 16–12.   Shows the appearance of the aorta at the time of operative exposure. The technique of primary repair is applicable in selected instances in which the injury has been minimal or the aortic ends are easily approximated.

are removed, and the tension required to approximate the vessel ends is assessed. A primary anastomosis can be utilized if undue tension can be avoided. This is accomplished by placing a running posterior layer of suture without tying any knots. The vessel ends can then be approximated, the suture pulled up, and the anterior row placed in running fashion as well. Small diameter aortas, such as those in women, can be relatively easily purse-stringed by the slippery Prolene sutures, resulting in inadequate caliber to the anastomosis. Therefore, care must be taken in tightening the suture. This can be done by tying the running suture medially and laterally after the posterior row is placed and placing interrupted anterior sutures or a second running suture anteriorly.

In most instances of traumatic disruption of the aorta, the simplest repair involves the use of a Dacron or Teflon graft. This has the advantage in that division of fewer intercostal arteries are necessary because the aorta does not have to be mobilized as extensively. The situation also may dictate utilization of a graft because a considerable resection of damaged aorta may be required. An appropriate graft, either nonporous, albumin-coated, or otherwise sealed, should be selected that is equivalent in size to the aorta. A proximal running suture line is placed starting posteriorly with the clamps placed in the anteroposterior direction. The medial and lateral suture line is placed and tied anteriorly. On completion of the proximal anastomosis, it is usually appropriate to test the integrity of the suture line because it is easier to reinforce the more tenuous proximal suture line before performing the second distal anastomosis. An alternate method for replacing the damaged aorta is to use an intraluminal graft, which has the advantage of easy and rapid insertion.[34]

Technical precautions to be considered in reconstruction of the aorta include dividing or sacrificing as few intercostal arteries as possible, thus ensuring blood supply to the spinal cord. Primary anastomosis may require temporary occlusion or division of one or two sets of upper intercostal arteries to permit mobilization of the aorta for approximation and suture. The ligamentum arteriosum usually requires division to facilitate exposure and repair of proximal descending aortic injuries.

When the injury lies in the distal descending aorta, the diaphragm may require division and retraction to permit enough exposure of the aorta to facilitate the repair. Again, as few intercostal arteries as possible should be divided because an anterior spinal artery syndrome, including paraplegia, may result from their interruption. Particularly critical are those at the T8-L1 area, where a large vessel supplying the anterior spinal artery often exists.[35] Those intercostal arteries in the operative field are better occluded temporarily by the application of silver clips.

Upon completion of the repair, the pleura is closed, if possible, which tends to reduce postoperative lymph seepage and protect the suture line. One or two chest tubes should be inserted into the pleural space, depending on the status of hemostasis and associated lung injury. Bypass, if used, is discontinued, and sites of bypass insertion are repaired. If full anticoagulation has been induced, heparin usually is reversed with protamine before closing the chest. The lung is reexpanded and the chest closed in standard fashion after placement of chest tubes for drainage.

POSTOPERATIVE CARE

Postoperatively, the patient is managed in an intensive care unit. In the absence of complications, the clinical course is usually benign and more related to associated injuries.

Cardiac failure or arrest can occur from hypovolemia or hypothermia. It also can occur after application of an occluding vascular clamp due to the sudden onset of proximal hypertension and the adverse effects on the heart. Attention to volume and pressure both during and after operation provides a means of prevention.

Cardiac depression resulting in cardiac failure may be due to myocardial contusion, long periods of hypotension, or hypovolemia. In addition, aortic cross-clamping with attendant acute hypertension may have an adverse effect on the myocardium. Serial monitoring, including ECGs, Swan-Ganz catheter monitoring, and accurate arterial monitoring, is essential for a smooth outcome. Trends are important and attention should be paid to both the preload and afterload dynamics. Normal cardiac indexes should be maintained as well as reasonable arterial blood gases.

Bleeding postsurgery, after adequate hemostasis has been obtained, should not be excessive. As transfused blood is deficient in platelets and when more than 5 U of blood have been required in the course of the operation, it is appropriate to order 5 to 10 U of platelet packs and administer them with the completion of the vascular anastomosis before closure of incisions.

Coagulation defects are rare, other than those occurring with consumption coagulopathy. Fresh frozen plasma occasionally may be of benefit should these defects occur. The prothrombin time and partial thromboplastin time provide screening tests for these transfusion-induced coagulopathies.

Hypothermia is another cause of diffuse oozing because it paralyzes the enzymatic reactions necessary for clotting and platelet aggregation. If the body temperature should decrease below 32° or 33°C, central warming is mandated using a heat exchanger with the pump oxygenator or warm saline solution poured into an accessible body cavity. Hypothermia can be prevented partially by warming all solutions before or during administration. In addition, a warming blanket should be placed and used on the operating table.

Bleeding occurring at an unacceptable rate, such as more than 2 U an hour for the first several hours or 1 U an hour for the first 6 hr, dictates reexploration if the clotting factors are corrected and a medical cause for bleeding ruled out by normal clotting tests. The suture line may require wrapping with Dacron, pericardium, or pleura. Large vessels, such as the internal mammary or intercostal artery, may be responsible for continued bleeding and should, of course, be ligated if found.

COMPLICATIONS

Postoperative complications are relatively rare but, when they occur, they are major. These complications fall into five categories: paraplegia, massive hemorrhage, hypertension, renal failure, and respiratory failure.

Paraplegia is the most feared complication. Its incidence is 5% to 20% after repair of blunt aortic trauma.[13,36] Prolonged hypotension, avulsion, or interruption of intercostal arteries often are found at operation in patients who have developed paraplegia preoperatively.

Direct injury to the spinal cord may occur in association with fracture or fracture dislocations of the thoracic vertebrae, secondary to thrombosis of intercostal artery at the time of injury or operation, or secondary to prolonged hypoxemia after shock. The fracture may be missed if the patient is comatose and, should paraplegia first be noted postoperatively, it may be inappropriately assumed to have resulted from the operation. The postoperative complication of paraplegia secondary to poor perfusion of the anterior spinal artery is not related to use or style of shunt, bypass, heparinization, or lack thereof. It does correlate with preexisting hypotension, as it is noted in more than three-fourths of patients who develop this complication. It also appears to relate to the length of aortic cross-clamp time[37–39] and is increased by ligation of intercostal vessels intraoperatively.[35,40] The fact that preoperative hypotension has been present when there is postoperative paraplegia may relate to the thrombotic tendency generated by shock.

The incidence of paraplegia may be diminished by rapid restoration of vascular volume to combat shock, shortened operative time occlusion, and avoidance of intraoperative division of intercostal vessels. In addition, the use of femoral-femoral bypass encompassing an oxygenator and heat exchanger now can be performed rapidly and allows better distal perfusion of the aorta, especially if extended periods of time are necessary to accomplish the repair. This technique allows for more accurate offloading of the proximal aortic pressure and can be used to supplement lost volume while maintaining the patient's temperature at acceptable levels.

New methods of monitoring spinal cord function during surgery offer promise that in the future it may be possible to identify impending ischemia and take corresponding steps to restore or improve perfusion.[41–43] In the future, the use of adjuncts during surgery such as lowering spinal fluid pressure with addition of steroids,[44] naloxone, an endorphin antagonist or intrathecal papaverin, administered during or after surgery, and the use of free radical antagonists may help to reduce the dreaded complication of paraplegia (see anesthesia management, Chapter 7).[45–48]

Massive bleeding, developing during the course of the operation and involving all portions of the wound including the anastomosis, most often is due to the consumption coagulopathy of disseminated intravascular coagulation. It results from a combination of shock and soft tissue injury but also may be the manifestation of a hemolytic transfusion reaction. Clotting factors are consumed intravascularly and fall to critical levels. Simultaneously, fibrinolysis is activated, resulting in secondary bleeding from areas in which there previously had been hemostasis. Management of this dreaded complication is difficult and the mortality rate is high. This condition is promoted by shock, and its correction requires the restoration and maintenance of normal blood volume. This may require massive transfusion and crystalloid administration. Adequate anticoagulation during vascular occlusion is the best means of preventing this complication. Once clotting is activated, the benefit of anticoagulation is controversial, because it is difficult to stop intravascular clotting with conventional doses of heparin. Nevertheless, in case of massive bleeding, reanticoagulation with heparin does not necessarily aggravate bleeding and may permit the build-up of clotting factors rather than allowing them to be consumed as rapidly as they are administered. At this point, platelets and fresh frozen plasma or warm, fresh, whole blood should be administered to restore adequate clotting factors to therapeutic levels while the dose of heparin wears off.

Persistent *hypertension* postoperatively may be precipitated by surgically induced coarctation through inadvertent purse stringing the anastomosis (pseudocoarctation). This also may occur despite restoration of adequate aortic luminal size and restoration of reasonable renal function and may be due to the basic injury to the aorta and the altered state of the baroreceptors in the arch and the involvement at the site of injury with an associated periaortic hematoma. Drug therapy is indicated to reduce the blood pressure toward normal and thus reduce the potential hazard to either the myocardium, brain, or suture line.

Renal failure after successful repair of traumatic aortic injury may be the result of a series of factors. The kidney is susceptible in injury by pre-, intra-, or postoperative hypotension, induction of anesthesia, decreased renal perfusion after cross-clamping of the aorta, and is heightened by preexisting renal disease. The incidence of renal failure in patients operated on without the use of a shunt or pump is approximately 5%.

Respiratory failure may follow either as a result of chest wall injury, pulmonary contusion, or the respiratory distress syndrome. Mechanical ventilation provides a means of support in the immediate postoperative period. This is best maintained postoperatively until there is assurance of adequate pulmonary function.[49]

RESULTS

Results of surgical treatment have improved progressively over the years. The mortality relates more to associated injuries than to the aortic surgery in the patient who is stable up to the period of control of the aortic injury. In the absence of shock and major associated injuries preoperatively, the operation mortality rate should not exceed 10%. When shock is present preoperatively, the operative mortality from bleeding complications and cardiac difficulties is high.

In the absence of paraplegia, full recovery is the rule. Late complications such as infection resulting in anastomotic breakdown or aneurysm are rare. Good healing of the aorta is the rule.

REFERENCES

1. Glinz W. *Chest Trauma. Diagnosis and Treatment*. Berlin: Springer-Verlag; 1981
2. Dshanelidze II. Manuscript, Petrograd, 1922. Cited by Lilienthal H: *Thoracic Surgery: The Surgical Treatment of Thoracic Diseases*. Philadelphia: Saunders; 1926.
3. Strassman G. Traumatic rupture of the aorta. *Am Heart J.* 1947;33:508.
4. Bahnsen HT. Definitive treatment of saccular aneurysms of the aorta with excision of the sac and aortic suture. *Surg Gynecol Obstet.* 1953;96:383.
5. Gerbode F, Baimbridge M, Osborn JJ, et al. Traumatic thoracic aneurysms: treatment by resection and grafting with the use of an extracorporeal bypass. *Surgery.* 1957;42:975.
6. Forsee JH, Blake HA. The recognition and management of closed chest trauma. *Surg Clin North Am.* 1958;38:1545.
7. Parmley LF, Mattingly TW, Manion WC. Nonpenetrating traumatic injury to the aorta. *Circulation.* 1958;17:1086.
8. Borman KR, Aurbakken CM, Weigelt JA. Treatment priorities in combined blunt abdominal and aortic trauma. *Am J Surg.* 1982;144:728.
9. Fleming AW, Green DC. Traumatic aneurysms of the thoracic aorta: report of 43 patients. *Ann Thorac Surg.* 1974;18:91.
10. Kirsh MM, Sloan H. *Blunt Chest Trauma*. Boston: Little, Brown; 1977.
12. Reul GR, Rubio RA, Beall AC. Surgical management of acute injuries of the thoracic aorta. *J Thorac Cardiovasc Surg.* 1974;67:272.
13. Van Niekerk JLM, Heijstraten RMJ, Goris RJA, et al. Spinal cord injury following surgery for acute traumatic rupture of the thoracic aorta. *Thorac Cardiovasc Surg.* 1986;34:30.
14. Eddy AC, Rusch VW, Fligner CL, et al. The epidemiology of traumatic rupture of the thoracic aorta in children: a 13-year review. *J Trauma.* 1990;30:989.
15. Haas GH. Types of internal injuries of personnel involved in aircraft accidents. *J Aviat Med.* 1944;15:77.

16. Shorr RM, Critten M, Indek M, et al. Blunt thoracic trauma: analysis of 515 patients. *Ann Surg.* 1987;(August):200.
17. Voigt CE. *Die biomechanik Stumfer brustverlet Zungen besonders von Thorax, Aorta, and Herz.* Stuttgart: Springer-Verlag; 1968.
18. Greendyke RM. Traumatic rupture of the aorta. *JAMA.* 1966;195:527.
19. Moran JM. Traumatic disruption of the thoracic aorta. In: Bergan JJ, Yao JST, eds. *Surgery of the Aorta and Its Branches.* New York: Grune & Stratton; 1979.
20. Zeldenrust J, Aarts JH. Traumatische aorta-ruptur bij verkeesongevallen. *Ned Tijdschr Geneeskd.* 1962;106:464.
21. Clark DE, Zeiger MA, Wallace KL, et al. Blunt aortic trauma: signs of high risk. *J Trauma.* 1990;30:701.
22. Wheat MW. Treatment of dissecting aneurysms of the aorta. *Prog Cardiovasc Dis.* 1973;16:87.
22. McLean, TR, Olinger, GN, Thorsen, MK. Computed tomography in the evaluation of the aorta in patients sustaining blunt chest trauma. *J Trauma.* 1991;31:254.
23. Fisher RG, Oria RA, Mattox KL, et al. Conservative management of aortic lacerations due to blunt trauma. *J Trauma.* 1990;30:1562.
24. Crawford ES, Fenstermacher JM, Richardson W, and Sandiford F. Re-appraisal of adjuncts to avoid ischemia in the treatment of thoracic aortic aneurysms. *Surgery.* 1970;67:182.
25. Crawford ES, Rukia P. Reassessment of adjuncts to avoid ischemia in the treatment of aneurysms of the descending aorta. *J Thorac Cardiovasc Surg.* 1973;66:693.
26. DelRossi AJ, Cernaianu AC, Madden LD, et al. Traumatic disruptions of the thoracic aorta: treatment and outcome. *Surgery.* 1990;108:864.
27. Grosso MA, Brown JM, Moore EE, Moore FA. Repair of the torn descending thoracic aorta using the centrifugal pump with partial left heart bypass: technical note. *J Trauma.* 1991;31:395.
28. Hug HR, Taber RE. Bypass flow requirements during thoracic aneurysmectomy with particular attention to the prevention of left heart failure. *J Thorac Cardiovasc Surg.* 1969;57:203.
29. Murray GF, Young WG. Thoracic aneurysmectomy utilizing direct left ventriculo-femoral shunt bypass. *Ann Thorac Surg.* 1976;21:26.
30. Roberts AJ, Michaelis LL. The use of bypass techniques and other forms of organ protection during thoracic aortic cross-clamping. In: Bergan JJ, Yao JST, eds. *Surgery of the Aorta and Its Branches.* New York: Grune & Stratton; 1979.
31. Molina JE, Cogordan J, Einzig S, et al. Adequacy of ascending aorta—descending aorta shunt during cross-clamping of the thoracic aorta for prevention of spinal cord injury. *J Thorac Cardiovasc Surg.* 1985;90:126.
32. Verdant A, Page A, Cossette R, et al. Surgery of the descending thoracic aorta: spinal cord protection with the Gott shunt. *Ann Thorac Surg.* 1988;46:147.
33. Ireland KW, Follette DM, Pollock ME, et al. Use of the Sci-med heat exchanger to prevent hypothermia during the repair of thoracic and thoracoabdominal aneurysms. *Ann Thorac Surg.* 1993;55:534.
34. Berger RL, Romero L, Chaudry AG, Dobnik DB. Graft replacement of the thoracic aorta with a sutureless technique. *Ann Thorac Surg.* 1983;35:231.
35. Pasternak BM, Boyd DP, Ellis HE. Spinal cord injury after procedures on the aorta. *Surg Gynecol Obstet.* 1972;135:29.
36. Marvasti MA, Meyer JA, Ford BE, et al. Spinal cord ischemia following operation for traumatic aortic transection. *Ann Thorac Surg.* 1986;42:425.
37. Adams HD, Van Geertruyden HH. Neurologic complications of aortic surgery. *Ann Surg.* 1956;144:574.
38. Krieger KH, Spencer FC. Is paraplegia after repair of coarctation of the aorta due principally to distal hypotension during aortic cross-clamping? *Surgery.* 1985;97:2.
39. Lynch C, Weingarden SI. Paraplegia following aortic surgery. *Paraplegia.* 1982;20:196.
40. Blaisdell FW, Cooley DA. The mechanism of paraplegia after temporary thoracic aortic occlusion. *Surgery.* 1962;51:351.
41. Coles JG, Wilson GJ, Sima AF, et al. Intraoperative detection of spinal cord ischemia using somatosensory cortical evoked potentials during thoracic aortic occlusion. *Ann Thorac Surg.* 1982;34:299.
42. Laschinger JC, Cunningham JN Jr, Nathan IM, et al. Interoperative identification of vessels critical to spinal cord blood supply. Use of somatosensory evoked potentials. *Curr Surg.* 1984;41:107.
43. Svenson LG, Patel V, Robinson MF, et al. Influence of preservation or perfusion of intraoperatively identified spinal cord blood supply on spinal motor evoked potentials and paraplegia after aortic surgery. *J Vasc Surg.* 1991;13:355.
44. Laschinger JC, Cunningham JN Jr, Cooper MM, et al. Prevention of ischemic spinal cord injury following aortic cross-clamping: use of corticosteroids. *Ann Thorac Surg.* 1984;38:500.
45. Archer CW, Wynn MM, Archibald J. Naloxone and spinal fluid drainage as adjuncts in the surgical treatment of thoracoabdominal and thoracic aneurysms. *Surgery.* 1990;108:755.
46. Faden AL, Jacobs TP, Holaday JW. Comparison of early and late naloxone treatment in experimental spinal injury. *Neurology.* 1982;32:677.

46. Van Norman GA, Parlin EG, Eddy AC, Parlin DJ. Hemodynamic and metabolic effects of aortic unclamping following emergency surgery for traumatic thoracic aortic tear in shunted and unshunted patients. *J Trauma.* 1991;31:1007.
47. Faden AL, Jacobs TP, Holaday JW. Opiate antagonist improves neurologic recovery after spinal injury. *Science.* 1981;211:493.
48. Svensson LG, Von Ritter CM, Groeneveld HT, et al. Cross-clamping of the thoracic aorta. Influence of aortic shunts, laminectomy, papaverine, calcium channel blocker, allopurinol and superoxide dismutase on spinal cord flow and paraplegia in baboons. *Ann Surg.* 1986;204:38.
49. Blaisdell FW, Lewis FR. *Respiratory Distress Syndrome of Shock and Trauma.* Philadelphia: Saunders; 1977.

17

Great Vessel Injury: Innominate, Right and Left Subclavian, and Right and Left Common Carotid

DONALD D. TRUNKEY, M.D.

HISTORY: Injuries to the great vessels as they exit the chest are inextricably linked to the history of traumatic aneurysms. This is undoubtedly due to the immediate lethality of any large wound of the great vessels and patients who sustained small wounds might survive if the bleeding tamponaded and eventually formed an aneurysm. The first description of an aneurysm was written in 1550 BC and is found in the Ebers Papyrus[1]:

> *Treatment of a swelling of the vessels. When thou considereth a swelling of the vessels on any part of the man's body, and thou findst it globular (and) firm under thine fingers when going, it is separated from the flesh, it is not large, it does not show the surface. Then thou shalt say: this is a vessels swelling, a disorder I will treat. It is the vessels that cause it. It originates from a injury upon the vessel. Then thou shall apply to it a treatment with the knife; this [knife] heated in fire, the bleeding will not be considerable.*

Galen was able to differentiate traumatic from fusiform aneurysms. Antyllus, who lived in the second or third century, operated on aneurysms of the arms, legs, or head but did not treat those in the axilla, groin, or neck. Paré introduced the concept of ligating the blood vessel above and below the aneurysm, expecting the contents to clot.

It was left to Larrey, the great French military surgeon, to treat large vessel injuries, including those of the thoracic outlet.[2] Although he did not treat wounds of the innominate left common carotid or left subclavian, he did treat injuries to the axillary arteries as they exited from underneath the clavicle. Two of these cases are particularly poignant. The first case, described in a letter to Alexis Larrey, involved a personal friend:

> *With regard to the unhappy Dupuy, my friend; his name is found inscribed in the list of heros who shed their blood for the conquest of Egypt and, in consequence, for the prosperity of the Republic. I had myself just passed through the bloodthirsty mob that*

had attacked him when I came upon him calling for my help. He was in the gravest danger as a lance thrust had caused a large wound which had cut the axillary artery and opened the left side of his chest. All his blood was gushing out. I gave him first aid, but nature made fruitless all my efforts to recall him to life. Several moments later he died asking me to remember him to his family. Will you, my dear uncle, console them and ease their grief.

His next case was more successful and occurred during the march on Moscow:

A peasant from one of the farms near Wilna, who was dangerously wounded in the left shoulder by a firearm at point blank range, was brought to the hospital shortly after the Polish officer. The Mother Superior begged me to see him and to help him. At the first glance I realized what great disorganization his wound had occasioned, but before examining him I sent for the surgeon of the hospital, professor Becu. The ball had passed through the arm from before backwards, very close to the shoulder joint. The muscles, brachial nerves, and axillary artery had been ruptured or torn, and the humerus and a large part of the shaft of the bone had been smashed to fragments below its head. The limb was cold, insensitive, incapable of movement and threatened with total gangrene and the shoulder and the whole of the side of the chest were covered with a deep ecchymosis. The wounds of entrance and exit were of no great size, and as they gave no hint of the derangement I had recognized, the consultants at first thought that the extirpation of the limb, which I had suggested, was unnecessary and the patient's arm might be preserved; but in the end they agreed to my observations and concluded that the operation should be done at once. In spite of the disordered state of the parts I was able to employ my own method. The operation was painful and difficult, since one fragment of the fractured head of the humerus was entangled amongst the cords of the brachial plexus below the subscapular muscle, and moreover the artery had been torn very high up and I was forced to look for it beneath the pectoral muscle in order to ligate it. Several months afterwards, by which time the patient had recovered completely, he succumbed to an internal malady the cause of which is unknown to me. I had obtained for him a provisional indemnity of 600 Francs.

Larrey was not intimidated by injuries to large vessels and his descriptions of tangential wounds, complete wound retraction, and clotting are classics that are as applicable now as they were then.

ANATOMY

The great vessels include the innominate, the left common carotid, and the left subclavian. In this chapter we also discuss the right subclavian and both axillary vessels.

Embryologically, the great vessels primarily represent a fusion or remnants of aortic arches three, four, and six. As a consequence of this complex embryologic development, there are many variations that occur, the most common of which is the fusion of the innominate and left carotid, which gives rise to the right subclavian, right common carotid, and left common carotid from the aorta below the sternal notch (Fig. 17–1). Occasionally there is fusion or common origin of the left common carotid and left subclavian arteries. The left vertebral artery also may share a common origin of the left subclavian. There are other less frequent variations that are encountered in the adult.

The innominate artery is the first branch of the aortic arch, usually arising at the apex of the arch. The artery then passes behind the left innominate vein obliquely to the right and cephalad. The typical innominate artery is 5 to 7 cm in length and immediately branches just behind the sternal clavicular joint. The right common carotid continues cephalad just lateral to the trachea, and the right subclavian passes obliquely to the right and at its apex gives off the right vertebral artery. The subclavian then arches over the apex of the pleura, giving off the thyrocervical trunk cephalad and the internal mammary artery rostrally. The artery then passes behind the scalenus anterior and anterior to the scalenus medius muscles. The artery then gives off the transversa colli or cervical artery and passes over the first rib, forming the axillary artery as it emerges from underneath the clavicle. Injuries to the subclavian artery as it is draped over the pleura and first rib are often associated with immediate exsanguination into the hemithorax.

Typically, the next branch of the aortic arch is the left common carotid. This artery arises directly behind the left innominate vein and just anterior to the esophagus. The trachea is to the right. The artery passes cephalad vertically, exiting the thoracic outlet almost directly behind the left protuberance of the manubrium. The next branch of the aortic arch is the left subclavian, which arises from the arch during its descent into the posterior mediastinum. This artery passes cephalad with a slightly oblique angle, draping itself over the left pleural apex and first rib almost as a mirror image of the right subclavian artery. The first branch is typically the left vertebral artery and the left thyrocervical trunk cephalad. The left internal mammary artery passes over the pleural cap rostrally, diving under the first rib. The left subclavian continues under the left scalenus anterior and anterior

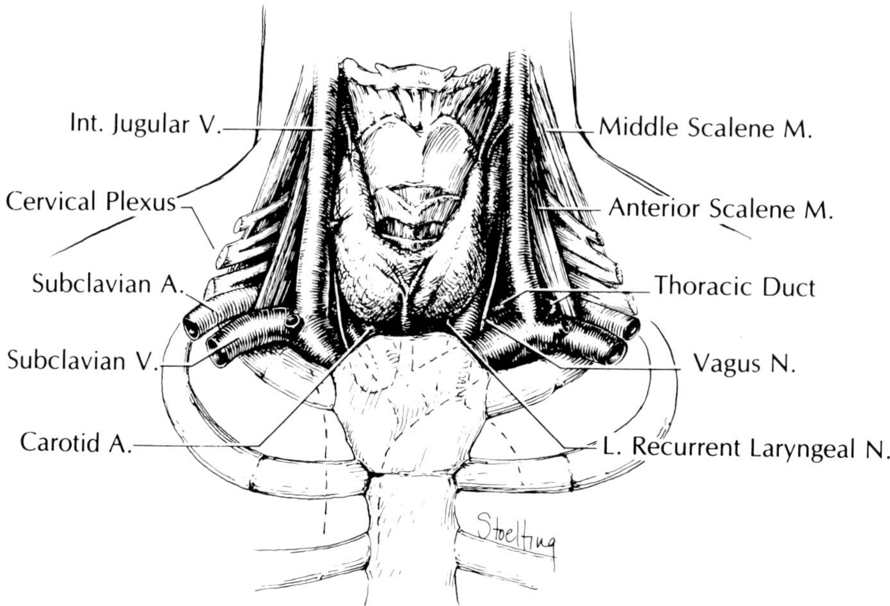

Figure 17–1.   The anatomy of the great vessels as they exit the thoracic outlet.

to the scalenus medius muscle, exiting over the first rib and forming the left axillary artery as it passes underneath the clavicle.

The venous drainage from the upper extremities and head are composed primarily of the left subclavian, left internal jugular, left vertebral, right internal jugular, and right subclavian veins. The latter two vessels unite at the base of the neck to form the innominate vein, which joins the left innominate vein, thus becoming the superior vena cava in the right upper thorax. Other important structures include the thoracic duct which, after passing cephalad up the chest near the esophagus, reaches its zenith behind the left common carotid and internal jugular vein and then turns rostrally to empty into the subclavian vein on its superior surface near the junction of the left internal and subclavian vein. The right vagus nerve also is in close proximity to the innominate artery, usually passing anterior to it midway between the primary branches and its origin off the arch. The vagus gives off the right recurrent laryngeal nerve, which passes backward and upward behind the subclavian artery. The left vagus usually is just lateral to the left common carotid. This nerve passes over the arch between the origins of the left subclavian and the left common carotid and then gives off the left recurrent laryngeal nerve, which passes underneath the ligamentum arteriosum inferior to the arch and then passes directly cephalad in the tracheoesophageal groove.

MECHANISM OF INJURY

Injury to the great vessels is due to either penetrating or blunt trauma. Penetrating trauma to the intrathoracic great vessels usually is not compatible with survival unless the missile or knife wound is quite small. Similarly, wounds to the subclavian and axillary vessels cause high mortality unless the wound is extrathoracic and is contained by the soft tissues of the neck and shoulder. Penetrating wounds to the veins, both intrathoracic and extrathoracic, are compatible with survival provided they are contained by the mediastinal structures or the soft tissues of the neck and shoulder. According to Rich and Spencer,[3] there were fewer than 20 survivors of intrathoracic arterial great vessel injuries before the Vietnam conflict. The few patients who did survive penetrating injuries most likely had small wounds caused by a knife or a low-velocity small caliber weapon such as a .22 or from pellets from a medium-range shotgun blast. In such instances, there is full thickness injury to the vessel wall but the adventitia or intima serves as a flap over the small hole, thus preventing exsanguinating hemorrhage. False aneurysm formation is not an uncommon complication after such low-velocity injuries (Fig. 17–2).

Injuries to the intrathoracic great vessels from blunt trauma most often are associated with direct compression, shear, or deceleration forces.[4,5] Direct compression of the anterior chest wall may force the innominate or left common carotid artery against the vertebral column, which then shears it from its origin. Deceleration also may cause injuries to the innominate artery at its origin, but, if such forces are involved, the aorta is also usually injured. Blunt trauma also can cause injury to the subclavian and axillary artery, but this is usually associated with fractures to the clavicle or first rib. It has been our impression that there has been a slight increase in such injuries, primarily due to shoulder harness seat belts. The subclavian artery, like the superior mesenteric artery, seems to lack as much collagen

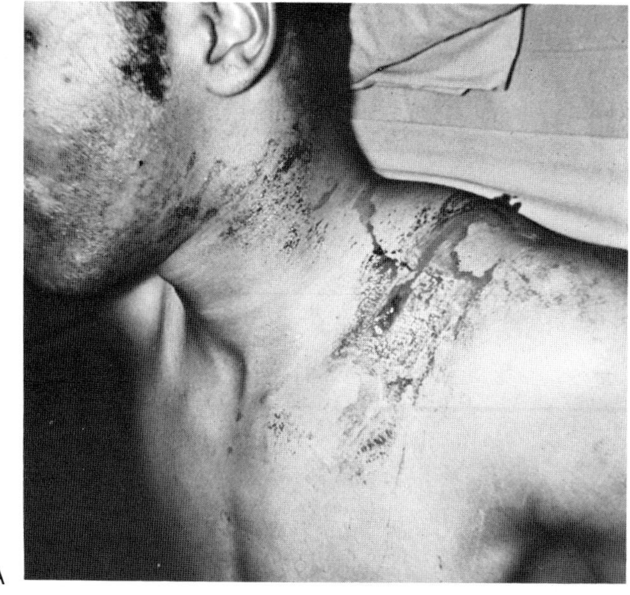

A

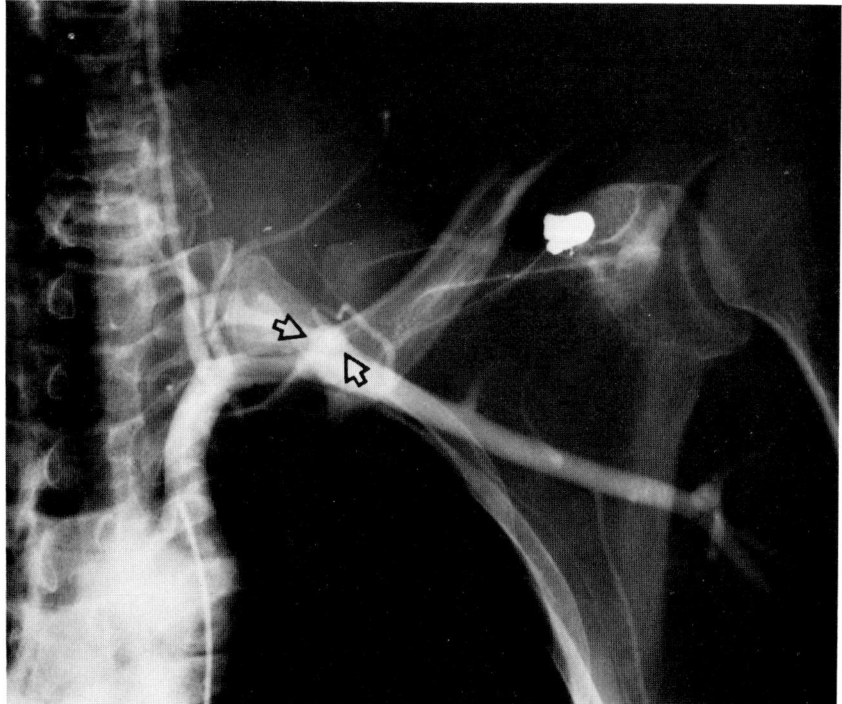

B

Figure 17–2.   A 38-year-old man sustained multiple gunshot wounds (**A**). There were no physical findings suggestive of a vascular injury; however, since the wound was in proximity to a major vessel, an arteriogram was done that shows a false aneurysm (**B**).

within the media compared with other vessels. This may contribute to avulsive and compressive-type injuries associated with blunt trauma to the apex of the chest.

RELATIVE INCIDENCES

Injuries to the thoracic great vessels are uncommonly reported because most patients exsanguinate at the time of injury. Patients with injuries to the distal left subclavian, right subclavian, and both axillary arteries may survive the initial insult, particularly if these arteries do not decompress into one of the hemothoraces or externally. The incidence of penetrating trauma to the great vessels is shown in Table 17–1. As one would imagine, most injuries that are reported occur in the subclavian and axillary arteries because these are most compatible with survival long enough to reach an emergency room or aid station.

Injuries to the great veins in the upper thorax probably are more common than is recognized. Undoubtedly, a widened mediastinum often is indicative of injury to a great vein that has tamponaded. In our experience, 85% of the arteriograms performed for widened mediastinum are negative for aortic or great vessel injury. How many of these represent venous injuries is unknown. Injuries to the subclavian and axillary vein also are relatively common, particularly with penetrating injuries. In most instances, these are associated findings at the time of exploration for arterial wounds, although in our experience we have had patients exsanguinate from penetrating injuries to the subclavian vein when it decompressed into the pleural cavity. During a 12-yr period, we treated five innominate vein injuries, nine subclavian vein injuries, and three axillary vein injuries. Eighty-three percent of these were due to penetrating trauma and 17% were due to blunt trauma.[6] Hewett and associates[7] treated 15 innominate, subclavian, and axillary vein injuries during a 13-yr period without a death.

SYMPTOMS AND DIAGNOSIS

If a patient sustains complete disruption of a great vessel secondary to blunt trauma, this is usually associated with massive hemorrhage and exsanguination. If, on the other hand, the injury causes disruption primarily of the media and intima with retraction of these two structures and the adventitia is still intact, survival is possible. These patients present with widened mediastinum, apical cap, lower neck hematoma, or swelling and hematoma formation in the infra- and supraclavicular spaces. Distortion of the airway with subsequent compromise of the airway often occurs. Although we and others[18,19] reported that fractures of ribs 1 and 2 are associated with an increased incidence of injury to aortic arch vessels, one report[6] showed no such correlation.

Penetrating injuries to the great vessels in the thorax should be obvious. The presence of a stab wound or gunshot wound in the neck or chest should alert the clinician to the possibility of arterial or venous injury. Even more remote wounds in the abdomen can transgress the diaphragm and cause injuries to the great vessels. Most patients with arterial injuries will have died at the scene. Those who arrive alive in an emergency room usually will be in profound shock with massive hemothorax. Injuries to the distal left subclavian, right subclavian, and axillary arteries usually will have compensated signs of shock and

Table 17–1. Incidence of Great Vessel Arterial Injury

WAR SERIES	TOTAL ARTERIES INJURED	INNOMINATE (%)	SUBCLAVIAN (%)	AXILLARY (%)
World War I	1191	0/0	45/3.8	108/9.0
World War II	2471	0/0	21/0.9	74/2.9
Korean	304	0/0	3/1.0	20/6.6
Vietnam	1000	3/0.3	8/0.8	59/5.9
Combined civilian series*	2642	31/1.1	127/4.8	154/5.8[†]

*Twelve series are included.[1,2,4,7,10–17]
[†]Axillary injuries are sometimes combined with subclavian injuries in civilian series.
Modified from ref. 3.

signs of swelling and occasionally airway obstruction. Because of the close proximity of the trachea and the esophagus to these vessels, associated hematemesis and hemoptysis are common. Associated neurologic injuries include those to the brachial plexus, vagus nerve, and recurrent laryngeal nerve, which may cause symptoms of hoarseness, dysphonia, and motor sensory deprivation in the involved extremity. Penetrating injuries to the great veins also may present with signs of hypovolemia if the injury has decompressed into the hemithorax. Venous injuries to the subclavian and axillary veins may be compressed by the surrounding tissues and not even be associated with hematoma formation because it is a low-pressure system. Bleeding is manifested in venous injuries only when not contained by tissues in the wound.

Low-velocity or small missile injuries to the great vessels sometimes are associated with missile embolization either in the ventricle, lungs, or systemic circulation (Fig. 17–3). Inability to find an exit wound and the missile on chest radiographs should alert one to the possibility of missile embolization, and a diligent radiographic search in peripheral veins or arteries should be carried out.

MANAGEMENT OF SPECIFIC INJURIES

The first priorities in any patient with great vessel injury, whether it be arterial or venous, are resuscitation of hypovolemia and control of airway. These have been described in previous chapters and will not be commented on further.

Many incisions have been described for gaining access to the great vessels, both intrathoracic and at the base of the neck (Fig. 17–4). Because the overwhelming majority of these patients are in shock or may have associated injuries, we strongly favor keeping the patient in a supine position and doing a midline incision. If a left anterior thoracotomy has not been performed in the emergency room, we prefer a midline sternotomy incision with the option of extending the incision more cephalad along the border of the stern-ocleidomastoid muscle on either side (Fig. 17–5). A second option is to carry the incision along the top of the clavicle with or without resecting the medial half of the clavicle to gain access to the proximal subclavian artery and vein. Axillary injuries usually are managed best by an infraclavicular incision or a combined supra- and infraclavicular incision in an S-type fashion, resecting the medial half of the clavicle to gain proximal control.

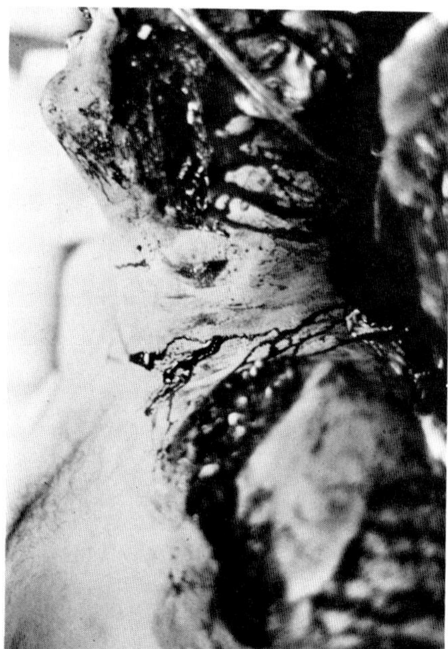

Figure 17–3.   This 29-year-old man sustained a shotgun blast through and through his left shoulder into the face (**A**). The chest radiograph (**B**) shows one missile in the right ventricle that did not require removal. A left ventricular missile of this size would require removal, since embolization to cerebral vessels has been reported. This patient had multiple injuries to the carotid and subclavian, all of which were repaired.

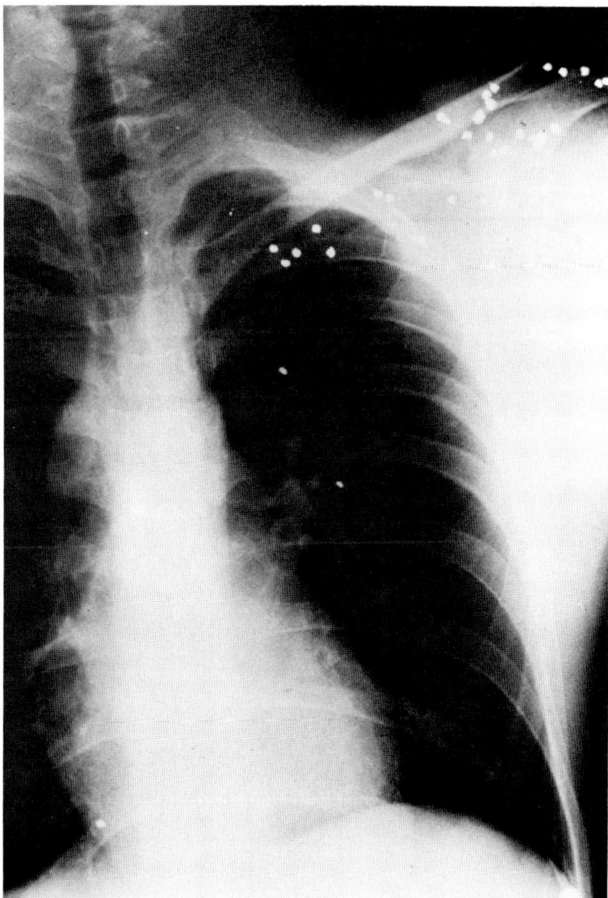

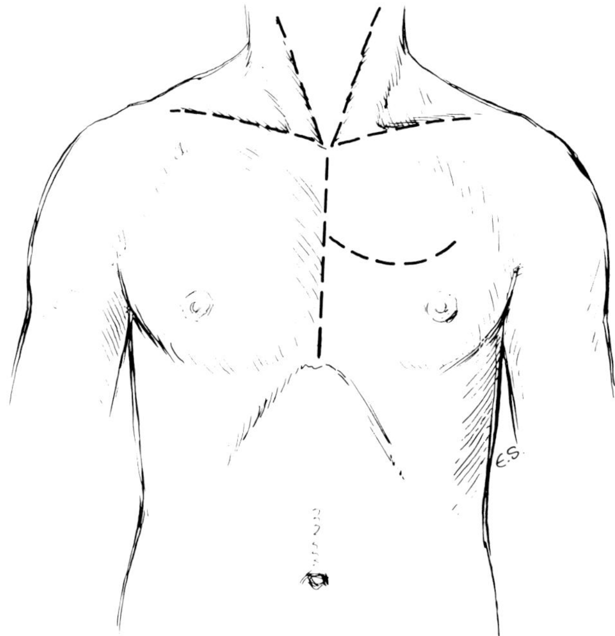

Figure 17–4.   Options for various incisions are shown and will depend on where the injury is and the need for proximal control.

Left subclavian injuries present a problem because the proximal vessel is posterior in the chest and it may be difficult to gain access through a median sternotomy. One option is to do a so-called trapdoor incision in which the left anterior chest is opened in the third or fourth intercostal space and is combined with a supraclavicular incision and resection of the clavicle. This incision allows the chest wall to be opened like a trapdoor (Fig. 17–6). This is a very morbid incision and postoperative pain is a problem. Another alternative is a left thoracotomy incision to obtain proximal control and then do a separate supraclavicular incision with or without clavicular resection (Fig. 17–7). Some investigators have described emergency access to the left subclavian at its origin by doing a third intercostal space left anterior thoracotomy in the emergency room. In our experience, it is never possible to diagnose without arteriograms such an injury even with a high index of suspicion when a penetrating wound is directly over the left subclavian. If the patient arrests or is dying, a standard left anterior lateral thoracotomy, as outlined in Chapter 21, is preferred. The options then include cutting the costal cartilage cephalad to gain access to the left subclavian artery if that is the injury or to extend it as a sternotomy and convert it into a trapdoor incision. Another option is to extend the incision into the right chest across the sternum, which gives excellent access to all vessels in the chest (Chapter 21).

Penetrating wounds occurring to the intrathoracic great vessels will almost invariably lend themselves to lateral repair (Fig. 17–8) because larger wounds are incompatible with survival, the exception being the great veins. With venous injuries, it is preferable to repair the innominate veins, but ligation can be tolerated by the patient. The latter would be done when there are extensive associated injuries demanding the surgeon's attention and venous

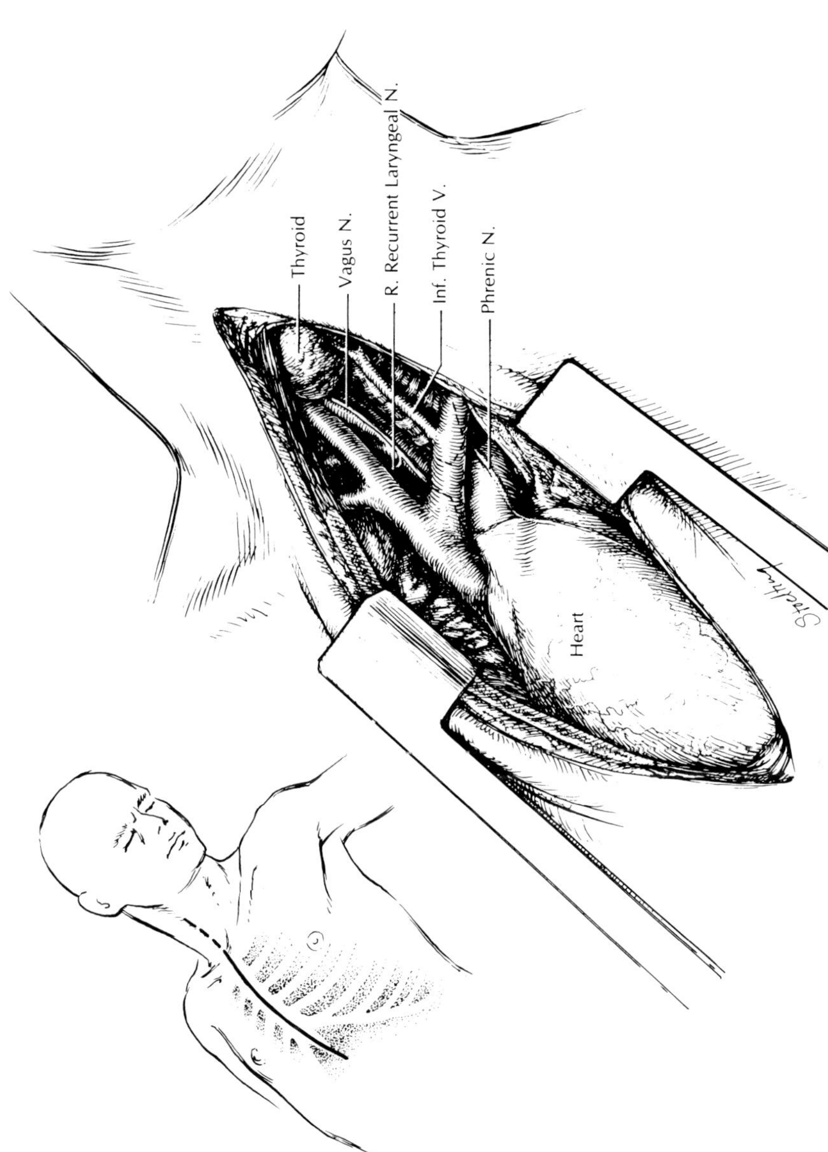

Figure 17–5.   The midline sternotomy with extension up the sternocleidomastoid exposes the heart and great vessels, allowing proximal control and repair of injuries.

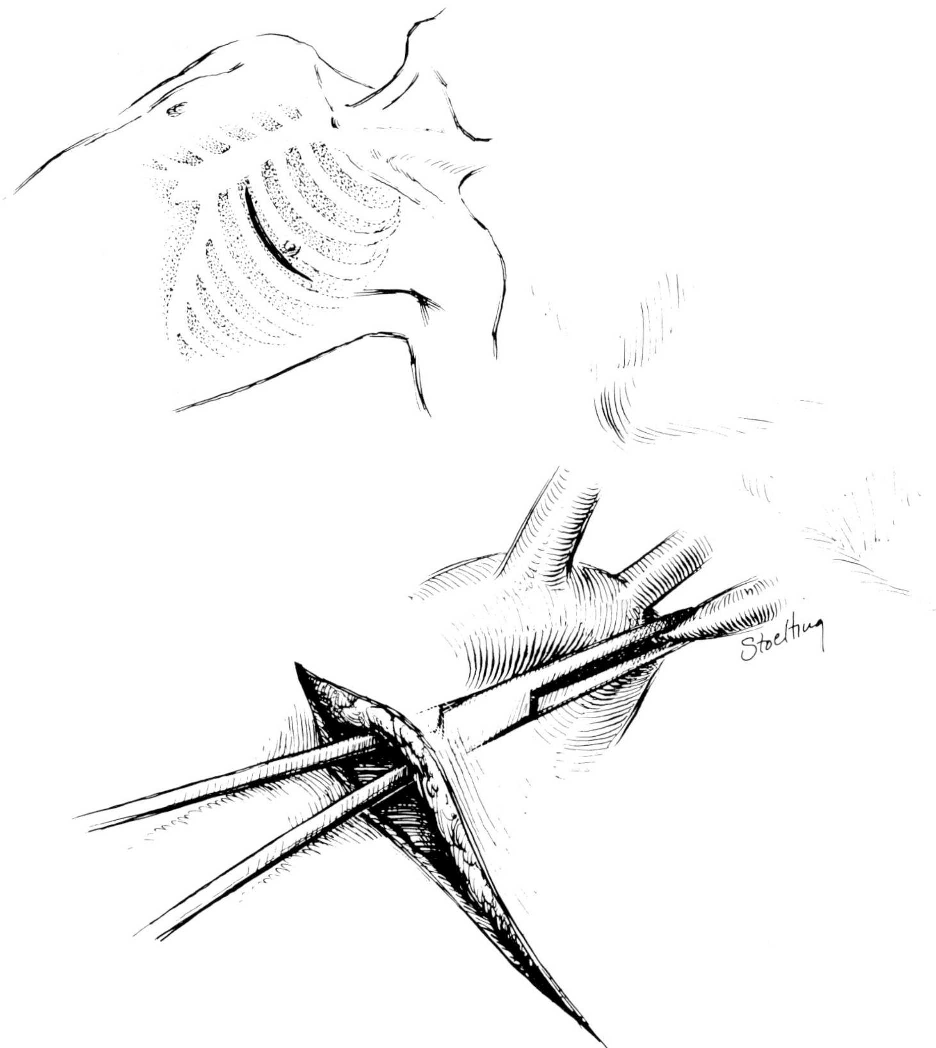

Figure 17–6. Control of the subclavian artery can be obtained in the unstable patient through a standard left anterior thoracotomy.

repair would take too long. Injuries to the subclavian and axillary vessels may be quite extensive and require either end-to-end anastomosis or even graft replacement. In our experience, the subclavian artery is one of the more difficult arteries to repair because of its relative lack of collagen. End-to-end anastomosis under any tension is doomed to failure, and it is better to do graft replacement, preferably with autogenous tissue, but it can be done with either polytetrafluoroethylene or Dacron. If there are associated hollow viscus injuries such as esophagus or trachea, then it is preferable to use autogenous tissue or ligate the vessel. If the vessel is ligated and the patient subsequently has signs of ischemia or claudication in the arm, extra anatomic bypass from the opposite extremity or neck may be done at a later date.

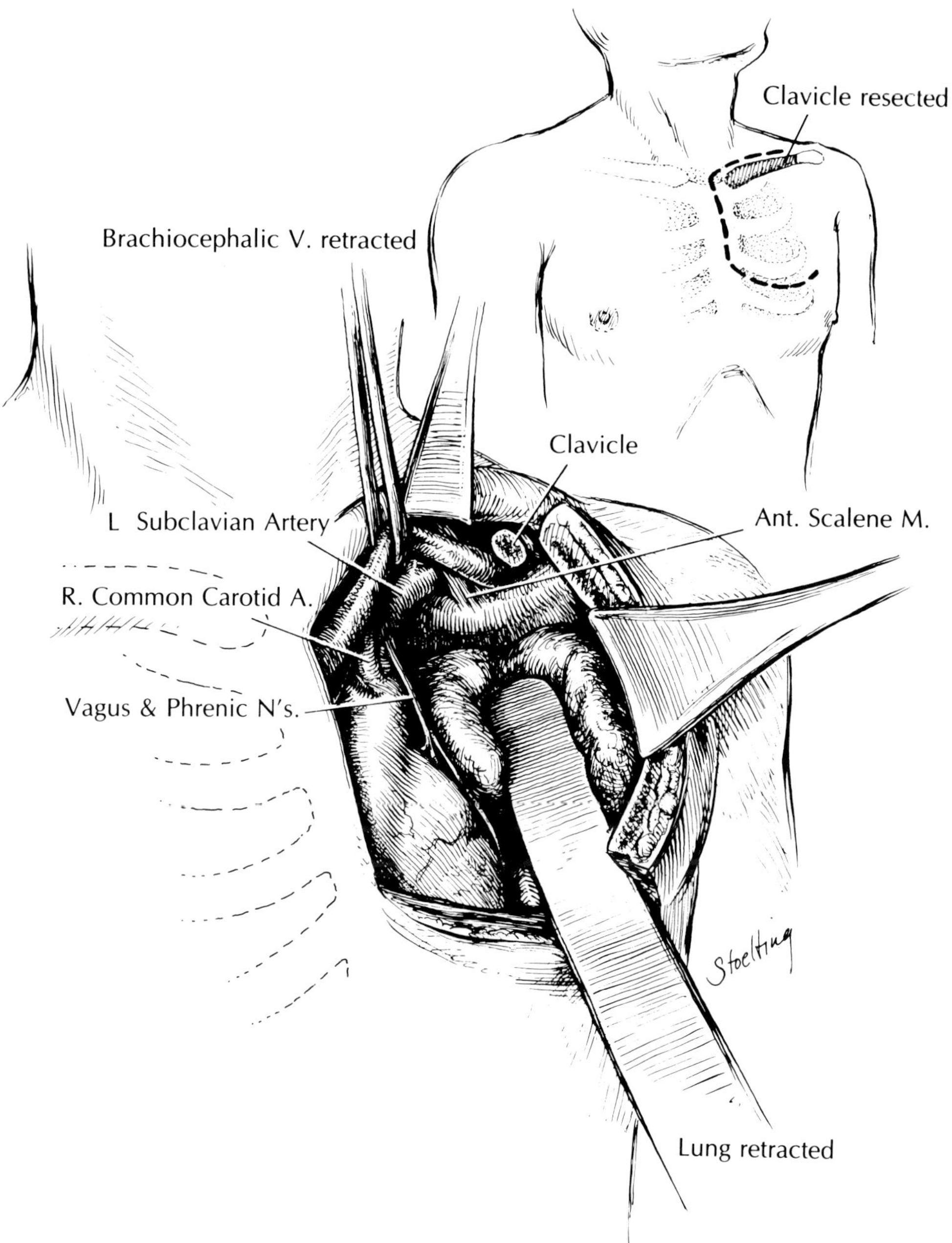

Figure 17–7.   If a left subclavian artery injury is found, access and control can be obtained through a trapdoor extension by resecting the medial clavicle and entering the third or fourth intercostal space.

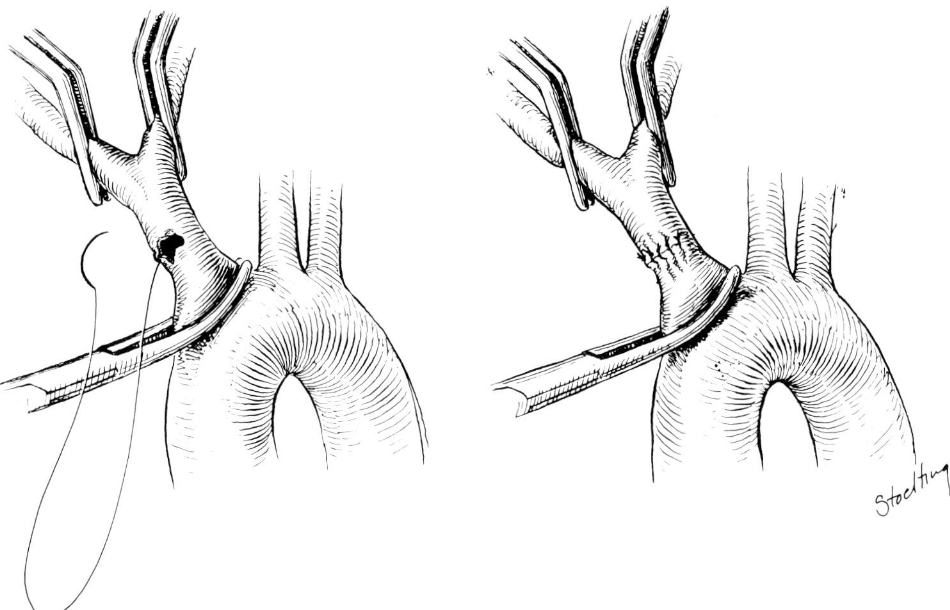

Figure 17–8.   Lateral repair is performed with temporary occlusion proximally and distally. In some instances repair can be done with a partial occluding clamp.

Blunt trauma injuries to the innominate, left common carotid, or subclavian may pose a more difficult operative management. In most of these instances the adventitia is the only intact portion of the vessel wall because the media and intima usually have retracted. Therefore, grafts often are necessary (Figs. 17–9, 17–10). If more than one of the great vessels is injured, heparin-bonded shunts or cardiac bypass should be considered. Full cardiac bypass may be contraindicated because of associated injuries (particularly closed head injuries) and increased risk of hemorrhage when the patient is fully heparinized. An alternative option is to use bypass using the Biomedicus or Sarnes pump without heparin, which gives excellent results.[8] Repair of the left subclavian artery is not mandatory and the patient will tolerate ligation. We also have ligated the common carotid successfully when the patient is a young healthy individual because the young usually have excellent collateral circulation.

POSTOPERATIVE CARE

The first priority in postoperative care is maintenance of the airway. Because of the close association of the great vessels to the trachea, postoperative airway intubation usually is required. We prefer either endotracheal or nasotracheal tubes with low-pressure, high-compliance cuffs. If tracheostomy has been indicated for any reason, the same type of cuff can be used with tracheostomy tubes.

Almost all patients with injuries to the great vessels within the thorax will require chest drainage with large-bore siliconized tubes. One of these tubes can be placed into the

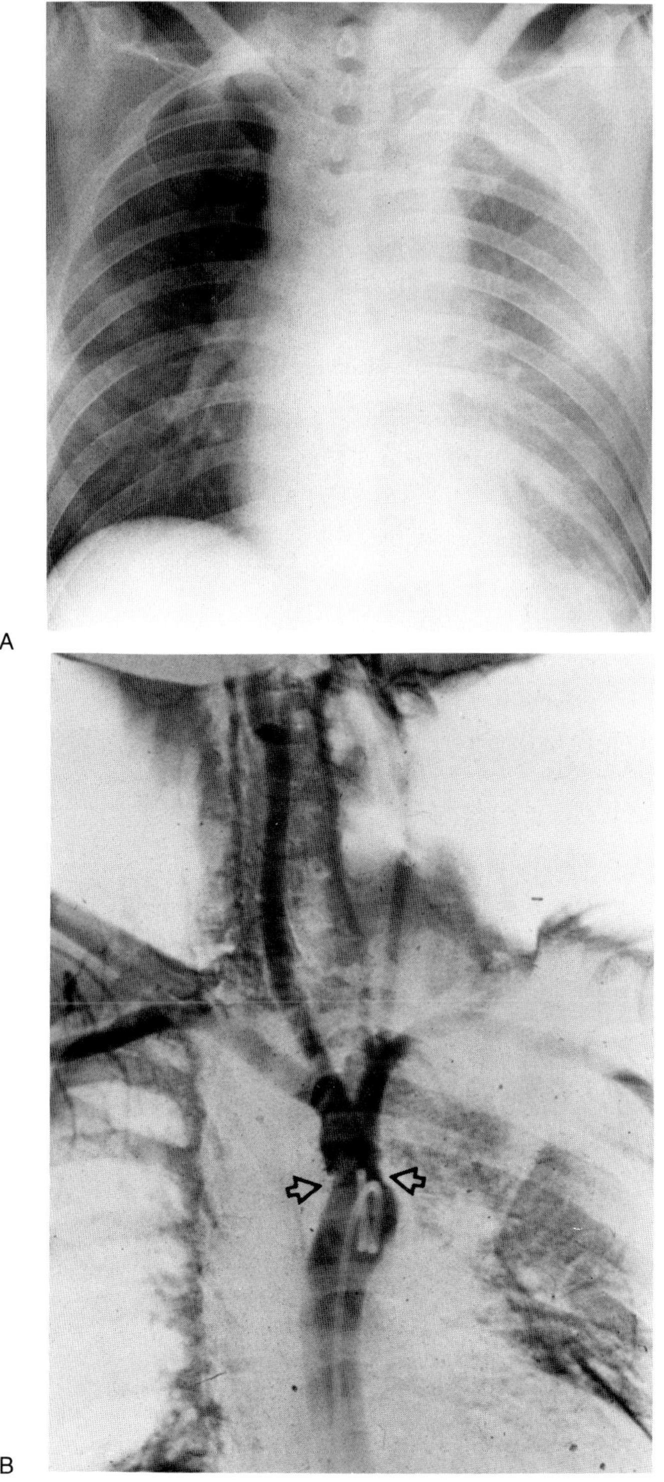

Figure 17–9. **A:** This is the chest radiograph of a 21-year-old man who sustained a severe compression injury when a truck pinned him to a brick wall. Because of the widened mediastinum and apical cap, an arteriogram was done. **B:** A filling defect at the takeoff of the innominate is seen. A similar injury to the common carotid was not appreciated but found at surgery. (Figure continued on next page.)

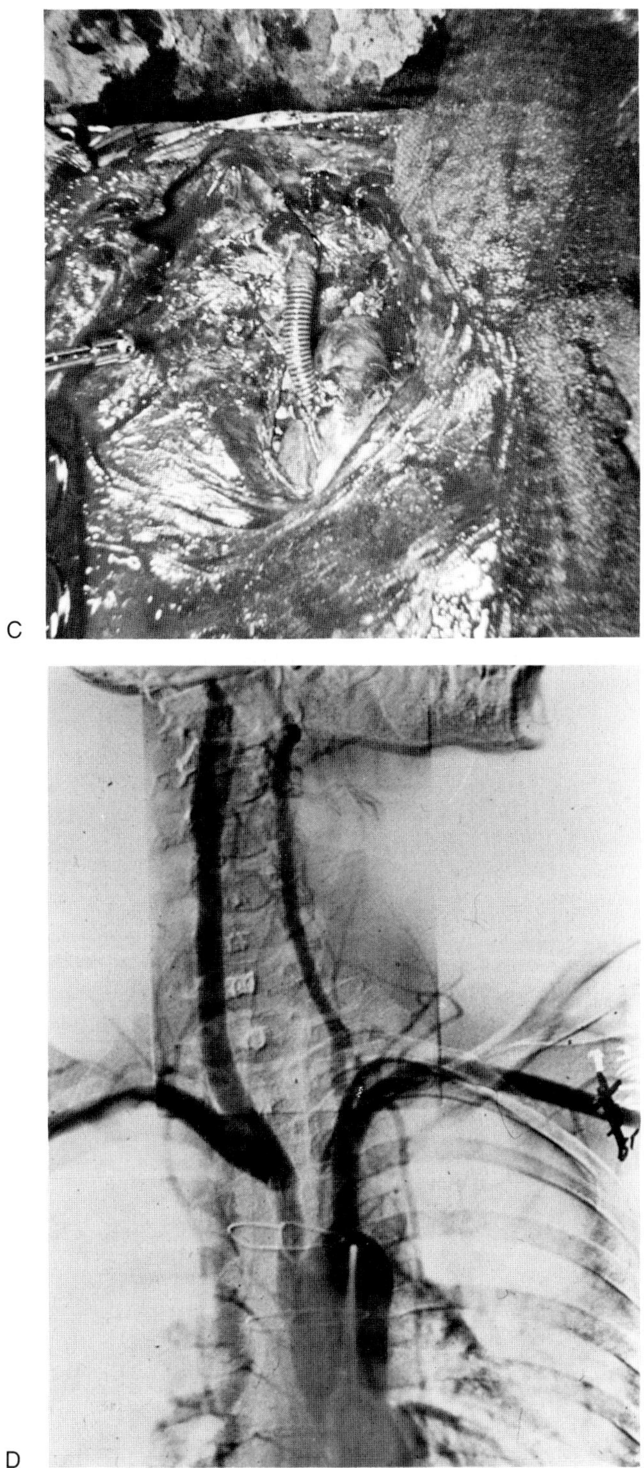

Figure 17–9, cont.   The left common carotid was ligated and a graft was substituted for the innominate (**C**) in less than 7 min. Postoperatively, the patient did well without neurologic deficit. **D:** The graft and absence of the left carotid are shown. The vessel on the left is the vertebral.

338

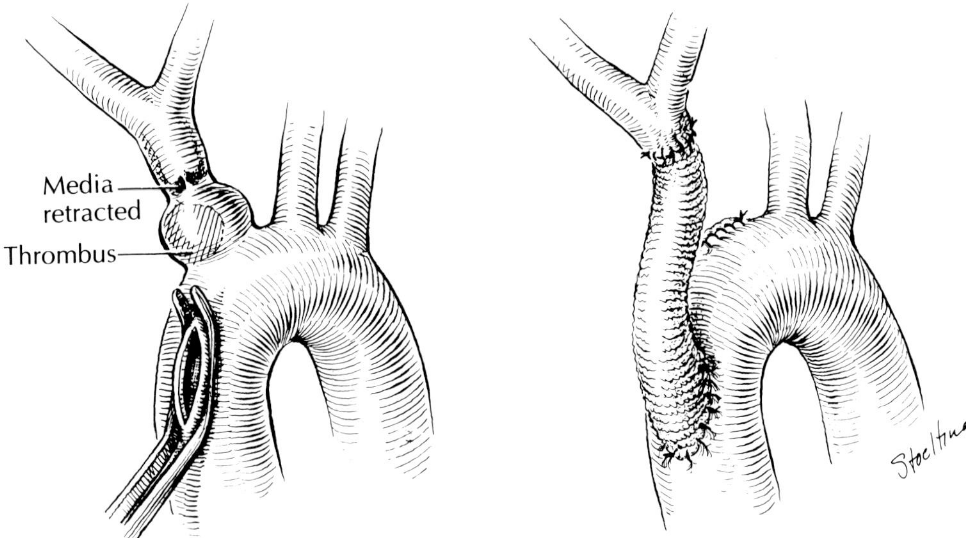

Figure 17–10.   Partial avulsion of the innominate or other great vessels can be repaired by oversewing the avulsed stump and performing a bypass from the arch to distal vessel.

mediastinum to maintain drainage and to monitor postoperative bleeding. Placement of drains next to the anastomosis should be avoided and drains should be removed within 24 hr or as soon as the risk of bleeding has subsided.

Some patients may develop postoperative hypertension, particularly those with head injuries. We prefer not to treat this hypertension unless the systolic blood pressure increases above 180 mm Hg. Although antibiotics have been advocated on a routine basis for chest injuries, we prefer to treat only those patients who require prosthetic grafts or have associated hollow viscus injury.

COMPLICATIONS

Hemorrhage is the most common postoperative complication after repair or ligation of one of the great vessels. Patients often have massive transfusions and the most common causes of hemorrhage are delutional thrombocytopenia or hypothermia.

In patients with chest tubes, careful monitoring of drainage is appropriate. Patients with blood loss of more than 300 ml per hour for 3 hr should be returned to the operating room for a second look. Similarly, if patients have had drains placed for repair of subclavian or axillary vessels and if there is ongoing hemorrhage of more than 200 ml in 2 to 3 hr, reexploration is indicated. We prefer closed drainage systems such as the Jackson-Pratt type.

Neurologic complications are intrinsic in great vessel injuries and also may occur during exposure and repair of them. The vagus or phrenic nerves can be injured. Arterial occlusion for the repair may precipitate or aggravate an ischemic cerebral injury and can follow thrombosis of the repair, although in our experience this has not been a problem because the vessels are quite large. Embolism from the suture line or graft also is an uncommon complication. If a prosthetic graft has been placed, infection is a remote possibility but, if antibiotics are used routinely, the incidence is minimized.

RESULTS

As Rich and Spencer have pointed out,[3] most injuries to the intrathoracic branches of the aortic arch are immediately fatal. The corollaries to this observation are that there are few reports of successful treatment, and that no single surgeon has much experience with these injuries. Nevertheless, two recent studies, one reporting blunt injuries and the other reporting predominantly penetrating injuries, showed far better results than previously reported.[5,9]

Rosenberg and colleagues[5] studied 30 patients with injuries to the aortic arch vessels secondary to blunt trauma. One patient died preoperatively and two died intraoperatively, a 6.7% operative mortality. The other patients did well, although two grafts occluded because of infection. The overall graft patency was 90% at 5 yr.

Weaver and colleagues[9] reported on 46 patients with 51 arterial injuries to the ascending aorta, aortic arch, and great vessels. Forty-two (82%) of the injuries were due to penetrating injuries. Three patients died (6.5%).

Neurologic sequelae after injuries to the great vessels are surprisingly low. A recent review from multiple trauma centers showed 1 deficit (9%) after innominate artery injury, 20 deficits (29%) after common carotid injury, and 1 deficit (5%) after vertebral artery injury.[10] It would thus appear that if the patient arrives alive in the emergency room, excellent operative results can be achieved with minimal to modest neurologic deficits and excellent graft patency.

REFERENCES

1. Meade R. *An Introduction to the History of General Surgery.* Philadelphia: Saunders; 1968.
2. Dible HJ. *Napoleon's Surgeon.* London: William Heinemann Medical Books; 1970.
3. Rich NM, Spencer FL. *Injuries of the Intrathoracic Branches of the Aortic Arch in Vascular Trauma.* Philadelphia: Saunders; 1978.
4. Marvasti MA, Parker FB, Bredenberg CE. Injuries to arterial branches of the aortic arch. *Thorac Cardiovasc Surg.* 1984;32:293.
5. Rosenberg JN, Bredenberg CE, Marvasti MA, et al. Blunt injuries to the aortic arch vessels. *Ann Thorac Surg.* 1989;48:508.
6. Mavroudis C, Roon AJ, Baker CC, Thomas AN. Management of acute cervical thoracic vascular injuries. *J Thorac Cardiovasc Surg.* 1980;80:342.
7. Hewitt RL, Smith AD, Becker ML, et al. Penetrating vascular injuries of the thoracic outlet. *Surgery.* 1974;76:715.
8. Grosso MA, Brown JM, Moore EE, Moore FA. Repair of the torn descending thoracic aorta using the centrifugal pump with partial left heart bypass. *J Trauma.* 1991;31:395.
9. Weaver FA, Suda RW, Stiles GM, Yellin AE. Injuries to the ascending aorta, aortic arch and great vessels. *Surg Gynecol Obstet.* 1989;169:27.
10. Richardson D, Obeid FN, Richardson D, et al. Cerebrovascular injury—neurologic consequences. *J Trauma.* 1992;32:755.
11. Busuttil RW, Acker B. Management of injuries to the brachiocephalic vessels. *Surg Gynecol Obstet.* 1982;154:737.

12. Drapanas T, Hewitt RL, Weichert RF, Smith AD. Civilian vascular injuries: a critical appraisal of three decades of management. *Ann Surg*. 1970;172:351.

13. Franz JL, Simpson CR, Penny RM, et al. Avulsion of the innominate artery after blunt chest trauma. *J Thorac Cardiovasc Surg*. 1984;67:478.

14. Graham JM, Feliciano DV, Mattox KL, et al. Management of subclavian vascular injuries. *J Trauma*. 1980;20:537.

15. Gubler KD, Wisner DH, Blaisdell FW. Multiple vessel injury to branches of the aortic arch: case report. *J Trauma*. 1991;31:1566.

16. Kirschner RL. Penetrating injury to vessels of the thoracic outlet. *Internat Surgery*. 1985;4:483.

17. Poole GV. Fracture of the upper ribs and injury to the great vessels. *Surg Gynecol Obstet*. 1989;169:275.

18. Strum JT, Dorsey JS, Olson FR, Perry JF Jr. The management of subclavian artery injuries following blunt thoracic trauma. *Ann Thorac Surg*. 1984;38:188.

19. Thomas AN, Goodman PC, Roon AJ. Role of angiography and cervical thoracic trauma. *J Thorac Cardiovasc Surg*. 1978;76:633.

18

Cervical Vascular Injury: Carotid, Vertebral, and Jugular

WILLIAM R. FRY, M.D.
R. STEPHEN SMITH, M.D.

HISTORY: In his collected works, published in 1568 and 1575, Ambroise Paré[1] relates two cases of vascular injuries involving the head and neck. The histories in the author's own words are quite descriptive. The first is:

> *A merchant grocer, living in the Rue Saint Denis, at the sign of Le Gros Tournois, named Le Juge, who fell upon his head where was made a wound near the temporal muscle, where he had an artery opened, from which the blood poured very impetuously, in such a manner that the ordinary measures for staunching the blood would not serve. I was called thither where I found Messieurs Rasse, Cointeret, Viard, sworn surgeons of Paris, staunching the blood; where promptly I took a threaded needle and tied the artery for him, and there was no bleeding afterwards and he was soon cured.*

The second history is equally dramatic:

> *A sergeant of the Chatelet, dwelling near Saint André des Arts, who had a sword thrust in the throat at the pre Aux Clercs, which cut completely through the external jugular vein. As soon as he was wounded, he placed his handkerchief on the wound and sought me at my house. When we lifted the handkerchief, the blood spouted forth with great impetuosity. I at once tied the vein towards its root. By this means it was staunched and he was cured, thanks to God.*

According to Garrison,[2] the first successful ligation of the common carotid artery for trauma was performed by David Fleming of H.M.S. Tonnant in October 1803. Cooper in 1808 ligated the common carotid for aneurysm.[2] Lord Parker in 1864 ligated a subclavian artery along with the common carotid and vertebral arteries for subclavian aneurysm. The patient died on the 42nd postoperative day.[2] Andrew W. Smith first successfully ligated the innominate artery together with the common carotid artery and subsequently the right vertebral for subclavian aneurysm in 1864, exhibiting his patient alive in 1869.[2]

Paré reintroduced and championed ligature of bleeding vessels, yet 312 years later Sir Frederic Treves[3] wrote, "I think the ligature of main arteries

*for the arrest of bleeding in distant parts is often somewhat blindly advised
and possibly too frequently carried out." He then reported on four patients of
his who had "temporary ligature" of the carotid artery to control hemorrhage, three of whom survived. He achieved this temporary control by
placing a chromic catgut loop around the injured arteries and removing
them at varying times after the operation. Sir Frederic hoped to achieve
control of the artery "without the artery being permanently closed." Despite
his case reports, ligature remained the primary treatment through World
Wars I and II.*

*In World War I, Americans had a carotid artery ligation mortality rate
of 44%, the same as reported by the British.[4] Of those successfully saved by
ligation, there was a 29.6% incidence of neurologic deficit secondary to the
ligation. As a result, Makins[4] advocated a nonoperative approach to penetrating neck wounds.*

*In World War II, similar mortality and morbidity results were demon-
strated, and there was only one successful repair of a carotid artery
reported.[4] It was not until the Korean conflict that definitive repair was
introduced.*

*In 1956, Fogelman[4] reported a comparison between conservative man-
agement and operative intervention; there was a 35% mortality in those
treated conservatively and a 10% mortality in those undergoing operative
repair. Bradley[5] reported deaths from hemorrhagic infarction after successful repair and advised against revascularization in patients with preexisting
neurologic deficits, as did Cohen and co-workers.[6] Liekwig and Greenfield,[7]
however, felt results were improved by revascularization of such patients. The
controversy remains today between those advocating selective and those
advocating routine repair.*

ANATOMY

Vascular anatomy is conveniently divided into the anterior circulation, consisting of the
carotid arteries and their branches and the jugular veins, and the posterior circulation, the
vertebral arteries and veins.

Anterior Vascular

Arterial

The cervical portions of the two common carotid arteries have similar anatomic relationships once the right common carotid artery emerges in the cervical region from behind the
sternoclavicular junction after having taken origin from the innominate (Fig. 18–1A). In the
lower part of the neck, the two common carotid arteries are separated from each other only
by the trachea. As they progress upward, the thyroid gland, the thyroid cartilage of the
larynx, and the pharynx project forward between the two vessels which, at this point, angle
slightly posteriorly.

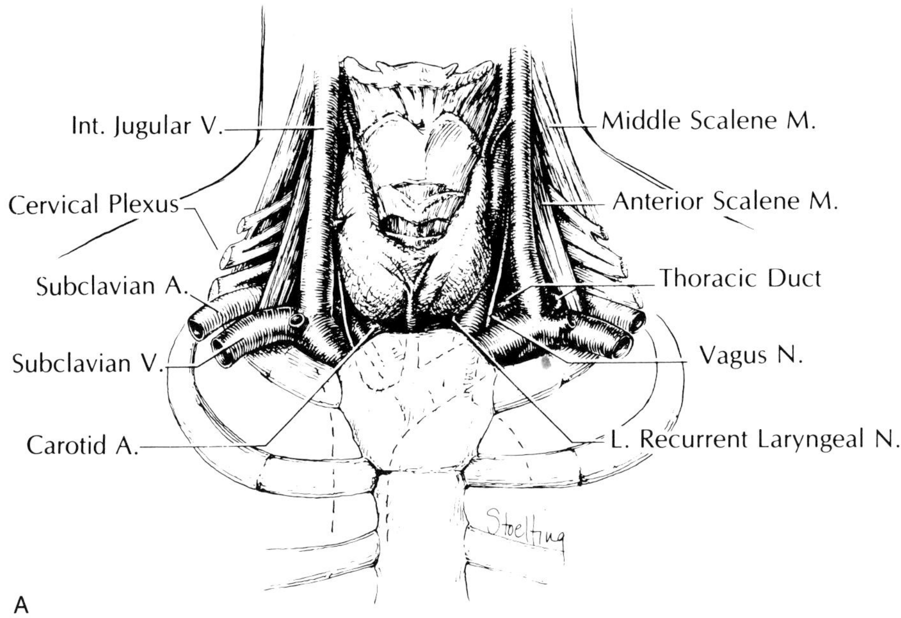

Figure 18–1.   Anatomy of the neck. Anterior view (**A**) demonstrates the relationship of the arteries and veins to the other structures of the neck.

A sheath derived from the deep cervical fascia surrounds the common and internal carotid arteries, internal jugular vein, and vagus nerve. The common carotid arteries divide into their terminal branches, the internal and external carotid arteries.

Due to the embryologic migration of the carotid bifurcation cephalad, the bifurcation can have a variable location. The most common location for the carotid bifurcation is 1 to 3 cm below the angle of the mandible (Fig. 18–1B). Up to 37% of bifurcations are located at other levels, from above the angle of the mandible to 6 cm below it.[8] This variation in locations of the carotid bifurcation must be kept in mind during cervical explorations done without the benefit of preoperative vascular studies, as the carotid bifurcation can lie high or low in the neck.

The common carotid arteries rarely have branches before their bifurcation, but occasionally the superior thyroid artery or the ascending pharyngeal artery will take origin at the level of the bifurcation.

The external carotid has eight branches. The *superior thyroid* artery is its first branch, which is covered by the sternocleidomastoid muscle and runs caudad and anterior under the omohyoid muscle to the thyroid gland. The *lingual* artery passes deep to the digastric and stylohyoid muscle to enter the sublingual space and immediately courses superior under the stylohyoid and digastric muscles to enter the submaxillary region. The *occipital* artery originates at the level of the facial artery but from the posterior surface of the external carotid. It courses deep to the superior belly of the digastric muscle and runs beneath the

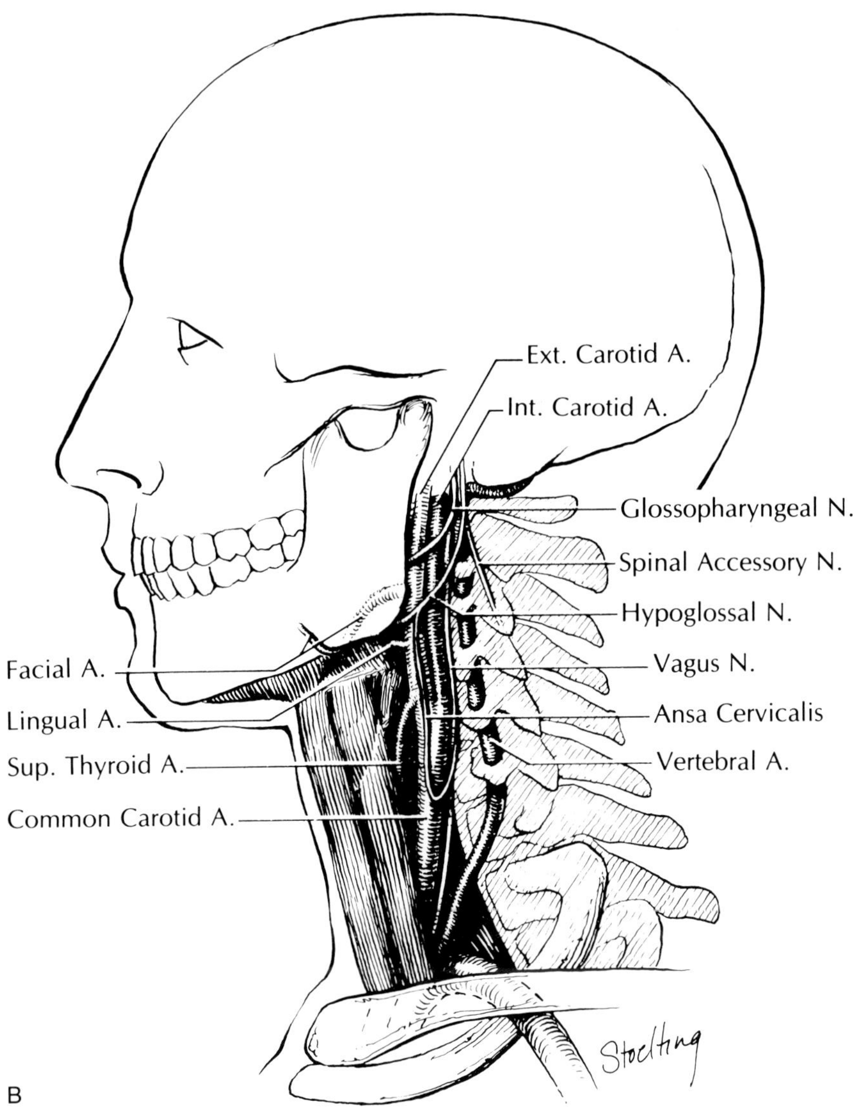

Figure 18–1, cont.   The lateral view (**B**) in particular shows the relationship of the vertebral artery to the vertebral canal in the transverse processes.

mastoid process. The *internal maxillary* and *superficial temporal* arteries are the terminal branches of the external carotid artery.

The internal carotid arteries at their origin are approximately the same size as the external carotids. They run vertically upward and in front of the transverse processes of the upper three cervical vertebrae to the carotid canal in the petrous portion of the temporal bone. The internal carotids are comparatively superficial at their origin and lie posterior and lateral to the external carotids, overlapped partially by the anterior border of the sternocleidomastoid muscle. As they pass beneath the parotid gland, they run under the hypoglossal nerve, the digastric and stylohyoid muscles, and the occipital and posterior auricular branches of the external carotids. Behind them lie the rectus capitis anticus major and the superior cervical ganglion of the sympathetic and superior laryngeal nerves. Posteriorly and externally lie the jugular veins and the vagus nerves, with the veins being on a plane posterior to the artery and the superior laryngeal nerve. The ascending pharyngeal artery is situated posteromedially. At the base of the skull, the glossopharyngeal, vagus, spinal accessory, and hypoglossal nerves lie between the arteries and the internal jugular veins.

Venous

The internal jugular veins, which collect blood from the cranium, face, and neck, commence at the base of the skull (jugular foramen). They course down the side of the neck in a vertical direction and lie on the lateral aspect of the internal carotid arteries. At the base of the neck they pass over the common carotid arteries, where they unite with the subclavian veins and form the innominate veins. The major tributaries that the veins receive on their way down the neck include the common facial veins that pass from medially to laterally over the bifurcation of the common carotid arteries, the largest branches received by the jugulars in the neck. Other tributaries that pass anterior to the arteries include the superior and middle thyroid veins.

In the anterior portion of the neck, the external jugular veins lie on top of the cervical fascia and deep to the platysma muscle. They are formed by the junction of the posterior auricular and temporomaxillary veins in the substance of the parotid gland. At approximately the level of the angle of the mandible, they run down the neck in an approximate line from the angle of the mandible to the middle of the clavicle. Here they penetrate the deep cervical fascia and enter the subclavian veins. The anterior jugular veins run from the upper border of the hyoid bone on the deep cervical fascia approximately in a line parallel to the anterior border of the sternohyoid muscles. In the lower part of the neck, they diverge laterally to join the external jugular veins just before they enter the subclavian.

Posterior Vascular

Arterial

The vertebral arteries originate on the superior posterior aspect of the first portion of the subclavian arteries in most cases, although in up to 5% of instances the left vertebral originates directly from the aorta. Accompanied by the vertebral veins, they enter the foramina of the transverse process of the sixth cervical vertebra. They remain in this intraosseus canal until between the second and first cervical vertebrae. Here, due to the small transverse process of C2 and the longer transverse processes of C1, the vertebral arteries are more accessible than in other areas within the transverse canal. After exiting the transverse process of the atlas, they pass beneath the posterior occipitoatlantal ligament to enter the skull through the foramen magnum. Except for tiny collaterals, the vertebral arteries have no major branches in the neck.

Venous

The vertebral veins are not discrete in the upper portion of the neck. They consist of a plexus of small veins that surround the artery and drain the adjacent spinal cord and cervical musculature. This plexus of veins unites to form the vertebral veins in the lower third of the neck. The vertebral veins then pass out of the sixth foramina with the vertebral arteries to enter the subclavian veins near their junction with the jugulars.

Cervical Nerves

Nerves encountered during exposure of the carotid arteries include the marginal mandibular vagus, hypoglossal, spinal accessory, posterior auricular, and the recurrent laryngeal.

The *ansa hypoglossus* is formed from branches of the hypoglossal nerve and branches from C1 and C2 from the cervical plexus. It originates from proximal on the hypoglossal, crosses the internal carotid, and then runs parallel to the carotid for a few centimeters before it curves downward over the internal jugular vein. This nerve supplies the strap muscles, including the sternohyoid, sternothyroid, and inferior belly of the omohyoid.

The *vagus* nerve runs within the carotid sheath from the jugular foramen to the thorax. Its position relative to the carotid artery and jugular vein is variable. Most commonly it courses posterolateral to the carotid. It may be found between the carotid and jugular, where it can be easily injured. Regardless of its position, the vagus nerve is closely applied to the internal carotid from the jugular foramen to the carotid bulb. Thus, dissection of the internal carotid should be performed in the adventitial plane, and complete circumferential dissection should be done before clamping of this vessel to avoid injury to the vagus.

The *recurrent laryngeal* nerve is best avoided in the lower neck by careful dissection of the jugular veins and common carotid artery out of the carotid sheath. Minimizing dissection of the vagus nerve will lessen the chance of injury to the vagus and recurrent laryngeal nerves. Injury to this nerve produces ipsilateral vocal cord paralysis.

The *hypoglossal* nerve becomes a surgical consideration when high dissection of the carotid bifurcation is necessary. Cephalad to a line between the mastoid process and the angle of the jaw, the hypoglossal nerve courses over the internal carotid artery and the external carotid artery. Careful mobilization will minimize injury during arterial exposure in this area. Injury causes tongue deviation to the ipsilateral side.

The *spinal accessory* nerve exits the skull through the jugular foramen. It then descends behind the digastric and stylohyoid muscles obliquely to enter the superior portion of the sternocleidomastoid muscle. The nerve can be injured when exploration for Zone III injuries are done. Injury causes paralysis of the trapezius muscle.

As with the spinal accessory nerve, the *glossopharyngeal* nerve can be at risk during internal carotid dissections near the base of the skull. After exiting the jugular foramen, the glossopharyngeal nerve crosses the internal carotid superficially. After crossing the internal carotid, the branch to the carotid sinus is seen running parallel to the artery. Injury to this nerve may result in dysphagia, discoordinate swallowing, and/or loss of the gag reflex.

The *marginal mandibular* nerve is a branch of the facial nerve. Coursing around the angle of the mandible, this nerve usually is injured by retractors placed against this area of the mandible. Injury results in ptosis of the ipsilateral lip.

The *posterior auricular* nerve is a superficial sensory nerve that usually is cut during initial exposure of the carotid sheath. Its loss causes a sensory deficit over the mastoid process.

The *transverse cervical* nerve crosses the sternocleidomastoid deep to the platysma. When using an incision along the anterior border of this muscle, branches of the transverse cervical nerve usually must be sacrificed. This results in numbness of the skin over the anterior neck.

The *cervical roots* may be encountered during exploration of the vertebral arteries. They usually lie posterior to the vertebral artery. Injury can occur when rongeuring off the lateral processes of the vertebra. Injury to these nerves will be manifested by deficits in the brachial plexus.

MECHANISM OF INJURY

Arterial injuries take a number of forms but are basically due to either blunt or penetrating trauma. *Penetrating trauma* that results in complete transection of an artery by a knife or bullet most often will cause retraction of the intima and media both proximally and distally and cessation of flow through the artery with a minimal amount of bleeding from the disrupted ends. Thrombus will form retrograde and prograde to the first major patent branch. In the case of the internal carotid artery, the thrombus tends to extend to the level of its first major branch, the ophthalmic artery.

In contrast, a partial transection, more often from a stab wound than a missile, often results in continued hemorrhage with variable compromise of distal blood flow. The intima and media are unable to retract and contract fully because of the remaining intact bridge of artery, thus preventing spontaneous cessation of bleeding.

Penetrating injuries with missiles of high or low velocity may cause significant injury without direct passage through the artery. Ballistic effects such as temporary cavitation and pressure waves developed by the bullet traversing through soft tissue produce a stretch type of injury that may disrupt the intima and/or media. This results in occlusion and thrombosis of the artery in proximity to the bullet's path (Fig. 18–2). Additionally, secondary missiles

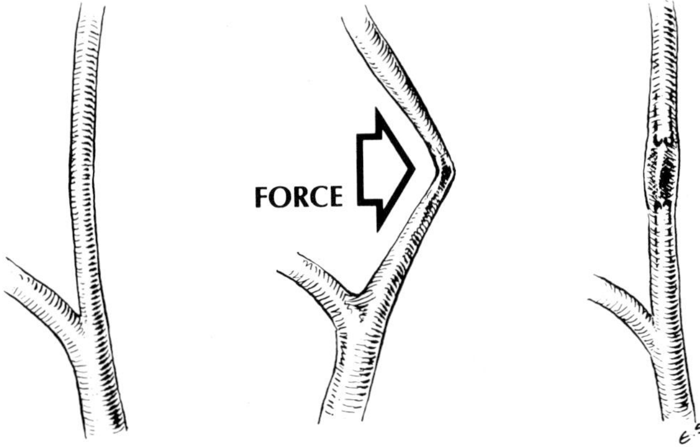

Figure 18–2.   Demonstration of the mechanism by which a bullet or blunt trauma produces a "stretch" lesion and intimal damage resulting in vessel thrombosis.

created by the bullet impacting bone (e.g., mandible, vertebrae) may cause penetrating injury to the vessel. Because of its size and length, the common carotid artery is the vessel injured most often by penetrating trauma (Table 18–1).

With *blunt injury,* the internal carotid artery is the cervical vessel most commonly injured. These injuries are far more subtle than penetrating trauma, as thrombosis rather than hemorrhage usually is the result of either a direct blow to the artery or hyperextension injury of the neck. The internal carotid can be injured by impingement on bony structures such as the styloid process, a fractured vertebral body, or (rarely) the mandible. A tear of the normal intima or a disruption at the site of atheromatous plaque becomes an entry point for distal dissection of the media and/or intima. These injuries can range from intimal flaps that may or may not be hemodynamically significant to complete thrombosis of the artery (Fig. 18–3). These arterial injuries may be present without external evidence of trauma or injury to surrounding structures.

It is appropriate to be aware of the potential for concomitant *venous injuries.* These usually are a result of penetrating trauma. A simultaneous internal jugular or common facial vein injury may lead to the development of an arteriovenous fistula with resultant venous hypertension in the area of injury. Arteriovenous fistulas may be encountered in up to 5% of vascular injuries.[9] Initial physical exam may not disclose these injuries, as the communication may require hours to days to develop fully, and results in the need for frequent reexamination of the injured area when diagnostic modalities or operative exploration are not undertaken.

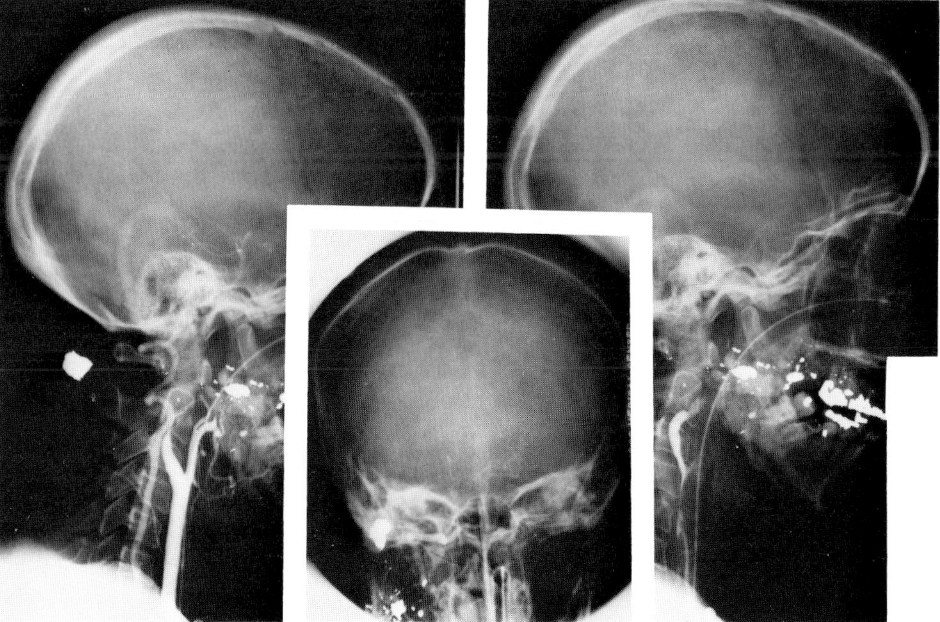

Figure 18–3.   The arteriogram of a patient who had a gunshot wound of the neck. Even though the artery was not hit directly, intimal damage resulted.

INCIDENCE OF CERVICAL VASCULAR INJURY

Cervical vascular injuries most often are due to penetrating trauma. Blunt injuries to the cervical vessels have been considered rare, but this may be because blunt vascular injuries usually result in thrombosis rather than bleeding and often occur with other injuries (e.g., head injury). Thus, it is likely that blunt cervical vascular injuries are much more common than are recognized.[10–12]

Mattox et al.[13] reviewed their 30-yr experience with cardiovascular injuries. Out of 5760 injuries suffered by 4459 patients, carotid artery injuries represented 3.2%, vertebral artery injuries 0.7%, and jugular vein injuries 5.1% of all cardiovascular injuries. This distribution is similar to that from the Korean and Vietnam wars.[4]

The artery most commonly injured by penetrating trauma is the common carotid artery. In our combined series, it was injured 72.7% of the time and the internal and external carotid arteries were injured 22.6% and 4.7% of the time, respectively (Table 18–1). External carotid injuries or injury to one of its branches usually occur more often than internal carotid injuries. When recognized, these injuries usually are treated by ligation. Lack of significant symptoms after external carotid branch injuries results in many of these injuries being undetected.

Blunt carotid trauma occurs more commonly than reported and frequently remains undiagnosed until neurologic symptoms appear.[11,12,24–29] These injuries usually result from a major force to the neck and often are associated with cervical dislocation or fracture. Most series contain at least one or two cases of blunt carotid artery injury that results from automobile, motorcycle, bicycle, snowmobile, or all-terrain vehicle accidents. However, blunt trauma from fall or forced extension or other apparent minor trauma can cause injury, particularly if preexisting disease is present. The most common location that produces clinical symptoms is that related to the internal carotid artery (Table 18–2). Lesions in this location appear as intimal fractures from excessive stretch injuries, with or without damage to the media.

Vertebral artery injuries may be one of the most underdiagnosed vascular injuries.[16] This is because these injuries are rarely symptomatic. The reason is that collateral flow

Table 18–1.   Location of Penetrating Carotid Artery Injuries

AUTHOR	COMMON	INTERNAL	EXTERNAL	TOTAL
Cohen	66	19	0	85
Bradley	17	7	2	26
Rubio	61	10	10	81
Thal	48	12	0	60
Unger	415	149	0	564
Ledgerwood	23	10	0	33
Fry	25	18	11	54
Brown	103	20	20	143
Karlin	38	9	3	50
Demetriades	104	10	10	124
Fabian	19	16	0	35
Sclafani	6	8	4	18
Totals	925 (72.7%)	288 (22.6%)	60 (4.7%)	1273 (100%)

Table 18–2. Location of Blunt Carotid Trauma

AUTHOR	MECHANISM	COMMON	INTERNAL	TOTAL
Perry	Assault	2	15	17
Zelenock	MVA	0	6	6
Mokri	MVA	0	18	18
Fabian	MVA	3	18	21
Davis	MVA	NS	NS	14
Martin	MVA	3	5	8
Totals		8 (11.4%)	62 (88.6%)	70 (100%)

MVA = motor vehicle accident; NS = not stated.

through the contralateral vertebral artery usually is sufficient to prevent posterior circulation symptomatology. The asymptomatic nature of most vertebral artery injuries results in the fact that they are rarely looked for. However, lesions initially asymptomatic can be associated with subsequent neurological problems, hemorrhage, or symptomatic arteriovenous fistulae.

Injuries should be suspected when vertebral fractures and/or dislocations potentially involve the transverse processes of the cervical spine. Vertebral artery injury also occurs with forced hyperextension.

Penetrating cervical venous injuries are recognized because of hemorrhage or the development of arteriovenous fistulas. The superficial and the internal jugular veins are the most frequently injured. Injuries to the vertebral veins are significant primarily when associated with a vertebral arteriovenous fistula, although bleeding from the vertebral veins can prove troublesome if they communicate with the surgical field.

INITIAL ASSESSMENT AND MANAGEMENT

Upon initial patient presentation, symptoms and physical signs may suggest cervical vascular trauma (Tables 18–3 and 18–4). New onset ipsilateral hemispheric symptoms including hemiplegia, hemiparesis, or monocular blindness should be assumed to be due to carotid artery injury until proven otherwise.[30] Deficits due to cranial nerves IX, X, XI, and/or XII may suggest the possibility of arterial injury because of their immediate proximity to the internal carotid artery.

Table 18–3. Penetrating Trauma: Symptoms and Signs

Arterial bleeding
Cervical hematoma
Delayed onset airway obstruction
IX, X, or XII nerve dysfunction
Hemiparesis or hemiplegia
Bruit or thrill

Table 18–4. Blunt Trauma: Symptoms and Signs

Cervical spine dislocation
Hyperextension neck injury
Transient hemiparesis
Hemiparesis or hemiplegia
Monocular visual symptoms
Bruit

Penetrating Trauma

Manifestation of penetrating trauma to the carotid artery usually consists of major hemorrhage that may temporarily subside when hypotension develops only to resume again when resuscitation is initiated. Bleeding from the neck that appears to be arterial should lead to the suspicion of major vascular injury. Venous bleeding is characteristically dark and, once it ceases, rarely recurs. However, increases in central venous or arterial pressure secondary to a Valsalva maneuver, such as occurs during endotracheal or nasogastric intubation, may dislodge a venous thrombus and cause bleeding to resume.

Clinically evident hematomas are frequently associated with arterial injury. Expanding cervical hematomas and/or active bleeding should prompt expedient cervical exploration. Because the cervical fascia is relatively nondistensible to acute pressure, it may contain arterial bleeding. Although little external evidence of hematoma may be present, the arterial hematoma may expand inward and dissect through the deep fascial planes of the neck and mediastinum. Unless decompressed, airway compromise often will follow. The extent of these injuries may not be apparent on initial examination. What appears to be only a simple cutaneous wound may be associated with a major underlying vascular injury tamponaded by the cervical fascia and/or musculature. Thus, particular attention must be paid to the airway in all patients who have wounds that penetrate the platysma muscle, as airway edema and obstruction may be the first overt manifestations of arterial injury (Fig. 18–4). Clinically evident hematomas are rarely produced by venous bleeding.

Early airway control, preferably via nasal or orotracheal intubation, should be instituted at the first sign of respiratory distress. If airway compromise is not present, prophylactic intubation is not indicated and intubation can be delayed until the patient has reached the operating room. Intubation done without neuromuscular blockade can result in the patient performing a Valsalva maneuver and activating venous hemorrhage. The surgical team should be immediately available at all times but especially during intubation. Neuromuscular blockade can assist intubation by preventing increased arterial and venous pressures; however, the neurologic exam is lost for a period of time depending on the neuromuscular blocker used. Although tracheostomy may be necessary as an emergency resuscitative procedure, opening the pretracheal fascia before control of vascular injuries in the carotid system at the thoracic inlet may decompress the tamponade produced by surrounding tissue with ensuing hemorrhage.

After the adequacy of the airway has been ensured and the patient is volume resuscitated, a careful neurological examination must be performed. The neurological status of the patient at the time of arrival in the emergency room should be documented, and any changes must be observed and recorded. Particular attention should be paid to cerebral function and also to the function of those cranial nerves that traverse the region of the carotid arteries—the glossopharyngeal, hypoglossal, and vagus nerves. Because of the

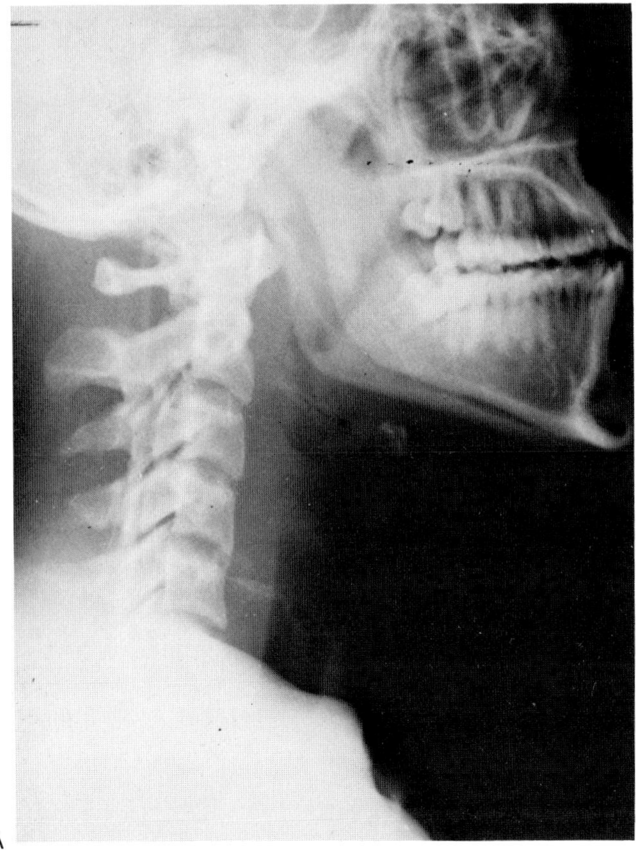

Figure 18–4.   Hemorrhage in the deep structures of the neck. **A:** The initial film was not remarkable, but when the patient developed respiratory distress a short time later, marked swelling of the prevertebral region was noted. (Figure continued on next page.)

high correlation between preoperative neurological function and complications after repair of carotid injuries,[4] accurate neurological assessment is mandatory before administration of pain medications and anesthetic agents.

Blunt Trauma

Because patients with blunt injury to the carotid arteries manifest symptoms of thrombosis rather than hemorrhage, their course is somewhat different from those with penetrating injuries.[10] A history of the patient being neurologically intact and lucid at the scene of the accident or at the time of arrival in the emergency room, followed by a transient or permanent hemiparesis or hemiplegia, strongly suggests blunt injury to the carotid artery. This sequence of events should not be mistaken for intracerebral injury or subdural or epidural hematoma.

Accurate neurological assessment in injured patients often is difficult due to alcohol or recreational drug use, associated fractures, or shock.[31] This indeterminate or equivocal

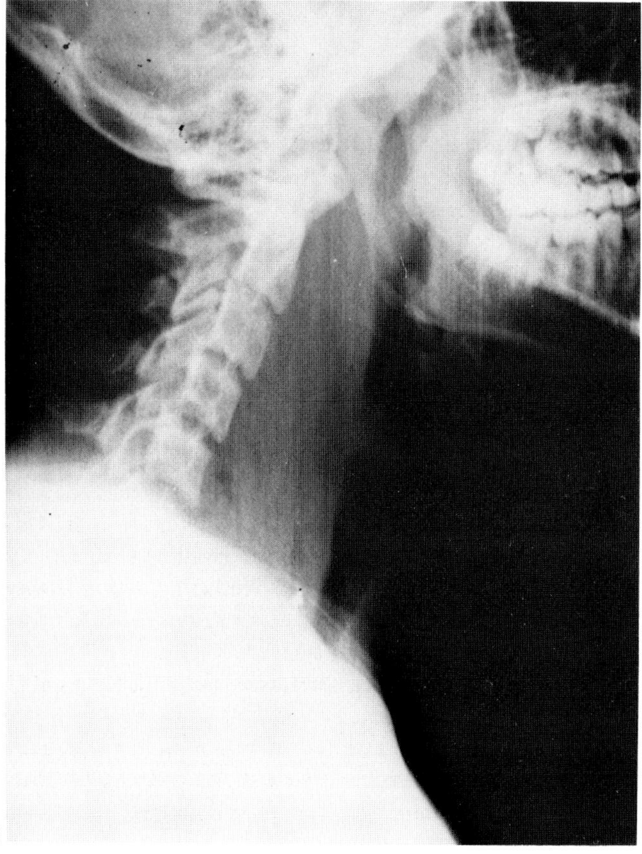

B

Figure 18–4, cont.   **B:** A previously unsuspected carotid artery lesion was found at operation and repaired.

neurological examination can be deceptively benign. Sympathetic dysfunction as manifested by Horner's syndrome must be looked for and noted if present. Sympathetic dysfunction may result from unsuspected cervical fracture or dislocation. Even though it may not seem necessary to perform a diagnostic work-up for minimal changes, the burden of proof is on the surgeon to prove no vascular injury has occurred. Close follow-up and special studies including noninvasive vascular laboratory exam, arteriograms, or computed tomography (CT) may be indicated to establish whether the changes are in the extracranial vessels or due to intracranial injury.[10]

Posterior Circulation

Injury to the vertebral artery can result in hemorrhage, arteriovenous fistulae, or thrombosis. Clinically significant vertebral artery injuries usually are the result of penetrating trauma. Hemorrhage or hematomas from a wound of the neck suggest the possibility of injury, especially if it passes medially near the transverse processes of the vertebrae.

The presence of an arteriovenous fistula can be diagnosed clinically if cervical auscultation reveals a bruit. Initially after injury, fistula flow may be minimal and increase to a clinically significant level only with the passage of days or weeks. The bruit will gradually develop a systolic and diastolic component and is not affected by carotid compression. Symptoms, when they occur, are related to the brain stem or occipital cortex and include visual symptoms, dizziness, lightheadedness, and vertigo.[19]

Thrombosis of the vessel, which usually is the complication from blunt injury, rarely produces symptoms because of parallel flow in the opposite vertebral. Thus, the possibility of thrombosis is rarely investigated. We believe that all anterior penetrating wounds that violate the platysma should have a Duplex scan, angiography, or operative exploration. As a result, vertebral injuries that are asymptomatic are being recognized. Unless bleeding, false aneurysm, or arteriovenous fistulas are present, no treatment is indicated.

Special Procedures

Wounds in the upper portion of the neck above a line drawn from the angle of the mandible to the mastoid process are difficult to expose. Wounds passing above this level in the vicinity of the carotid arteries should be evaluated preoperatively by Duplex scanning or angiography if the patient is stable. If the presumed lesion is at the base of the neck below the level of the cricoid cartilage and if the patient is stable, angiography also should be used. Simple local cervical exploration may result in a catastrophe unless the chest has been opened to ensure proximal control of injured vessels (Chapter 17).

Immediate examination with Duplex scanning can reliably identify carotid injury, including disruption of the intima and media or complete thrombosis. We have used Duplex scans to assess for arterial injury at our institution and have found excellent correlation between the scan and angiographic or operative findings. Angiography may provide further anatomic information in those cases with injury initially diagnosed by Duplex scanning. If the Duplex scan does not reveal carotid injury, CT of the brain should be obtained to rule out intracranial pathology.[11,20,21]

In the case of gunshot wounds, when a foreign body is present in the neck, anteroposterior and lateral films are of value to locate the probable course of the missile. Probing a wound deep to the platysma with a sterile applicator stick can precipitate bleeding or dislodge an embolus. False passages also can misrepresent the true course of the missile or knife unless the wound is quite large or the position of the head and neck as well as the direction of entry is known. Duplex scanning can provide information regarding vascular integrity and remove any need for wound probing.

A high index of suspicion must be present if blunt carotid injuries are to be diagnosed before the development of neurological symptoms. More than half of the patients with asymptomatic carotid injuries have signs of major injury of the neck as manifest by hematomas or cervical fractures and 75% of the patients have had head trauma. Therefore, intracranial injury often is the initial diagnosis. The diagnosis may be made inadvertently when angiography is used to evaluate intracranial disease but, with the advent of CT scanning, angiography is being used less frequently and there is the resultant increased risk of missing this diagnosis. Duplex scanning provides an accurate noninvasive method of assessing suspected blunt carotid injury; however, soft tissue swelling or hematomas may render the diagnosis unreliable. Should these be present or should an injury be shown by Duplex scan, angiographic evaluation may further delineate anatomic abnormalities. Duplex scanning also is useful for reevaluation of questionable abnormalities or for postoperative follow-up.

OPERATIVE EXPOSURE

The primary guiding principle in dealing with vascular injuries is to obtain proximal and distal control of the injured artery or its parent artery before entering the hematoma at the level of injury.

For diagnostic purposes, the neck is commonly divided into three zones. Zone I includes the thoracic outlet. This zone has its boundaries from the sternal notch to the level of the cricoid cartilage. Zone II encompasses the central area of the neck where most carotid artery injuries occur. Its boundaries are the cricoid cartilage to the level of the angle of the mandible. Zone III spans the area bounded by the angle of the mandible to the base of the skull.

Exposure of Zone II *carotid* and *jugular* injuries will be dealt with first because exposure of Zones I and III are extensions of Zone II exposure.

Exposure of Zone II is accomplished by an incision on the anterior border of the sternocleidomastoid muscle from the clavicular head to the level of angle of the mandible. This incision is carried down through the platysma to the sternocleidomastoid muscle. The transverse cervical nerve usually is sacrificed at this point. The sternocleidomastoid is then reflected posterolaterally to expose the carotid sheath. After incising the carotid sheath, the internal jugular vein is dissected laterally and posteriorly away from the carotid artery. If needed, further exposure can be gained by division of the facial vein and ansa cervicalis and omohyoid muscle (Fig. 18–5).

When dealing with carotid artery injuries, the principles used in the dissection of the artery for carotid endarterectomy should be followed. Attempts should be made to dissect structures away from the carotid artery rather than dissecting the carotid artery away from the surrounding structures. Minimal manipulation of the artery, when possible, minimizes the chances of distal embolization and intraoperative cerebral infarction. The common carotid should be controlled first, well proximal to the area of injury, followed by control of the internal and then the external carotid distal to the area of injury. Should hemorrhage occur before distal control, the common carotid artery should be cross-clamped and residual bleeding controlled by pressure while distal exposure is obtained. This sequence of vascular control will help minimize hemorrhage and potential cerebral embolization.

Zone I exposure usually requires median sternotomy to ensure proximal control. Initially this can be accomplished by carrying the incision on the anterior border of the sternocleidomastoid down to the sternal notch. At this point, more proximal exposure is gained by median sternotomy. The phrenic nerve can come into the field of dissection when hematomas distort the normal anatomy or when dissecting out the origin of the common carotid. Injury to the vagus nerve and/or recurrent laryngeal nerve should be avoided by careful dissection and awareness of their probable location.

Exposure of Zone III is achieved by extension of the anterior sternocleidomastoid incision to the inferior margin of the mastoid process (Fig. 18–6). The incision should then be carried over the posterior aspect of the mastoid process to minimize injury to the posterior auricular nerve. The major artery in Zone III is predominantly the internal, as the external carotid usually has divided into its smaller divisions in this sector.

The carotid artery in Zone III is contained within a triangle with two bony edges. The posterior border includes the mastoid process and the sternocleidomastoid muscle. The anterior border consists of the posterior aspect of the mandibular ramus. To gain access effectively to this portion of the carotid artery, this triangle must be converted into a

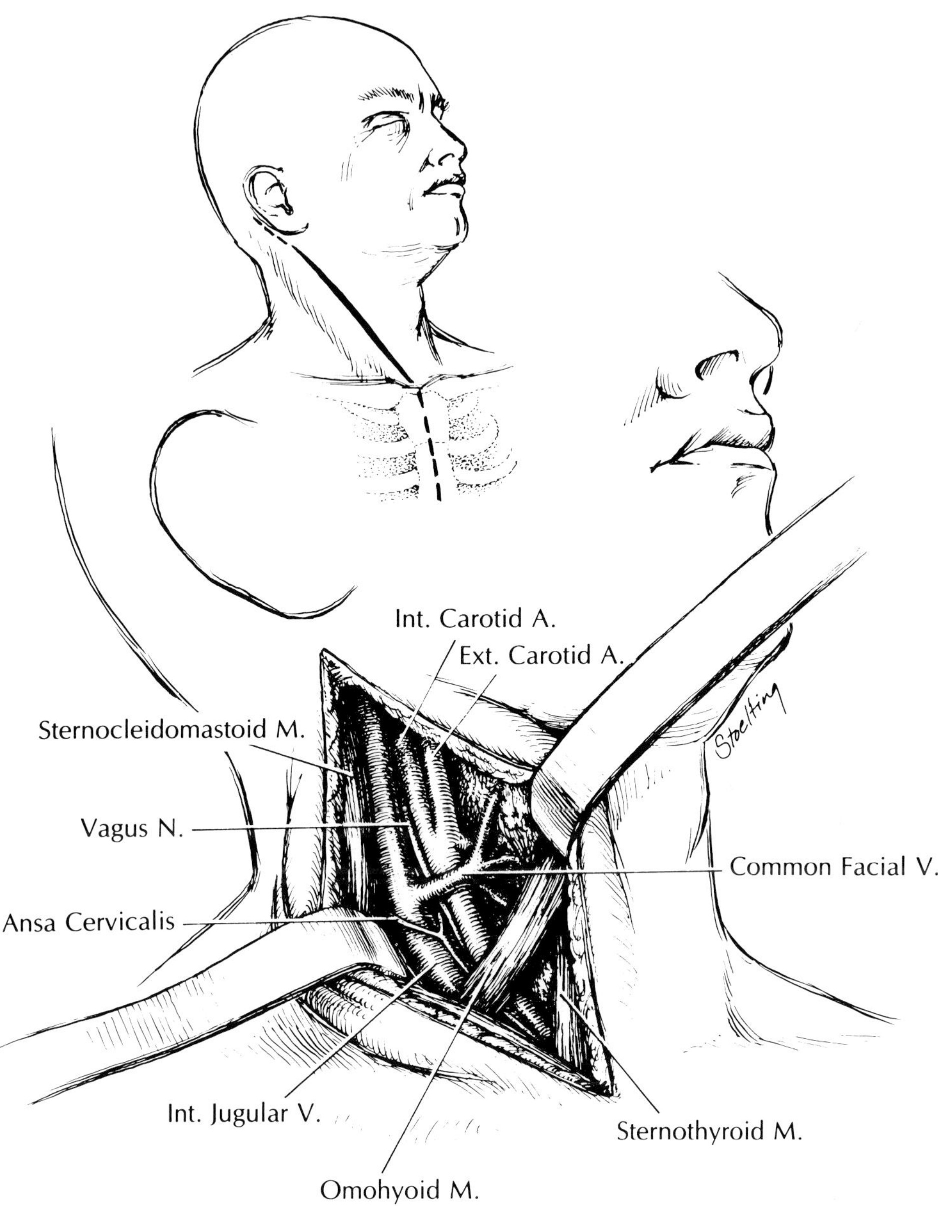

Figure 18–5. Location of the incision for carotid artery and jugular vein exploration is shown. The incision can be extended upward behind the ear for lesions located near the base of the skull or extended downward as a median sternotomy to control proximal injuries.

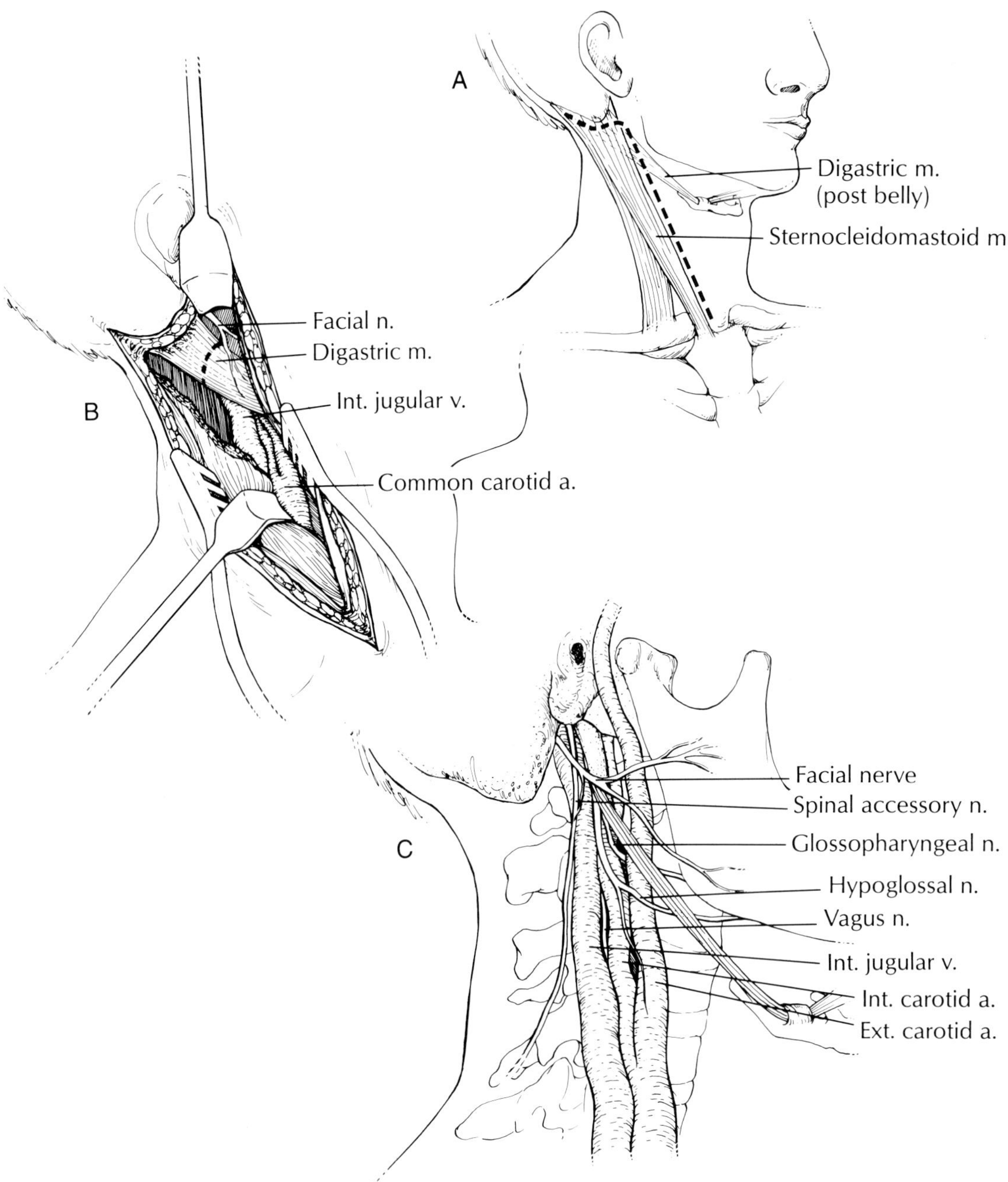

Figure 18–6. Exposure of the carotid artery in Zone III. **A:** The incision should be extended up the anterior edge of the sternocleidomastoid muscle, then across the base of the skull, detaching the muscle. **B:** The digastric muscle is transected. **C:** The cranial nerves should be identified, preserved, if possible, and distal control of the artery obtained.

rectangle. In the setting of a stable patient with a known Zone III injury, subluxation of the mandible can be done. Division of the mandibular ramus is an alternative but may take longer to accomplish.

As with the carotid artery, the *vertebral artery* has three anatomic zones. The first zone includes the origin to the transverse foramina of the sixth cervical vertebra. Zone II spans the intraosseus segment from C6 to C1. Zone III has boundaries from C1 to the base of the skull. Thus, the first and third sections of the vertebral artery are most easily accessible for surgical intervention.

Exposure of the third section is accomplished in a similar way to exposure of Zone III carotid artery injuries (Fig. 18–7). An incision along the anterior border of the sternocleidomastoid is made to the inferior portion of the mastoid process. At this level, the incision is carried posterior to the border of the mastoid, detaching the sternocleidomastoid from its insertion as well as the splenius capitis attachment to the mastoid. The spinal accessory nerve enters the sternocleidomastoid 2 to 3 cm below the mastoid process and should be carefully exposed. By staying *posterior* to the transverse processes, the internal jugular vein can be avoided.

After location of the transverse process of the atlas, the prevertebral fascia is divided from the transverse process parallel to the spinal accessory nerve. The levator scapulae is then encountered just below the atlas. Careful division of the levator scapulae reveals the vertebral artery in the relatively wide intervertebral space (1–2 cm). At this level, the anterior ramus of the second cervical nerve crosses the artery. By mobilization of the anterior ramus, the vertebral artery can be ligated at this location. Distal to the C1 transverse foramina, the vertebral artery courses medially to the foramen magnum.

The proximal portion of the vertebral artery is most easily reached through an incision 2 to 3 cm above the clavicle over the clavicular portion of the sternocleidomastoid (Fig. 18–8). Division of the clavicular head exposes the anterior scalene fat pad, phrenic nerve, and anterior scalene muscle. With mobilization of the phrenic nerve and division of the anterior scalene muscle, the subclavian artery is exposed. Following the course of the subclavian artery medially, the vertebral artery origin is encountered.

Exposure also can be obtained through an incision on the anterior border of the sternocleidomastoid carried down to the clavicular head. Reflection of the jugular vein and carotid artery laterally allows identification of the vertebral artery. The artery can be palpated between the longus colli and anterior scalene muscles.

Exposure of the intraosseus portion of the vertebral artery is rarely needed if interventional neuroradiologic support is available for embolization therapy. In some cases, though, acute exsanguinating hemorrhage from this portion of the vertebral artery can mandate operative exploration (Fig. 18–9).

Exposure from the C2 to C6 level again can be gained through an incision placed over the anterior or posterior border of the sternocleidomastoid and medial reflection of the jugular vein, carotid artery, and vagus nerve. Posterior and medial to these structures lie the longus coli and longus capitus muscles. These muscles then can be dissected off the transverse processes at the desired level and reflected medially. The roof of the transverse canal should be gently rongeured off, exposing the vertebral artery. The cervical nerves lie directly posterior to the vertebral artery and must be protected. Thus, ligatures must be placed carefully around the vertebral artery alone to avoid injury to the cervical nerves. Depending on the location of the injury on the vertebral artery, operative interventions

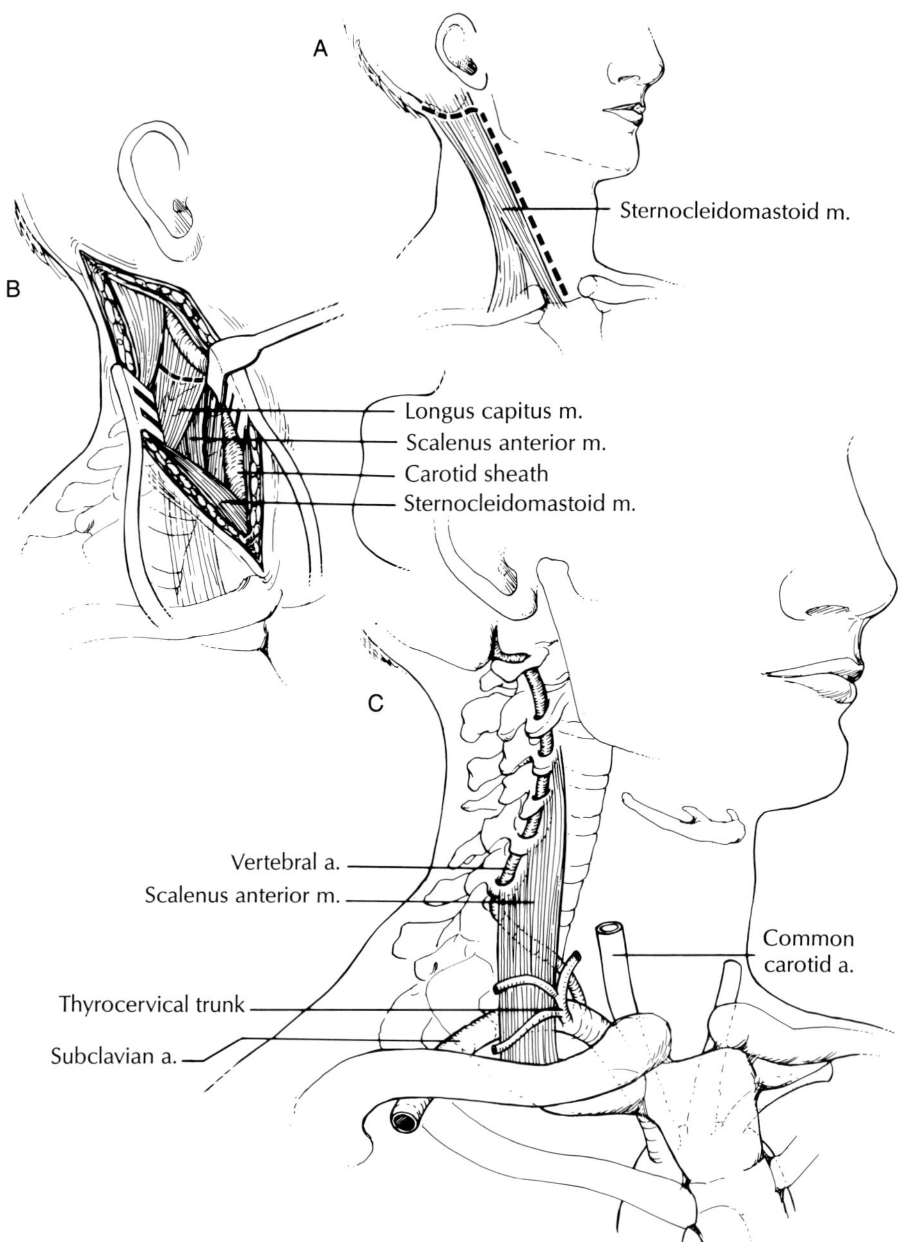

Figure 18–7.   Exposure of the distal third of the vertebral artery. **A:** The initial incision is similar to that used for the distal internal carotid artery. **B:** The longus capitus muscle is divided while the carotid sheath is retracted medially. **C:** The transverse process of the atlas is located and the prevertebral fascia divided, followed by that of the levator scapulae exposing the vertebral artery.

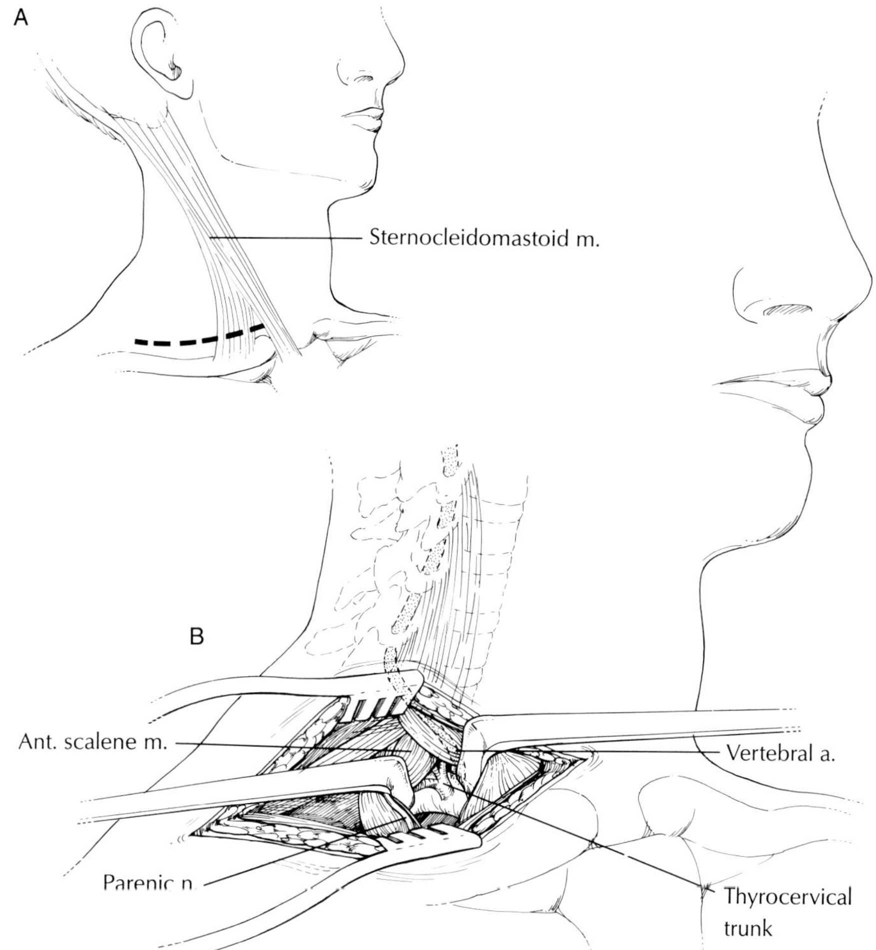

Figure 18–8.   Approach to proximal vertebral artery. **A:** Location of incision. **B:** Retraction of anterior scalene muscle to expose vertebral artery origin.

including ligation, reimplantation (if necessary), or passage of a balloon for tamponade can be accomplished.[35]

OPERATIVE TREATMENT

Although injuries to the external carotid artery may be ligated, injuries to the common or internal carotid artery should be repaired if technically feasible. Continued experience with carotid reconstructions in patients with carotid artery injury and suffering neurologic ischemia including transient ischemic attacks, hemiparesis, or hemiplegia and even coma has revealed that an aggressive approach to reconstruction is justified.

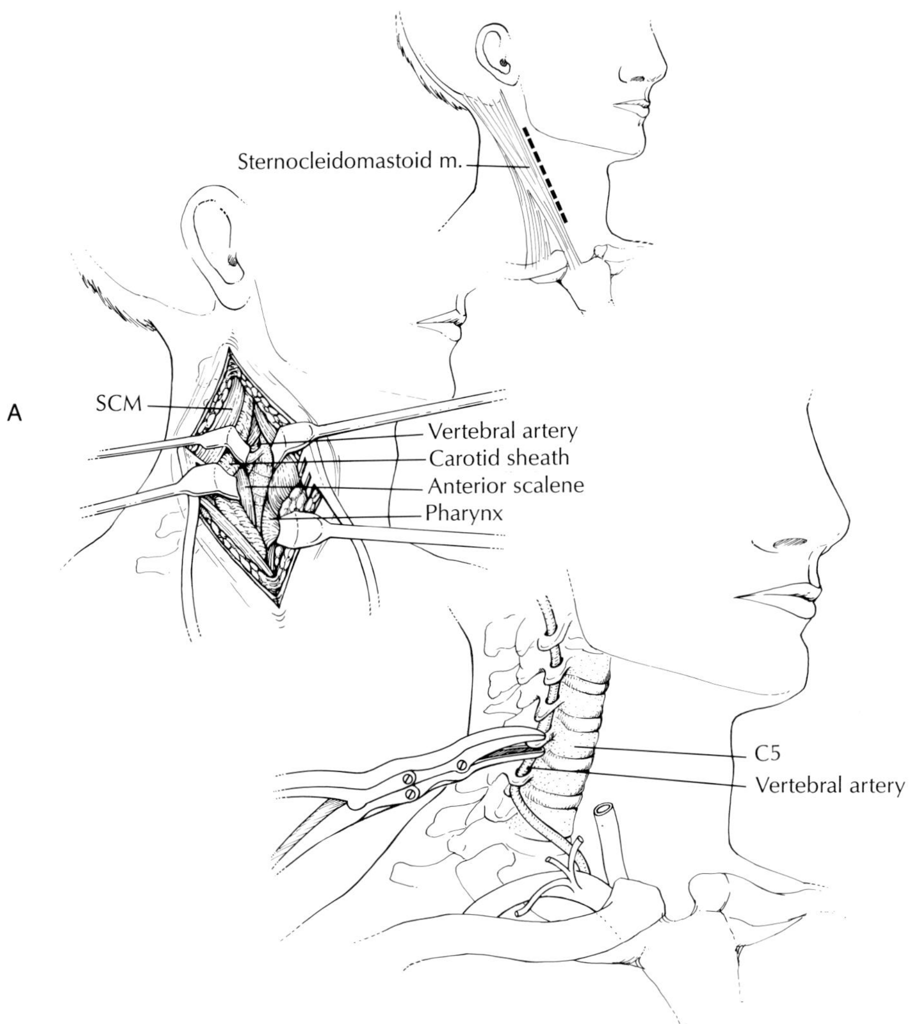

Figure 18–9.   Exposure of the vertebral artery in midneck. **A:** The incision is carried medial to the carotid artery and jugular vein and the longus coli and capitus muscles exposed and dissected medially off the transverse process. **B:** The roof of the transverse process is rongeured to expose the vertebral artery.

To this end, the American Association for the Surgery of Trauma (AAST) conducted a multicenter retrospective review of cerebrovascular injuries. Richardson et al. reviewed these data and found that sufficient numbers existed for penetrating trauma analysis only.[30] Common carotid injuries had the highest rate of neurologic deficits (29%) on presentation. Internal carotid injuries had a 15% rate of neurological deficits on presentation, innominate artery injuries had a 9% rate, and vertebral artery injuries had a 5% rate. Analysis of the data suggested that conscious patients with weakness or paralysis had favorable results with arterial repair. When global symptoms of cerebral ischemia were present, the results were indeterminate. When internal carotid artery injuries caused neurologic deficits, ligation resulted in worsening of symptoms or death. The one patient who underwent repair did well.

With these data in mind, the exact approach to the patient with cerebrovascular injury and neurological deficits has been clarified. Even though few surgeons have a wealth of experience in dealing with cerebrovascular injury, most agree that arterial repair should be attempted for patients suffering cerebrovascular injury and having lateralizing hemispheric symptoms. In patients with extracranial cerebrovascular injury and coma due to neurologic ischemia and not drugs or alcohol, ligation or repair produce equally dismal results at present.

After gaining control of the arterial injury, anticoagulation should be used if no contraindications such as head injury exist. Heparin in dosages of 5000 to 10,000 U intravenously is appropriate in these circumstances. If systemic anticoagulation is contraindicated due to other injuries, local anticoagulation can be instituted to prevent proximal and distal thrombosis. This can be accomplished by injecting 3 to 5 ml of saline containing 1000–2000 U of heparin into the proximal and distal artery with a fine-gauge needle. To minimize heparin from going into the systemic circulation, the arteries should be vented both proximally and distally just before completion of the anastomosis.

One goal of operative repair of *carotid artery* injuries is minimizing the complications of cerebral ischemia. When injuries are limited to the common carotid artery, the external carotid will provide collateral flow to the internal carotid. The collateral flow available intracranially when the internal carotid artery is occluded is more speculative. To this end, intraluminal shunting of the internal carotid artery during repair remains unaddressed in the literature. Even though shunting can increase the technical difficulty of carotid artery repair, it should be used when the injured artery had been functioning before occlusion for repair and the surgeon is comfortable with its application. When backbleeding from the distal end of the common or internal carotid is minimal, collateral cerebral blood flow may be insufficient to prevent cerebral ischemia. This can be particularly true when contralateral carotid injury or occlusive disease is present. If a carotid artery injury reconstruction requires a saphenous vein interposition graft, intraluminal shunting can allow more time for vein harvesting and preparation. When injuries to the internal carotid occur at or near the base of the skull, intraluminal shunting, particularly with a balloon-tipped shunt, allows control of the distal arterial segment without the need for arterial clamping. The shunt occasionally can be used for judicious traction of the distal internal carotid. This allows the distal end to be pulled below the base of the skull and facilitates repair. Conversely, when dealing with completely occluded arteries, neurologic damage, if any, should have already occurred.

The devastating effects of postoperative thrombosis or embolization from sites of residual injury mandate the debridement of all areas of intimal injury. Although techniques of endarterectomy as performed in carotid atherosclerotic disease may be applicable for some patients with intimal disruptions, they usually are inadequate because of the absence of the cleavage plane within the media created by atherosclerotic lesions. Moreover, trauma patients often are hypercoagulable, and raw surfaces of blood vessels thrombose readily.

If the repair of an arterial injury requires an interposition graft, autogenous tissue is preferred. The external carotid artery is an easily accessible substitute for injuries to the internal carotid near the bifurcation. Ligation of its branches, division, and transposition of the distal end of the external to the distal end of the internal with primary anastomosis creates a durable repair (Fig. 18–10). Likewise, the external carotid artery or its branches

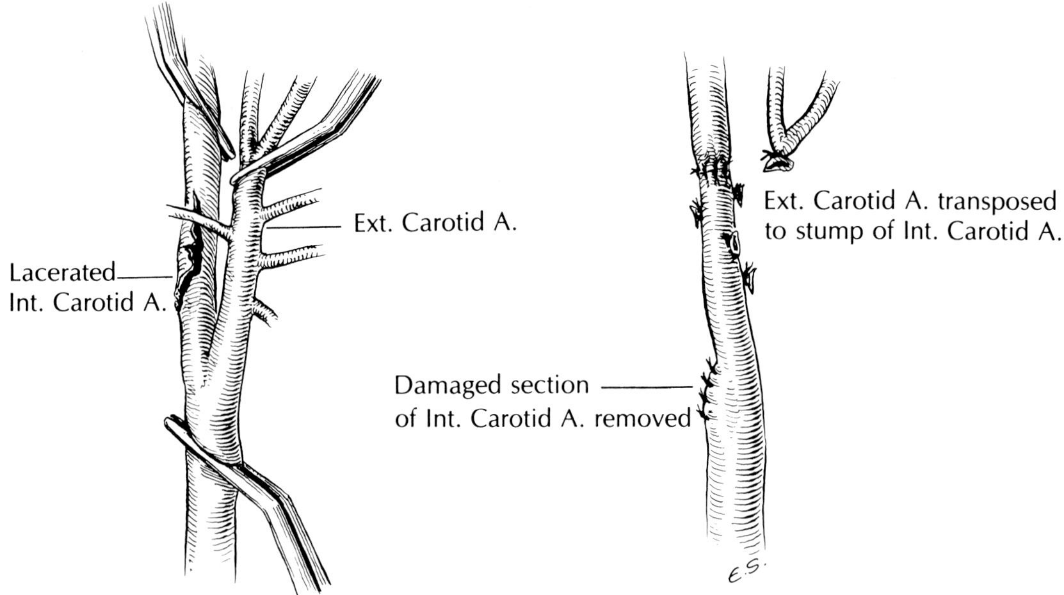

Figure 18–10. The technique of internal carotid replacement utilizing the external carotid artery.

function well when used for patch angioplasty to repair partial disruptions of the common or internal carotid artery.

In those instances where arterial defects cannot be repaired using local tissue, saphenous vein grafts are appropriate conduits for reconstruction. The saphenous vein is most suitable for reconstruction and is the first choice for venous substitution of the carotid artery. If this is unavailable, then consideration should be given to use the internal iliac artery. This can be harvested through an extraperitoneal lower quadrant incision.

Prosthetic materials should be viewed as an option of last resort for repair of carotid injuries. The high incidence of pharyngeal penetration and wound contamination from external debris raises significant concerns regarding prosthetic graft infection. Although the use of autologous tissue does not ensure the prevention of infection, native tissue appears to heal with fewer complications than prosthetic grafts. If simultaneous arterial and pharyngeal or esophageal injuries occur, we have used a pedicle of the sternocleidomastoid to protect the vascular repair.

Anastomoses should be performed with fine (5-0, 6-0), monofilament sutures in the standard way coapting intima to intima. Although running suture repair is appropriate for the common carotid artery, interrupted sutures produce less risk of narrowing the lumen in a smaller artery such as the internal carotid or vertebral. Lateral repairs of arterial injuries should be performed using the same suture in either an interrupted or running fashion, and care should be taken so as not to restrict the lumen diameter of the artery. If it appears that this may happen, a patch of external carotid artery or saphenous vein is best used to ensure an adequate lumen.

After control and repair of arterial injuries, a continued exploration of the path of the missile is mandatory. Injuries to major veins such as the jugular should not be overlooked. Jugular venous injuries may be ligated without significant sequelae, although small lateral defects should be repaired to optimize jugular venous flow. The surgeon must be aware of the potential for pulmonary air embolism resulting from aspiration of air into the open veins of the neck. This is best avoided by keeping the patient in a slight Trendelenburg position during venous exposure and repair.

Thorough investigation of the pharynx and esophagus must be undertaken, and repair of injuries to these structures must be performed. Failure to recognize injuries sets the stage for catastrophic cervicomediastinal infections (Chapter 9).

Most *vertebral artery* injuries do not require operative intervention. If the contralateral vertebral artery is patent, then vertebral artery trauma resulting in stenosis, pseudoaneurysm, or arteriovenous fistula can be treated by interventional neuroradiologic modalities to occlude the artery.[37] If thrombosis of a vertebral artery has occurred with the contralateral side remaining patent, no further interventions are indicated.

The indication for operative intervention with vertebral artery injuries is external bleeding or arteriovenous fistulae. These injuries can occur at any level of the vertebral artery, but lack of experience with exposure of the vertebral artery can make control of these lesions difficult. Except under rare circumstances (e.g., absent contralateral vertebral artery), vertebral artery injuries need only ligation rather than reconstruction.

A technique that is simpler than direct exposure of Zone II injuries, when urgent treatment is required, is to approach the vertebral artery near its origin and ligate the vessel proximally. The distal vessel is then cannulated with a Fogarty catheter of appropriate size and caliber, and the balloon advanced to the level of the injury or fistula[30] (Fig. 18–8). The Fogarty catheter balloon is then inflated with contrast media and, after inflation is completed and the catheter is satisfactorily placed using radiologic control, the catheter lumina should be crushed with a needle holder as it emerges from the vertebral artery, divided, and then secured with a fast-setting glue before the clamp or needle holder is removed. The foreign body in this instance is left in place to ensure permanent thrombotic obliteration of any arteriovenous communication that may be present. An alternative is to inject fast-setting glue directly into the defect through the catheter (Fig. 18–11).

Lacerations of the vertebral veins are best controlled by direct pressure, either forceps, finger, sponge, or peanut dissector. While the vessel is dissected proximally and distally for ligation, nothing should be clamped and ligated until all of the relevant structures, particularly the nerves, have been identified.

Intraoperative arteriography after carotid artery repair is useful to confirm vascular patency and, if it is normal, ensures that the vessel will remain free of thrombotic complications. This is performed with a 20- or 21-gauge scalp vein needle inserted into the common carotid artery well below the repair. Ten milliliters of contrast material is injected while a radiograph is exposed.

Drainage of vascular wounds is not required. Drainage should be dictated by the presence of oral, pharyngeal, or esophageal injuries and the degree of soilage of the wound. Drains should be routed away from the area of arterial injury and every attempt made at interposition of viable tissue between the injured artery and hollow viscus injuries. All patients should be given preoperative antibiotic coverage with a broad-spectrum drug appropriate for oral and upper gastrointestinal organisms.

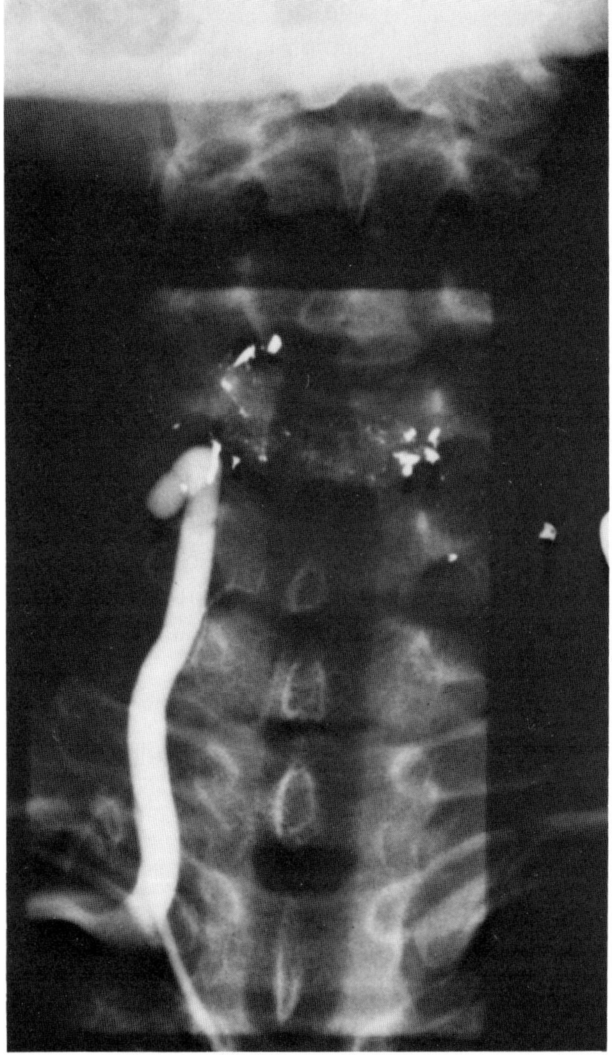

Figure 18–11.   **A:** This vertebral arteriogram shows an abrupt cutoff of the vertebral artery in the midneck and the initial filling of the vertebral vein.

POSTOPERATIVE CARE

The postoperative care required for these patients is dictated by the extent of associated injuries more than by the arterial injury itself. It is important to maintain adequate oxygenation and adequate perfusion pressure to the brain. Postoperative anticoagulation is generally contraindicated because of the risk of bleeding into the fresh wound as well as other sites of injury. However, infusion of low molecular weight dextran may be useful in selected cases that are high risk for thrombotic complications.

When there has been major soft tissue damage, particularly around the airway,

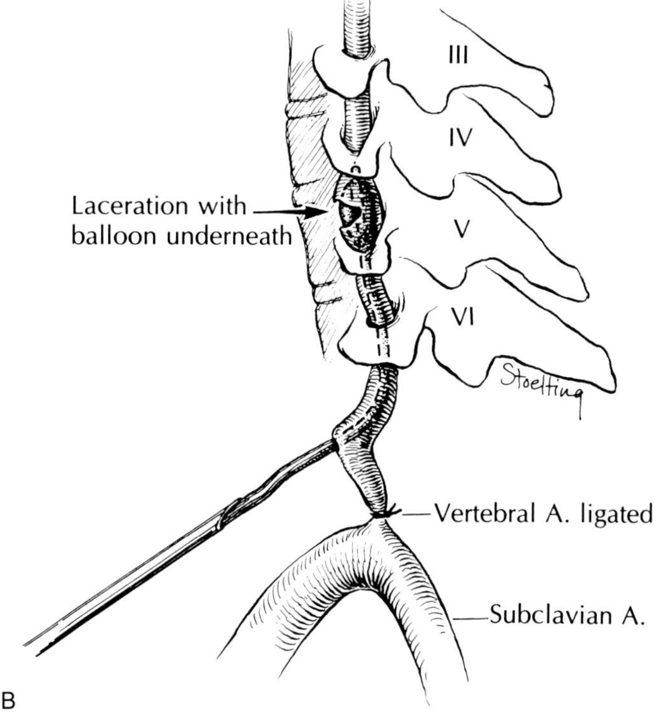

B

Figure 18–11, cont.   **B:** The arteriovenous fistula was successfully managed by embolization with cyano-acrylate glue.

laryngeal edema is a frequent accompaniment, and endotracheal tubes should not be removed until the patient is fully awake and in a setting where reintubation can be promptly carried out, should this be necessary. For associated major laryngeal or maxillofacial injuries, a tracheostomy may be appropriate, although this puts any vascular repair at added risk for chronic contamination from this stoma.

Antibiotic prophylaxis that should have been initiated preoperatively should be stopped within 24 hr after the operation if there is no evidence of oral, laryngeal, or esophageal contamination and no suspicion of infection or fistula.

COMPLICATIONS

There are three major, early postoperative complications associated with arterial repair in the neck. The first is continued bleeding, the second is thrombosis of the repair, and the third is infection surrounding the repair. Bleeding may occur anywhere along the area of tissue injury and, as noted earlier, bleeding in the deep cervical space may result in airway compromise or set the stage for either or both of the next two complications, thrombosis and infection.

A thorough postoperative examination to determine baseline neurological status should be conducted as soon as the patient has adequately awakened from anesthesia. A subsequent deterioration of the neurological status should alert the surgeon to possible failure of the vascular repair. The patient's postoperative neurological status should be the same or better than the preoperative neurological status. If this is not the case, or if the patient regains neurological function and then it subsequently deteriorates, thrombosis of the repair is likely. At this point the patient should be returned directly to the operating room for assessment of the repair status. This may be facilitated by an operative angiogram. Declotting of a thrombosed repair with resolution of the problem causing the thrombosis may salvage the outcome. Duplex scan also is a useful method to study the arterial repair in the immediate postoperative setting if there is a question of thrombosis being present.

The third major complication is a deep wound infection in the tissue surrounding the repaired artery.[26] These infections often are difficult to control and predispose the repair to disruption or thrombosis. All of the steps mentioned previously regarding preoperative antibiotics, drainage, and the use of autogenous tissue for repairs are aimed at the prevention of this complication. Treatment of this complication may require rerouting of the repair away from the infected tissue or ligation of the infected artery if breakdown of the anastomosis and hemorrhage occurs.

Further complications such as false aneurysm or arteriovenous fistula in the absence of infection are exceedingly rare after repair of the carotid arteries. Peripheral nerve injury that was not present preoperatively should not occur if careful attention is paid to adequate exposure, proximal control, and careful identification of the relevant nerves. Particular care must be exercised in retraction of the hypoglossal nerve because it often spans the operative field. Undue tension will cause a neuropraxis with tongue paralysis or paresis. Injury to the vagus nerve is possible, and an injury to the main trunk produces vocal cord paralysis in slight abduction. As a result, airway obstruction usually is not a problem. The primary manifestation will be the loss of volume of the voice or a hoarse voice. Vocal cord function should be checked at extubation when bilateral neck explorations are done.

Air embolism, which is a complication of major venous injury, may be recognized during the course of the operation. A sudden onset of unexplained hypotension, cardiac arrhythmias, or arrest should lead to the suspicion that air embolism is present. The patient should be placed in the left lateral decubitus position with the head downward to trap air in the right ventricle. Pressor agents should be administered to force air bubbles through the coronary circulation. Should arrest occur, the chest should be opened with an intercostal thoracotomy and open cardiac massage performed. Air should be aspirated from the ventricles as the apex of the heart is elevated.

RESULTS

The results of treatment of carotid artery injuries are generally good. The exceptions are those patients with preexisting neurological deficits.[5,6] In patients with any type of neurological deficit, the blood pressure should be carefully controlled, preferably at slightly hypotensive levels, with the administration of nitroprusside and ganglionic blocking agents.

Beall and co-workers[40] reported 25 injuries to the carotid arteries in 1963. Three patients died before definitive therapy was performed and the overall mortality was 20%. Two of the 22 patients in whom carotid artery repair was possible died, a mortality rate of 9%; both patients had cerebral damage at the time of admission. Among 20 long-term survivors, 16 were asymptomatic and 4 had neurologic deficits after operations.

Cohen and associates[6] in 1970 reported a mortality rate of 15% in 82 patients with carotid artery injuries, although the mortality was only 6% if death from associated injuries was excluded. Eight of these 82 patients had neurologic deficits on admission; after repair of the vessel, two of these eight were normal, two were worse, one remained unchanged, and three patients died. As a result, Cohen et al. recommended that patients with neurological deficits should not have repair done but instead have their vessels ligated.

The Vietnam Vascular Registry reported that of 14 penetrating carotid artery injuries in patients who were normal on admission, three developed neurologic deficits post-operatively.[4] Of 14 who presented with neurologic deficits, 2 were normal after operation and 12 had residual deficits.

Richardson et al. in a 1992 multicenter review[36] found that of 27 patients who presented with neurologic deficits after common carotid injury, 4 died before receiving specific treatment and 1 of 5 treated by ligation died. The outcome in 19 patients who had repair of the injury was as follows: 5 were normal, 4 improved, 2 were unchanged, 3 were worse, and 5 died. Five patients had injuries of the internal carotid artery and had neurologic deficits on presentation. One treated by repair had a normal outcome. Of four treated by ligation, one was normal, one unchanged, and two died.

As opposed to penetrating trauma, the results of treatment of blunt traumatic carotid injury were poor if diagnosis was not made and treatment was not initiated until neurologi-cal symptoms developed.[34] Yamada and associates[41] described results in 21 patients in 1967. Of those operated on, 3 died, 12 had a persistent serious neurological deficit, 2 had moderate deficits, and only 4 were asymptomatic. In 31 patients who were not operated on, 17 died and 14 had a severe deficit, the overall mortality rate was 40%, and severe neurologic residue occurred in 52% of the patients with such injuries. In the report by Towne[42] in 1972, two of the three patients operated on died. None of the three improved. The fourth patient who was treated by nonoperative management recovered without neurological residual.

REFERENCES

1. Packard FR. Apology and treatise. In: *Life and Times of Ambroise Paré*. New York: Paul B. Hoeber; 1926.
2. Garrison EH. *History of Medicine*. Philadelphia: Saunders; 1929.
3. Treves F. The treatment of carotid haemorrhage. *Proc Med Soc (Lond)*. 1887/88;11:115.
4. Rich N, Spencer FC. Carotid and vertebral artery injuries. In: Rich N, Spencer FC, eds. *Vascular Trauma*. Philadelphia: Saunders; 1978.
5. Bradley EL. Management of penetrating carotid injuries. *J Trauma*. 1973;13:49.
6. Cohen A, Brief D, Mathewson CJ. Carotid artery injuries: an analysis of 85 cases. *Am J Surg*. 1970;120:210.
7. Liekweg WG, Greenfield LJ. Management of penetrating carotid arterial injury. *Ann Surg*. 1978;188:581.
8. *Gray's Anatomy*. 37th ed. New York: Churchill Livingstone; 1989.
9. Hewitt RL, Smith AD, Drapanas T. Acute traumatic arteriovenous fistulas. *J Trauma*. 1973;13:901.
10. Crissey MM, Bernstein EF. Delayed presentation of carotid intimal tear following blunt craniocervical trauma. *Surgery*. 1974;75:543.
11. Davis JW, Holbrook TL, Hoyt DB, et al. Blunt carotid artery dissection: incidence, associated injuries, screening and treatment. *J Trauma*. 1990;30:1514.
12. Lee C, Woodring JH, Walsh JW. Carotid and vertebral artery survivors of atlanto-occipital dislocation: case reports and literature review. *J Trauma*. 1991;31:401.
13. Mattox KL, Feliciano DV, Burch J, et al. Five thousand seven hundred sixty cardiovascular injuries in 4459 patients. *Ann Surg*. 1989;209:695.
14. Rubio PA, Reul GJ Jr, Beall AK Jr, et al. Acute carotid artery injury: 25 years experience. *J. Trauma* 1974;14:967.
15. Thal ER, Snyder WH, Haus RA, et al. Management of carotid artery injuries. *Surgery* 1974;76:955.

16. Unger SW, Tucker WS Jr, Merdeza MA, et al. Carotid artery trauma. *Surgery* 1980;87:477.
17. Ledgerwood AM, Mullins RJ, Lucas CE. Primary repair vs. ligation for carotid artery injuries. *Arch Surg* 1980;115:488.
18. Fry RE, Fry WJ. Extracranial carotid artery injuries. *Surgery* 1980;88:581–587.
19. Brown MF, Graham JM, Feliciano DV, et al. Carotid artery injuries. *Am J Surg* 1982;144:748–753.
20. Karlin RM, Marks C. Extracranial carotid artery injury: Current surgical management. *Am J Surg* 1983;146:225–227.
21. Demetriades D, Skalkides J, Sofianos C, et al. Carotid artery injuries: Experience with 124 cases. *J Trauma* 1989;29:91.
22. Fabian TC, George SM, Croce MA, et al. Carotid artery trauma: Management based on mechanism of injury. *J Trauma* 1990;30:953–963.
23. Sclafani SJA, Cavaliere G, Atweh N, et al. The role of angiography in penetrating neck trauma. *J Trauma* 1991;31:557.
24. Perry MO, Snyder WH, Thal ER. Carotid artery injuries caused by blunt trauma. *Ann Surg* 1980;192:74–77.
25. Zelenock GB, Kazmers, A, Whitehouse WM Jr, et al. Extracranial internal carotid artery dissection. *Arch Surg* 1982;117:425–432.
26. Mokvi B, Piepqras DG, Houser OW. Traumatic dissections of the extracranial internal carotid artery. *J Neurosurg* 1988;68:189–197.
27. Martin RF, Eldrup-Jorgensen J, Clark DE, Bredenberg CE. Blunt trauma to the carotid arteries. *J Vasc Surg* 1991;14:789–795.
28. Jernigan WR, Gardner WC. Carotid artery injuries due to closed cervical trauma. *J Trauma*. 1971;11:429.
29. Krajewski LP, Hertzer NR. Blunt carotid artery trauma. Report of two cases and review of the literature. *Ann Surg*. 1980;191:341.
30. Weaver FA, Wagner WH, Yellen AE, Cohen JL. Monocular blindness after penetrating trauma to the carotid artery. *J Vasc Surg*. 1989;10:89.
31. Ward RE, Flynn TC, Miller PW, Blaisdell FW. Effects of ethanol ingestion on the severity and outcome of trauma. *Am J Surg*. 1983;144:153.
32. Berguer R, Feldman J, Wilner HI, Lazo A. Arteriovenous vertebral fistulae. *Ann Surg*. 1982;196:65.
33. Meissner M, Paun M, Johansen K. Duplex scanning for arterial trauma. *Am J Surg*. 1991;161:552.
34. Fabian TC, George SM Jr, Croce MA, et al. Carotid artery trauma: management based on mechanism of injury. *J Trauma*. 1990;30:953.
35. Scalea TM, Sclafani SJA. Angiographically placed balloons for arterial control: a description of a technique. *J Trauma*. 1991;31:1671.
36. Richardson R, Obeid FN, Richardson JD, et al. Neurologic consequences of cerebrovascular injury. *J Trauma*. 1992;32:755.
37. Higashida RT, Halbach VV, Tsai FY, et al. Interventional neurovascular treatment of traumatic carotid and vertebral lesions: Results in 234 cases. *AJR* 1989;153:577–582.
38. Binkley FM, Wylie EJ. A new technique for obliteration of cerebrovascular arteriovenous fistulae. *Arch Surg*. 1973;106:525.
39. Ward RE, Hudson M, Flynn TC. Gram-negative infections of arterial injury. *Ann Surg*. 1978;188:581.
40. Beall AC Jr, Shirkey AL, DeBakey ME. Penetrating wounds of the carotid arteries. *J Trauma*. 1963;3:276.
41. Yamada S, Kindt GW, Youmans JRJ. Carotid artery occlusion due to nonpenetrating injury. *J Trauma*. 1967;7:333.
42. Towne JB. Thrombosis of the internal carotid artery following blunt trauma. *Arch Surg*. 1972;104:565.

19

Phrenic Nerve and Diaphragmatic Injuries

JOHN T. OWINGS, M.D.

HISTORY: Sennertus, in 1541, was the first to describe a diaphragmatic injury. He reported a patient who suffered a self-inflicted stab wound to the chest, with herniation of the stomach into the left chest. In 1580, Paré described herniation of abdominal contents through a penetrating diaphragmatic wound. Paré additionally classified the clinical progression of these injuries from asymptomatic, to vague symptoms, then on to obstruction and strangulation.[1] The first report of diaphragmatic injury in the American literature was by Bowditch in 1853.[2] In 1938, Harrington classified diaphragmatic hernias into traumatic and nontraumatic, noting that there was a tendency of blunt injuries to herniate through embryologic points of fusion.[3]

The incidence of injuries, both to the phrenic nerve and diaphragm, have progressively increased during this century. Blunt diaphragmatic rupture is indicative of the dissipation of a large amount of energy and the incidence has paralleled the rise in high-speed motor vehicle accidents. Plus, with improvement in prehospital care, patients with more serious injuries are surviving to reach the hospital.

Most phrenic nerve injuries probably are iatrogenic, produced by surgical dissection, placement of monitoring devices in central veins, or the result of myocardial cooling during cardiac surgery. Fortunately, injuries to the phrenic nerve are rare, as they can cause serious long-term disability. Phrenic nerve transections cause immediate ipsilateral diaphragmatic paralysis and, when the phrenic nerve is injured, atrophy or thinning of the diaphragm can occur. This may stretch the diaphragm further, resulting in herniation of abdominal contents upward into the ipsilateral chest as the atrophic diaphragm continues to thin and stretch (eventration).

The most treacherous aspect of the management of diaphragmatic injuries is their timely diagnosis. After blunt trauma, injuries often are a minor component of a devastating complex of injuries and may be missed while the more obvious immediate life-threatening injuries are dealt with. After penetrating trauma, the diaphragmatic laceration may be relatively occult and may even be missed if laparotomy is performed. In any case, with early diagnosis, treatment becomes relatively simple. If the diagnosis is missed, the potential for late morbidity and even mortality is quite high.

ANATOMY

The phrenic nerves arise from the fourth and fifth cervical nerve roots, with a few contributions from the third and, rarely, the second or sixth. The nerves run obliquely downward, superficial to the anterior scalene muscle and deep to the sternocleidomastoid and omohyoid muscles. The nerves then enter the thoracic cavity, passing posteriorly to the subclavian vein and anteriorly to the subclavian artery where they cross over the origin of the internal mammary artery. The nerves then are joined by the pericardiophrenic branches of the internal mammary artery and vein. The right phrenic nerve descends on the lateral aspect of the superior vena cava, and then continues down the lateral surface of the pericardium, where it gives off pain fibers to the pericardium (Fig. 19–1). The left phrenic nerve passes downward between the common carotid and left subclavian artery and then travels down the lateral aspect of the pericardium (Fig. 19–2).[4]

Both phrenic nerves travel extrapleurally anterior to the pulmonary hili on the pericardium. The nerves then course to the central tendon where they divide into three to five branches at the pericardiodiaphragmatic angle. The most posterior branch pierces the diaphragm immediately and runs posterior on the undersurface of the diaphragm to supply the crura. The other branches also penetrate the diaphragm and run on its undersurface to innervate both the diaphragm and its overlying peritoneum.

The function of the phrenic nerve is to supply motor, sensory, and some sympathetic innervation to the diaphragm. Motor supply to the diaphragm is required for normal

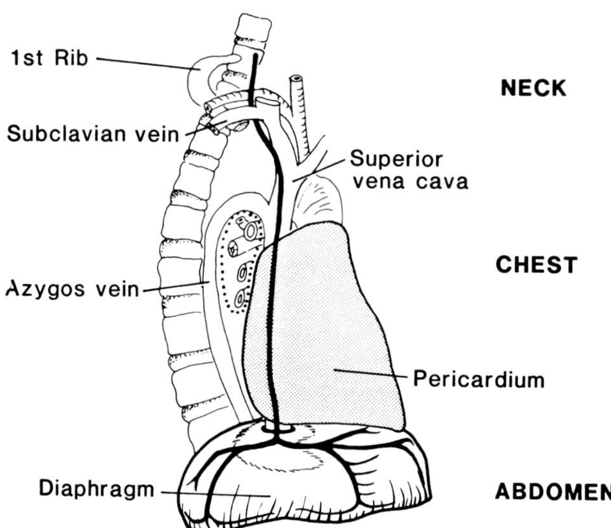

Figure 19–1. Right phrenic nerve course and diaphragm innervation.

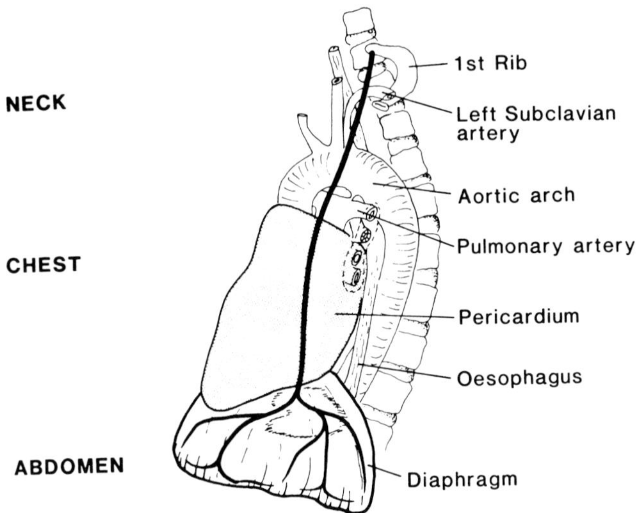

Figure 19–2. Left phrenic nerve course and diaphragm innervation.

respiration. This is true especially in children, where breathing is almost completely diaphragmatic. The sensory component derives pain fibers from the pericardium, mediastinum pleura, and peritoneum. Because of the origin of these nerves, the pain from these surfaces may be felt (referred) anywhere from the lower shoulder (C6) up to the tip of the ear (if C2 fibers are present).

The diaphragm is comprised of the central tendon and radially oriented muscle fibers connecting it to the chest wall. There are three openings in the diaphragm: the aortic, esophageal, and caval hiatuses. There are several structures that traverse the diaphragm via small discrete openings. The internal mammary artery, originating from the subclavian artery, becomes the superior epigastric artery as it passes through the anterior diaphragm just lateral to the xiphisternal articulation. The phrenic nerves cross the diaphragm in the central tendon, then run on its inferior aspect. The aortic hiatus is the most inferior and posterior hiatus and is separated from the vertebral bodies by only the prevertebral fascia. On either side of the aorta, the diaphragmatic crura originate inferiorly from L3 on the right and L2 on the left. Fibers of the crura cross as they pass anterior to the aorta. A portion of these fibers continue anteriorly to cross in front of the esophagus, thereby creating the more anterior superior esophageal hiatus. These two openings are in a direct anterior posterior plane. The aortic hiatus allows passage of the aorta, splanchnic nerves, and azygos vein. The esophageal hiatus contains the esophagus and vagus nerves. The caval hiatus allows passage of the inferior vena cava and, occasionally, branches of the phrenic nerves and vessels[4] (Fig. 19–3).

The diaphragm has three muscular portions arranged radially about the central tendons. These are the sternal, costal, and vertebral; their names are based on their origin. The location of origin and insertion are critically important when assessing the likelihood of thoracic versus abdominal penetrating injury. The vertebral origin, as noted above, is the lowest at roughly L3 (Fig. 19–4). Anteriorly the costal portion arises from the lower six ribs. The sternal portion is fixed at the xiphoid. The central portion of the diaphragm in the

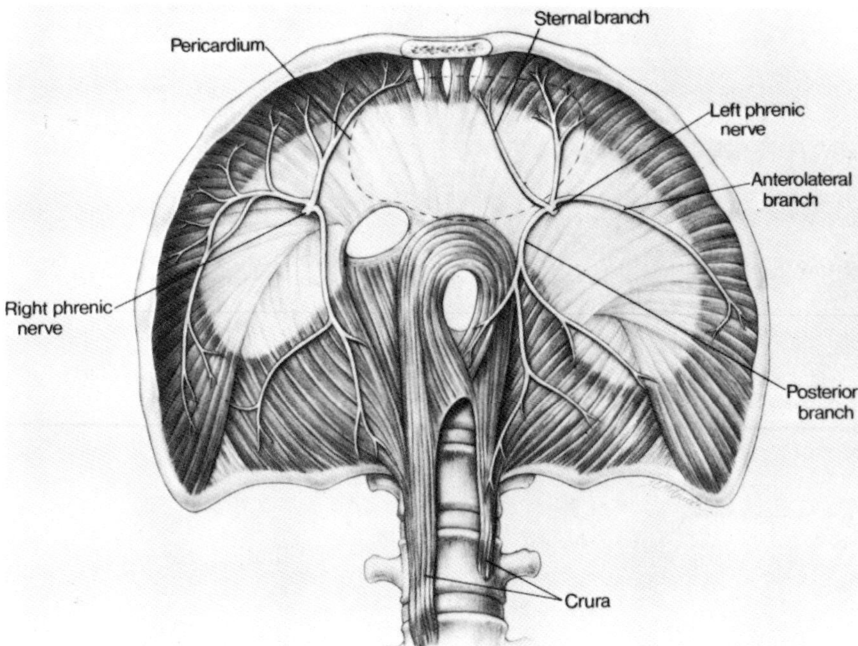

Figure 19–3. Anatomy of the under surface of the diaphragm. (Reprinted with permission from Van Trigt.[28])

relaxed state is dome-shaped, drawn upward by negative intrathoracic pressure. With active inspiration, muscular forces draw it taut and downward, resulting in respiratory exchange. At full expiration, the dome and therefore the border between the peritoneum and thorax may rise as high as the fifth interspace. This corresponds to roughly one interspace below the nipple.

MECHANISM OF INJURY

Injury to the *phrenic nerve* may occur as a result of thermal, blunt, or penetrating trauma (Table 19–1); in most cases, the etiology is iatrogenic. Thermal injury has drawn increasing attention during the past 15 years because the use of topical iced saline for myocardial protection has become routine in maintaining myocardial hypothermia during cardioplegic arrest. In one study, the incidence of roentgenographically documented phrenic nerve injury was from 18% to 32% when no insulating techniques were used.[5] Unless bilateral injury occurred, the morbidity usually was inconsequential; however, if a bilateral injury did occur, the morbidity was severe, although no increase in mortality was experienced.[6] Blunt trauma may result in stretch injury. Crush injury has been used historically in the treatment of tuberculosis and requires no specific treatment. In these cases, recovery of nerve function is the rule. When phrenic dysfunction occurs after blunt trauma, it should alert the clinician to the possibility of aortic or subclavian injury.

Penetrating injury to the phrenic nerve may occur anywhere along the course of the nerve. Of particular interest are case reports of iatrogenic phrenic nerve injury due to

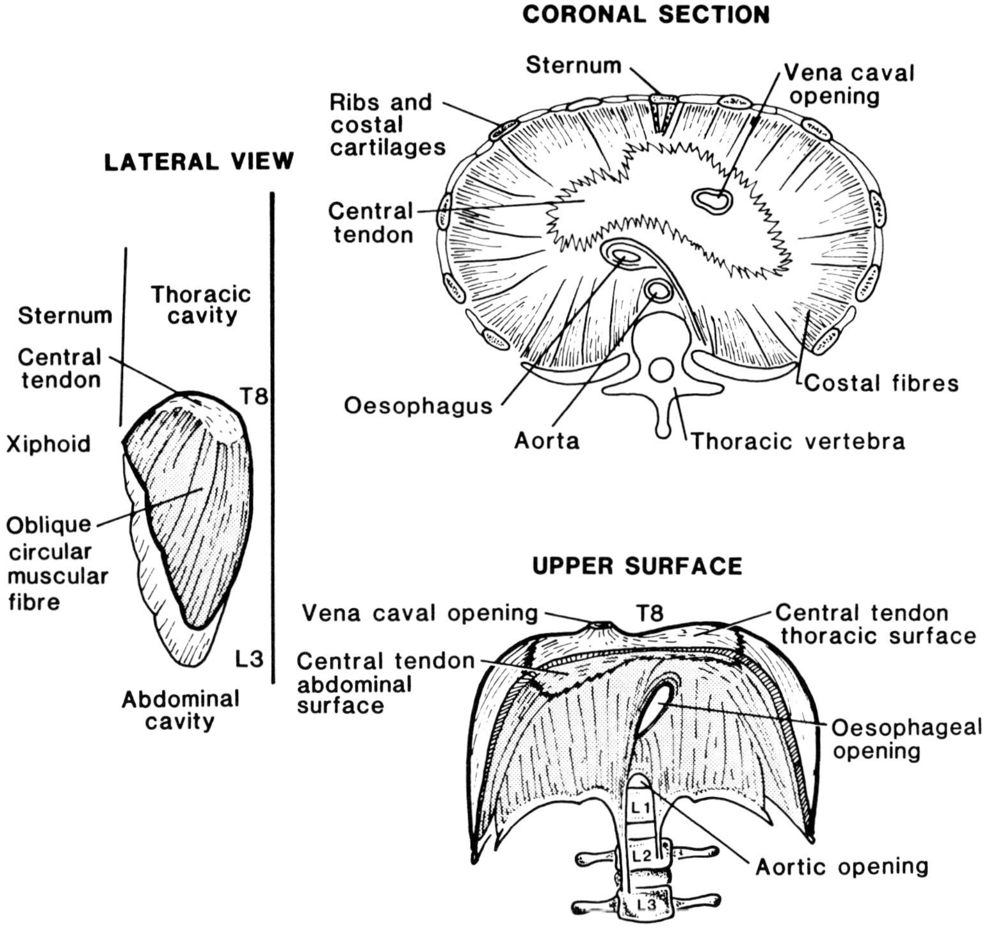

Figure 19–4.   Anatomy of the lateral and upper surface of the diaphragm.

attempts at internal jugular venous cannulation.[7] Use of central venous catheters has increased significantly during the past 10 to 20 years, and as indications for catheters have increased (TPN, monitoring of right heart pressures, and long-term venous access), the complications of their placement, which include phrenic nerve injury, have risen in parallel.

The types of injury to the *diaphragm* are quite different from those to the phrenic nerve. The basic mechanisms of injury are blunt and penetrating trauma. *Blunt trauma* usually results from a forceful blow to the abdomen or thorax that produces a bursting type of injury. This type of diaphragmatic injury is almost always associated with other severe injuries as a result of the high degree of force required to produce the diaphragmatic rupture.[8,9]

Kearney et al., in reviewing 30 patients with blunt diaphragmatic injury secondary to motor vehicle accidents, reported that victims of side impact collisions were three times more likely to suffer diaphragmatic rupture than victims of frontal impact. Further, they found that a frontal impact with a severe thoracic blow resulted in a downward burst type of

Table 19–1. Mechanism of Phrenic Nerve Injuries

Thermal
   Topical iced solutions
Blunt
   Stretch
      Accident (cervical)
      At pericardiotomy (thoracic)
   Crush
      Intentional (therapeutic)
      Inadvertent
Penetrating
   Iatrogenic (cervical, thoracic)
   Stab
   Missile

injury. Lateral and side impact resulted in abdominal compression with upward burst. All of these tears tended to occur at weak points in the diaphragm, which consist primarily of the embryological points of attachment, especially at the costosternal region or paravertebral region.

Penetrating trauma such as a stab or gunshot injury results in a laceration at the point of injury. Blunt trauma also may result in penetrating injury to the diaphragm from a fractured rib. Each of these may be initially small and asymptomatic; however, with time they tend to enlarge and have all the potential hazards of larger diaphragmatic hernias.

INCIDENCE

The true incidence of *phrenic nerve injuries* is difficult to assess because the adult patient with unilateral nerve injury is rarely symptomatic and most injuries probably are not recognized. There is a wide range of reported incidences after cardiac surgery in which local hypothermia is used; the incidence of injuries, based on prospective studies, is between 20% and 40%.[5,6] Phrenic nerve injury after penetrating trauma is rare due to the relatively small amount of space the nerve occupies. Although the true incidence is low, prospective studies are not available, nor are they practical to pursue. Stretch injuries to the phrenic nerve also are quite rare, and the true incidence equally undocumentable.[10]

Blunt diaphragmatic injuries are somewhat easier to track because they tend to be larger and, therefore, more evident, more often symptomatic, and easier to identify at operation. Patients with these injuries usually are critically ill and, if the diaphragmatic injury is not found at operation, it may be identified at post mortem after death from associated injuries. Beal and McKennan[9] reported on 1280 seriously injured, blunt trauma victims admitted to our trauma service. There were 39 patients with ruptured diaphragms, for an incidence of 3%. Other authors have reported an incidence of between 0.08% and 3%.[8,11] There is a strong predilection for injury to the left hemidiaphragm, with roughly a two-thirds to one-third left-to-right ratio. This is likely due to the dispersion of force by the dome of the liver on the right. Bilateral injuries occur in approximately 2% to 3% of blunt diaphragmatic ruptures.

Penetrating diaphragmatic injury, in contrast, often is the patient's only significant injury. As the management of abdominal stab wounds has shifted toward observation and indirect assessment of possible internal injury, these lesions frequently are missed until complications occur. This is because neither peritoneal lavage nor computed tomography (CT) scanning will pick up a small lesion. Diaphragmatic laceration represents an injury that may be asymptomatic for an extended period but, months or years later, present with complications.[12] Of all penetrating abdominal injuries, diaphragmatic injuries constitute roughly 6%.[13]

With penetrating trauma, especially stab wounds, the likelihood of diaphragmatic injury is related to the area of entry wound. Given a zone of proximity, Madden et al. found the incidence of diaphragmatic injury with thoracoabdominal stab wounds to be 19%[14]; Mariadason et al. found the incidence to be 11%.[12] As with blunt trauma, the left diaphragm is involved more often than the right. It has been theorized that this is because most assailants are right-handed and they attack face to face.

DIAGNOSIS

As noted in the introductory comments, the manifestations of both phrenic nerve and diaphragmatic injuries may be quite subtle. The *phrenic nerve* may be injured in a number of ways. The diagnosis of injury or dysfunction may be obvious if transection is found during a neck exploration or exploratory thoracotomy or if the patient has a high quadriplegia with respiratory distress. The diagnosis may be quite subtle as in a stretch injury resulting from a flexion extension injury of the neck. The possibility of, and hence diagnosis of, phrenic nerve injury may never even occur to the treating surgeons. Because of this, it is important that the trauma surgeon be sensitive in all cases to the possibility of phrenic nerve injury.

Most patients will be asymptomatic initially, as unilateral paralysis of the diaphragm is relatively well tolerated. Signs and symptoms range from an asymptomatic patient with elevated hemidiaphragm on x-ray to the inability to wean a patient from the ventilator. When a bilateral injury is present, the patient usually is symptomatic with dyspnea, chest pain, or hypercarbia. When associated with quadriplegia, the phrenic nerve injury usually represents an incomplete lesion that results in diaphragm weakness. Patients with quadriplegia and complete bilateral phrenic nerve loss are unable to breathe and rarely survive the acute accident.

Patient manifestations are primarily those of shortness of breath due to diaphragmatic paralysis. On chest x-ray, there may be an elevated hemidiaphragm. If inspiratory and expiratory films are taken, the diaphragm will move very little with respiration on the affected side. If the patient has required intubation with positive pressure ventilation, the hemidiaphragm will not be elevated. These patients may first show signs of dysfunction when there is difficulty weaning them from the ventilator. They may have a persistent lobar collapse on the side of injury.

There have been several tests used to document phrenic nerve dysfunction. The most sensitive and specific is the measurement of phrenic nerve conduction time (phrenic latency).[15,16] With this method, an electrical stimulus is applied to the phrenic nerve in the neck. Diaphragmatic electromyographic signals are then measured with abdominal surface electrodes. Absent or delayed activity is indicative of phrenic nerve injury. X-ray studies, such as the Sniff test, use fluoroscopy to watch the diaphragm as the patient is asked to sniff. The paralyzed hemidiaphragm will show paradoxical motion, up on inspiration and down on expiration. Although this is quicker and easier to document with fluoroscopy, plain radiography usually will suffice. These latter methods have the disadvantage of requiring patient cooperation and being unsuitable for the patient on positive pressure ventilation.

In cases of blunt trauma or high velocity penetrating *diaphragm trauma,* the associated injuries may provide sufficient distraction to result in diaphragmatic injuries going unnoticed, even at operation, where they are easily missed unless specifically sought.[10] Passing an examining hand along the undersurface of the diaphragm at laparotomy is not sufficient. The diaphragm must be inspected visually if these injuries are to be ruled out. With stab wounds, there may be no other injuries, and these penetrating lesions may be asymptomatic for months or years if an operation is not performed.[14,17]

Because the mechanism of blunt and *penetrating* diaphragmatic injuries is so different, their presentations are quite different. Most patients with diaphragmatic stab wounds are asymptomatic. The most suggestive sign of diaphragmatic laceration is proximity of the entry wound to the diaphragm. Both Mariadason et al. and Madden et al. defined specific anatomical zones with graded probability of diaphragmatic injury.[12,14] This somewhat intuitive approach does prove to be statistically valid. The area of concern is anteriorly below the fourth intercostal space, laterally below the sixth, and posteriorly below the eighth. Those patients who are symptomatic may manifest a number of signs and symptoms, as shown in Table 19–2. Although the symptoms of diaphragmatic laceration due to gunshot or knife are similar, the proximity of the entry wound as a predictor of injury is not. Diaphragmatic injury may be present in the gunshot victim regardless of location of bullet entry. Demetriapes found ". . . no correlation . . . between site of entrance and presence of diaphragmatic injury."[18]

As previously emphasized, *blunt trauma* victims with diaphragmatic rupture tend to be severely injured. One study reported that 75% of patients with blunt diaphragmatic rupture had some other intraabdominal injury that required correction. Beal and McKennan reported that 37 patients with blunt diaphragmatic rupture had a total of 179 associated injuries (Table 19–3), and only 1 patient had an isolated diaphragmatic rupture.[9] The average injury severity score was 34. These patients usually manifest a number of signs and symptoms all related to the underlying associated injuries.

A multitude of *diagnostic tests* have been recommended for the assessment of diaphragmatic injuries (Table 19–4). Most trauma patients undergo routine *chest radio-*

Table 19–2.   Signs and Symptoms of Diaphragmatic Injury

None (asymptomatic)
Proximity of stab wound
Shoulder or ear pain
Pleuritic chest pain or rib pain
Tachypnea, tachycardia
Dyspnea
Acute abdomen
Continued bleeding from chest or
    drainage of bile, enteric con-
    tents, or urine from a chest tube

Table 19–3. Associated Injuries in 37 Patients with Blunt Diaphragmatic Rupture[9]

INJURY	NO. OF INJURIES
Head	24
Rib fracture	18
Pulmonary contusion	18
Spleen	18
Liver	18
Hemothorax	16
Pelvic fracture	14
Renal contusion	10
Hollow viscus	7
Lung laceration	6
Tibia-fibula fracture	6
Femur fracture	5
Pneumothorax	5
Humerus fracture	3
Cervical spine fracture	2
Bladder rupture	2
Myocardial contusion	2
Lumbar spine fracture	1
Pancreas	1
Shoulder dislocation	1
Clavicle fracture	1
Aortic laceration	1

graph on admission because it is inexpensive, easy to obtain, and has high yield as a screening test for thoracic injury. The chest x-ray should serve only to facilitate the diagnosis of diaphragmatic rupture and never be used to rule out the lesion. This is because of the high rate of false negative studies. After penetrating injury, diagnostic radiologic evidence of diaphragmatic injury is rare: the chest x-ray is normal in roughly one-third of cases, shows nonspecific changes in nearly two-thirds, and is diagnostic in less than 5%.[19,20] With blunt injuries, the chest x-ray is rarely normal; however, it is diagnostic in only one-third to two-thirds of cases. Findings that should alert the trauma surgeon to the possibility of diaphragmatic injury are hemothorax, elevated hemidiaphragm, eventration of diaphragm, blunted costophrenic angle, abnormal gas pattern, a clear outline of hollow

Table 19–4. Diagnostic Studies for Diaphragmatic Injury

Chest x-ray
Computerized tomography
Magnetic resonance imaging
Diagnostic peritoneal lavage
Thoracoscopy, laparoscopy
Contrast GI study
Pneumo, contrast peritoneography
Exploratory laparotomy

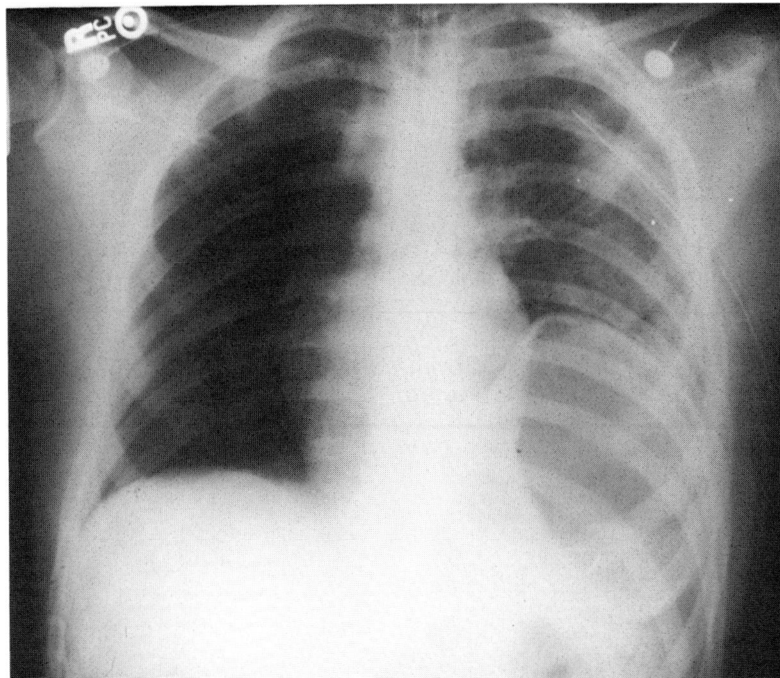

Figure 19–5.   Chest radiograph showing blunt diaphragmatic rupture. Note gastric bubble with the nasogastric tube displaced into the left hemothorax.

viscus in hemithorax, or an abnormally located nasogastric tube (Fig. 19–5).[17] If an abdominal organ has herniated through the defect, then the radiologic diagnosis will be relatively easy. More often, this is not the case, but the hydrostatic forces, negative in the chest and positive in the abdomen, tend to result in blood or fluid from an injured abdominal organ flowing through the defect into the chest. This causes blunting of the costophrenic angle and leads to a nonspecific abnormality in chest x-ray.

Computerized tomographic (CT) scanning is becoming an increasingly prominent part in the diagnostic work-up of the trauma patient. As a result, there has been debate regarding the best screening modality for blunt abdominal trauma, CT scan, or lavage.[21] Unfortunately, CT scans rarely identify a specific diaphragmatic injury.[19] The CT is of value in its ability to pick up the patients with associated intraabdominal injury (75%) and thus direct the treatment to laparotomy. The cost of obtaining this information in the acutely injured patient is their removal from an area where they are well monitored, with immediate access to critical care personnel, and placement in relative isolation, frequently with suboptimal monitoring.

Magnetic resonance imaging (MRI) has been used recently in selected cases to identify diaphragmatic defects.[22] Even though this does give a superior image of the soft tissue, there are a number of drawbacks. MRI requires an extended period of patient isolation. Also, the imaging systems in many centers are incompatible with ventilators and many monitoring devices. Because a large percent of those patients with diaphragmatic injury will have severe, even life-threatening associated injuries, the compromises needed to get the study usually are not warranted. As scanning times decrease and ability to monitor and support patients undergoing this type of exam improve, the role of MRI likely will expand.

Peritoneal lavage is used frequently at our institution for screening in blunt trauma and others have recommended its use in penetrating trauma.[23] Even though 100,000 red blood cells per cubic millimeter is generally accepted as a positive lavage in blunt trauma, there is no such consensus with penetrating trauma. Thal[23] has recommended using 100,000 RBC per mm^3; Oreskovich and Carrico[24] have recommended 1000 RBC/mm^3. This is a published disagreement of 100-fold, and there are proponents for numbers in between. In all of these studies, even when the lowest threshold is used, lavage is insensitive for diaphragmatic injury. Peritoneal lavage poses a unique and interesting diagnostic problem in patients with diaphragmatic injury such that lavage is more often negative when there has been abdominal organ injury and diaphragm injury than when there has been abdominal injury alone. The most commonly injured organs, and those most often identified by peritoneal lavage after blunt trauma, are the liver and spleen. These are identified by quantifying red blood cells in the peritoneal cavity. If a simultaneous diaphragmatic defect exists, then the flow of liver or splenic hemorrhage will be into the chest (due to the pull of negative intrathoracic pressures), leaving the abdomen relatively dry. Despite significant bleeding, the lavage fluid, placed in the pelvis, may return with few red cells. Alternatively, the lavagate may be pulled up into the thoracic cavity, causing little lavage fluid to be returned. When the latter occurs, the lavage should be considered positive. Freeman and Fisher found a 29% false negative peritoneal lavage rate in blunt diaphragmatic injury when using 100,000 RBC/mm.[25] Further, they had 100% false negative rate in those cases where the diaphragm was an isolated abdominal injury. Without diaphragmatic injury, the expected false negative rate of peritoneal lavage in blunt trauma is less than 2%.[13] This illustrates why the diaphragmatic disruption is difficult to diagnose by peritoneal lavage and also may mask other potentially lethal injuries.

Recently, there has been increased interest in *thoracoscopic* and *laparoscopic* evaluation. Both of these methods will likely be very sensitive and specific for diaphragmatic disruption. These techniques, however, present at least two major drawbacks as diagnostic tools. First, they both require a general anesthetic, which is a high price to pay for diagnosis alone. This will become less of a deterrent as endoscopic suturing techniques improve and these become not only diagnostic but therapeutic procedures. The second drawback relates to the issue of the safety of positive pressure pneumoperitoneum in the trauma patient. In cases of major hepatic or hepatovenous injury (found in 35–45% of diaphragmatic injuries),[8,25] there is potential for CO_2 embolism. Patients with hypovolemic shock will have decreased venous return and may deteriorate rapidly as the peritoneum is insufflated. Further studies of the safety of these techniques are needed. Once these issues are resolved and as endoscopic suturing continues to be refined, this modality will hold promise for future diagnostic and therapeutic intervention.

Several radiologic and nuclear medicine tests have been used. These include contrast gastrointestinal (GI) studies, contrast and pneumoperitoneography, and radiolabeled peritoneography. Contrast GI studies are sensitive only if herniation of a hollow viscus into the thorax has already occurred. Conversely, all of the studies that place a substance (CO_2, contrast material, or a labeled substance) in the peritoneal cavity and look for passage into the chest will be unreliable if herniation has occurred. This is because the herniated organ frequently will occlude the diaphragmatic defect, thus not allowing passage of the study fluid into the chest.

The gold standard for diagnosis and treatment of diaphragmatic injury is *exploratory laparotomy*. This method is by no means infallible, however, and depends on its proper use. When palpation alone is used to make the diagnosis, a significant number of injuries will be missed.[17] This occurred in Feliciano et al.'s experience and accounted for one-third of missed diaphragm injuries.[17] For this reason, we and others feel that exploratory laparotomy should be used liberally with penetrating injuries that raise the suspicion of diaphragmatic injury. At exploration, palpation alone is unacceptable; the visual inspection of both hemidiaphragms is needed to adequately rule out injury.

TREATMENT

Treatment of *phrenic nerve injuries* clearly depends on the mechanism of injury. Most blunt traumatic injuries to the phrenic nerve are the result of stretch or contusion. If the nerve is grossly intact, most of these patients will experience full, or near full, return of phrenic nerve function and, therefore, diaphragmatic function. An historical illustration of this is the use of phrenic nerve crush in tuberculosis; most of such patients had return of function within 6 months.[10] If complete transection of the phrenic nerve has occurred, it is unlikely that return of function will occur without intervention. Merav et al.[26] described the successful repair of a phrenic nerve transection occurring during a pericardiotomy for a cardiac stab wound. In this case, a graft of a sural nerve was used to perform a microscopic, fascicle-to-fascicle repair. This led to radiographic return of diaphragmatic function. Although other authors have not all experienced full success, if complete transection is identified, direct repair is worth attempting.

Fortunately, most adults with unilateral diaphragmatic paralysis will tolerate the lesion well. Adults with coexisting pulmonary disease and young children clearly do not tolerate these injuries as well. This prompted Shoemaker et al. to recommend early diaphragmatic plication in children with diaphragmatic paralysis.[27] If complete disruption of the nerve is not suspected, that is, return of function is eventually expected, most would advocate expectant management. Should this result in continued disability at 4 to 6 months, diaphragmatic plication may be in order. Patients with a high quadriplegia have diaphragmatic dysfunction due to a cord lesion and have an intact lower motor neuron (phrenic nerve). The chance for return of their function is nil, and almost all cases have bilateral diaphragm paralysis. Additionally, these patients have lost most of the associated muscles of respiration. With all these factors combined, many of these patients, even with plication, are permanently ventilator dependent.

Diaphragmatic pacing was originally described more than 200 years ago when an electrical stimulus was applied to the phrenic nerve of a criminal who had been recently hung. Respiratory movements were observed to resemble those of the premorbid state. This method has shown some promise during the past decade for providing long-term phrenic nerve stimulation that maintains diaphragm function. With the present technique, an electrode is placed around the phrenic nerve and connected to a receiver. The pacing signal is generated from an external transmitter. Once the diaphragm has been conditioned with one system on each nerve, each side is stimulated alternately for 12 hr, then rested 12 hr.[28] This system has been used with long-term success in some centers, rendering the patient ventilator independent. Unfortunately, this technique is not acceptable for all patients. Patients must have normal anterior horn cells and intact phrenic nerves that respond to electrical stimulation. Those with anterior horn cell disease or phrenic nerve transection cannot be paced electrically. Also, these patients must have permanent tracheostomies, 24-hr availability of ventilatory support with apnea alarm, and strong family support.[29]

In cases where the diaphragm has lost its innervation and pacing is not possible, gradual wasting of the muscle will occur. This progresses to eventration, which may compromise the patient's ability to ventilate as the abdominal contents are gradually displaced upward. This also may lead to recurrent lobar collapse and pneumonias. In these cases, diaphragmatic plication can be performed with good success. The object of this operation is to return the diaphragm and, thereby, the abdominal contents to a more normal position allowing the associated respiratory muscles to function more effectively.

An accepted technique for diaphragmatic plication is shown in Figure 19–6A. The diaphragm is approached through the chest, and a thinned hemidiaphragm leaf is incised in a curvilinear fashion. Then, using a pants-over-vest technique with 0 or 00 nonabsorbable suture, the leaf is doubled over on itself. This tightens the hemidiaphragm and drops its height of maximal excision.[30]

Diaphragmatic injuries usually are relatively simple to repair. As noted in the previous section, recognizing them is the primary challenge. If a diaphragmatic injury is found by diagnostic studies before laparotomy, it is best approached with a vertical, midline abdominal incision. This approach gives excellent exposure to the injured hemidiaphragm, it allows for visual examination of the contralateral side, and it allows for diagnosis and repair of any associated intraabdominal injuries. If there are combined thoracic and abdominal injuries requiring surgical intervention, separate incisions will reduce morbidity.

Regardless of the mechanism, blunt or penetrating, any defect, even if quite small, should be repaired. Small defects, like small inguinal hernias, may incarcerate and occasionally strangulate a loop of bowel. After reduction of any displaced abdominal viscus, which is most easily accomplished transabdominally, the edges of the defect are exposed. Defects are closed with 0 or 00 nonabsorbable or P.D.S. suture in an interrupted fashion. If exposure is difficult, the first suture is placed most posteriorly, then is used to elevate the diaphragm to facilitate exposure and the next stitch. When the injury is in the muscular portion of the diaphragm, simple sutures may tend to pull through, so an interrupted horizontal mattress suture is optimal, with an associated simple running or interrupted suture used as needed for hemostasis (Fig. 19–6B). If the injury is directly adjacent to a rib, then the suture should be placed in a figure-eight style, with one loop about the rib and the other through the diaphragm.[31] When the wound is secondary to a knife injury and there are no signs of intrathoracic injury, the diaphragm may be repaired without placement of a chest tube. Before placement of the final stitch, a red Robinson Catheter is passed through the defect into the hemithorax. A "U" stitch is placed about the catheter and then suction is applied to evacuate any blood, fluid, or air. The "U" stitch is then snugged down and tied as the catheter is removed. This technique must be checked with a postoperative chest x-ray to ensure that reaccumulation of a hemo- or pneumothorax does not occur. In cases of blunt diaphragmatic rupture or where there has been bleeding or possible thoracic contamination, a large-bore (36F) chest tube should be placed.

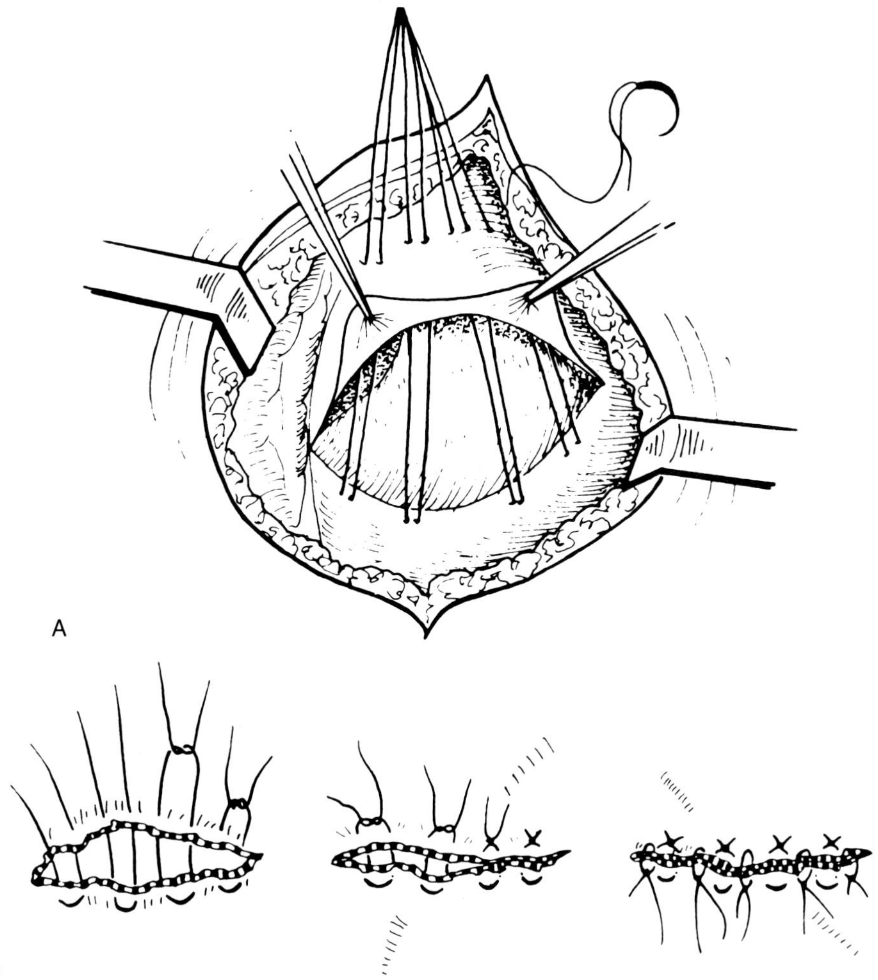

Figure 19–6.   **A:** Repair of eventration of the diaphragm. **B:** Repair of diaphragmatic laceration.

POSTOPERATIVE MANAGEMENT

The postoperative management of most phrenic nerve injuries is supportive. If ventilatory support is required to maintain adequate pulmonary function and expansion, then this is provided as needed. When a direct nerve repair has been performed, regeneration will occur at roughly 1 mm per day, although, as previously noted, most unilateral phrenic nerve injuries will not require ventilatory support. Those patients in whom diaphragmatic pacing has been employed will require 4 to 6 months of hospitalization with rigorous diaphragmatic training to allow for ventilator-independent living. The scope of this training is beyond this chapter but is well described in a number of references.[28,29]

Those injuries associated with diaphragmatic injury usually dictate the postoperative course. As previously mentioned, with penetrating trauma, the diaphragmatic injury may be an isolated injury; therefore, once the patient has recovered from the immediate surgical procedure, discharge is expected. Patients with blunt diaphragmatic trauma, however, have associated injuries and often need longer hospitalization.

Postoperatively, for both phrenic nerve and diaphragmatic injuries, it is important to follow serial chest x-rays in order to follow pulmonary aeration. If the patient is not on positive pressure ventilation, then it is critical that he/she be mobilized early and encouraged to cough and breathe deeply. All patients should be instructed on the use of the incentive spirometer.

COMPLICATIONS AND RESULTS

Complications of *phrenic nerve injury* pertain to ventilation inadequacy, atelectasis, and pneumonia. These conditions may result in prolonged or recurrent ventilator dependency (Table 19–5).[9]

There are no large series documenting primary phrenic nerve repair, but the early complications are those mentioned above. Primary concern clearly relates to failure of nerve regeneration and the presence or absence of ventilatory insufficiency. Phrenic nerve pacing has several potential complications. Complete failure to respond, implying primary phrenic nerve dysfunction, occurs 10% to 30% of the time. Late failure of the pacing device has occurred and has caused the proponents of this method to require that the patients receive constant availability of positive pressure ventilation and apnea monitoring. As methods for pacing have become more refined, the incidence of phrenic nerve burnout has decreased and long-term successes are more common.

If a patient suffers an isolated *diaphragmatic injury* and the diagnosis is made promptly and treatment carried out, the results are uniformly good. This scenario, however, is rare with blunt trauma. As has been described earlier, the most difficult aspect of these cases is the diagnosis. When diaphragmatic injury is missed, a diaphragmatic hernia results. The most commonly herniated organs are stomach, colon, spleen, small bowel, liver, kidney, and omentum, in descending order of frequency. Reports on the morbidity and mortality of missed diaphragmatic injuries vary. Madden et al. reported a mortality

Table 19–5. Complications in 37 Patients with Blunt Diaphragmatic Rupture[9]

COMPLICATIONS	NO. (%) OF COMPLICATIONS
Lobar collapse requiring bronchoscopy	15 (68)
Pleural effusion	5 (23)
Pneumonia	4 (18)
Sepsis	3 (14)
Small bowel obstruction	1
Wound infection	2
Traumatic vocal cord granulations	1
Intraabdominal abscess	1
Rectus muscle necrosis	1
Flank abscess	1
Urinary tract infection	1
Pleural peel	1

mortality of 36% when these hernias were missed and led to incarceration.[14] Complications that occur even with immediate repair include pulmonary lobar collapse in 68%, atelectasis in 23%, and pneumonia in 18%. Table 19–5 shows complications of 37 patients with blunt diaphragmatic rupture.[9] As noted above, such patients generally have outcomes reflective of their associated injuries.

The key to the successful outcome of the injuries discussed in this chapter is an aggressive approach. Operative intervention is the cornerstone of this approach. Operation provides the best means of diagnosing and the only means of repairing diaphragmatic injuries or phrenic transections. With an early, aggressive, operative approach, the morbidity and mortality caused by these injuries will be minimal.

REFERENCES

1. Paré A. *Oeuvres completes.* vol. 2. Malaigne JF, ed. Paris: Bailliere; 1840:94–100.
2. Bowditch HI. Diaphragmatic hernia. *Buffalo Med J.* 1853;9:1–39, 65–94.
3. Harrington SW. Clinical and roentgenological manifestations and surgical treatment of diaphragmatic hernia. *Radiology.* 1938;30:147.
4. Gardner E, Gray DS, O'Rahilly R. *Anatomy: A Regional Study of Human Structure.* Philadelphia: Saunders; 1975.
5. Efthimiou J, Butler J, Woodham C, et al. Diaphragm paralysis following cardiac surgery: role of phrenic nerve cold injury. *Ann Thorac Surg.* 1991;52:1005–1008.
6. Laub GW, Muralidharan S, Chen C, et al. Phrenic nerve injury: a prospective study. *Chest.* 1991;100:376–379.
7. Hadeed HA, Braun TW. Paralysis of hemidiaphragm as a complication of internal jugular vein cannulation: report of a case. *Am Assoc Oral Maxillofac Surg.* 1988;46:409–411.
8. Kearney PA, Rouhana SW, Burney RE. Blunt rupture of the diaphragm mechanism, diagnosis and treatment. *Ann Emerg Med.* 1989;18:1326–1330.
9. Beal SL, McKennan M. Blunt diaphragm rupture: a morbid injury. *Arch Surg.* 1988;123:828–832.
10. Iverson LIG, Mittal A, Dugan DJ, Samson PC. Injuries to the phrenic nerve resulting in diaphragmatic paralysis with special reference to stretch trauma. *Am J Surg.* 1976;132:263.
11. Brearly S, Tubbs N. Rupture of the diaphragm in blunt injuries of the trunk. *Injury.* 1980;12:480.
12. Mariadason JG, Parsa MH, Ayuyao A, Freeman HP. Management of stab wounds to the thoracoabdominal region. *Ann Surg.* 1988;207:335–340.
13. Blaisdell FW, Trunkey DD. *Abdominal Trauma.* New York: Thieme-Stratton; 1982.
14. Madden MR, Paull DE, Finkelstein JL, et al. Occult diaphragmatic injury from stab wounds to the lower chest and abdomen. *J Trauma.* 1989;29:292–298.
15. Russell RIJ, Mulvey D, Laroche C, et al. Bedside assessment of phrenic nerve function in infants and children. *J Thorac Cardiovasc Surg.* 1991;101:143–147.
16. Markland ON, Kincaid JC, Pourmand RA, et al. Electrophysiologic evaluation of diaphragm by transcutaneous phrenic nerve stimulation. *Neurology.* 1984;34:604–614.
17. Feliciano DV, Cruse PA, Mattox KL, et al. Delayed diagnosis of injuries to the diaphragm after penetrating wounds. *J Trauma.* 1988;28:1135–1144.
18. Demetriades D, Kakoyiannis S, Parekh D, Hatzitheofilou C. Penetrating injuries of the diaphragm. *Br J Surg.* 1988;75:824–826.
19. Chen JC, Wilson SE. Diaphragmatic injuries: recognition and management in sixty-two patients. *Am Surg.* 1991;57:810–815.
20. Wise L, Connors J, Hwang YH, et al. Traumatic injuries to the diaphragm. *J Trauma.* 1973;13:946–950.
21. Kearney PA, Vahey T, Burney RE, Glazer G. Computed tomography and diagnostic peritoneal lavage in blunt trauma. *Arch Surg.* 1989;124:334–337.
22. Boulanger BR, Mirvis SE, Rodriguez A. Magnetic resonance imaging in traumatic diaphragmatic rupture: case reports. *J Trauma.* 1992;32:89–93.
23. Thal ER. Peritoneal lavage: reliability of RBC count in patients with stab wounds to the chest. *Arch Surg.* 1984;119:579–584.
24. Oreskovich MR, Carrico J. Stab wounds to the anterior abdomen: analysis of a management plan using local wound exploration and quantitative peritoneal lavage. *Ann Surg.* 1983;198:411–419.
25. Freeman T, Fisher RP. Inadequacy of peritoneal lavage in diagnosing acute diaphragmatic rupture. *J Trauma.* 1976;16:538–542.

26. Merav AD, Attai LA, Condit DD. Successful repair of a transected phrenic nerve with restoration of diaphragmatic function. *Chest*. 1983;84:642–644.
27. Shoemaker R, Palmer G, Brown JW, King H. Aggressive treatment of acquired phrenic nerve paralysis in infants and small children. *Ann Thorac Surg*. 1982;32:251.
28. Van Trigt P. Diaphragm and diaphragmatic pacing. In: Sabiston DC, Spencer FC, eds. *Surgery of the Chest*. Philadelphia: Saunders; 1990:957–973.
29. Miller JI, Farmer JA, et al. Phrenic nerve pacing of the quadriplegic patient. *Thorac Cardiovasc Surg*. 1990;99:35–40.
30. Shields TW. The diaphragm. In: *General Thoracic Surgery*. Philadelphia: Lea and Febiger; 1989:572–573.
31. Ward RE. Repair of diaphragmatic injury. In: Champion HR, Robbs JV, Trunkey DD, eds. *Operative Surgery*. 4th ed, pt 1. *Trauma Surgery*. Boston: Butterworths; 1989:449–451.

20

Thoracic Duct Injury

MARC POLLOCK, M.D.

> *HISTORY: The thoracic duct was involved in an aura of mystery for some time. It was felt that thoracic duct drainage was essential for life because the sequelae of injury, namely empyema or chyle fistula, led to cachexia and death.[1,2]*
>
> *Thoracic duct surgery began and was made possible by a detailed account of its anatomy described by Mascagni in 1787.[3] Until Lampson's report in 1948, it was believed that thoracic duct continuity was necessary for survival.[1,4] In the decade that followed, this was disproved by successful treatment of ductal fistulae after both medical and surgical management.[5,6]*

EMBRYOLOGY AND ANATOMY

In 1916, Sabin demonstrated that the original lymph sacs arose from the endothelium of the adjacent veins.[7] Six original lymph spaces were recognized. These consisted of paired jugular sacs, paired iliac sacs, a single retroperitoneal sac, and a sac that later became known as the cisterna chyli.

Enlargement and fusion of small vessels that communicate between the sacs leads to the formation of two distinct symmetric ducts with multiple anastomoses between them. With maturation, the upper third of the right duct and the lower two-thirds of the left duct are obliterated, but the main communication between them persists, giving the configuration of the adult thoracic duct[8] (Fig. 20–1). However, variations in this anatomic structure occur in more than 50% of patients.[3]

The thoracic duct arises from the cisterna chyli, which overlies the anterior surface of the first or second lumbar vertebra and lies posterior and to the right of the aorta. The cisterna chyli continues upward as the thoracic duct. The duct then ascends through the aortic hiatus on the anterior surface of the vertebral bodies between the aorta and azygous vein, usually anterior to the right intercostal branches of the aorta. Injury in this lower region generally results in right chylothorax. Between the seventh and fifth thoracic vertebra, the thoracic duct crosses to the left and ascends behind the arch of the aorta and subclavian artery into the base of the neck, where it empties at or near the junction of the left subclavian and left internal jugular veins.[9–11] Injury to the thoracic duct above the fifth thoracic vertebra will most frequently cause a left chylothorax.

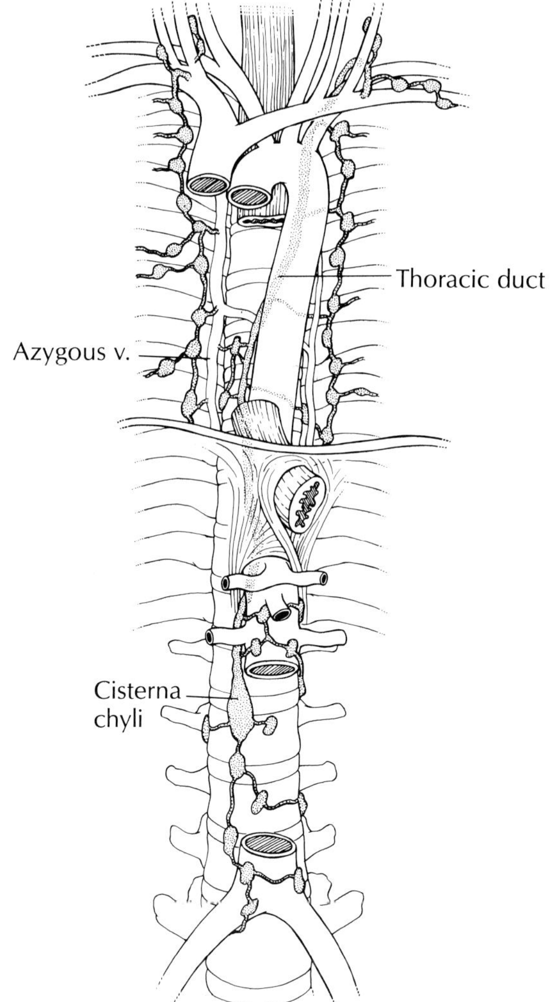

Figure 20–1.   Anatomy of the thoracic duct. The thoracic duct takes origin at the cysterna chyli, which overlies the first and second thoracic vertebrae, and extends upward through the chest to enter the left subclavian vein just proximal to the jugular vein.

PHYSIOLOGY

The word *chyle* literally means "juice." Chyle is typically thought of as a milky, alkaline exudate containing 0.4 to 3 g/dl of fat.[11] Staats et al. found less than 50% of chylous effusions to be milky in appearance.[12] Particularly in blunt chest trauma, the initial appearance of chyle is often sanguinous and low in fat content as a result of fasting. The same report found a triglyceride value of more than 110 mg % in the pleural fluid was associated with a chylous effusion in more than 99% of cases. If the value for the triglyceride level in the effusion is less than 50 mg %, there is no more than a 5% chance of it being chylous.[12] Fat droplets are characteristically red when stained with sudan III dye,

Table 20–1. Characteristics of Chyle[2]

Milky appearance
pH 7.4–7.8
Specific gravity, 1.012
Sterile
Fat globules seen on staining with Sudan III
Lymphocytes, 0.4–6.8 × 10^9/L
Erythrocytes, 0.05–0.6 × 10^9/L

Table 20–2. Composition of Chyle[2,13]

Total protein, 22–59 g/L
  Albumin, 12–41.6 g/L
  Globulin, 11–30.8 g/L
  Fibrinogen, 160–240 mg/L
Total fat, 4–60 g/L
  Triglycerides, plasma value
  Cholesterol, plasma value
Sugar, 2.7–11.1 mM/L
Urea, 1.4–3.0 mM/L
Electrolytes similar to plasma values
Fat-soluble vitamins present
Pancreatic exocrine enzyme present

and lipoprotein analysis demonstrates the presence of a chylomicron band (Tables 20–1 and 20–2).

The chyle flows from the lacteal system of the intestine to the confluence of the jugular and left subclavian veins and transports tissue fluids, ingested fats, extravascular plasma proteins, and cellular elements of blood (Table 20–3). In adults, a flow rate of 14 to 110 cc/hr has been measured.[14] The thoracic duct pressure at the time of maximal flow is 10 to 28 cm H_2O. The normal daily volume is 1500 to 2400 cc.[14,15] Aspiration of the pleural cavity after ductal injury demonstrated that in some cases there may be a loss of between 2 and 3 L of chyle per day from a chylous fistula. Water taken by mouth can increase the flow of chyle by 20%, and an ordinary meal causes a threefold increase in flow.[11]

Table 20–3. Biochemical Analysis of Chyle and Serum[13,16]

CONTENT	CHYLE	SERUM
Total protein (g/L)	30	66
Albumin (g/L)	27	31
Globulin (g/L)	3	35
Triglycerides (mm/L)	13.4	0.98
Cholesterol (mm/L)	2.6	3.9
Free fatty acids (mm/L)	8070	347

The average daily output of lymphocytes from the thoracic duct in man has been estimated at 10×10^9 to 50×10^9.[6,10] Hypoproteinemia associated with ongoing lymphatic leakage is associated with a number of physiologic responses, including increased blood renin concentration and reduced vascular to interstitial protein transfer.[6,17,18] Despite activation of these protective mechanisms, which help maintain the circulatory status, prolonged drainage of plasma proteins from the thoracic duct results in progressive hypoproteinemia and decreased cell-mediated immunity. This is manifested by nutritional wasting, extended skin graft survival, and loss of responsiveness to primary and secondary antigens after 4 to 6 weeks of ongoing drainage.[6]

MECHANISM OF INJURY

Closed trauma such as falls from a height, compression or hyperextension spinal injuries, and blunt abdominal trauma are the most likely causes of ductal rupture and fistulae. This occurs most commonly in the region of the ninth or tenth thoracic vertebra, resulting in either chylous ascites or right chylothorax. Sudden hyperextension of the spine, the most common cause, results in the rupture of the duct just above the diaphragm. In some instances, it may be sheared across the right crus of the diaphragm. Should the duct be full after a fatty meal, it is considerably more susceptible to injury. In one-fifth of closed injuries of the chest, there is an associated spinal fracture or fractures of the posterior parts of the ribs, which may endanger the thoracic duct.[19,20]

Injury to the duct from gunshot or stab wounds does occur but this is associated with injuries to the adjacent large, major vascular structures (which are more vulnerable) and are immediately lethal. Isolated injury to the duct from a penetrating wound is rare but has been reported.[17]

Chylothorax can occur as a complication in almost every known thoracic operation. Several large review series estimated a prevalence of 0.2% to 0.5% in postoperative cardiothoracic patients.[21,22] Catheterization of the subclavian veins, dissections in the left supraclavicular region, and thoracic procedures such as repair of coarctation of the aorta, patent ductus ligation, and esophageal operations can result in chylothorax or extrapleural chyloma. Bilateral chylothorax can develop if the injury occurs between the third and sixth thoracic vertebra.[23]

FINDINGS

A chylous effusion can present itself at the time of the injury or the manifestation can be delayed for 7 to 10 days. This variable latent period relates to the formation of an extrapleural collection of lymph after initial duct disruption known as a "chyloma."[24] Rupture of this chyloma results in a low-grade fever and evidence of a pleural effusion. A large pleural effusion can embarrass respiration and occasionally results in a shock-like state. Aspiration of the effusion characteristically produces milky white fluid or, when mixed with blood, a cocoa-colored fluid. Aspiration results in symptomatic relief and permits analysis of the nature and composition of the chyle so it can be differentiated from other types of effusion. Pseudo-chyle, for example, contains no triglycerides and has less protein and cholesterol than chyle (Tables 20–1, 20–2, 20–3).

DIAGNOSIS

Bipedal lymphography to demonstrate leakage of lipiodol from the thoracic duct was first described in 1963.[25] A number of imaging techniques have since become available to diagnose and localize thoracic duct injury.[15,25,26] Ductography or injection of methylene blue into the esophagus is generally not advised, as the leaking blue chyle tends to stain all the tissues in the surgical field.

Computed tomography (CT) scanning with opacification of thoracic duct by oral ingestion of ethiodized oil and a 50% fat emulsion has been used with some success.[12] Nuclear lymphangiography with ingested ^{123}I heptadecanoic acid offers a lower resolution evaluation of anatomic variations and level of thoracic duct disruption, but in a less invasive manner than subcutaneous injection of $^{99}NT_c$ sulfur colloid in the interdigital spaces of the feet.[15] These methods need to be evaluated clinically in terms of the efficacy of diagnosis and influence on method of treatment.

Recently, Ngan et al. found lymphography to be useful in nine patients, not only in identifying the precise site of leakage (including collateral lymphatics) but also demonstrating in two cases complete occlusion of the thoracic duct.[26] In these two latter patients, thoracic duct occlusion resolved without operative intervention. In patients with large leaks that require surgical intervention, lymphangiography can identify the location of the leak and facilitate the operation.

TREATMENT

A wide variety of methods have been used to treat thoracic duct injury. Those patients whose fistula did not close spontaneously developed severe cachexia and were associated with a 50% mortality rate. The turning point was in 1948 when Lampson first successfully ligated the thoracic duct in the chest for the control of chylous fistula.[11] Today, with selective expectant treatment including intravenous hyperalimentation followed by operative ligation, the mortality rate is small.[16,27,28]

The general plan of management consists of the following principles (Table 20–4). One, large-bore chest tubes should be inserted and high negative pressure used to prevent tubal obstruction from the gelatinous chyle. Two, full expansion of the lung should be ensured to encourage pleural symphysis; the obliteration of the pleuromediastinal space is vital and will assist in facilitating closure of the chylous fistula. Three, flow of chyle should be reduced by giving patients nothing by mouth. Four, total parenteral nutrition with accurate replacement of water and electrolytes should be initiated to prevent serious metabolic consequences from prolonged drainage of chyle. Finally, the loss of dietary fat

Table 20–4. Principles of Management

Large-bore chest tubes with high negative pressure
Ensure full lung expansion
Nothing by mouth
Total parenteral nutrition (TPN)
Medium chain triglycerides in TPN

should be substituted for by administration of medium-chain triglycerides that are absorbed directly into the portal venous system. This conservative management should be followed for 7 to 14 days. During this period, plasma protein, serum electrolytes, white cell count, and chest radiographs should be monitored daily.

The primary controversy in management of thoracic duct injury is how long to continue conservative management. There is no consensus on this issue, but most would agree that it should be no longer than 3 to 4 weeks (Table 20–5).[27–29] Operative intervention should proceed when the amount of chyle drainage in an adult is in excess of 1500 ml per 24 hr for 5 days or when the amount of chyle drainage exceeds 100 cc per 24 hr for every year of a child's age or if the flow of chyle has not disappeared after 14 days and exceeds 200 ml/day with institution of duct.

Low thoracic duct ligation at the level of the diaphragm should be the procedure performed regardless of the site of chylous effusion.[21,28,29] When the location of the fistula can be identified, the duct should be ligated above as well as below the fistula. Extensive animal experiments and clinical experience have shown that because of the tendency of the lymphatics to develop collaterals, the ligation of the thoracic duct does not produce any permanent clinical abnormality.[30]

Double cream or olive oil given through a nasogastric tube 4 hr before the operation will cause marked increase in the flow of chyle, thus facilitating the identification of the site of leakage.[11] If the duct cannot be located, all tissues between the aorta and the azygous vein should be mass ligated at the level of the esophageal hiatus. This approach has been successful in controlling persistent chylothorax in more than 90% of patients. Pleurodesis, irrespective of the agent used, has met with little success.[27]

Other techniques involving the shunting of chyle have been used, the most promising of which has been pleuroperitoneal shunting. Millisom et al., in a nonrandomized series comparing ligation of the thoracic duct with pleuroperitoneal shunting after a minimal trial of nonoperative therapy, found good results with both approaches.[21] On the basis of their experience, the authors found chylothorax is a self-limiting disease. Eight of 14 patients were treated with shunting and 6 were cured as a result of spontaneous fistula closure. If this is true, then rationale exists for the use of pleuroperitoneal shunting as a stage between failed nonoperative management and operative ligation, thus avoiding a thoracotomy in a significant percentage of cases.

POSTOPERATIVE CARE

After thoracotomy and ductal ligation, one or more large-bore chest tubes should be used to drain the pleural space. Any tubes draining the space ipsilateral to the thoracotomy should be left in place until control of the fistula has been verified. This is assumed when chest drainage through the chest tubes decreases below 50 to 100 cc for at least 24 hr and a chest radiograph documents a dry thorax.

Table 20–5. Indications for Operation

Chyle drainage >1500 ml/day for 5 days
Chyle drainage >200 ml/day after 14 days
Metabolic complications from prolonged drainage

Prophylactic antibiotics initiated preoperatively are continued for 24 hr. It is probably prudent to limit oral fluid intake and diet for 3 to 4 days postoperatively until the result of the surgical intervention can be assessed. Theoretically, this will limit pressure in the ligated duct and decrease the risk of secondary disruption.

COMPLICATIONS

The clinical consequences of duct ligation have been minimal presumably because of the rich collateral pathways for lymphatic return to the vascular system.[11,14] Lymphatic congestion of the gut has not been a problem. Postoperative problems relate primarily to the extent of surgical dissection during the thoracotomy and whether or not lung decortication has been required. Difficult dissections with attendant complications are best avoided by timely interventions using the criteria previously described. Recurrent chylothorax is most unusual. Should this occur, an aggressive approach to management of the recurrence with lymphangiography and repeat operative intervention is advisable.

RESULTS

There has been a great deal of controversy in the literature about whether or not operative or nonoperative management is appropriate and most importantly the timing of and indications for each form of treatment for chylous fistulae. In 1955, Goorwitch reported no mortality in a group of 15 patients treated operatively compared with a 19% mortality rate in those treated nonoperatively.[11] In 1956, Maloney and Spencer published a series in which 11 of 13 children had resolution of their chylothoraces with aspiration alone.[6]

Since then a number of large series have been published.[6,8,11,20,22,29] With increasing experience with injuries of the thoracic duct, it has become clear that iatrogenic trauma is far more frequent as a cause of chylous effusion than either blunt or penetrating trauma. Also, irrespective of the etiology of the chylous effusion or the age of the patient, an operative approach should be undertaken before serious metabolic, nutritional, or immunological sequelae result.[23,27,28,31] When criteria previously given for surgical intervention are used and nutrition has been restored or maintained through the venous route, mortality is low compared with historic series when conservative management alone was used.[5,6]

REFERENCES

1. Bonet T. Sepulchetrum, sive anatomia practica ex cadaveribus morbo denatis. Fol. Lib IV, Sect III, Observ. XXIV, 5 p 360. L Chouet, Genevae, 1679.
2. Tauber L. Die verletzungen des ductus thoracus. *Langenbecks Arch Chir.* 1956;284:188.
3. Forster E, Maguet A, Cinqualbre J, Piombini JL, Schiltz E. A propos d'un cas de cyclothorax consecutif à un traumatisme ferme vertebro-costal. *J Chir (Paris).* 1975;101:605.
4. Lampson RS. Traumatic chylothorax. *J Thorac Surg.* 1948;17:778.
5. Crawford C. A contribution to thoracic duct surgery. *Acta Chir Scand.* 1963–1964;85:99.
6. Maloney JV, Spencer FC. The nonoperative treatment of traumatic chylothorax. *Surgery.* 1956;40:121.
7. Sabin ER. The origin and development of lymphatic system. *Johns Hopkins Hosp Rep.* 1916;17:347.
8. Bessone LB, Ferguson TB, Burford TH. Chylothorax. *Ann Thorac Surg.* 1971;12:527.
9. Glenn WWL. The lymphatic system. *Arch Surg.* 1981;116:989.
10. Glinz W. *Chest Trauma.* New York: Springer-Verlag; 1981.

11. Goorwitch J. Traumatic chylothorax and thoracic duct ligation. *J Thorac Surg*. 1955;29:467.
12. Klepser RG, Berry JF. The diagnosis and surgical management of chylothorax with the aid of lipophilic dyes. *Dis Chest*. 1954;25:409.
13. Staats BA, Ellefson RD, Budahn LL, et al. The lipoprotein profile of chylous and non-chylous pleural effusions. *Mayo Clin Proc*. 1980;55:700–704.
14. Crandall LA, Barker SB. A study of the lymph flow from a patient with thoracic duct fistula. *Gastroenterology*. 1943;1:1040.
15. Hvid-Jacobsen K, Thomsen H, Nielsen SL, et al. Scintigraphic demonstration of the thoracic duct following oral ingestion of ^{123}I-heptadecanoic acid. *Gastrointest Radiol*. 1989;14:212–214.
16. Hesseling PB, Hoffman H. Chylothorax. *S Afr Med J*. 1981;60:675.
17. Pollack CV, Kolb JC, Griswold JA, et al. Chylous drainage from a stab wound to the neck. *Ann Emerg Med*. 1990;19:1450–1453.
18. Wantanabe A, Jeffery R, Brook W. Chylothorax diagnosis of traumatic rupture of cisterna chyli. *J Comput Assist Tomogr*. 1987;11(1):175–176.
19. Engevik L. Traumatic chylothorax. *Scand J Thorac Cardiovasc Surg*. 1976;10:77.
20. Williams KR, Burfurd TH. The management of chylothorax related to trauma. *J Trauma*. 1963;3:317.
21. Millsom JW, Kroni L, Rheuban KS, Rodgers BM. Chylothorax: an assessment of current surgical management. *J Thorac Cardiovasc Surg*. 1985;89:221–227.
22. Cevese PG, Vecchioni R, R'Amico DF, et al. Postoperative chylothorax. *J Thorac Cardiovasc Surg*. 1975;69(6):966.
23. Reilly KM, Tsou E. Bilateral chylothorax. *JAMA*. 1975;223:536.
24. Sinclair D, Woods E, Saibel EA, et al. Chyloma: a persistent post-traumatic collection in the left supraclavicular region. *J Trauma*. 1987;27(5):567–569.
25. Sachs PB, Zelch MG, Rice TW, et al. Diagnosis and localization of laceration of the thoracic duct: usefulness of lymphangiography and chylothorax. *Am J Radiol*. 1991;157:703–705.
26. Ngan H, Fok M, Wong J. The role of lymphography in chylothorax following thoracic surgery. *Br J Radiol*. 1988;61:1032–1036.
27. Ross JK. A review of the surgery of the thoracic duct. *Thorax*. 1961;16:12.
28. Nacrevio EA. *Chest Injuries*. New York: Grune & Stratton; 1971.
29. LeCoultre C, Oberhansli I, Mossaz A, et al. Postoperative chylothorax in children: differences between vascular and traumatic origin. *J Pediatr Surg*. 1991;26(5):519–523.
30. Valenzuela GJ, Hewitt CW, Kramer GC, et al. Effects of sustained lymph drainage on cardiovascular lymph in sheep. *Am J Physiol*. 1989;256(4):R867–875.
31. Machleder HI, Paulus H. Clinical and immunological alterations observed in patients undergoing long-term thoracic duct drainage. *Surgery*. 1978;84:157.

21
Surgical Procedures

DONALD D. TRUNKEY, M.D.
JAMES M. GUERNSEY, M.D.
F. WILLIAM BLAISDELL, M.D.

TRACHEOSTOMY AND CRICOTHYROIDOTOMY

HISTORY: It is not known when the first tracheostomy was performed.[1] It was first mentioned by Asclepiades, but it is unlikely that he actually did one. It is documented that Galen performed a tracheostomy, but it was done infrequently through the Greco-Roman period. During the second century Antyllus gave the following description of tracheostomy:

> *We slit open a part of the arteria aspera (for it is dangerous to divide the whole) below the top of the windpipe, about the third or fourth ring. This is a convenient location, as being free from flesh, and because the vessels are placed at a distance from the part which is divided. Wherefore, bending the patient's head backwards, so as to bring the windpipe better in view, we are to make a transverse incision between two of the rings so that it may not be the cartilage which is divided, but the membrane connecting the cartilages. If one be more timid in operating, one may stretch the skin with a hook and divide it, and then moving the vessels aside, if they come in the way, make the incision.*

There were further descriptions by Paulus Aeginata (625–690) and throughout the Middle Ages. Although the procedure had many names, it was finally called tracheotomy by Trousseau in the mid-18th century.[1]

Anatomy

The anatomy of the trachea has been described in Chapter 11. For purposes of tracheostomy and cricothyroidotomy, review of the topical anatomy is now appropriate.

The cricoid membrane can be palpated easily in both children and adults. It is located directly in the midline approximately one-third of the distance rostrally from the upper neck to the manubrial notch. It is an elliptical concave depression formed by the thyroid cartilages above and the cricoid ring below (Fig. 21–1).

With the neck extended, using the same landmark, the cricothyroid membrane, it usually is possible to count tracheal rings except in the patient with an obese neck or who has fresh hemorrhage or swelling. In general, it is appropriate to make a transverse skin

396

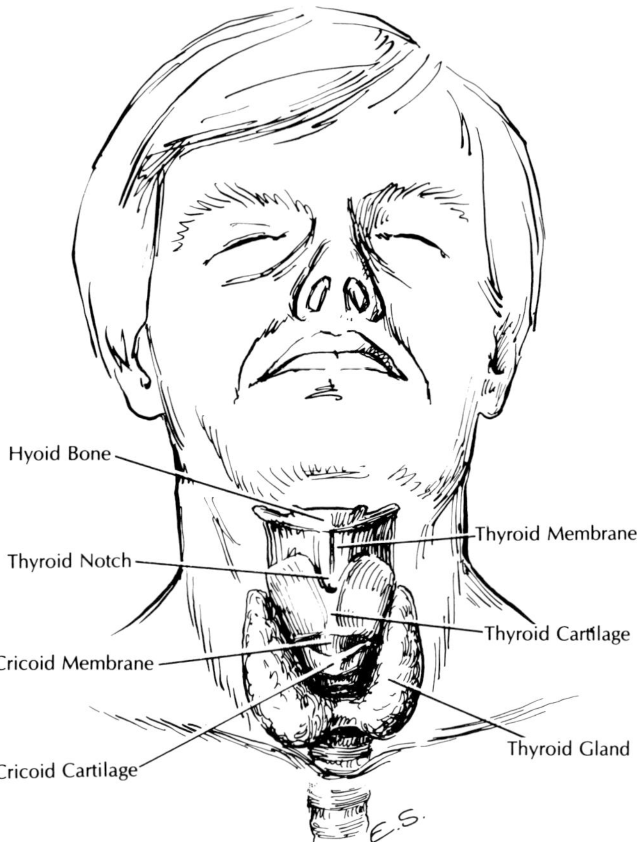

Figure 21–1. Normal anatomy, trachea area.

incision for tracheostomy directly over the first cartilaginous ring, which will place the incision between the thyroid isthmus and the cricothyroid membrane. Two layers of fascia must be penetrated to reach the plane of the trachea proper. These are the deep cervical fascia that enclose all the critical structures of the neck except the superficial veins and the pretracheal fascia, a thin layer enclosing the trachea. By staying in the midline, most serious bleeding can be avoided, unless one inadvertently dissects into the thyroid isthmus, whose superior margin crosses the trachea at the level of the first or second ring or lacerates the thyroidea ima vein, which can be in the midline.

Indications

In general, any patient who is hemodynamically unstable, is unconscious or cannot protect the airway, or has ventilatory insufficiency will require immediate intubation of the airway. In almost all these patients, airway access with oral or nasal intubation of the trachea is successful in the emergency department. The occasional patient, however, because of severe maxillofacial injury, bleeding, distortion of anatomy, or foreign body will require emergency tracheostomy or cricothyroidotomy. Cricothyroidotomy has an advantage because it can be performed rapidly and requires minimal technical skill.[2-6] Tracheostomy takes longer to perform and is more ideally suited to be done in the operating room with its full lighting and support facilities.[7]

The one contraindication to cricothyroidotomy is blunt laryngeal trauma. In a few instances, there may be complete tracheal laryngeal separation and cricothyroidotomy might place the airway outside the trachea. If the patient presents with blunt laryngeal trauma and an emergency airway is indicated, tracheostomy is the procedure of choice.

Cricothyroidotomy

Technique

If the patient's condition permits, extension of the chin and the neck is optimal to stretch the tissues overlying the cricothyroid membrane and make it readily palpable. Care should be taken to ensure that the interval between the thyroid cartilage and the cricoid cartilage is clearly identified. This can be done by palpation with the chin extended. If the patient is conscious, the neck can be prepared quickly with iodine and the skin of the anterior neck infiltrated in a transverse direction with a small amount of local anesthetic corresponding to the location of the cricothyroid membrane below. The knife can be passed directly through the cricothyroid membrane without further dissection, and the small opening dilated with the knife handle or hemostat sufficiently to permit the introduction of a 4- or, preferably, a 6-mm cuffed endotracheal or tracheostomy tube. Any bleeding in the skin or subcutaneous tissue can then be controlled by cautery or suture ligature. If bleeding should occur at the level of the trachea, placement of a larger bore tube through the opening usually will provide compression hemostasis at the tracheal level (Fig. 21–2).

Should a tube be required for more than 24 to 48 hr, a conventional nasotracheal or orotracheal tube can be passed, if circumstances permit. If this is not possible, the cricothyroidotomy should be converted to a conventional tracheostomy (see next section).

Complications

Complications of cricothyroidotomy primarily relate to inadvertent placement of the incision above rather than below the thyroid cartilage, with resultant damage to the vocal cords during tube placement. Hemorrhage can occur if an anterior jugular vein is lacerated. This usually is readily controllable with simple sutures. The cricoid cartilage can be injured, with subsequent compromise of laryngeal function or development of a frank laryngeal stenosis. It is possible to damage the recurrent laryngeal nerves or the intrinsic laryngeal musculature. Nonetheless, it is an underutilized procedure and is relatively safe even in unskilled hands and, provided it is used only for 1 or 2 days, late complications such as airway stenosis are rare.

Tracheostomy

Technique

The tracheostomy should be performed with the patient's head and neck in the hyperextended position. This is best accomplished by placing a rolled towel or other suitable pad

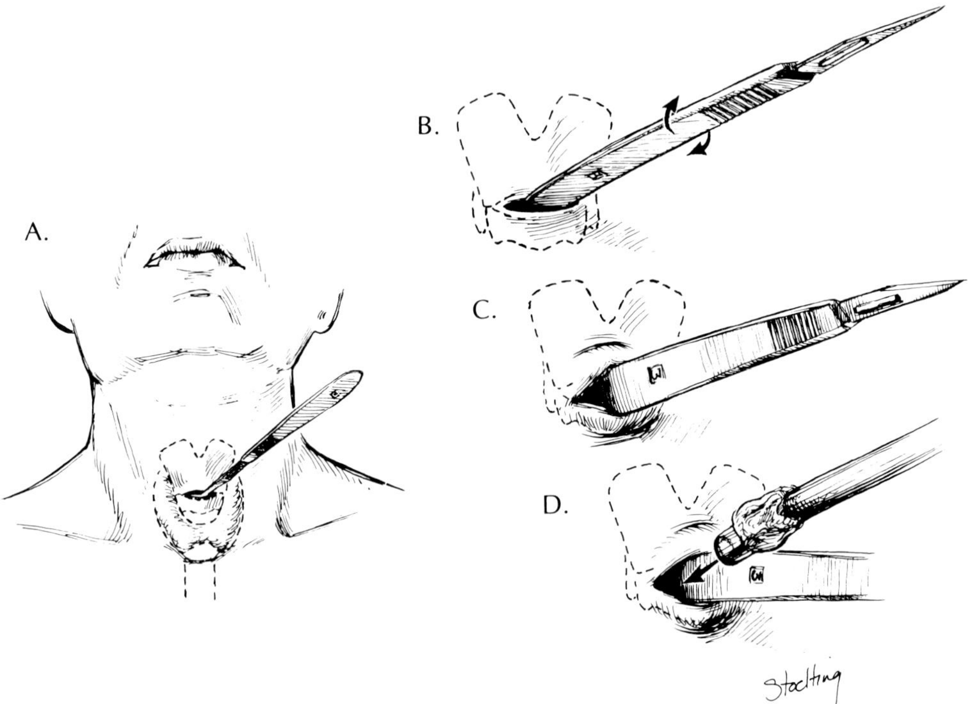

Figure 21–2. Cricothyroidotomy is performed by making an incision 1.5 cm through the skin and cricoid membrane (**A**). The knife handle is then inserted horizontally (**B**) and turned vertically (**C**). A 5F endotracheal tube is then passed through the stoma alongside the handle (**D**).

between the patient's scapulae and extending the head and neck. The level of the cricoid cartilage should be palpated because, when the neck returns to a neutral position, a portion of the skin will come to overlie the second to third tracheal cartilage. The skin incision should be centered just below the cricoid cartilage and can be either transverse or longitudinal. A small transverse incision has the advantage of leaving minimal scar, although in the critically ill patient this is of little consequence. The area of the proposed incision should be at least two finger breadths long and, if the patient is conscious, the area should be infiltrated with a local anesthetic containing epinephrine (Fig. 21–3).

The incision is carried down through the skin and platysma muscle in the midline and the cervical fascia identified. This requires that the neck and head be absolutely straight and that the sternal notch be identified and location of incision be verified by repeated palpation of the trachea.

If a transverse incision is used, the incision should be spread when the deep cervical fascia is reached and the two skin flaps held longitudinally with a self-retaining retractor or by two small retractors held by the first assistant. The anterior jugular veins that course along the medial edges of the strap muscles should be avoided if possible. The tendency for venous bleeding can be modified by performing the tracheostomy with the patient in a slightly upright position (too much of an upright position risks an air embolism).

The cricoid cartilage is identified by a step-off or shelf between it and the first tracheal cartilage. The midline fascia between the strap muscles is opened with a knife or scissors

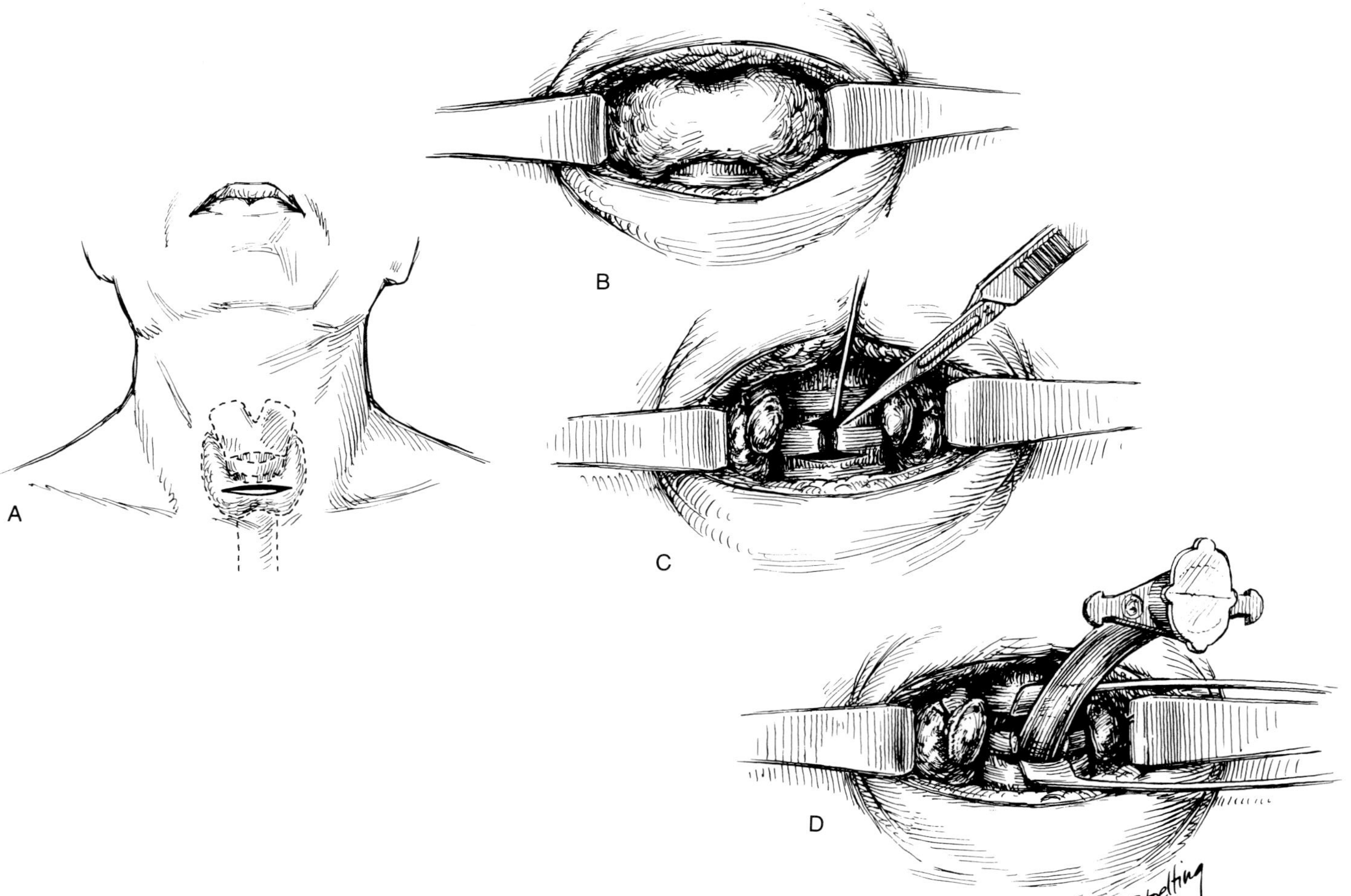

Figure 21–3.   Tracheostomy is performed by making an incision one finger breadth below the cricoid membrane (**A**). The midline is dissected exposing the thyroid isthmus (**B**) and dissecting just above the isthmus, the second tracheal ring is incised and a small piece removed (**C**). A tracheal hook provides stability and traction as the tracheostomy tube is inserted (**D**).

just below the cricoid. The dissection to identify the tracheal rings should be done just below the palpable edge of the cricoid, and this can be done by spreading a pointed hemostat longitudinally. Until the last fascial plane overlying the trachea has been opened, care should be taken to avoid the thyroid isthmus. At this point, the isthmus usually can be retracted downward with a vein retractor. The dissection is carried partially under the thyroid isthmus to identify the second thyroid cartilage. If necessary, the thyroid isthmus can be divided between hemostats and the raw surface oversewn with a suture ligature behind the hemostat.

The first, second, and third tracheal rings should be located by counting down from the cricoid. The optimal location for the incision in the trachea is the second or third tracheal ring, depending on the ease of access.

Once the optimal tracheal ring has been exposed and cleared of overlying fascia but before opening the trachea, tension on the incision should be relaxed and complete hemostasis ensured. The attachments of any inlying endotracheal tube should be loosened and a sterile suction tubing, which should be available on the tracheostomy tray, connected to wall suction. A tracheostomy tube should be selected; an appropriate size is usually #6 or 8 for women and #8 or 10 for men. The cuff on this tube should be tested to ensure its patency.

All of the emergency instruments for the final entrance into the trachea should be at hand. This includes a tracheal hook and a tracheal stoma dilator (a large, blunt, Mayo-type hemostat will suffice). Lighting should be adequate. Ventilator-dependent patients should be placed on 100% oxygen. In the conscious patient, it is appropriate to infiltrate the trachea at the site of the proposed incision above and below the cartilage selected for removal. At the time of infiltration, the surgeon should be prepared to move rapidly because the insertion of the needle into the trachea may rupture the balloon on the endotracheal tube. Should the patient be ventilator dependent, the loss of seal will result in respiratory distress and requires that the operation proceed rapidly.

Removal of a piece of cartilage facilitates dilation of the trachea and also facilitates replacement of the tracheostomy tube should it become dislodged soon after placement. Using a #15 blade or the tip of a cautery, an incision is made above and below the cartilage to be removed so that this section of tracheal ring can be secured with an Allis-type forceps or a blunt hemostat. A section of cartilage, approximately 1 cm long, is then removed, providing access to the trachea. Any inlying endotracheal tube should be backed above the stoma at this point. The stoma should then be dilated with the tracheal dilator or with a suitable hemostat sufficiently to accommodate the tracheostomy tube. If the secretions are abundant or bleeding into the trachea is present, the trachea should be suctioned and the tracheotomy tube inserted with its blunt trocar in place. The trocar is removed, tracheostomy tube liner is placed, and ventilation tubing is attached to the tracheostomy tube (with newer polypropylene tubes, the inner liner is absent). The patient is then ventilated with 100% oxygen for a few minutes after placement. Suction should be used as necessary. The tracheostomy tube should be stabilized manually while the tapes to secure it in place are tied around the neck. Alternatively, in high-risk cases, the tracheostomy tube can be sutured in place to prevent premature dislodgement.

Usually, sutures to approximate the skin are not necessary unless the skin incision has been unusually large. At this point, a dressing should be placed under the tracheostomy tube. Should there be bleeding from the tracheostomy stoma, it is often from the skin incision and will generally respond to an injection of lidocaine with epinephrine. If the patient is not receiving humidified gas via ventilator, humidified air or oxygen should be provided through the tube using a cupula.

Removal of the Tracheostomy Tube

Whenever the tracheostomy tube is replaced or changed, adequate light should be available and the patient positioned as for a tracheostomy. When the tube is no longer needed, a large tube is traded progressively for one of smaller size, usually by changing a #8 or 9 tube to a #6. Then a few days later, the #6 can be exchanged for a #4 fenestrated tube through which the patient can talk. When the #4 tube is removed, the stoma is closed with a dry dressing and secretions and encrustations cleared several times a day with moist sponges. The stoma usually closes spontaneously within 3 to 4 days.

Complications

Tracheostomy is used less frequently now than in the past.[3] This is because it is apparent that the tracheostomy wound in the seriously ill patient becomes a subsequent source of contamination of the airway and increases the risk of pulmonary infection. However, it is much more comfortable for the patient than a nasotracheal or endotracheal tube and, should chronic access to the airway be necessary, it can be used to great advantage. Moreover, in ventilator-dependent patients, inadvertent extubation is easily corrected as opposed to that associated with orotracheal or nasotracheal tubes.

If the tracheotomy tube is poorly placed, the top of the tube may erode the trachea. The balloon itself, even though a soft cuff, may cause pressure necrosis of the trachea and erosion of adjacent vascular structures. Stenosis of the trachea is a late complication as well.

Carefully done, there should be minimal complications. Hastily done, life-threatening complications are possible, consisting of bleeding, airway compromise, and esophageal injury.

PRINCIPLES OF CHEST TUBE INSERTION AND CHEST DRAINAGE

> *HISTORY: It is to Hewson and Larrey that we owe the credit for the principle of closing chest wounds.[1] Despite their observations, however, this was not practiced until the American Civil War, and then only sporadically. Closing the chest wound did not treat the retained blood or pneumothorax. Paré had handled this problem by leaving the chest wound open for 2 or 3 days and then closing it when all blood loss ceased. During the Civil War, an assistant surgeon, A.H. Smith, invented a valve that permitted blood and other fluid to escape but prevented the inflow of air. The valve was made from intestine and placed into the middle of a circular piece of leather. By placing this into the chest wound, air and fluid could escape and the lung could reexpand.*
>
> *In 1875, a German internist, Buelau, introduced the concept of a closed underwater drainage system for the treatment of empyema. It was this concept plus introduction of positive pressure ventilation that led to modern concepts of tube drainage for hemothorax and pneumothorax.*
>
> *Although there had been a gradual reduction in mortality with penetrating chest wounds before World War I, a dramatic reduction occurred midway through World War I secondary to a standardized approach to these injuries.*

Wounds were closed, frequent thoracocentesis was carried out, and even thoracotomy to remove retained clot was performed. During World War II, closed drainage was used routinely to treat intrapleural complications of chest injury and mortality correspondingly dropped.

Anatomy

The anatomy of the chest wall has been discussed in Chapter 8. The topical anatomy for placement of a chest tube concerns two areas: the infraclavicular and the axillary regions. Any area of the chest wall 2 cm lateral to the sternum and anterior to the posterior axillary line from the second to sixth interspace can be used. The preferred anatomic location for tube thoracostomy after trauma is the interval between the anterior and posterior axillary lines. It is the thinnest part of the chest wall and allows easy and rapid placement of a chest tube. It also allows maximum dependent drainage for both air and fluid. In general, the tube placement should be in the fifth to seventh intercostal space in the midaxillary line that corresponds to a level just above the pectoral or inframammary groove (Fig. 21–4). A lower intercostal space can be used provided care is taken not to perforate the diaphragm and enter the abdominal cavity. This mandates careful exploration of the wound before insertion of the chest tube. Latitude also can be exercised in placing the chest tube between the posterior and the anterior axillary lines, depending on the location of the penetrating wound, and to avoid having the chest tube on the bedline. This latter problem will cause extra pain to the patient from bed pressure, particularly with movement.

A second choice, and one that we consider less optimal for trauma management, is the second intercostal space in the midclavicular line. The primary indication is for pneumothorax, but, in our experience, pneumothorax is almost always accompanied by some degree of hemorrhage. When the pneumothorax is spontaneous, there may be preexisting

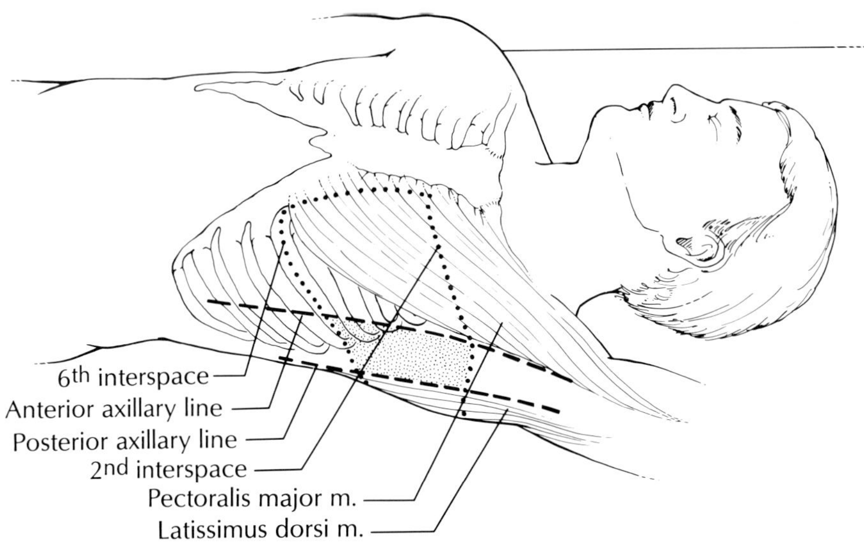

Figure 21–4.   Optimal location for insertion of chest tube is shown in gray stipled area. Acceptable sites are enclosed by the dotted line.

adhesions in the area as well. Other disadvantages to placement of a chest tube in the second intercostal space is that the bulky pectoralis major muscle must be transgressed and, in women, the subsequent thoracostomy scar may be objectionable.

Indications

Chest tube utilization is fundamental in treating most chest trauma as it permits continuous monitoring of the pleural space. A chest tube is used to drain air, blood, and chyle. It can identify foreign fluids in the pleural space such as sputum or gastric juice from an unsuspected esophageal injury or gastric or intestinal contents secondary to hollow viscus injury and diaphragm perforation. It is useful to monitor the status of the pleural space after severe chest wall trauma to prevent pneumothorax or permit early recognition of bleeding. Chest tubes are placed in the pleural space at the completion of thoracotomy to ensure pulmonary expansion and to remove blood.

Tube thoracostomy is indicated for all open chest wounds, pneumothorax greater than 10%, and hemothorax that is visible by radiography. Other indications that require selective judgment include patients with chest injury who have no obvious pneumothorax or hemothorax but who will require positive pressure ventilation either for operation or management of their injuries. These patients are at risk for lung collapse and bleeding, which, if not promptly recognized, could result in serious morbidity or death.

If a patient with penetrating or blunt trauma presents to the emergency room dead or dying, the immediate placement of bilateral tube thoracostomies may be appropriate. A rush of air, heard from either hemithorax, is diagnostic of a tension pneumothorax. A gush of blood when placing a tube thoracostomy permits immediate diagnosis of major hemorrhage, and placement of a tube allows the clinician to collect the blood and give it back immediately as an autotransfusion. Because the risk of tube thoracostomy is minimal and the benefit potentially lifesaving, it should be used liberally in critical trauma patients.

In most instances, large-bore (#30–40F) siliconized chest tubes are used in adult patients in the acute trauma setting. Because all tubes tend to plug with fibrin and clot, the larger the tube, the more certain it will continue to function. Although in theory air can be removed adequately by using a small tube, it is necessary to ensure that the air can be removed from the pleural space more quickly than it leaks from the lung. This is best accomplished with a large-bore tube. Infants and children, of course, should have proportionately smaller tubes.

It is important to be absolutely certain that the chest tube is in the pleural space. For this reason, an adequate opening must be made in the chest wall and, in particular, the intercostal muscles to ensure the ready entry of the tube. Because an occasional patient will have unsuspected, preexisting pulmonary pleural synthesis or, more rarely, previous surgical removal of a lung, an important safeguard is to palpate the pleural space with a finger before inserting the tube to ensure that a pleural space does exist. An opening of this size permits the lung to collapse briefly during placement of the tube so that the tube can be directed to an appropriate location anteriorly, posteriorly, or inferiorly within the pleural space.

Technique

If the patient is stable and only a small pneumothorax or hemothorax exists and the reason for surgery is an abdominal, orthopedic, or central nervous system problem, the chest tube can be placed immediately after the induction of general anesthesia. In almost all other circumstances, the chest tube is placed under local anesthesia. In theory, the skin incision should be one interspace below the interspace used to enter the pleural cavity; this is optimally done when the tube is placed as part of chest surgery. However, when placed through the intact chest, oblique placement is risky because the tube may slide upward over the rib and come to lie in the areolar space between the ribs and the thoracic musculature. In an anteroposterior chest radiograph, the tube may appear to lie in the pleural space, even though it is actually extrapleural.

In emergency circumstances, the tube is best placed directly through the skin and intercostal musculature in a more or less direct line. Unless contraindicated, the site for insertion is the midaxillary line in the fifth to seventh interspace at or above the level of the nipple line anteriorly.

The skin should be infiltrated with 1% or 2% lidocaine in a transverse direction that will correspond to the skin incision. The needle should be advanced until an underlying rib is encountered and then the needle advanced over the top of the rib with infiltration of lidocaine preceding the needle (Fig. 21–5). The patient will experience sharp discomfort when the pleura is encountered. This depth should be noted and the needle advanced at least two additional times in anterior and posterior direction off the top of the rib to penetrate an area of pleura corresponding to extent of the proposed skin incision. Using a #15 knife

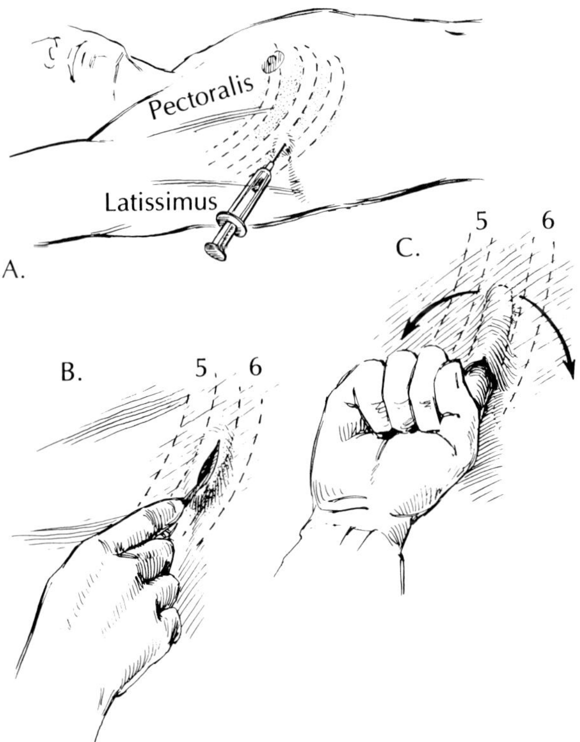

Figure 21–5. Tube thoracostomy is done in the fifth to seventh intercostal space in the midaxillary line. The skin is infiltrated with local anesthetic (**A**) and an incision approximately 2 cm in length is made (**B**). The pleural cavity is then explored with the digit (**C**). (Figure continued on next page.)

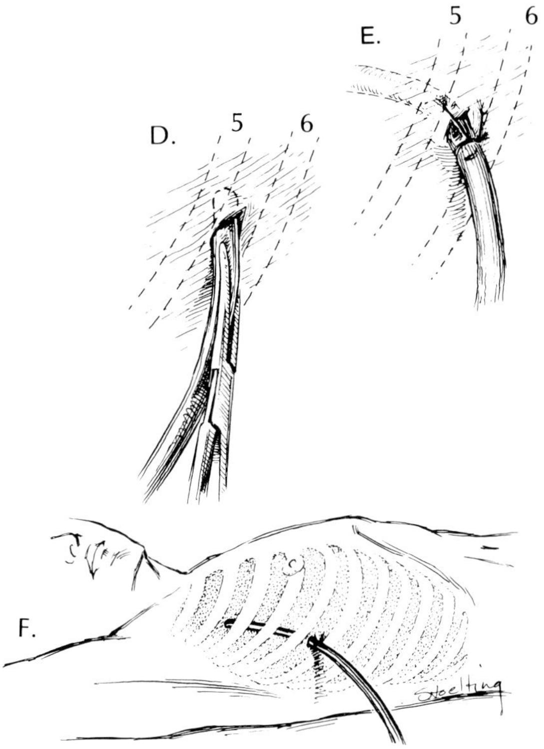

Figure 21–5, cont.   A chest tube is inserted with the aid of a clamp (**D**), and a suture secures the tube to the chest wall (**E** and **F**).

blade, a 2-cm incision should be made in the skin in transverse direction corresponding to the direction of the rib. If the patient has minimal subcutaneous tissue, the knife blade can be advanced in the direction of the previously located intercostal musculature over the top of the rib and the intercostal fascia incised sharply. A safer, less traumatic technique is to advance the knife until it hits the rib and then cut transversely to give a generous skin and fascial incision.

In most instances, however, a pointed hemostat is best used to make the hole in the intercostal musculature and pleura. The tip of the clamp should be passed over the top of the rib until it pops through the intercostal fascia. This is usually associated with some immediate discomfort for the patient. The clamp is then spread vigorously and quickly parallel to the course of the rib in order to minimize the time of the discomfort. At least a 1.5-cm opening should be made in the intercostal musculature and underlying pleura.

It is perfectly appropriate to allow air to enter the incision, because slight collapse of the lung will facilitate chest tube insertion. The index finger or, if this is not possible, the little finger is advanced through the drain tract until the pleural space is encountered and the absence of pleural adhesions verified. A #30 up to a #40 straight chest tube then can be directed easily through the tract into the pleural space. The tube is directed posteriorly and inferiorly for hemothorax or hemopneumothorax. For pneumothorax alone, the tube should be directed, if at all possible, anteriorly and superiorly (Fig. 21–5F).

The tube should pass easily and extend the entire length of the perforated portion of the tube. If this is not possible, the tube should be removed and redirected or a straight tube changed for a right-angle tube or vice versa. Allowing more air to enter the pleural space also may facilitate directing the tube in an appropriate manner. The tube can be left unclamped to facilitate the pneumothorax, if needed. Obviously, if the patient already has bilateral pneumothoraces or is in severe respiratory distress, the addition of more air should be avoided and the tube should be clamped near its distal end before insertion.

After insertion, the tube should be sutured in place, preferably with heavy nylon or polypropylene such as 2-0. In instances of trauma, the skin should not be sutured tightly around the tube, and the suture is best placed through either the superior or inferior lip of the skin incision. By leaving the skin incision open, subcutaneous air, if present, can dissect its way out along the chest tube site. Moreover, any peritube infection that might follow inadvertent contamination induced during an emergency placement can drain along the tube rather than into the chest. Should the tube, for some reason, be placed in an extrapleural position or an intrapleural position where it becomes plugged or does not drain effectively, a tension pneumothorax can still dissect out along the tube and decompress outside.

Antibiotic ointment should be placed around the tube. This is followed by a notched piece of 4 × 4 sterile gauze sealed around its edges with adhesive tape. A tight seal with nonporous tape will prevent drainage along the tube, and this drainage is desirable, as noted previously. The tube then is best supported by a strap of three-tailed tape to prevent the entire weight of the tube being carried by the suture. If the patient is on positive pressure ventilation during placement of the tube, there is no rush to connect the patient to underwater drainage because simply opening the clamp will permit decompression of the pneumothorax and intrapleural blood. The only problem of an open system is potential contamination of the interior of the tube. As soon as possible, closed water seal drainage should be instituted with one of the conventional commercial tube draining systems or with standard three-bottle drainage.

Chest Tube Removal

Because tubes placed under emergency circumstances outside the operating room should always be considered potentially contaminated, they are managed differently than chest tubes placed in the operating room where, with removal of the tube, the skin can be closed with preplaced sutures. With emergency placement, it should always be assumed that the tube tract is infected, and closure of the skin or tight wound compression by a sealed dressing will force any contaminated secretions from the tube tract back into the pleural space, with risk of empyema. Therefore, as the chest tube is removed, the chest tube hole should be closed with two layers of petrolatum gauze, followed by a larger 4 × 4 gauze dressing. The dressing should be sealed by tape only at the edges. This permits a type of flap valve so that any fluid remaining in the chest can decompress past the petrolatum gauze. Should a tension pneumothorax develop subsequently, air can still decompress because the tube drainage site usually remains functionally patent for as long as 24 to 48 hr.

The patient should be told that there will be slight discomfort with removal of the tube and that he/she should take a deep breath and do a Valsalva maneuver as the tube is rapidly removed. The surgeon removing the tube should have a piece of petrolatum gauze in a sterile gloved hand. This should be placed over the tube drainage site as soon as the tube is removed by the opposite hand. Alternatively, the petrolatum gauze can be placed in the center of a 4 × 4 gauze pad that is held in the left hand in such a way as not to contaminate the petrolatum gauze and the 4 × 4 gauze placed over the chest tube site as the tube is removed.

Both after placement of the chest tube and withdrawal of the chest tube, posteroanterior and lateral chest films should be obtained, in the first instance to ensure proper intrapleural placement of the tube and in the latter instance to verify the absence of pneumothorax induced during removal of the tube. Should the patient develop a pneumothorax during tube removal and if there is less than 1 cm rim of air, this usually can be ignored. However, should major collapse be present, a smaller tube placed anteriorly for an additional few hours is appropriate. Alternatively, an attempt to aspirate the pneumothorax with a needle or small trocar may be done.

Complications

The complications of chest tubes are minimal. They consist of perforation of the diaphragm and pneumothorax from partial dislodgement of a tube so that one air hole lies outside the skin. It includes laceration of the lung, particularly if the lung is adherent to the chest wall; bleeding, should an intercostal artery be injured; and infection of the tube tract or pleural space. Almost all complications can be avoided by good technique as described previously.

PERICARDIOCENTESIS AND PERICARDIOTOMY

> *HISTORY: In 1650, Riolanus suggested that the sternum be trephined for aspiration of fluid from the pericardial cavity. The rationale for this was clarified by Morgagni in 1761, who demonstrated the fatal effect of cardiac tamponade.[8]*
>
> *In 1935 Bright and Beck reported a case treated by C.W. Mansell in 1895 of a boy injured in the chest playing football. Twenty-five days later he was critically ill. It was found that the area of cardiac dullness was increased, heart sounds were distant, and he was cyanotic. Incision and drainage of the pericardium released 6 pints of fluid and was followed by rapid recovery of the patient.[9]*
>
> *Biggers[10] in 1934 reported on 17 cases of cardiac injury. When there was evidence of tamponade, he inserted a cannula into the pericardium. If bleeding was rapid, he proceeded with operation; if bleeding was minimal, he treated the wound nonoperatively.*
>
> *In 1943, Blalock and Ravitch[11] advocated nonoperative treatment of cardiac wounds. In four survivors, one was treated with plasma alone and three were treated successfully initially by pericardiocentesis, one of whom was subsequently successfully operated on.*

Anatomy

The anatomy of the heart and pericardium is provided in Chapter 15. It is sufficient to point out that the heart and its pericardial enclosure occupy the anterior one-half of the chest cavity and are in intimate contact with the diaphragm (Fig. 21–6). Although the heart

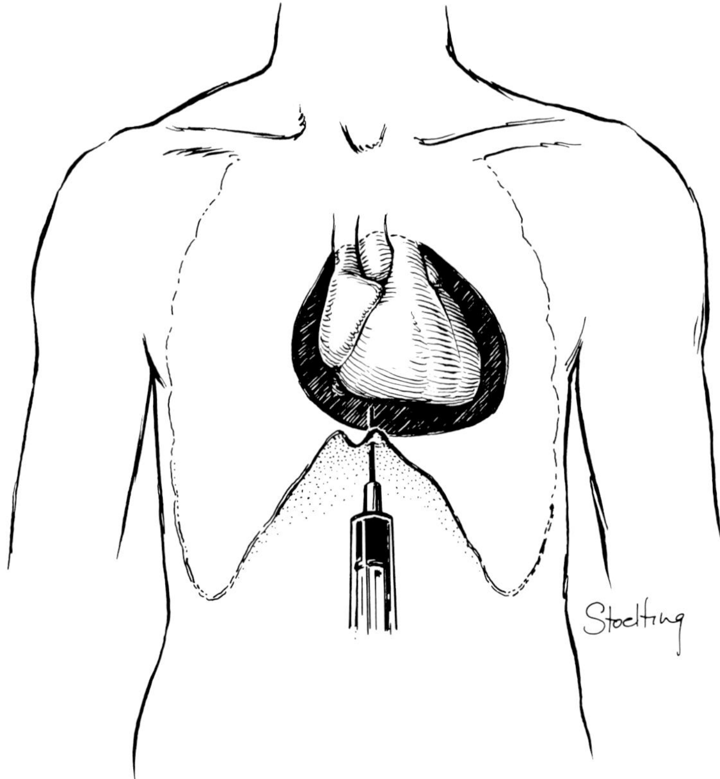

Figure 21–6. Technique of pericardiocentesis. The aspirating needle is advanced upward from the paraxiphoid area toward the sternal notch at an angle of 45° to the skin.

projects into the left pleural space, it is a midline structure and lies on the diaphragm centering at the level of the xiphisternal joint.

Indications

In most emergency circumstances where pericardial tamponade is suspected, emergent thoracotomy in the emergency room or operating room is appropriate as the urgency of circumstances dictate. However, if surgical expertise is not immediately available or there is a delay in operation room availability, pericardiocentesis, leaving an inlying catheter in the pericardium, may temporarily decompress the pericardium and buy time.[12] In other circumstances, particularly in the older patient in whom a primary cardiac problem may be suspected, pericardiocentesis can be diagnostic.

Although pericardiotomy can be done via the subxiphoid route, this approach is of primary value in the chronic compression syndromes. However, transdiaphragmatic pericardiotomy may be of great value in the patient with thoracic abdominal blunt or penetrating trauma when the abdomen has already been opened to deal with an infradiaphragmatic problem. In this circumstance, if there is any question of intrapericardial injury, it is a simple matter to make a small opening in the diaphragm to investigate the possibility of intrapericardial injury. If such is found, a median sternotomy incision can be done to obtain immediate access to the heart.

Pericardiocentesis

Technique

Pericardiocentesis is easily accomplished with an 18- or 20-gauge spinal needle or equivalent-sized plastic-sheathed needle. This is advanced directly upward from the left paraxiphoid position aiming 45° posteriorly (Fig. 21–6). Blood coming from the hub of the needle or with aspiration using a small syringe may be either from the pericardial space or a cardiac chamber. Regardless, 25 to 50 ml of blood should be aspirated, if obtainable. A prompt improvement in vital signs is diagnostic of an intrapericardial location of the needle and that tamponade has been present.

Although a failure of the aspirated blood to clot also is a manifestation of pericardial blood, this requires 5 to 10 min of observation, which is not practical in urgent life-threatening circumstances.

An alternative to ascertain if aspirated blood came from a cardiac chamber is to connect the hub of the exploring needle to the chest lead of the electrocardiogram and constantly record the electrocardiogram as the needle is advanced. A giant electrocardiographic complex (current of injury complex) indicates contact of the needle tip with the myocardium, whereas aspiration of blood and no change in the electrocardiographic reading indicates that the needle tip is in the pericardial space. The use of a plastic catheter is advantageous if thoracotomy may be delayed because it permits repeated or continuous decompression of the pericardial space.

Transabdominal Pericardiotomy

Technique

After laparotomy and assessment of the need for pericardial exploration, the left lobe of the liver is retracted downward and the membranous portion of the diaphragm just to the left of the midline exposed (Fig. 21–7). The diaphragm just above the liver is grasped firmly with two Allis clamps and a 1- to 2-cm opening made in the diaphragm between the clamps. A second layer, the pericardium, is then encountered and grasped with a clamp and incised with scissors. The release of a small amount of fluid and the visualization of the beating heart confirms entrance into the pericardium. If the exploration is negative, the diaphragm is approximated with one or two synthetic collagen sutures.

Complications

Complications after both procedures are minimal. As noted, the exploring needle used for pericardiocentesis can be advanced into a cardiac chamber with minimal risk. However, with both procedures, the possibility of myocardial laceration with intrapericardial bleeding and cardiac tamponade theoretically exists and progressive signs of tamponade in the posttreatment period dictate ultrasonic assessment or reoperation.

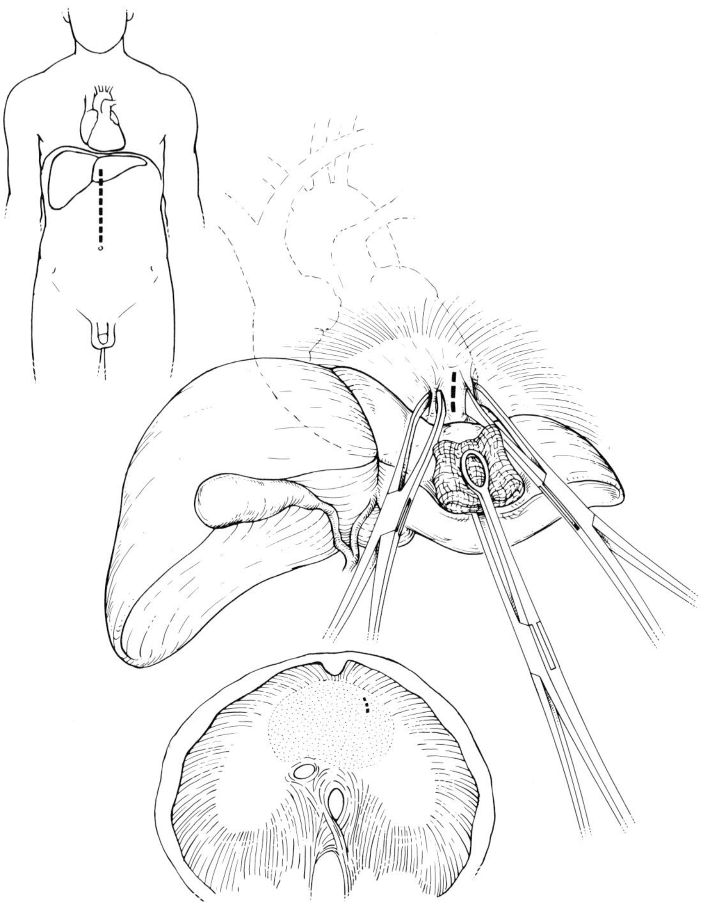

Figure 21–7. After laparotomy (when indicated to rule out abdominal trauma), the left lobe of the liver is retracted downward and the subxiphoid membranous diaphragm is opened just to the left of the midline.

CHEST WALL STABILIZATION

HISTORY: In speaking of fractured ribs, Theodoric said that ". . . if the fractures were depressed and punctured the pleura no amount of manual dexterity will avail to reduce it. If one should have to make an incision, then it is necessary to cut at the point of injury and disclose the broken rib . . . by placing an instrument under the rib . . . it is easy to excise that part of the bone which is penetrating the pleura."[11]

Before the advent of ventilators, the patient who presented with multiple rib fractures that resulted in a flail chest presented an almost insurmountable problem. Treatment of moderate flails such as those involving four to six ribs unilaterally could be managed by splinting the ipsilateral thorax with sandbags and by positioning the patient flail side down. This, combined with pain relief by administration of repeated nerve blocks or judicial use of narcotics, resulted in salvage of most good-risk cases with flail chest.

In cases with more extensive injury, various traction devices were instituted to stabilize the chest wall. These consisted of towel clips around involved ribs with traction weights applied through overhead pulleys, wires placed around the ribs, or devices such as cup hooks screwed into the ribs to provide a source for traction. Although the use of mechanical ventilators has supplanted most of these devices, the occasional case whose primary problem relates primarily to instability of the chest wall will benefit from operative fixation.

Indications

The indications for operative fixation of the chest wall consist of two groups of patients. The first consists of that group who require operative intervention to deal with open wounds or bleeding from the chest wall or those requiring thoracotomy to deal with parenchymal injuries. Closure of the chest wall in these circumstances may be facilitated by rib stabilization. The second group of patients are those whose injuries are so extensive that multiple weeks of ventilatory support may be required or those who have preexisting pulmonary disease in whom ventilation weaning may be difficult.

Technique

Posterolateral thoracotomy is the approach of choice, although anterolateral thoracotomy also can be used depending on the location of the rib injury. Ribs 1 and 2 rarely need stabilization as they are short, move very little with normal ventilation, and rarely contribute significantly to the flail. This is also true of the floating ribs 11 and 12 so that for practical purposes the need for stabilization involves ribs 3 through 10.

The thoracic incision is best centered over the area of injury—this usually involves the standard location, the fifth to sixth interspace.

In these severe injuries, the status of the structures inside the chest wall should be initially assessed and bleeding, air leaks, lacerations, and mediastinal injuries dealt with as appropriate. If pulmonary resection is required, the patient will benefit from resection of at least one of the most badly damaged ribs to lessen the dead space.

At this point, the extent of rib damage should be assessed. A significant injury usually will involve four or more ribs, each having three or more fractures. Stabilization of all injured ribs is not required; stabilization of alternate ribs is all that is necessary.

A light orthopedic plate is selected long enough to overlap the area of rib fracture by 2 cm on each side (Fig. 21–8). The plates are then bent to match the curvature of the chest wall; the plate is then laid over the appropriate rib and fixed at both ends to stable ribs by monofilament, plastic, nonabsorbable wire, or synthetic collagen passed around the rib or through small drill holes placed through the rib. The intervening loose segments of rib are approximated and stabilized to the plate by similar sutures. All ribs do not need stabilization. Stabilizing alternate ribs is sufficient. After placement of the plates on alternate ribs, the stability of the chest wall is then verified and chest wall closed in the standard fashion with tube drainage of the pleural space.

Long-acting narcotics can be injected into the nerve bundles before closure or, preferably, epidural analgesia induced for long-term pain control to facilitate early extubation.

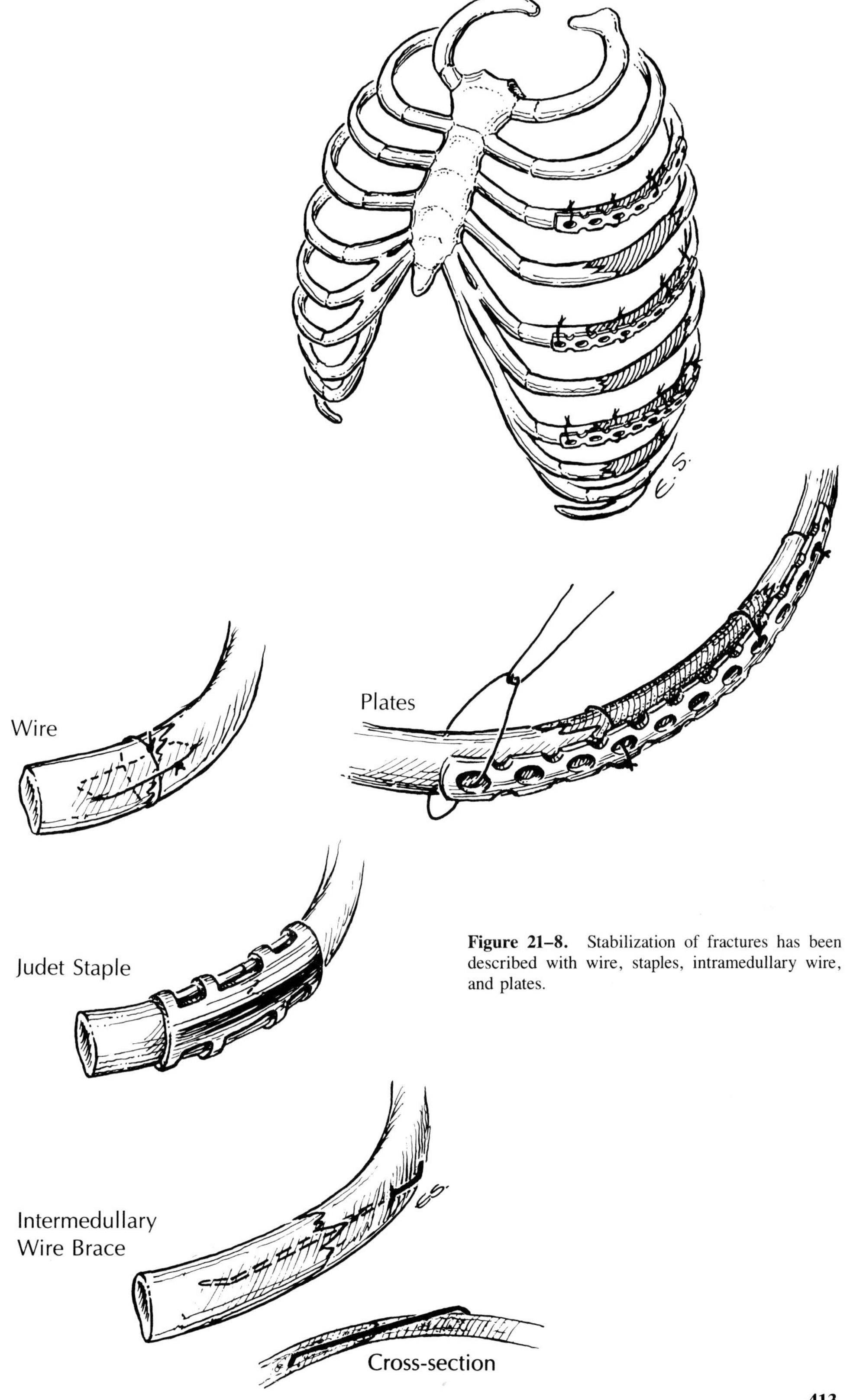

Figure 21–8. Stabilization of fractures has been described with wire, staples, intramedullary wire, and plates.

Prophylactic antibiotics should be instituted preoperatively and should be continued for 24 to 48 hr postoperatively.

Complications and Results

In our experience, the complications of stabilization are in themselves negligible and relate primarily to associated injuries. In theory, infection could be a problem but this has not occurred in our experience. With the advent of epidural anesthesia, it is rarely necessary to continue ventilatory support for more than 24 hr when lung injury has been minimal. Because the procedure of internal fixation is required only occasionally in all series, experience is anecdotal. However, in our opinion, chest wall stabilization is an under-utilized procedure and should be applied more frequently.

MINI-LAPAROTOMY

HISTORY: All methods of indirect assessment of abdominal injury have their limitations and the "gold standard" regarding assessment for abdominal injury remains laparotomy. In certain situations, such as thoracic cardiovascular injuries where anticoagulation may be necessary for pump bypass, even a minor bleeding source in the abdomen may create potential life-threatening problems during prolonged thoracic procedures. In other situations where prolonged orthopedic procedures are about to be instituted, there may be an unsuspected minor abdominal injury. Under these circumstances, the "minor lesion" may be responsible for continual blood loss and instability during operation.

In circumstances such as these when there is a high index of suspicion, laparotomy may be appropriate as the initial operative intervention to rule out associated abdominal injury. In situations where the probability of injury is low or where wound bleeding after anticoagulation parallels the size of the wound, a small exploratory incision combined with suction evaluation of the four corners of the abdomen (mini-laparotomy), may be the exploratory procedure of choice. It will be more accurate than CT and peritoneal lavage, the alternative techniques available, in picking up a minimal bleeding source or a significant retroperitoneal injury.

Technique

Depending on the depth of subcutaneous tissue, a midline incision two to three finger breadths long is made in the epigastrium (Fig. 21–9). With retraction of the wound, the first maneuver is to mobilize the omentum downward using sponge sticks so as to identify the anterior wall of the stomach. This is then depressed downward with the same sponge sticks until the gastrohepatic ligament is identified. This may require retraction of the left lobe of the liver upward. The area is then inspected for evidence of a central retroperitoneal hematoma (Fig. 21–9B), the primary area of clinical significance in the absence of other gross evidence of injury (Chapter 20).

In the absence of pathology, a Yankauer (tonsil) sucker is advanced sequentially into the four abdominal quadrants with suction temporarily clamped, then removed with suction

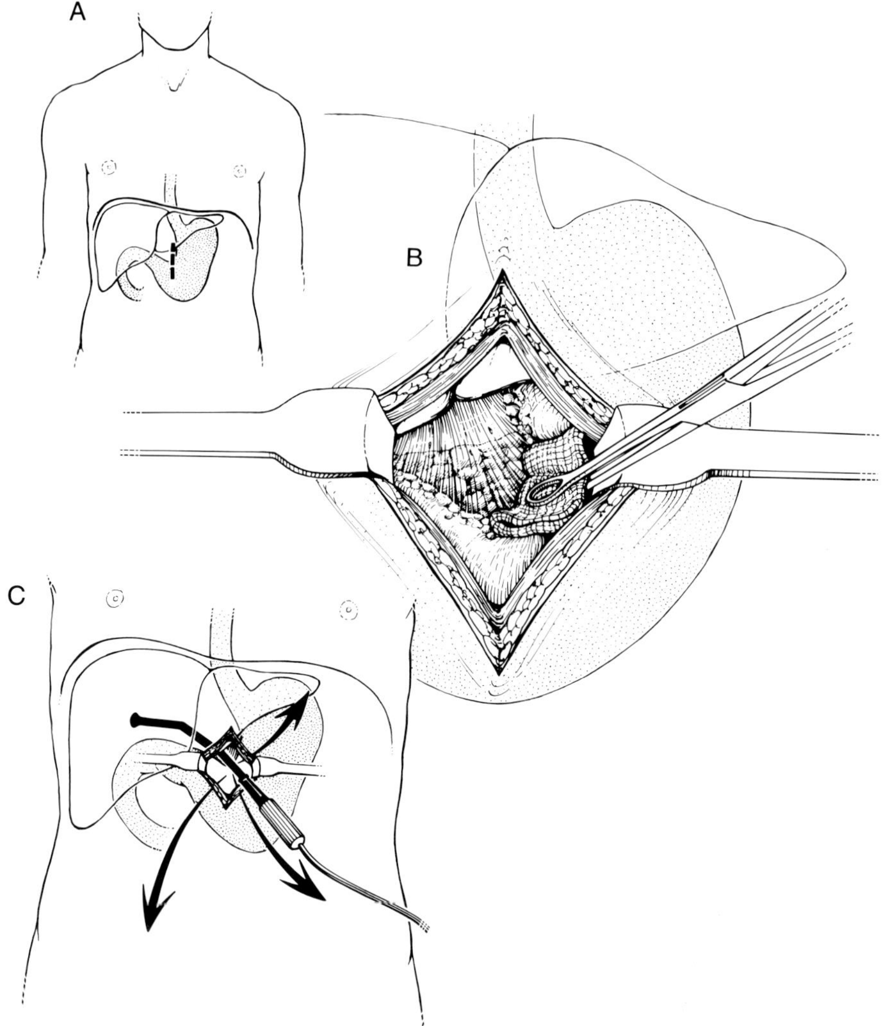

Figure 21–9.   Technique of mini-laparotomy. **A:** A 2–3 finger-breadths incision is made through skin and fascia and the peritoneum opened. **B:** The stomach is then retracted downward as the liver is elevated upward with sponge sticks and the gastrohepatic area is inspected for evidence of a central hematoma. **C:** A suction tip is passed successively into all four quadrants of the abdomen, assessing for fluid or blood.

applied (Fig. 21–9C). A final advance to the pelvis completes the evaluation. The absence of blood or fluid in the areas sampled provides reassurance that no abdominal injury exists. After this, the incision is closed tightly and the previously planned surgical procedure carried out.

The presence of blood will or will not dictate subsequent management depending on the assumed risk in that individual case. This may require formal laparotomy. At the very minimum, it will alert all involved about potential bleeding risk, resulting in the recognition of need for operative intervention should any secondary problems develop.

Complications

Under the circumstances just described, morbidity is minimal. Because the procedure is done in the operating room in an anesthetized patient, the complications in our experience have been nonexistent, as opposed to peritoneal lavage, whether done by the direct or indirect technique, where there may be an occasional problem related to bowel injury, bleeding, and a false positive or negative result. The morbidity of the incision has not been much greater than open peritoneal lavage regarding discomfort or subsequent ileus.

REFERENCES

1. Meade RH. *An Introduction to the History of General Surgery.* Philadelphia: Saunders; 1968.
2. Boyd AD, Romita MC, Conlan AA, et al. A clinical evaluation of cricothyroidotomy. *Surg Gynecol Obstet.* 1979;149:365.
3. Brantigan CD. Cricothyroidostomy, aye or nay. *Plast Reconstr Surg.* 1981;67:97.
4. Committee on Trauma. *Advanced Trauma Life Support Course Manual.* Chicago: American College of Surgeons; 1980.
5. Morain WD. Cricothyroidostomy in head and neck surgery. *Plast Reconstr Surg.* 1980;65:424.
6. Sise MJ, Shackford SR, Cruckshank JC, et al. Cricothyroidotomy for long-term tracheal access. *Ann Surg.* 1984;200:13.
7. El-Kilany SM. Complications of tracheostomy. *Ear Nose Throat J.* 1980;59:59.
8. Meade RH. *A History of Thoracic Surgery.* Springfield, IL: Charles C Thomas; 1961.
9. Bright EF, Beck CS. Contusions of the heart. *JAMA.* 1935;104:109.
10. Biggers IA. Wounds of the heart. *Int Clin.* 1934;1:135.
11. Blalock A, Ravitch MM. A consideration of nonoperative treatment of cardiac tamponade resulting from wounds of the heart. *Surgery.* 1943;14:157.
12. DeGennaro VA, Bonfils-Roberts EA, Ching N, Nelson TF. Aggressive management of potential penetrating cardiac injuries. *J Thorac Cardiovasc Surg.* 1980;79:833.

Index

(Italic page numbers indicate a table or figure)

AAST, *see* American Association for the Surgery of Trauma
Abdominal injury, 6, 193–194, 230, 284, 309, 383
Absorption atelectasis, 17
Acid-base electrolytes, 115–116
Acromium, 129
Acute cardiac injury, 271
Adrenergic nervous system, 22
Adult respiratory distress syndrome (ARDS), 113, 114, 187–188
Adventitia, 305, *308*, 317, 336
AIDS, *see* Autoimmune deficiency syndrome
Air embolism, 36, 240, 259–260, 290, *291*, 368
Air leaks, 12, 60, 231, 256, 258
Airway
  blood in, 16, 111, 128, 181, 184, 243
  difficult situations, 117–119
  establishment of, 135–136, 169, 186, 203, 352, 397
  evaluation of, 133
  management of, 110–111
  obstruction, 141, 175
  postoperative care, 336
  pressure in, 244
  stenosis, 188
  upper and lower, 121–122
Alimentary canal, 144
Alveolar capillary membrane, 17–18
Alveolar ventilation, 16
American Association for the Surgery of Trauma (AAST), 362
Amnesia, 110
Amrinone, 31
Anastomosis, 318, 334, 364
Anesthesia
  angiography, 93
  thoracic trauma, 108–110
    acid-base electrolytes, 115–116
    airway, 110–111, 117–119, 121–122
    aorta, 123–125
    chest wall, 122, 405

    circulatory support, 114–115
    heart, 122–123
    history, 105
    induction, 110, 125
    pleura, 122
    postanesthesia, 119–121
    preanesthetic evaluation, 106–108
    spinal cord, 125–126
    transfusion, 117
    ventilation, 111–113
Aneurysm, 279, 307
  false, *306*, 327, *328*, 368
Angiogram, 50, 308
Angiography, 86–94, 99
  complications, 92
  contraindications, 89–91
  findings, 93–94
  history, 86
  indications, 87–88
  technique, 91–94
Ansa hypoglossus nerve, 347
Anterior cervical spine view, 69, *70*
Anterior vascular anatomy, 343–346
Anterior vertebral line, 72
Antibiotics, 231, 394, 407, 414
Aorta, 298–299, *300*, 302
Aortic injury, 11, 96, 97, 146, 265, 298–321
  anatomy, 298–302
  complications, 319–321
  diagnosis, 304–310
  history, 298
  management of, 310–313
  mechanism, 302–304
  postoperative care, 318–319
  results, 321
  rupture, 305, 307, 316
  surgical treatment, 313–318
  valve, 281, 298
Aortogram, *303*, *306*, 307, *311*
Apical capping, *12*
ARDS, *see* Adult respiratory distress syndrome
Arrhythmias, 115, 278
Arterial blood gases, 29
Arterial cannula, 29

Arterial injuries, 25–26, 136
Arteries, 255, 343–346
Arteriogram, 89, *328*, 349
Arteriography, 136, 365
Arytenoid cartilages, 161
Ascending aorta, 298–299, *300*, 302
Asphyxia, 181
Aspiration, 60, 108, 110, 113, 259–260
Asystole, 38, 43
Atelectasis, 17, 60, 175, 187, 204, 385
Atlas, 359
Atrial injuries, 287
Atrium, 265
Autogenous graft, 139
Autoimmune deficiency syndrome (AIDS), 117
Automobile accidents, 267, 277, 279, 302, 304

Babcock clamp, *288*
Balloon catheter, 27, *28*, 287, *289*, 365, *367*
Barium, 65, 151, 157
Beck's triad, 271, 275
Biopsy, 148
Bipedal lymphography, 392
Blast injury, 239, 244–245
  see also Traumatic asphyxia
Bleeding
  abdomen, 230
  airway, 111
  aortic, 319
  cardiac, 294
  chest, 60, 62, 222–224, 256
  lung, 247
  neck, 128, 137, 367
  pulmonary, 257
  thoracotomy, 45, 229
  see also Hemorrhage
Blood gases, 292, 294
Blood pressure, 30–31, 108, 123
Blood vessels, 87
Blood volume, 114, 256
Blunt trauma, 3, 6, 9, 13, 87, 99